The Essential Guide to Prescription Drugs

The Essential Guide to
PRESCRIPTION DRUGS

1987 EDITION

James W. Long, M.D.

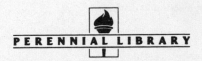

PERENNIAL LIBRARY

Harper & Row, Publishers, New York
Cambridge, Philadelphia, San Francisco, Washington
London, Mexico City, São Paulo, Singapore, Sydney

Designed by C. Linda Dingler

Library of Congress Cataloging-in-Publication Data

Long, James W.
  The essential guide to prescription drugs.

  Bibliography: p.
  Includes index.
  1. Drugs.   2. Chemotherapy.   I. Title.
[DNLM: 1. Drugs—handbooks.   2. Drugs—popular
works. QV 39 L848e]
RM302.5.L66   1987   615′.1   86-45125
ISBN 0-06-181552-7   87 88 89 90 91 HC 10 9 8 7 6 5 4 3 2 1
ISBN 0-06-096037-X (pbk.)   87 88 89 90 91 HC 10 9 8 7 6 5 4 3 2 1

Contents

SECTION SIX:
Tables of Drug Information

Author's Note for the 1987 Edition

The innovations in this edition of the Guide reflect two notable changes in our society that have occurred over the past 15 years. Opposing views within the health care professions regarding drug information for patients have been largely reconciled. And ever increasing numbers of consumers are coming to recognize the importance of being better informed in matters of health and medical care. The remarkable proliferation of books for the layman and news media coverage devoted to health and medicine are clear testimony to the meeting of minds that is evolving between health care providers and consumers.

In keeping with growing public awareness of the need to be better informed about drugs in current use, this edition of the Guide introduces several new features. Information regarding the usefulness and importance of measuring drug levels in the patient's blood has been added to Section One. A new Section Two provides an overview of how drugs are used to treat the 20 most common chronic disorders in this country. New information categories covering dosage ranges and dosing instructions have been added to each Drug Profile in Section Three. Also new to each Profile is a side-by-side presentation of the principal benefits and risks that accompany the use of the drug. Ten new terms have been added to the Glossary (Section Five), and selected tables of drug information have been expanded (Section Six).

In an effort to remain current and still provide useful information to the greatest number of readers possible, we have focused the always difficult task of drug selection on retaining the best of the old and adding the most important of the new. The 200 Drug Profiles in Section Three are a considered blend of the most widely used and needed of the prescription and over-the-counter drugs available at the time the manuscript was submitted for publication. We have added 34 new Drug Profiles to provide information on drugs that have gained wider use or become available since the last edition of the Guide was published.

As noted in each previous edition, no claim is made that all known side-effects, adverse effects, interactions, precautions, etc., for a drug are included in the information provided in the Drug Profiles. While diligent care has been taken to ensure the accuracy of the information provided during the preparation of this revision, the continued accuracy and currentness are ever subject to change relative to the dissemination of new information in drug development and research.

1
HOW TO USE THIS BOOK

2
GUIDELINES FOR SAFE
AND EFFECTIVE DRUG USE

1

How to Use This Book

Your physician has advised you to take a drug (or drugs), or you have been directed to administer a drug (or drugs) to someone under your care. The kind and amount of information you have been given about how to use these drugs, and what to expect from them, will vary tremendously. In many instances it will not be practical or possible for the physician to provide you with *all* the information that could be considered appropriate and useful, or it will be difficult for you to remember it. From time to time you will find it desirable—even necessary—to seek clarification and guidance about some aspect of drug action or drug use. The aim of this book is to give you the kind of information you may need to supplement the direction and guidance you receive from your physician.

The book consists of six sections. The first section will give you the orientation and insight necessary to appreciate the complexities of modern drug therapy and help you to make the best use of the information contained in Sections Two through Six.

Section Two presents useful information regarding the role of drugs in treating 20 common chronic disorders that require long-term drug therapy. A synopsis of each disorder is followed by information categories that cover drug selection, the goals of drug treatment and an overview of drug management during the period of therapy. A list of the disorders reviewed is found in the introduction to the section.

Section Three is a compilation of Drug Profiles covering 200 prescription (and several nonprescription) drugs used widely in the United States and Canada. The selection of each drug was based upon three considerations: the extent of its use; the urgency of the conditions for which it is prescribed; the volume and complexity of the information essential to its proper utilization. The Drug Profiles are arranged alpha-

3

betically by generic name. (Some generic names have spellings similar to other generic names; be careful not to confuse one with another.)

The Profile of each drug is presented in a uniform sequence of information categories. (When you become familiar with the format, you will be able to find quickly specific items of information on any drug, without having to read the entire Profile.) Each Drug Profile contains 42 (or more) separate categories of information. The principal categories include the following.

Year Introduced

This tells you how long the drug has been in general use. The older the drug, the more likely its full spectrum of actions is known and the less likely its continued use will produce new surprises. The date given represents the year the drug was introduced for human use anywhere in the world.

Drug Class

This identifies the principal therapeutic class(es) to which the drug belongs. When appropriate, the chemical and/or pharmacological class designations are also given. You will find it helpful to recognize the class of the drug you are taking because many actions, reactions and interactions with other drugs are often shared by drugs of the same class. Throughout this book (and in most literature on drug information) you will find reference to drugs by their class designation. (Section Four provides alphabetically arranged listings of the classes of drugs referred to in this guide.)

Prescription Required

This indicates whether a drug is a prescription or a nonprescription (over-the-counter) purchase. Because there are significant differences in prescription requirements between the United States and Canada, the designation for each country is given when appropriate.

Controlled Drug

Drugs subject to regulation under the Controlled Substances Act of 1970 (those with potential for abuse) are so designated by the particular schedule that governs their dispensing in the United States. A corresponding schedule is also given for Canada when applicable. A description of the Schedules of Controlled Drugs is found inside the back cover of this guide.

Available for Purchase by Generic Name

Increasing interest in the availability of prescription drugs for purchase by their generic names has been prompted by two issues of major significance. The first is concerned with the cost of prescription drugs. The comparison shopper realizes that in general the cost of prescription medication is significantly less when a generic equivalent of a brand name product is purchased. The second issue relates to what is termed "bioavailability and bioequivalence"—the comparative composition, quality and effectiveness of the generic versus the brand name drug product. Further discussion of bioavailability and bioequivalence of drug products will be found in the Glossary, Section Five.

Brand Names

These are provided to confirm that you are consulting the correct Drug Profile. They may also help you to recognize a brand name that identifies this drug as one that produced in you an unfavorable reaction on previous use. Brand names are listed for the United States and for Canada (✤). A combination drug (a drug product with more than one active ingredient) is identified by [CD] following the brand name.

In a few instances a particular brand name in current use in both the United States and Canada will represent entirely different generic drugs (in a single drug product), or a significantly different mixture of generic ingredients (in a combination drug product). The generic composition of such brand name products is identified by country in the index. Travelers between the two countries who obtain their medications by brand name in either country are advised to ascertain that they are being provided the intended generic drug(s) in every instance.

Benefits versus Risks

A deliberate attempt is made here to crystallize the "pros" and "cons" for each drug. The format adopted for this category utilizes capital letters to give weight (emphasis) to the drug's principal benefits and risks, and lower case letters are used for benefits and risks of lesser significance. A glance reveals the comparative "weights" of the two columns and provides an initial and tentative impression as to whether a drug's benefits exceed its risks, or vice versa, or whether its benefits and risks seem to be roughly equivalent.

This presentation is not intended to be the principal basis for decision on whether or not to use the drug. Its purpose is to enjoin the reader to be more circumspect and discriminating in his or her use of drugs. The failure to give adequate attention to the individualization of drug selection and dosage is perhaps the greatest weakness seen in the current management of drug therapy.

Principal Uses

A drug may be available as a single drug product or in combination with other drugs. In this section of the Profile under the designation As a Single Drug Product, you will find the primary use(s) of the drug when used alone. Under the designation As a Combination Drug Product [CD], you will find the primary use(s) when combined with other active drugs within the same tablet, capsule, etc. The uses stated are those determined by consensus within the medical community and substantiated by current scientific study. Combination drugs have been developed because some conditions that warrant drug therapy have more than one cause, are characterized by a variety of symptoms or may be treated in more than one way. Where appropriate, in this guide, the logic for combining certain drugs to enhance their therapeutic value is explained. When you find the designation for Combination Drugs [CD] in the Brand Name list at the beginning of the Drug Profile, read under the Principal Uses section to learn more about the drug's use in combination products.

How This Drug Works

This simplified explanation is limited to consideration of how the drug acts to produce its principal (intended) therapeutic effect(s). If a specific method of action has not been established, the currently held theory is given.

Available Dosage Forms and Strengths

This represents a composite of available manufacturers' dosage forms (tablets, capsules, elixirs, etc.) and strengths, without company identification. Included are those dosage forms appropriate for use by outpatients and in extended care facilities and nursing homes. Dosage forms limited to hospital use are not included. Refer to Dosage Forms and Strengths in the Glossary for an explanation of those few abbreviations used to designate the strengths of each dosage form.

Usual Adult Dosage Range

The dosage information given represents a carefully derived consensus by appropriate authorities and is the currently recommended standard. It is provided as a guide that indicates the amount of the drug that is reasonably expected to be both effective and safe when properly used for its intended purpose. Under certain circumstances, your physician may elect to modify this "standard" dosage scheme. Adhere strictly to his or her prescribed dosages and schedules.

Dosing Instructions

Specific guidance is given here regarding the timing of oral medication with regard to food intake. In addition, there are occasions when an individual finds it difficult or impossible to swallow a tablet or a capsule, and the drug to be taken is not available in a liquid dosage form. On those occasions when the patient's condition urgently requires the medication, one may wish to crush the tablet or open the capsule and mix the contents with a palatable food or beverage for administration. Many of today's drugs are available in a bewildering array of solid dosage forms, some of which should *not* be altered to accommodate administration. This information category identifies those dosage forms of each drug that may be and those that should not be altered for administration. In addition, your pharmacist can provide appropriate guidance if you should need it.

Usual Duration of Use

Many factors influence the period of time required for any drug to exert beneficial effects. Among them are the nature and severity of the symptoms being treated, the formulation and strength of the drug, the presence or absence of food in the stomach, the ability of the patient to respond and the concurrent use of other drugs. The information in this category is helpful in preventing premature termination of medication in treatment situations where improvement may seem to you to be unreasonably delayed. Where appropriate, limitations in the duration of use are given.

This Drug Should Not Be Taken If

This category consists of the *absolute* contraindications to the use of the drug (see Contraindications in Glossary). It is most important that you alert your physician or dentist if any information in this category applies to you.

Inform Your Physician Before Taking This Drug If

This category lists the *relative* contraindications to the use of the drug. Here again, it is important that you communicate all relevant information to your physician or dentist.

Possible Side-effects

This category describes the natural, expected and usually unavoidable actions of the drug—the normal and anticipated consequences of taking it. It is important that you maintain a realistic perspective that balances properly the occurrence of side-effects and the goals of treatment. Consult your physician for guidance whenever side-effects are troublesome or distressing, so that appropriate adjustments of your treatment program can be made.

Possible Adverse Effects

This category includes those unusual, unexpected and infrequent drug effects that are commonly referred to as adverse drug reactions. For the sake of evaluation, adverse effects are classified as mild or serious in nature. It is always wise to inform your physician as soon as you have reason to suspect you may be experiencing an adverse drug effect. Serious adverse reactions usually announce their development initially in the form of mild, unthreatening symptoms. It is important that you remain alert to significant changes in your well-being when you are taking a drug that is known to be capable of producing a serious adverse effect. It is also possible to experience an adverse reaction that has not yet been reported. Do not discount the possibility of an adverse effect just because it is not listed in this category. Following standard practice, some adverse reactions (and interactions) of certain drugs are listed, as a precaution, because these reactions are associated with the use of a particular class of drugs. Although the literature may not document such reactions in connection with the use of an individual drug within that class, the possibility of their occurrence must be considered.

A word of caution is appropriate here. You have consulted your physician for medical evaluation and management. He or she has advised you to take a drug (or administer it to someone else). It is important that you recognize and understand that *in the vast majority of instances a properly selected drug has a comparatively small chance of producing serious harm.* Most of the drugs included in this book produce serious adverse effects rarely. Knowledge that a drug is capable of causing a serious adverse reaction should not deter you from using it when it has been properly selected and its use will be carefully supervised.

Adverse Effects That May Appear Similar to Natural Diseases or Disorders

The failure to recognize that a given symptom or disorder is actually drug induced occurs with surprising frequency. Quite often this inadvertent error is compounded by the administration of yet another drug to relieve the "symptoms" (unrecognized manifestations) of a drug being taken on a regular basis. For milder symptoms (*e.g.*, the nasal congestion and diarrhea caused by reserpine), the oversight may not be too serious. But in the case of parkinsonlike effects of some drugs, the mistake can be devastating. This category can alert you to this common flaw in the management of drug therapy.

Natural Diseases or Disorders That May Be Activated by This Drug

Similar to the situation described in the previous category, many drugs in common use are capable of "activating" latent disorders that may not be recognized as drug induced. The development of a new and seemingly unrelated disorder during the course of any treatment program should arouse suspicion that it may be drug related.

Caution

This category provides information on certain aspects of drug action and/or drug use that require special emphasis. Occasionally these warnings may relate to information provided in other categories. When included here, such entries are of sufficient importance to warrant repetition.

Precautions for Use by Infants and Children

In addition to mandatory adjustments of drug dosage for infants and children under twelve years of age, some drugs and/or treatment situations call for special precautions. This category provides such information for selected drugs. When administering *any* drug (whether prescription or over-the-counter drug), it is advisable to ask the attending physician about precautions to observe or procedures to follow.

Precautions for Use by Those over 60 Years of Age

Changes in body composition and function occur naturally as part of normal aging. As would be expected, there is enormous individual variation in the speed with which such changes occur and the degree of these changes. With regard to medical management—and to drug therapy in particular—the assessment of one's "age" must be based upon the individual's mental and physical condition and never upon years alone. In general, however, it should be recognized that changes that accompany aging may affect the actions of the body on the drug, as well as the actions of the drug on the body. Appropriate precautions are outlined in this category.

Advisability of Use During Pregnancy: Pregnancy Categeory

Information regarding the safe use of a particular drug during pregnancy was one of the most forceful concerns that led to the formal petitioning of the Food and Drug Administration in 1975 for the provision of such guidance to the public. Most category designations are labeled "tentative" at this time in recognition of the fact that data not readily available now may be advanced by pharmaceutical manufacturers as they negotiate with the FDA to eventually determine final category assignments. The FDA definitions of the five Pregnancy Categories are listed inside the back cover of the book. It should be noted that the FDA does not make the initial category assignment; this is the responsibility of the manufacturer that markets the drug. The initial designation is then subject to review and modification by the FDA as deemed appropriate. The Pregnancy Category designations presented in each Profile were determined by the author after thorough review of pertinent literature and consultation with appropriate authorities. They are offered at this time for initial guidance only. They are in no sense "official" and do not have the endorsement of either the manufacturer or the FDA.

Advisability of Use If Breast-Feeding

Information presented here includes what could be ascertained regarding the effects of the drug on milk production, the presence of the drug in human milk and the possible effects of the drug on the nursing infant. Prudent recommendations are given where appropriate.

Suggested Periodic Examinations While Taking This Drug

This category lists those examinations your physician may recommend you undergo while taking the drug(s) he or she has prescribed, in order to monitor your reaction to them and the course of your condition. You should remember that the advisability of performing such examinations varies greatly from one situation to another, and is best left to the judgment of your physician. The selection and timing of examinations are based on many variables, including your past and present medical history, the nature of the condition under treatment, the dosage and anticipated duration of drug use and your physician's observations of your response to treatment. There may be many occasions when he or she will feel no examinations are necessary.

To assure optimal results from drug treatment, it is important that you keep your physician informed of all developments you think may be drug related.

While Taking This Drug, Observe the Following: Marijuana Smoking

The widespread "social" use of marijuana by virtually all age groups has led to inquiries regarding the possibility of interactions between the pharmacologically active chemicals in marijuana smoke and medicinal drugs in common use. Currently available literature on the health aspects of marijuana use contains very little practical information concerning the potential for drug interactions. The limited information presented in this category of selected Drug Profiles represents those *possible interactions* that are considered likely to occur in view of the known pharmacological effects of the principal components of marijuana and of the medicinal drug reviewed in the Profile. In most instances, the interaction statements are not based on documented evidence since very little is available. However, the conclusions stated— derived by logical inductive reasoning—represent the concurrence of authorities with expertise in this field.

While Taking This Drug, Observe the Following: Other Drugs

For clarification of this confusing and often controversial area of drug information, this category is divided into five subcategories of possible interactions between drugs. Observe carefully the wording of each subcategory heading (see also Interaction in Glossary). Some of the drugs listed as possible interactants do not have a representative Profile in Section Three. If you are using one of these drugs, consult your physician for guidance regarding potential interactions. A brand name (or names) that follows the generic name of an interacting drug is given for purposes of illustration only. It is not intended to mean that the particular brand(s) named have interactions that are different from other brands of the same generic drug. If you are taking the generic drug, *all* brand names under which it is marketed are to be considered as possible interactants.

Driving, Hazardous Activities

In addition to driving motor vehicles, the information in this category applies to any activity of a dangerous nature such as operating machinery, working on ladders, using power tools and handling weapons.

Aviation Note

Until the publication of Dr. Stanley Mohler's *Medication and Flying: A Pilot's Drug Guide* in 1982, there was no authoritative source of current drug information written specifically to serve the needs of civil aviation. The military airman enjoys the expert guidance and surveillance provided by the flight surgeon, but no tightly structured control system exists for his civilian counterpart. However, the need for practical information regarding the possible effects of medicinal drugs on flight performance is the same for pilots in all settings. This category is designed to inform the civilian pilot how a particular drug may affect his or her eligibility to fly and when it is advisable or necessary to consult a designated Aviation Medical Examiner or an FAA medical officer.

Occurrence of Unrelated Illness

This category relates to those drugs that require careful regulation of daily doses to maintain a constant drug effect within critical limits. Anticoagulants, antidiabetic medication and digitalis are examples of such drugs. Emphasis is given to those interim illnesses, separate from the condition for which the drug has been prescribed, that might affect the established schedule of drug use.

Discontinuation

This aspect of drug use is often overlooked when a plan of drug therapy is first discussed. However, for some drugs it is mandatory that the patient be fully informed on *when* to discontinue, when *not* to discontinue and precisely *how* to discontinue use of the drug.

Another consideration in discontinuation is the need to adjust the dosage schedules of other drugs being taken concurrently. The physician who is primarily responsible for your overall management must be kept informed of *all* the drugs you are taking at a given time.

The remaining information categories in the Drug Profile are self-explanatory.

Section Four is a presentation of Drug Classes arranged alphabetically according to their chemical or therapeutic class designation. The drugs within each class are listed alphabetically by their generic names. Because of their chemical composition and biological activities, some drugs will appear in two or more classes. For example, the drug product with the brand name Diuril will be represented by its generic name, chlorothiazide, in three drug classes: the Thiazide Diuretics (a chemical classification), the Diuretics (a drug action classification) and the Antihypertensives (a disease-oriented classification).

Frequently in the Drug Profiles in Section Three you are advised to "See (a particular) Drug Class." This alerts you to a possible contraindication for drug use, or to possible interactions with certain foods, alcohol or other drugs. In each case, you can determine the more readily recognized brand names for each drug listed generically within a drug class by consulting the appropriate Drug Profile. Timely use of these references will enable you to avoid many possible hazards of medication.

Section Five is a glossary of drug-related terms used throughout the book. The preferred use of each term is explained. Frequent references to the Glossary are made in the Drug Profiles. Use of the Glossary will increase your understanding of how to recognize and interpret significant drug effects.

Section Six consists of tables of drug information. The title and introductory material explain the content and purpose of each table. The information in the tables is drawn from certain information categories in the Profiles and is rearranged to emphasize pertinent aspects of drug behavior. The tables are intended to provide another source of ready reference.

The index of Brand and Generic Names in the back of the book is a single alphabetical listing that provides page references to the appropriate Drug Profile(s) for all drugs found in this book. Its usefulness will be enhanced if you read first the introductory explanation of the special features of this combined index.

2

Guidelines for Safe and Effective Drug Use

DO NOT

- pressure your physician to prescribe drugs that, in his or her judgment, you do not need.
- take prescription drugs on your own or on the advice of friends and neighbors because your symptoms are "just like theirs."
- offer drugs prescribed for you to anyone else without a physician's guidance.
- change the dose or timing of any drug without the advice of your physician (except when the drug appears to be causing adverse effects).
- continue to take a drug that you feel is causing adverse effects, until you are able to reach your physician for clarification.
- take *any* drug (prescription or nonprescription) while pregnant or nursing an infant until you are assured by your physician that no harmful effects will occur to either mother or child.
- take any more medicines than are absolutely necessary. (The greater the number of drugs taken simultaneously, the greater the likelihood of adverse effects.)
- withhold from your physician important information about previous drug experiences. He or she will want to know both beneficial and undesirable drug effects you have experienced in the past.
- take any drug in the dark. Identify every dose of medicine carefully in adequate light to be certain you are taking the drug intended.
- keep drugs on a bedside table. Drugs for emergency use, such as nitroglycerin, are an exception. It is advisable to have only one such drug at the bedside for use during the night.

DO

- know the name (and correct spelling) of the drug(s) you are taking. It is advisable to know both the brand name and the generic name.
- read the package labels of all nonprescription drugs to become familiar with the contents of the product.
- follow your physician's instructions regarding dosage schedules as closely as possible. Notify him or her if it becomes necessary to make major changes in your treatment routine.
- thoroughly shake all liquid suspensions of drugs to ensure uniform distribution of ingredients.
- use a standardized measuring device for giving liquid medications by mouth. The household "teaspoon" varies greatly in size.
- follow your physician's instruction on dietary and other treatment measures designed to augment the actions of the drugs prescribed. This makes it possible to achieve desired drug effects with smaller doses. (A familiar example is the reduction of salt intake during drug treatment for high blood pressure.)
- keep your personal physician informed of all drugs prescribed for you by someone else. Consult him or her regarding nonprescription drugs you intend to take on your own initiative at the same time that you are taking drugs prescribed by him or her.
- inform your anesthesiologist, surgeon and dentist of *all* drugs you are taking, prior to any surgery.
- inform your physician if you become pregnant while you are taking any drugs from any source.
- keep a written record of *all* drugs (and vaccines) you take during your entire pregnancy—name, dose, dates taken and reasons for use.
- keep a written record of *all* drugs (and vaccines) to which you become allergic or experience an adverse reaction. This should be done for each member of the family, especially the elderly and infirm.
- keep a written record of *all* drugs (and vaccines) to which *your children* become allergic or experience an adverse reaction.
- inform your physician of all known or suspected allergies, especially allergies to drugs. Be certain that this information is included in your medical record. (Allergic individuals are four times more prone to drug reactions than those who are free of allergy).
- inform your physician promptly if you think you are experiencing an overdose, a side-effect or an adverse effect from a drug.
- determine if it is safe to drive a car, operate machinery or engage in other hazardous activities while taking the drug(s) prescribed.
- determine if it is safe to drink alcoholic beverages while taking the drug(s) prescribed.

- determine if any particular foods, beverages or other drugs should be avoided while taking the drug(s) prescribed.
- keep all appointments for follow-up examinations to determine the effects of the drugs and the course of your illness.
- ask for clarification of any point that is confusing or difficult to understand, at the time the drug(s) are prescribed or later if you have forgotten. Request information in writing if circumstances justify it.
- discard all outdated prescription drugs. This will prevent the use of drugs that have deteriorated with time.
- store all drugs to be retained for intermittent use out of the reach of children to prevent accidental poisoning.

PREVENTING ADVERSE DRUG REACTIONS

Our knowledge of the mechanisms of adverse reactions is very limited. For the most part, we cannot identify with certainty the person who is at greater risk of experiencing a true adverse effect. Available tests for the early detection of toxicity are of definite value, but they do not provide as full a measure of protection as we could wish.

As our understanding of drug actions and reactions expands, it becomes more apparent that there *is* a sizable proportion of adverse effects that are, to some extent, predictable and preventable. The exact percentage of preventable reactions is yet to be determined, but several contributing factors are now well recognized, and specific recommendations are available to guide both physican and patient. These fall into eleven categories of consideration.

Previous Adverse Reaction to a Drug

There is evidence to indicate that an individual who has experienced an adverse drug reaction in the past is more likely to have adverse reactions to other drugs, even though the drugs are unrelated. This suggests that some individuals may have a genetic (inborn) predisposition to unusual and abnormal drug responses. *The patient should inform the physician of any history of prior adverse drug experiences.*

Allergies

Individuals who are allergic by nature (hayfever, asthma, eczema, hives) are more likely to develop allergies to drugs than are nonallergic individuals. The allergic patient must be observed very closely for the earliest indication of a developing hypersensitivity to any drug. Known drug allergies must be noted in the medical record. The patient must inform every physician and dentist consulted that he or she is allergic by nature and is allergic to specific drugs by name. *The patient should provide this information without waiting to be asked.* The physician will then be able to avoid those drugs that could provoke an allergic reaction, as well as those related drugs to which the patient may have developed a cross-sensitivity.

Contraindications

Both patient and physician must strictly observe all known contraindications to any drug under consideration. *Absolute contraindications* include those conditions and situations that prohibit the use of the drug for any reason. *Relative contraindications* include those conditions that, in the judgment of the physician, do not preclude the use of the drug altogether, but make it essential that special considerations be given to its use to prevent the intensification of preexisting disease or the development of new disease. Such conditions and situations usually require adjustment of dosage, additional supportive measures and close supervision.

Precautions in Use

The patient should know about any special precautions to observe while taking the drug. This includes the advisability of use during pregnancy or while nursing an infant; precautions regarding exposure to the sun (or ultraviolet lamps); the avoidance of extreme heat or cold, heavy physical exertion, etc.

Dosage

The patient must adhere to the prescribed dosage schedule as closely as possible. *This is most important with those drugs that have narrow margins of safety.* Circumstances that interfere with taking the drug as prescribed (nausea, vomiting, diarrhea) must be reported to the physician so that appropriate adjustments can be made.

Interactions

Much is known today about how some drugs can interact unfavorably with certain foods, alcohol and other drugs to produce serious adverse effects. *The patient must be informed regarding all likely interactants that could alter the action of the drug he or she is using.* If, during the course of treatment, the patient has reason to feel he or she has discovered a new interaction of importance, the physician should be informed so that its full significance can be determined. (It is through such observations that much of our understanding of drug interactions has come.)

Warning Symptoms

Experience has shown that many drugs will produce symptoms that are actually early indications of a developing adverse effect. Examples include the appearance of severe headaches and visual disturbances *before* the onset of a stroke in a woman taking oral contraceptives; the development of acid indigestion and stomach distress *before* the activation of a bleeding peptic ulcer in a man taking phenylbutazone (Butazolidin) for shoulder bursitis. *It is imperative that the patient be familar with those symptoms and signs that could be early indicators of impending adverse reactions.* With this knowledge he or she can act in his or her own behalf by discontinuing the drug and consulting the physician for additional guidance.

Examinations to Monitor Drug Effects

Certain drugs (less than half of those in common use) are capable of damaging vital body tissues (bone marrow, liver, kidney, eye structures, etc.)—especially when these drugs are used over an extended period. Such adverse effects are relatively rare, and many of them are not discovered until the drug has been in wide use for a long time. As our knowledge of such effects accumulates, we learn which kinds of drugs (that is, which chemical structures) are most likely to produce such tissue reactions. Hence, we know those drugs that should be monitored periodically to detect as early as possible any evidence of tissue injury resulting from their use. *The patient should cooperate fully with the physician in the performance of periodic examinations for evidence of adverse drug effects.*

Advanced Age and Debility

The altered functional capacity of vital organs that accompanies advancing age and debilitating disease can greatly influence the body's response to drugs. Such patients tend not to tolerate drugs with inherent toxic potential well; it is usually necessary for them to use smaller doses at longer intervals. *The effects of drugs on the elderly and severely ill are often unpredictable.* The frequent need for dosage adjustments or change in drug selection requires continuous observation of these patients if adverse effects are to be prevented or minimized.

Appopriate Drug Choice

The drug(s) selected to treat any condition should be the most appropriate of those available. Many adverse reactions can be prevented if both physician and patient exercise good judgment and restraint. *The wise patient will not demand overtreatment.* He or she will cooperate with the physician's attempt to balance properly the seriousness of the illness and the hazard of the drug.

Polypharmacy

This term refers to the concurrent use by an individual of several drugs prescribed separately by two (or more) physicians for different disorders—often without appropriate communication between patient and prescriber. This frequent practice is conducive to potentially serious drug/drug interactions. *The patient should routinely inform each physician (and dentist) consulted of all the drugs—prescription and nonprescription—that he or she may be taking at the time.* It is mandatory that each physician have this information before prescribing additional drugs.

DRUGS AND THE ELDERLY

Advancing age brings changes in body structure and function that may alter significantly the action of drugs. An impaired digestive system may interfere with drug absorption. Reduced capacity of the liver and kidneys to metabolize and eliminate drugs may result in the accumulation of drugs in the body to toxic levels. By impairing the body's ability to maintain a "steady state" (homeostasis), the aging process may increase the sensitivity of many tissues to the actions of drugs, thereby altering greatly the responsiveness of the nervous and circulatory systems to standard drug doses. If aging should cause deterioration of understanding, memory, vision or physical coordination, people with such impairments may not always use drugs safely and effectively.

Adverse reactions to drugs occur three times more frequently in the older population. An unwanted drug response can render a functioning and independent older person whose health and reserves are at marginal levels, confused, incompetent or helpless. For these reasons, drug treatment in the elderly must always be accompanied by the most careful consideration of the individual's health and tolerances, the selection of drugs and dosage schedules and the possible need for assistance in treatment routines.

Guidelines for the Use of Drugs by the Elderly

Be certain that drug treatment is necessary. Many health problems of the elderly can be managed without the use of drugs.
Avoid if possible the use of many drugs at one time. It is advisable to use not more than three drugs concurrently.

- Dosage schedules should be as uncomplicated as possible. When feasible, a single daily dose of each drug is preferable.
- In order to establish individual tolerance, treatment with most drugs is usually best begun by using smaller than standard doses. Maintenance doses should also be determined carefully. A maintenance dose is often smaller for persons over 60 years of age than for younger persons.
- Avoid large tablets and capsules if other dosage forms are available. Liquid preparations are easier for the elderly or debilitated to swallow.
- Have all drug containers labeled with the drug name and directions for use in large, easy-to-read letters.
- Ask the pharmacist to package drugs in easy-to-open containers. Avoid "child-proof" caps and stoppers.
- Do not take any drug in the dark. Identify each dose of medicine carefully in adequate light to be certain you are taking the drug intended.
- To avoid taking the wrong drug or an extra dose, do not keep drugs on a bedside table. Drugs for emergency use, such as nitroglycerin, are an exception. It is advisable to have only one such drug at the bedside for use during the night.
- Drug use by older persons may require supervision. Observe drug effects continuously to ensure safe and effective use.
- Remember the adage: "Start low, go slow and (when appropriate) learn to say no."

Drugs Best Avoided by the Elderly Because of Increased Possibility of Adverse Reactions

antacids (high sodium)*
barbiturates*
cyclophosphamide
diethylstilbestrol
estrogens
indomethacin

monoamine oxidase inhibitors
  (MAOI's)*
oxyphenbutazone
phenacetin
phenylbutazone
tetracyclines*

Drugs That Should Be Used by the Elderly in Reduced Dosages Until Full Effect Has Been Determined

anticoagulants (oral)*
antidepressants*
antidiabetic drugs*
antihistamines*
antihypertensives*
anti-inflammatory drugs*

barbiturates*
beta-blockers*
colchicine
cortisonelike drugs*
digitalis preparations*
diuretics* (all types)

*See Drug Class, Section Four.

ephedrine
epinephrine
haloperidol
isoetharine
nalidixic acid
narcotic drugs

prazosin
pseudoephedrine
quinidine
sleep inducers (hypnotics)*
terbutaline
thyroid preparations

Drugs That May Cause Confusion and Behavioral Disturbances in the Elderly

amantadine
antidepressants*
antidiabetic drugs*
antihistamines*
anti-inflammatory drugs*
atropine* (and drugs containing
   belladonna)
barbiturates*
benzodiazepines*
carbamazepine
cimetidine
digitalis preparations*
diuretics*
ergoloid mesylates

levodopa
meprobamate
methocarbamol
methyldopa
narcotic drugs
pentazocine
phenytoin
primidone
reserpine
sedatives
sleep inducers (hypnotics)*
thiothixene
tranquilizers (mild)*
trihexyphenidyl

Drugs That May Cause Orthostatic Hypotension in the Elderly

antidepressants*
antihypertensives*
diuretics* (all types)
phenothiazines*

sedatives
tranquilizers (mild)*
vasodilators*

Drugs That May Cause Constipation and/or Retention of Urine in the Elderly

amantadine
androgens
antidepressants*
antiparkinsonism drugs*
atropinelike drugs*
epinephrine

ergoloid mesylates
isoetharine
narcotic drugs
phenothiazines*
terbutaline

Drugs That May Cause Loss of Bladder Control (Urinary Incontinence) in the Elderly

diuretics* (all types)
sedatives

sleep inducers (hypnotics)*
tranquilizers (mild)*

*See Drug Class, Section Four.

THERAPEUTIC DRUG MONITORING
(Measuring Drug Levels in Blood)

The routine use of measuring drug levels in blood as an aid in managing drug therapy has evolved gradually over the past 20 years. Because individuals vary so greatly in the nature and degree of their response to drugs, it became apparent that greater precision in determining optimal dosage for the individual was needed. For many drugs, th responses observed by the physician (clinical changes) clearly indicate that the drug is working as intended and that the dosage scheme i satisfactory. However, for some drugs—especially those with narrow safety margins—the toxic reactions closely resemble the symptoms o the disorder for which the drugs are prescribed. In many instances th patient's response is not in keeping with his or her clinical condition o program of drug therapy. By measuring the blood levels of certain drugs at appropriate times, the physician can adjust dosage schedule more accurately, predict drug response more precisely, reduce the ris of toxicity and achieve greater benefit.

The timing of the blood samples is an important consideration. As general rule, the best time for sampling is just before the next sched uled dose of the drug to be measured (the "trough" level). Samplin should be avoided during the two hours following oral administration during this absorption period, blood levels do not represent tissue level of the drug.

The following drugs are those most suitable for therapeutic dru monitoring. If you are using any of these on a regular basis, consu your physician regarding the advisability or need for periodic measure ment of drug levels in your blood.

Generic Name	Brand Name(s)
acetaminophen	Datril, Tylenol, etc.
amikacin	Amikin
amitriptyline	Amitril, Elavil, Endep, etc.
aspirin (other salicylates)	Bufferin, Ecotrin, etc.
carbamazepine	Tegretol
chloramphenicol	Chloromycetin
chlorpromazine	Thorazine
clonazepam	Clonopin
desipramine	Norpramin, Pertofrane
digitoxin	Crystodigin
digoxin	Lanoxin
disopyramide	Norpace
doxepin	Adapin, Sinequan
dyphylline	Brophylline, Neothylline, etc.
ethosuximide	Zarontin

ethotoin	Peganone
gentamicin	Garamycin
gold salts	Auranofin, Myochrisine, etc.
imipramine	Imavate, Tofranil, etc.
isoniazid	INH, Niconyl, etc.
lidocaine	Xylocaine, etc.
lithium	Lithobid, Lithotabs, etc.
mephenytoin	Mesantoin
mephobarbital	Mebaral
methotrexate	Mexate
methsuximide	Celontin
nortriptyline	Aventyl, Pamelor
paramethadione	Paradione
phenobarbital	Luminal, etc.
phensuximide	Milontin
phenytoin	Dilantin
primidone	Mysoline
procainamide	Pronestyl
propranolol	Inderal
protriptyline	Vivactil
quinidine	Cardioquin, Quinaglute, etc.
theophylline	Aminophylline, Theo-Dur, etc.
thioridazine	Mellaril
tobramycin	Nebcin
trimethadione	Tridione
valproic acid	Depakene

THE USE
OF DRUGS IN TREATING
CHRONIC DISORDERS

Chronic Disorders Reviewed in This Section

Alzheimer's Disease
Angina Pectoris
Asthma
Congestive Heart Failure
Crohn's Disease
Depression
Diabetes
Epilepsy
Glaucoma
Gout
High Blood Pressure
Hypothyroidism
Menopause
Osteoarthritis
Osteoporosis
Parkinson's Disease
Peptic Ulcer
Rheumatoid Arthritis
Schizophrenia
Ulcerative Colitis

INTRODUCTION

Of the 200 drugs prescribed most frequently by physicians in the United States from July 1, 1985, to June 30, 1986, 108 (54%) are used in the treatment of chronic disorders. This section provides an overview of the management of some of the more common disorders that require drug therapy for long periods of time, some of them for life. As you read this section, you will become familiar with important principles in the use of selected drugs and will gain perspectives that can help you to understand what your physician is attempting to accomplish with the therapy recommended. Since the lack of reasonable compliance by the patient is one of the major causes of failure in today's use of drugs, your greater understanding will encourage you to cooperate fully with your physician's instructions so that together you can achieve the greatest benefit with the least risk from the drugs prescribed.

Although drugs are essential to the rational treatment of most chronic disorders, proper attention must also be given to other treatment procedures, of equal importance. Examples include adherence to the appropriate diet in the management of diabetes, cessation of smoking in the treatment of angina (coronary artery disease), weight control in the treatment of high blood pressure (hypertension) and the use of "allergy shots" (immunotherapy) in the management of asthma. The intelligent use of drugs can make a significant contribution, but it must be recognized that drugs have their limitations and should be looked upon as but one part of a comprehensive and integrated treatment program.

WARNING: Each physician develops his or her own favored approach to the use of drugs. This is based upon knowledge of the drug's characteristics plus personal experience and observation of drug performance. The treatment program recommended by your physician may vary somewhat from the guidelines provided in this book. It is important that you follow your physician's instructions precisely as given—that you comply fully. If you question any aspect of drug selection, dosage schedule, drug effects, etc., consult your physician before attempting any modification of your drug treatment program on your own. *Under no circumstances should you attempt to initiate prescription drug therapy for yourself or others without the full knowledge and guidance of a qualified physician.*

ALZHEIMER'S DISEASE

Other Names: Alzheimer's Presenile and Senile Dementia, Senile Dementia (Alzheimer Type)

Prevalence in USA: Approximately 2.5 million; the cause of 50% of all progressive dementias.

Age Group: Occurs occasionally under 50 years of age; uncommon before 65 years; the majority occurs over 65 years: mild dementia in 5% and moderate to severe in 10–20%. Moderate to severe dementia occurs in 20% of all over 80.

Male to Female Ratio: More common in women.

Principal Features
Insidious onset leading to progressive and permanent decline of all intellectual functions.
Mood changes: apathy, depression, irritability, anxiety, paranoia.
Loss of recent memory, inability to recall facts of common knowledge, disorientation, confusion, all worse at night.
Impaired attention, understanding, judgment. Loss of ability to think abstractly, to use language correctly, to calculate.
Eventual gait disturbances, incoordination of movements.
Social skills may be retained until late in course of disease.
Course is from 3 to 20 years, with mean duration of 7 years.

Causes: Degeneration of nerve cells in the areas of the brain that control intellectual functions. Actual cause of degeneration is unknown. Genetic predisposition appears probable; Alzheimer type dementia is four times more frequent among family members than in the general population. There is a history of previous head injury in 15% to 20% of cases. One common feature is a marked deficiency of the nerve transmitter acetylcholine.

Drugs That Can Cause This Disorder: No drugs cause true Alzheimer's dementia. However, 3% of all dementias are drug induced. The following drugs can cause symptoms in the elderly that resemble Alzheimer's disease (see Drug Classes, Section Four):

antidepressants	butyrophenones
atropinelike drugs	cortisonelike drugs
barbiturates	digitalis preparations
benzodiazepines	MAO inhibitors

Drugs Used to Treat This Disorder

No specific or truly effective drug treatment is available at this time.

Ergoloid mesylates (Deapril-ST, Hydergine) are tried during the early stages to relieve symptoms; benefits are infrequent, negligible and fleeting. (See Drug Profile, Section Three.)

Experimental drugs: choline, lecithin, physostigmine (none are curative or significantly beneficial).

Goals of Drug Treatment

Temporary improvement of alertness and memory.

Relief of confusion, depression and behavioral disturbances.

Drug Management

Keep all medications to a minimum.

If any drug is used, start treatment with small doses, increase the dosage cautiously and monitor the response very closely.

Avoid drugs with strong atropinelike effects and strong sedative effects.

Ergoloid mesylates may act as a mild antidepressant and may improve mood. If it is tolerated well, a trial of 6 months is justified.

Lecithin may increase the acetylcholine content of brain tissue and temporarily improve memory in some individuals. It is available in health food stores without prescription. It is safe to try. Ask your physician for guidance.

Use antipsychotics (Haldol, Mellaril, etc.) and sedatives (chloral hydrate, Benadryl, etc.) only when clearly needed. Use the smallest dose that proves to be effective.

Ancillary Drug Treatment (as required)

Condition	Drug Treatment
For agitation, confusion:	haloperidol (Haldol)
	thioridazine (Mellaril)
For insomnia:	chloral hydrate (Noctec, Somnos, etc.)
	diphenhydramine (Benadryl)
For depression:	trazodone (Desyrel)
For constipation:	docusate (Colace, Doxinate, Surfak, etc.)

Note: Drug selection, dosage and administration schedule must be determined by the physician for each patient individually.

ANGINA PECTORIS

Other Names: Coronary Artery Insufficiency, Coronary Artery Disease, Coronary Heart Disease, Ischemic Heart Disease

Prevalence in USA: Approximately 6 million; coronary artery disease is the leading cause of death in the USA.

Age Group: Under 45 years—0.2% of population; 45 to 64 years—6.5% of population; over 65 years—11% of population.

Male to Female Ratio: Under 45 years—1.5 to 1; 45 to 64 years—3 to 1; 65 to 74 years—1.8 to 1; over 75 years—1 to 1.

Principal Features
Classical Angina-of-Effort (Exertional Angina): A moderate to severe discomfort (pain, pressure, tightness, fullness, squeezing or burning sensation) usually located deeply behind the breastbone (but may be felt in the jaw, neck, shoulder, arms, upper back or pit of the stomach). It is characteristically brought on by physical exertion, a large meal, emotional stress or exposure to cold; it usually lasts 1 to 3 minutes and disappears with rest.
Variant (Prinzmetal's) Angina: Usually occurs at rest, and is unpredictable and unrelated to the situations that provoke effort angina. It often occurs between midnight and 8 A.M. The two types of angina can coexist. Acute anginal pain may be accompanied by weakness, sweating, shortness of breath or nausea.

Causes
Exertional Angina: Due to atherosclerosis (thickening and hardening) of segments of coronary arteries. Contributory causes of these arterial changes include heredity (genetic susceptibility), hypertension, high blood cholesterol, diabetes and smoking.
Variant (Prinzmetal's) Angina: Due to spontaneous spasm of segments of coronary arteries; the cause of the spasm is not known. Anemia, hyperthyroidism, aortic valve disease and heart rhythm disorders predispose to angina.

Drugs That Can Cause This Disorder: The following drugs do not cause coronary artery disease per se, but they can affect heart function adversely and induce or intensify angina in susceptible individuals:

amphetamines	isoproterenol
bromocriptine	metaproterenol
cocaine	methysergide
epinephrine	oral contraceptives
ergot preparations	phenylpropanolamine
hydralazine	prazosin
indomethacin	terbutaline
isoetharine	thyroid

Drugs Used to Treat This Disorder

Nitrate Preparations
- nitroglycerin lingual aerosol (Nitrolingual Spray).
- nitroglycerin sublingual tablets (Nitrostat).
- nitroglycerin buccal tablets (Susadrin).
- nitroglycerin prolonged action forms (Nitro-Bid, etc.).
- nitroglycerin ointment (Nitrol, etc.).
- nitroglycerin patches (Nitrodisc, Nitro-Dur, etc.).
- isosorbide dinitrate (Isordil, Sorbitrate).
- erythrityl tetranitrate (Cardilate).
- pentaerythritol tetranitrate (Peritrate).

Beta-blocker Drugs
- propranolol (Inderal).
- nadolol (Corgard).

Other beta-blockers are used but have not yet been approved by the FDA for specific use in the management of angina.

Calcium Blocker Drugs
- nifedipine (Adalat, Procardia).
- diltiazem (Cardizem).
- verapamil (Calan, Isoptin).

Others
- aspirin (for its antiplatelet action).
- dipyridamole (Persantine).

Goals of Drug Treatment

Prompt relief of acute anginal attack.

Prevention of anticipated angina by use of nitroglyerin just before physical activity.

Long-term prevention of angina; reduced frequency, severity and duration of recurrent anginal episodes.

Prevention of heart rhythm disturbances.

Prevention of heart attack (myocardial infarction).

Drug Management

For Stable Exertional Angina

Frequency and severity of angina-of-effort remain at a constant level.

Nitroglycerin spray or sublingual tablet for relief of acute attacks.

Long-acting nitrates and/or a beta-blocker.

If control is not adequate, add a calcium blocker.

For Unstable Angina

Frequency and severity of angina increase over time; angina occurs with exertion and at rest, is less responsive to treatment.

Hospitalization in coronary care unit.

Mild sedation with benzodiazepines (Valium, etc.).

Combined use of nitrates, beta-blocker and calcium blocker.

Aspirin, for antiplatelet effect.

For Variant (Prinzmetal's) Angina
Anginal attacks primarily at rest.
Nitroglycerin spray or sublingual tablets.
Long-acting nitrates.
Calcium blocker.
Avoid beta-blockers (unless it is established that both types of angina are present).

Use of Nitroglycerin
1. Nitroglycerin is the mainstay of managing angina. Always have a supply of fresh, active tablets available. Keep them in the original dark glass bottle, tightly closed, no cotton added. Do not transfer them to a metal or plastic container.
2. The sublingual tablet will produce a mild stinging sensation under the tongue, flushing of the face and throbbing in the head. These reactions are normal and indicate that the drug is active and you are having a good response.
3. Use nitrolycerin promptly and as often as necessary, no matter how often. Unless instructed otherwise, do not consciously keep count of the tablets used.
4. If the lingual spray or sublingual tablet causes weakness, dizziness or faintness, sit down or lie down until the sensation passes.
5. Use the spray or tablet to prevent an attack by taking it just before starting a specific physical activity that is known to induce angina.
6. If anginal pain persists after taking 3 successive sublingual tablets (1 tablet at 3-to-5-minute intervals for 3 doses), consult your physician immediately or seek assistance at the nearest hospital emergency room.
7. Nitroglycerin ointment may be used at bedtime to prevent angina during sleep. Follow the instructions for application carefully. Do not use your fingers. Do not rub the ointment into the skin.
8. Nitroglycerin patches (discs) may induce tolerance to the drug and cause it to be less effective with continuous use. The intermittent use of oral dosage forms may be more effective for long-term treatment. Ask your physician for guidance.
9. If you have glaucoma, consult your physician regarding the periodic measurement of your internal eye pressures while using long-term nitrates for angina.
10. Following long-term use, nitrates should be discontinued gradually to prevent symptoms of withdrawal.

Use of Beta-blocker Drugs
1. Do not use this type of drug without your physician's knowledge and guidance.
2. Beta-blockers are not recommended for mild angina that is well controlled by nitrates. Their use is generally reserved for severe and unstable angina.
3. Beta-blockers are not recommended for variant (Prinzmetal's) vasospastic angina.
4. If your angina worsens with the use of a beta-blocker drug, notify your physician promptly.

5. Atenolol (Tenormin) and metoprolol (Lopressor) are preferred for individuals with asthma, emphysema, diabetes or peripheral circulatory disorders.
6. Atenolol (Tenormin) and nadolol (Corgard) are effective with once-daily dosage and tend to cause less depression and insomnia.
7. Beta-blocker drugs must not be discontinued suddenly. Abrupt withdrawal can cause severe angina and increase the risk of heart attack (myocardial infarction).

Use of Calcium Blocker Drugs
1. A calcium blocker is the drug of choice for treating variant (Prinzmetal's) angina.
2. Nifedipine (Adalat, Procardia) is the most potent antianginal calcium blocker. However, angina may worsen if the heart rate increases excessively.
3. Verapamil (Calan, Isoptin) can delay the excretion of digoxin and increase the risk of digoxin toxicity. Dosage adjustments may be necessary.
4. These drugs can be used initially by individuals who should not use beta-blockers.

Ancillary Drug Treatment (as required)

Condition	*Drug Treatment*
For anxiety:	benzodiazepines (Valium, etc.) (See Drug Class, Section Four.)
For hypertension:	see Profile of Hypertension in this section
For congestive heart failure:	see Profile of Congestive Heart Failure in this section
For hyperthyroidism:	methimazole (Tapazole) propylthiouracil propranolol (Inderal)
For anemia:	iron preparations

Note: Drug selection, dosage and administration schedule must be determined by the physician for each patient individually.

ASTHMA

Other Names: Bronchial Asthma, Reversible Airway Disease, Reversible Obstructive Airway Disease

Prevalence in USA: Approximately 7 million, 3% of population (includes 1.5 million school-age children).

Age Group: Under 18 years—2.5 million; 18 to 44 years—2.7 million; 45 to 64 years—1.6 million; 65 to 74 years—726,000; 75 years and over—308,000.

Male to Female Ratio: About equal.

Principal Features: Recurring acute attacks of shortness of breath, wheezing (labored breathing), a sensation of tightness in the chest and cough, with symptom-free intervals between attacks. Episodes of active asthma may last an hour to several days. The acute attack begins with tightening of muscles in the walls of bronchial tubes (airways), which causes constriction and reduced air flow. This is followed by swelling of the lining of bronchial tubes and the excessive production of mucus, both of which cause additional narrowing of the airways, forced breathing and coughing. Severe asthma may be accompanied by sweating, insomnia and bluish discoloration of the face and extremities (cyanosis). Asthma that begins in infancy (under 2 years of age) may persist into adulthood. With onset after 2 years, 50% of asthma cases will "outgrow" the disorder by 16 years. Asthma with onset in adulthood is often severe and persistent.

Causes

Extrinsic (Allergic) Asthma: Due to a true allergy (allergen-antibody reaction); hereditary susceptibility to the development of allergies. Common allergens are house dust (and mites in house dust), pollens, animal danders, feathers, wool, molds.

Intrinsic (Idiosyncratic) Asthma: Due to an unusual individual sensitivity (not a true allergy). Onset usually 35 to 45 years of age; 10% to 15% are sensitive to aspirin and have nasal polyps.

Exercise-induced Asthma: Usually in children and young adults; occurs alone or with other types of asthma; often worse 15 minutes after exercise.

Asthma "Triggers": Cold air, smoke, cooking odors, respiratory infections, emotional stress.

Drugs That Can Cause This Disorder

acetaminophen
aspirin (and substitutes)
beta-blocker drugs
erythromycin
griseofulvin
hydralazine
ibuprofen
indomethacin
ketoprofen
mefenamic acid

monoamine oxidase inhibitors
nitrofurantoin
oral contraceptives
penicillin
pentazocine
phenothiazines
phenylbutazone
procainamide
propoxyphene
reserpine

Drugs Used to Treat This Disorder

Xanthine Preparations
• aminophylline (Aminophyllin, Aminodur, etc.).
• oxtriphylline (Brondecon, Choledyl).
• theophylline (Bronkodyl, Slo-bid, Theo-Dur, etc.).

Beta-Adrenergic Drugs (in Order of Preference)
• albuterol (Proventil, Ventolin).
• terbutaline (Brethine, Bricanyl).

- metaproterenol (Alupent, Metaprel).
- isoetharine (Bronkometer, Bronkosol).
- isoproterenol (Isuprel, Medihaler-Iso, etc.).

Cortisonelike Steroids
- beclomethasone aerosol (Beclovent, Vanceril).
- prednisolone (Delta-Cortef, Sterane, etc.).
- prednisone (Deltasone, Meticorten, etc.).

Others
- cromolyn (Intal).
- oxygen.

Goals of Drug Treatment

Prompt relief of acute asthmatic attacks.

Prevention of recurrent acute attacks.

Stabilization of lung function: freedom from asthma to the greatest degree possible, with a minimal use of drugs.

Prevention of later complications: bronchiectasis, emphysema, heart disease (cor pulmonale).

Drug Management

For Extrinsic (Allergic) Asthma

For occasional and predictable acute attacks, start treatment with beta-adrenergic inhalers.

For attacks of increasing frequency and duration, add albuterol or terbutaline tablets or a long-acting oral theophylline preparation.

For severe acute attacks or aggravation of chronic asthma, add beclomethasone aerosol inhaler.

If control is not adequate, use albuterol (or terbutaline) tablets and a theophylline preparation concurrently.

If control is still inadequate, add cromolyn on a regular basis.

If an adequate trial of all of the above fails to produce satisfactory relief and control, add cortisonelike steroids (tablets by mouth).

For Intrinsic (Idiosyncratic, Late-onset) Asthma

Attacks may be less responsive to the use of the bronchodilators (beta-adrenergics and theophylline) as outlined above.

Earlier control may require the use of cromolyn and steroid preparations on a regular schedule.

For Exercise-induced Asthma

Try cromolyn on a regular schedule for prevention of attacks that follow exercise.

Use albuterol or terbutaline inhalation 5 to 10 minutes before exercise and following exercise for prevention.

Long-acting theophylline preparations may be effective in children for prevention.

Use of Theophylline Preparations
1. Theophylline elixir and uncoated tablets are used for prompt relief of acute asthma.
2. Theophylline sustained-release forms (Slo-bid, Slo-phyllin, Theo-Dur)

are used for smooth maintenance therapy of chronic asthma. Theo-phylline blood levels are helpful in determining optimal dosage sched-ules.

3. Theophylline potentiates beta-adrenergic bronchodilators and increases their effectiveness.
4. See the Drug Profile of Theophylline in Section Three for important drug interactions.

Use of Beta-Adrenergic Bronchodilators
1. These presssurized inhalers are potent drugs that must be used cau-tiously. Avoid excessive use; follow dosage schedules precisely.
2. They are most effective at the beginning of an asthmatic attack and before exercise that induces asthma.
3. For the most effective use of aerosol bronchodilators, learn the correct procedure: exhale through the mouth to empty lungs; squirt and inhale the first dose at the same time; hold your breath and count to 10, then exhale. If necessary, use a second inhalation in 10 to 15 minutes.
4. Limit inhalations to 1 or 2 at a time, and at least 3 to 4 hours apart.
5. Do not use isoproterenol (Isuprel) aerosol and epinephrine (Adrenalin) aerosol concurrently.

Use of Cortisonelike Steroids
1. Steroids are not bronchodilators; they will not relieve acute asthma. This includes beclomethasone.
2. Their use should be restricted to the treatment of severe acute and chronic asthma that is not controlled by conventional drugs.
3. Steroids should never be used as the sole drug for managing asthma.
4. For short-term use: when an acute attack is prolonged and fails to respond to bronchodilators; steroids are very effective when used for 7 to 10 days of a "burst and taper" schedule—high initial dose followed by gradual dose reduction and withdrawal.
5. For long-term use: when asthma becomes severe and continuous and cannot be controlled by other drugs; a trial period of 2 to 4 weeks of steroids will determine effectiveness. The optimal long-term use con-sists of a relatively large single dose of prednisone (or prednisolone) every other morning (alternate-day schedule). This provides adequate asthma control with minimal adverse effects of long-term steroid use.
6. The steroid beclomethasone, inhaled in aerosol form, is used to control asthma as steroid tablets are withdrawn.

Use of Cromolyn
1. Cromolyn is not a bronchodilator; it will not relieve acute asthma.
2. It is used only by inhalation; powder and liquid aerosol forms are avail-able.
3. A trial of cromolyn (as an asthma preventive) should begin while you are free of asthma, before acute attacks occur.
4. When used on a regular schedule, cromolyn is 70% to 75% effective in preventing recurrences of acute asthma.
5. Cromolyn is most effective in preventing extrinsic (allergic) asthma, and least effective in preventing intrinsic (idiosyncratic) asthma. It may or may not prevent exercise-induced asthma but is worth a trial.

6. Cromolyn should be used on a regular basis for 8 to 10 weeks to evaluate its protective benefit.
7. For best results, a beta-adrenergic aerosol should be used 10 minutes before inhaling cromolyn.

Ancillary Drug Treatment (as required)

Condition	*Drug Treatment*
For anxiety:	promethazine (Phenergan) Note: Avoid *all* sedatives in active asthma.
For pain, mild to moderate:	acetaminophen (Tylenol, etc.)
For pain, severe:	methotrimeprazine (Leroprome) This does not depress respiration.
For bacterial infection of respiratory tract (complicating asthma):	ampicillin amoxicillin trimethoprim and sulfamethoxazole tetracycline (avoid during pregnancy and under 8 years of age)
For viral infection of respiratory tract (triggering asthma):	steroids: prednisone, methylprednisolone

Note: Drug selection, dosage and administration schedule must be determined by the physician for each patient individually.

CONGESTIVE HEART FAILURE

Other Names: Chronic Heart Failure, Cardiac Decompensation, Myocardial Decompensation

Prevalence in USA: 2.3 million; 400,000 new cases annually.

Age Group: 45 to 54 years—2.6/1000 population; 55 to 64 years—7/1000 population; 65 to 74 years—15/1000 population.

Male to Female Ratio: 1.5 to 1.

Principal Features: The designation "congestive heart failure" refers to a condition in which the heart is unable to pump enough blood to satisfy the needs of the body. Diseased heart muscle loses its contracting power, allowing increased filling pressures inside the heart chambers (ventricles); further stretching and weakening of muscle tissue leads to muscle exhaustion and reduced pumping capacity; the forward flow of blood is impaired and excessive volumes of blood accumulate in vital areas throughout the body, producing congestion. Resulting symptoms include shortness of breath (dyspnea), first with exertion and later at rest; inability to breathe comfortably while lying down (orthopnea); fatigue and weakness, especially in the legs; a dry cough; night urination; swelling of the feet and ankles at the end of the day; and vague discomfort in the chest and abdomen.

Causes: Primary causes of heart disease that ultimately lead to congestive heart failure:

hypertension (75%)   myocarditis
coronary heart disease (10%)   diabetes (16%)
valvular heart disease (10%)   emphysema
congenital heart disease

Precipitating causes in predisposed individuals: reduction of therapy (most common), heart rhythm disorders, severe infections, obesity, pregnancy, anemia, hyperthyroidism, excessive heat and humidity.

Drugs That Can Cause This Disorder: In individuals with borderline heart function, the following drugs can precipitate congestive heart failure:
beta-adrenergic blocking drugs (see Drug Class, Section Four)
cortisonelike steroids (see Drug Class, Section Four)
disopyramide (Norpace)
nonsteroidal anti-inflammatory drugs (see Drug Class, Section Four)

Drugs Used to Treat This Disorder
- digitalis preparations: digitoxin, digoxin.
- diuretics (see Drug Class, Section Four).
- vasodilators: arterial dilators—hydralazine, prazosin.
              venous dilators—isosorbide dinitrate, nitroglycerin.
- calcium channel-blocking drugs: ditiazem, nifedipine, verapamil.
- ACE inhibitors: captopril, enalapril.
- milrinone (investigational only).
- oxygen.

Goals of Drug Treatment
Improvement of the heart's pumping performance by the use of digitalis.
Reduction of the heart's workload by the use of arterial and venous vasodilators.
Removal of excess salt and water from the body by the use of diuretics.
Relief of symptoms—fatigue, shortness of breath, ankle swelling, etc.—by means of the above procedures.

Drug Management

For Early, Mild Congestive Heart Failure

Two variations of initial treatment are used widely:

1. Treatment is started with digitalis (digoxin or digitoxin). This may be the only drug used if response is satisfactory. If necessary, a thiazide diuretic (or equivalent) is added.
2. Treatment is started with a thiazide diuretic (or equivalent), given alone. This may give a very adequate response, especially in the elderly. If necessary, digoxin (or digitoxin) is added.

For Moderate to Severe Congestive Heart Failure

Digoxin (or digitoxin) and thiazide diuretics are used in maximal tolerated dosage.

As necessary, a stronger diuretic, such as furosemide or ethacrynic acid, is added.

If the response is inadequate, vasodilators are started: isosorbide dinitrate or nitroglycerin patches for venous dilation; hydralazine for arterial dilation.

If additional improvement is sought, captopril (or enalapril) may be tried as a replacement for the nitrates (isosorbide dinitrate or nitroglycerin).

For long-term maintenance, a combination of hydralazine and nitrates or hydralazine and captropril may be tried.

For congestive heart failure with angina and/or hypertension, a trial of nifedipine is justified.

Use of Digitalis

1. Should be started only when there is a firm diagnosis of heart failure. Periodic reassessment is necessary to determine continued need. Maintenance digitalis may not be necessary for life.
2. Digoxin is the forms of digitalis most frequently used. Because digoxin products vary in their absorbability, refill your prescriptions with the same brand to ensure uniform drug effects.
3. Take the exact dose at the same time each day.
4. Learn to count your pulse and check its regularity. Notify your physician if your pulse rate is below 60 beats/minute or your pulse rhythm changes significantly.
5. The elderly and individuals with hypothyroidism often have a reduced tolerance for digitalis; smaller doses are advisable.
6. Digitalis toxicity (overdosage) occurs in 20% of users; it is more common in the elderly. The earliest indications of toxicity are usually loss of appetite, nausea and vomiting; other indications include headache, facial pains, blurred vision, seeing "snowflakes" or yellowish-green halos, fatigue, weakness and disturbances of heart rhythm. The elderly may show confusion; rarely, seizures may occur.
7. Periodic blood levels can help to determine optimal dosage, especially if kidney function is impaired. The blood sample should be taken no less than 6 hours after the last dose.

8. See the Drug Profile of Digoxin in Section Three for important drug interactions.

Use of Diuretics ("Water Pills")

1. Thiazide (or equivalent) diuretics may suffice as the only drug treatment for mild heart failure in many elderly patients.
2. When possible, diuretics should be taken in the morning to minimize nighttime urination.
3. If your diuretic is one that increases the excretion of potassium in the urine, it is important that your blood level of potassium be checked periodically. An abnormally low potassium level can increase the risk of digitalis toxicity. Consult your physician regarding the advisability of omitting your diuretic every third day to minimize the loss of potassium.
4. If your diuretic is one that does not increase the excretion of potassium (amiloride, spironolactone, triamterene), you should not take a potassium supplement or eat excessive amounts of high-potassium foods.
5. If you use diuretics on a regular basis, consult your physician regarding the degree of salt restriction he or she recommends for you.
6. Many salt substitutes have a high potassium content. Ask your physician for guidance regarding the selection and use of commercially available salt substitutes.
7. In advanced congestive heart failure, you may be advised to use a thiazide diuretic concurrently with furosemide (or ethacrynic acid) and a potassium-saving diuretic; the combined actions of the three types of drugs give a maximal diuretic effect.

Use of Vasodilators

1. These are generally used when heart failure does not respond adequately to digitalis and diuretics.
2. These may be used earlier for those who cannot tolerate digitalis, and for those who need a vasodilator to treat hypertension (hydralazine) or angina (nifedipine).
3. Nitrate vasodilators (primarily venous dilators) contribute to the relief of shortness of breath.
4. Hydralazine (primarily an arterial dilator) contributes to the relief of fatigue and weakness.
5. Isosorbide dinitrate (venous) and hydralazine (arterial) vasodilators can be used concurrently to advantage; they are quite effective in the majority of cases of chronic congestive failure.
6. Prazosin (both an arterial and a venous dilator) is an alternative choice. However it causes fluid retention and requires increasing doses and additional diuretics with continued use.

Use of Oxygen

1. Oxygen must be properly humidified to prevent drying of tissues of the respiratory tract.
2. Administer by nasal prongs; avoid a mask.

Ancillary Drug Treatment (as required)

Condition	Drug Treatment
For anxiety:	diazepam (only as needed)
For insomnia:	chloral hydrate (Noctec, Somnos)
For anemia:	iron preparations
For hypertension:	see Profile of Hypertension in this section

Note: Drug selection, dosage and administration schedule must be determined by the physician for each patient individually.

CROHN'S DISEASE

Other Names: Regional Enteritis, Regional Ileitis, Granulomatous Colitis, Inflammatory Bowel Disease

Prevalence in USA: 1 million (includes 100,000 children); 15,000 new cases annually.

Age Group: Onset from infancy to 25 years of age; 15% to 30% have onset before puberty. Peak incidence is from 10 to 25 years of age.

Male to Female Ratio: Slightly more common in females.

Principal Features: An intermittent to chronic disorder of the small intestine and colon; one third of cases occur in the lower segment of the small intestine (the ileum), one third in the colon and one third in both. Less than 50% of cases involve the rectum. The onset is usually insidious, but may be rapid and resemble acute appendicitis. Symptoms include loss of appetite, fatigue, fever, loss of weight, abdominal cramps and pain after eating, nausea, vomiting, diarrhea (occasionally bloody), anal sores and retarded growth in children. There may also be inflammatory disorders in the skin, eyes, mouth and large joints. Children may experience fever and joint pains before any indications of disease in the intestine or colon. Adults may have a higher incidence of gallstones or kidney stones. This disorder often recurs throughout life.

Causes: The primary cause is unknown. There is a familial clustering in 15% to 20% of cases. It is thought that an inherited susceptibility may predispose to unknown environmental factors capable of inducing the disorder.

Drugs That Can Cause This Disorder: By altering the normal balance of bacteria in the intestine, several antibiotics can cause a form of enteritis that might resemble Crohn's disease. These include some of the tetracyclines, penicillin and chloramphenicol. Antibiotic-induced enteritis is transient and easily corrected; no permanent damage occurs.

Drugs Used to Treat This Disorder

- sulfasalazine (Azulfidine).
- cortisonelike steroids, principally prednisone.
- azathioprine (Imuran); 6-mercaptopurine (Purinethol).
- metronidazole (Flagyl).
- antidiarrheals: diphenoxylate (Lomotil), loperamide (Imodium).
- antispasmodics: belladonna (Donnatal), dicyclomine (Bentyl).
- antibiotics: ampicillin (Amcill, etc.), tetracycline (Achromycin, etc.); used when appropriate for bacterial infections of intestine.

Goals of Drug Treatment

Induction of a remission (return to normal) during the active phase of the disease.

Relief of symptoms.

Protection of bowel, avoidance of complications.

Maintenance of general nutrition.

Drug Management

General Principles

For initial treatment of mild disease: sulfasalazine.

For moderate to severe disease: prednisone, used concurrently with sulfasalazine.

For acute recurrences: prednisone.

For long-term maintenance: sulfasalazine; avoid use of cortisonelike steroids (prednisone).

For active disease that fails to respond to combined use of sulfasalazine and prednisone: (1) a trial of metronidazole as replacement for sulfasalazine; (2) a trial of azathioprine or 6-mercaptopurine added to sulfasalazine and prednisone programs.

Use of Sulfasalazine

1. Used to initiate treatment in active disease.
2. About 50% effective when used with prednisone.
3. Most beneficial in treating Crohn's disease of the colon.
4. Usually not effective in preventing recurrences; however, it may be tried for long-term maintenance until a better treatment is developed.
5. Common adverse effects are headache, nausea and vomiting; take with or immediately following food.

Use of Cortisonelike Steroids (Prednisone, etc.)

1. Usually 60% to 70% effective during first 6 months of treatment; if use is extended to 12 months, only 20% to 30% remain in remission.
2. Good initial response in treating Crohn's disease of the colon, but the majority relapse within 1 year.
3. Long-term use for mild disease or to prevent recurrences is usually ineffective and is not advised.
4. Use primarily to control worsening symptoms and to suppress acute flare-ups. Continue use until a sustained improvement is established. Try to use the lowest effective dose.

5. When possible, an alternate-day dosing schedule is recommended: a single morning dose every 48 hours.
6. When appropriate, taper dose very slowly over a period of 4 to 12 months.
7. Repeated intermittent short courses are preferable to continual long-term use.
8. Crohn's disease of the rectum should be treated with steroid suppositories and retention enemas.

Use of Antidiarrheals
1. Use very cautiously and as sparingly as possible.
2. Excessive use can induce two complications: (1) paralytic (adynamic) ileus, a paralysis of the small intestine that results in a functional obstruction; (2) toxic megacolon, a marked distention of the colon with air, and a danger of perforation.

Use of Adsorbents
1. Cholestyramine (Questran) and aluminum hydroxide (Amphojel) can adsorb bile in the intestine and reduce bile-induced diarrhea.
2. These adsorbents can also adsorb other drugs being used concurrently. Schedule all dosages to ensure maximal effectiveness—adequate spacing between adsorbents and other active drugs.

Use of Immunosuppressants
1. Azathioprine (Imuran) and 6-mercaptopurine (Purinethol) may be tried when sulfasalazine and prednisone have failed to control the disease after an adequate trial.
2. Either one may be tried as an adjunct to the established treatment program.
3. A trial of 4 to 6 months of treatment is often necessary to determine effectiveness.
4. These drugs make it possible to reduce the dose of steroids or withdraw them completely in some individuals.

Use of Antibiotics
1. Appropriately selected antibiotics may be used to treat a diarrhea due to specific bacterial overgrowth (superinfection).
2. Antibiotics should not be taken concurrently with sulfasalazine.

Ancillary Drug Treatment (as required)

Condition	Drug Treatment
For anemia (common):	iron preparations, vitamin B-12, folic acid (as required)
For malnutrition:	multiple vitamins and the minerals calcium, magnesium, zinc
For depression:	see Profile of Depression in this section

Note: Drug selection, dosage and administration schedule must be determined by the physician for each patient individually.

DEPRESSION

Other Names: Depressive Reaction (Reactive Depression, Secondary Depression), Depressive Illness (Biologic Depression, Major Depressive Disorder), Affective Disorder: Depressive Phase of Manic-Depressive Disorder

Prevalence in USA: Approximately 30 million; 5% to 8% of general population. One third of all depressions are severe enough to require medical treatment.

Age Group: Can occur at any age. Peak occurrence is between 25 and 44 years of age.

Male to Female Ratio: 1 male to 2 females; 25% of women and 10% of men will experience depression during their lifetime.

Principal Features

Depressive Reaction: a situational (exogenous) reactive depression that represents an understandable adaptive response to a significant loss or stressful life situation; a sense of despondency and distress, comparatively mild to moderate, usually self-limiting with a duration of 2 weeks to 6 months.

Depressive Illness: a spontaneous (endogenous) unexplained and seemingly unprovoked depression of moderate to severe degree; characterized by (1) a depressed mood—sadness, dejection, hopelessness, despair; (2) reduced energy level—loss of interest, fatigue, inability to function effectively; (3) negative self-image—sense of inferiority, incompetence, exaggerated guilt. Common features include loss of appetite, broken sleep, early morning awakening, constipation. Often clears spontaneously in 6 to 12 months, even without treatment.

Causes: Depressive reactions are normal mood responses to the stresses and strains of daily life. The primary cause of major depressive illness is unknown. Research indicates that in many cases there appears to be a genetic (constitutional) predisposition to depression. The actual onset of depressive illness is attributed to a deficiency of certain brain chemicals—the neurotransmitters norepinephrine, dopamine and/or serotonin. What initiates the deficiency is not known.

Drugs That Can Cause This Disorder: Drug-induced depressions are more likely to occur in those who are genetically susceptible to depression. The following drugs are known to cause depression:

benzodiazepines (in excess)	levodopa
certain beta-blocking drugs	methyldopa
clonidine	oral contraceptives
cortisonelike steroids	some phenothiazines
digitalis (toxicity)	reserpine (and related drugs)
indomethacin	

Drugs Used to Treat This Disorder

Tricyclic Antidepressants (TCA's)
- amitriptyline (Elavil, Endep).
- amoxapine (Asendin).
- desipramine (Norpramin, Pertofrane).
- doxepin (Adapin, Sinequan).
- imipramine (Imavate, Presamine, Tofranil).
- nortriptyline (Aventyl, Pamelor).
- protriptyline (Vivactil).

Tetracyclic Antidepressant
- maprotiline (Ludiomil).

Monoamine Oxidase Inhibitors (MAOI's)
- phenelzine (Nardil).
- tranylcypromine (Parnate).

Other Drugs
- alprazolam (Xanax)
- lithium (Eskalith, Lithane, Lithobid, Lithotab)
- methylphenidate (Ritalin)
- trazodone (Desyrel)

Goals of Drug Treatment

Alleviation of symptoms.

Termination of depression, restoration of normal mood.

Prevention of recurrence.

Prevention of swing from depression to manic psychosis (in manic-depressive disorder).

Drug Management

For Depressive Reactions: Reactive depressions are often mild and self-limiting; they usually respond well to supportive psychotherapy. Drug treatment is not necessary for everyone who is depressed. If this type of depression becomes severe or is unreasonably prolonged, a tricyclic antidepressant (or a new generation equivalent) may be tried for 1 month to determine its effectiveness.

For Depressive Illness: Major endogenous depressions are usually very responsive to an appropriate and adequate trial of antidepressant drug therapy. Spontaneous remissions often occur within 6 to 12 months, but recovery can be initiated earlier and greatly accelerated by proper medication. Adequate dosage and a sufficient period of treatment are essential to a successful outcome.

Treatment is usually started with a tricyclic antidepressant or one of the newer equivalents. If response is inadequate after a reasonable trial, another tricyclic or similar antidepressant should be tried. If this fails, a monoamine oxidase inhibitor may be considered. Some cyclic depressions respond better to lithium than to tricyclic antidepressants.

Not all depressions are recurrent. For a first episode, the antidepressant drug may be gradually reduced and discontinued after 3 to 6 months of a stable mood, free of depression.

For the 50% of depressions that are recurrent, the optimal maintenance dose of the most effective drug should be determined and continued indefinitely.

Use of Tricyclic Antidepressants (TCA's)

1. These are the drugs of choice when drug treatment is deemed necessary.
2. They are 60% to 75% effective in treating major endogenous depressive illness. They may also be effective in treating severe reactive depressions.
3. Continual use on a regular schedule for 2 to 5 weeks is necessary to determine a drug's effectiveness in relieving depression.
4. Treatment with all antidepressants is necessarily empirical; a period of trial and error is unavoidable for both the selection of the best drug and the determination of optimal dosage.
5. If one TCA (or equivalent) shows no significant benefit after 3 weeks of adequate dosage, it is advisable to try another drug of the same or similar class.
6. During drug trials, and during maintenance treatment later, stay with the same brand (manufacturer) to ensure uniform results.
7. Periodic measurement of blood levels of the drug can be helpful in determining optimal dosage. (See Therapeutic Drug Monitoring in Section One.)
8. Most drugs of this class cause drowsiness, especially during the first several weeks of use. Avoid alcoholic beverages and use extreme caution in driving and engaging in all hazardous activities.
9. When the correct total daily dose has been determined, it can usually be taken as a single dose at bedtime.
10. Use these drugs cautiously if you have glaucoma, prostatism or a heart rhythm disorder.
11. Avoid rapid withdrawal of TCA's; abrupt discontinuation may cause restlessness, headache, anxiety, insomnia, muscle aches, nausea. Withdraw gradually over a period of 10 to 14 days.
12. See the Drug Profiles of respective TCA's in Section Three for important drug interactions.

Use of Newer ("Second Generation") Antidepressants

1. Maprotiline (Ludiomil) may act more rapidly than TCA's; it is quite sedating. Avoid if you have a seizure disorder.
2. Alprazolam (Xanax) is sedating. After long-term use, withdraw gradually to avoid possible seizures.
3. Amoxapine (Asendin) is less sedating. It can cause parkinsonlike symptoms, restlessness and tardive dyskinesia (rarely). Do not use longer than 3 to 4 months.
4. Trazodone (Desyrel) is also sedating, but it has little or no atropinelike effects. It is very useful in the elderly and for those with glaucoma or prostatism.

Use of Monoamine Oxidase Inhibitors (MAOI's)

1. Used to treat biologic endogenous depressions that do not respond to TCA's.
2. Also useful for treating "atypical" and neurotic depressions that are

characterized by marked anxiety, phobias, hypochondriasis, excessive eating and excessive sleeping.

3. Continual use on a regular schedule for 2 to 5 weeks is necessary to determine effectiveness in relieving depression.
4. Avoid concurrent use of over-the-counter diet pills, nose drops and cold and allergy preparations.
5. Avoid foods and beverages that contain tyramine and similar compounds. (See Tyramine in Glossary.)
6. If switching from a TCA to a MAOI, allow a "washout" period of 7 to 10 days before starting the MAOI.
   If switching from a MAOI to a TCA, allow a "washout" period of 14 days before starting the TCA.
7. MAOI's can cause low blood pressure, overstimulation, insomnia, confusion, nausea, vomiting, diarrhea and fluid retention.
8. MAOI's can provoke an abrupt swing from depression to manic psychosis in manic-depressive disorder.
9. MAOI's can activate psychosis in those with schizophrenia.
10. Do not discontinue these drugs suddenly. A rebound depression can follow abrupt withdrawal.
11. See the Drug Profiles of respective MAOI's in Section Three for important drug interactions.

Use of Lithium

1. Can be 70% effective in stabilizing mood, especially in bipolar manic-depressive illness; reduces the frequency and severity of attacks of both mania and depression.
2. Often effective in preventing recurrences of depression in unipolar (depression only) disorders.
3. Must be taken in divided doses to avoid stomach irritation and excessively high (toxic) blood levels.
4. When lithium proves to be effective in preventing recurrence of depression, it is very important to continue maintenance treatment when feeling well and free of depression.
5. Periodic measurements of blood levels are mandatory to maintain effective concentrations and to prevent toxicity. Blood samples should be taken 12 hours after the last dose.
6. Mild side-effects (not toxicity) include loss of appetite, metallic taste, indigestion, nausea, thirst, fatigue, tremor, fluid retention, acne.
7. Early toxic effects include vomiting, dizziness, unsteadiness, weakness, slurred speech, muscle twitching, confusion.
8. While taking lithium, maintain a high liquid intake, but avoid excessive coffee, tea and cola drinks.
9. Do not restrict your salt intake.
10. Use lithium cautiously if you have heart disease, kidney disease or a thyroid disorder.
11. Check thyroid and kidney functions before and during lithium therapy.

Use of Other Antidepressant Drugs
1. Methylphenidate (Ritalin) may be tried for long-term treatment of selected elderly persons with depression.
2. Alprazolam (Xanax), a benzodiazepine tranquilizer, may be useful for short-term treatment of minor depression.

Ancillary Drug Treatment (as required)

Condition	Drug Treatment
For mild anxiety:	alprazolam (Xanax)
For severe anxiety and agitation:	thioridazine (Mellaril)
	thiothixene (Navane)
For psychosis:	amitriptyline and perphenazine (Etrafon, Triavil)
For constipation:	docusate (Colace, Doxinate, etc.)

Note: Drug selection, dosage and administration schedule must be determined by the physician for each patient individually.

DIABETES

Other Names: Diabetes Mellitus; Insulin-Dependent Diabetes Mellitus (IDDM), Type I; Non-Insulin-Dependent Diabetes Mellitus (NIDDM), Type II

Prevalence in USA: Approximately 10 million: 6 million known, 4 million undiagnosed; 2% to 4% of the population, with a 6% increase (new cases) annually.

Age Group: Under 18 years—90,000; 18 to 44 years—880,000; 45 to 64 years—2.6 million; 65 to 74 years—1.6 million; 75 years and over—800,000.

Male to Female Ratio: Type I—same incidence in men and women. Type II—greater incidence in women.

Principal Features: A disorder of carbohydrate, protein and fat metabolism that renders the body unable to convert foods properly into energy for vital functions.
Type I (10% to 15% of All Diabetes): Occurs most commonly in children and adolescents, with peak onset from 11 to 14 years; can begin at any age. Individuals are usually thin or normal weight (nonobese). Requires life-long insulin for control of blood sugar and prevention of acidosis.
Type II (85% to 90% of All Diabetes): Most common after 40 years of age, with peak onset from 45 to 64 years. Up to 90% of individuals are obese. Does

not require lifelong insulin for control; not prone to development of acidosis.

Characteristic symptoms include excessive hunger and thirst, excessive urination, unexplained weight loss, blurred vision, fatigue, itching of skin, anal and vaginal yeast infections and delayed healing of wounds.

Causes: Primary causes are unknown, but a genetic (hereditary) predisposition appears certain for both types of diabetes. In addition, some individuals who develop type I diabetes may have a genetic susceptibility to viral infection of the pancreas that initiates destruction of the tissue cells that produce insulin. In type I diabetes the pancreas produces very little or no insulin. In type II diabetes insulin production may be normal or partially reduced, but not absent; the diabetes is due to insulin resistance in body tissues.

Drugs That Can Cause This Disorder: In susceptible individuals and those with latent diabetes, the following drugs may induce diabetic manifestations; these are usually mild in nature and reversible:

cortisonelike steroids
ethacrynic acid
furosemide
indomethacin
lithium
oral contraceptives

phenothiazines
phenytoin
propranolol
thiazide diuretics
tricyclic antidepressants

Drugs Used to Treat This Disorder
The Insulins: see Drug Profile of Insulin in Section Three
The Sulfonylureas (Oral Hypoglycemic Drugs)
- acetohexamide (Dymelor).
- chlorpropamide (Diabinese).
- glipizide (Glucotrol).
- glyburide (Diabeta, Micronase).
- tolazamide (Tolinase).
- tolbutamide (Orinase).

Goals of Drug Treatment
Normalization of carbohydrate, protein and fat metabolism insofar as possible; control of blood sugar; elimination of acidosis.
Elimination of symptoms; restoration of well-being.
Prevention of hypoglycemia (insulin "shock").
Prevention of recurrent acidosis.
Promotion of normal growth and development in diabetic children.
Prevention or minimization of late complications.
Achievement of normal life expectancy.

Drug Management
General Principles
"Good control" consists of the optimal balance of properly selected foods, exercise and drugs—either insulin or a sulfonylurea in correct dosage.

The degree of control is estimated by periodic measurement of blood-sugar levels or urine sugar content.

"Tight control" consists of maintaining a fasting blood sugar between 100 and 140 mg, and a 2-hour (after eating) blood sugar betweeen 100 and 200 mg. Consideration must be given to the possible benefits of "tight control" versus the possible risks of inducing hypoglycemia.

"Tight control" is appropriate for the young diabetic who is otherwise healthy, free of coronary artery and cerebral circulatory disease, capable of excellent self-care and not living alone. It is not appropriate for the elderly, those with circulatory disorders of the brain or heart, those with established complications of long-standing diabetes and those with other serious disorders.

Although more expensive and inconvenient, the home monitoring of blood-sugar levels is the method of choice for managing diabetic control. The blood-sugar strips Chemstrip bG and Visidex II are recommended for this purpose.

The use of urine-testing strips for the detection of urine sugar and ketones is a useful and practical alternative to the use of blood-sugar strips. Regular testing of urine before meals and at bedtime provides adequate information for the proper adjustment of insulin dosage schedules and the prevention of hypoglycemia and acidosis. Accuracy is improved when the bladder is first emptied and the urine for testing is collected 30 minutes later; the sugar content of this second voiding is more representative of the current blood-sugar level.

If urine testing reveals the repeated presence of ketones, consult your physician promptly.

The following drugs can cause a *false positive* test result for urine sugar when using Clinitest: aspirin (with doses larger than 2400 mg/day), ascorbic acid (vitamin C), cephalosporins, chloral hydrate, chloramphenicol, isoniazid, levodopa, methyldopa, nalidixic acid, penicillin G, probenecid, streptomycin.

The following drugs can cause a *false negative* test result for urine sugar when using Diastix or Testape: aspirin (with doses larger than 2400 mg/day), ascorbic acid (vitamin C), levodopa, methyldopa.

The following drugs can cause a *false positive* test result for urine ketones when using Acetest or Ketostix: aspirin (in moderate to high doses), levodopa, phenazopyridine (Ketostix only).

Learn to recognize the early indications of hypoglycemia and what to do to correct it. Signs that warn of a developing insulin reaction include hunger, sweating, headache, dizziness, nervousness, trembling, blurred vision, drowsiness, confusion, inability to think, sense of inebriation. At the first indication of impending hypoglycemia, take sugar immediately: 5 small sugar cubes; or 2 teaspoonsful or 2 packets of granulated sugar; or 1/2 to 1 cup of fruit juice; or 1 candy bar. An alternative treatment is the injection of 1 mg of glucagon, repeated in 5 to 10 minutes if necessary. Glucagon is a pancreatic hormone that increases the level of blood sugar.

Learn to recognize the early indications of acidosis. These include the slow development of increasing thirst, excessive urination, drowsiness, fatigue, nausea, vomiting, stomach pain.

The use of beta-blocking drugs (especially in high doses) may predispose to hypoglycemia and mask its symptoms.

For Type I, IDDM

Insulin is a lifelong requirement for control. Sulfonylureas (oral hypoglycemics) are not effective and should not be used.

Insulin requirements will vary continually throughout a lifetime. Therefore, you must learn how to manage your diabetes on a day-by-day basis, modifying insulin types and dosage schedules as necessary, according to the results of regular blood- or urine sugar testing.

For the newly diagnosed diabetic who is not acutely ill and is without complications, the usual American procedure for initiating treatment is to give a single morning dose of 15 to 30 units of an intermediate-acting insulin (NPH or Lente) before breakfast; the dose is then increased by 5 units every 48 hours as required to achieve normal blood-sugar levels. The British method is to start with 6 to 10 units of an intermediate-acting insulin given twice daily, before the morning and evening meals. Either method will relieve most symptoms in 90% of cases within 4 days.

The optimal schedule of insulin injections for regulating the disordered metabolism is determined by periodic monitoring of blood-sugar levels at appropriate times during the 24-hour day. In this way individual patterns of blood-sugar fluctuation and response to insulin can be studied so that the most appropriate types and doses of insulin are given in proper relationship to eating.

A most effective and practical method of providing adequate insulin for the average diabetic is to give a mixture (1 injection) of a rapid-acting insulin (Regular) and an intermediate-acting insulin (NPH or Lente) 20 to 30 minutes before the morning and evening meals, just 2 injections daily. This scheme provides for easy modification of doses of each type of insulin as necessary to obtain smooth control throughout 24 hours.

During periods of stress—infections, injuries, surgery—insulin requirements will increase. Consult your physician for guidance if you have difficulty in making the necessary adjustments of insulin dosage, food intake, etc.

Even during periods of fasting, small amounts of insulin are necessary to control blood sugar and prevent acidosis.

For Type II, NIDDM

Diet is of primary importance and should be tried diligently before starting drugs. Dietary goals are reduction of blood sugar and correction of obesity. Seventy-five percent of cases of Type II diabetes can be controlled by diet alone.

If an adequate trial of dietary management fails, either sulfonylurea drugs (oral hypoglycemics) or insulin may be added to the treatment program. If the blood sugar is only moderately above normal, a sulfonylurea may be tried. If the blood sugar is quite high and the individual is thin, it is best to initiate drug treatment with insulin. After the blood sugar has

been stabilized for 3 to 4 weeks, the insulin may be withdrawn and a
sulfonylurea may be started to determine its effectiveness.

The major reaction to sulfonylureas is hypoglycemia. It is most likely to
occur in the elderly, in alcoholics and in those with significant impairment of liver or kidney function. Hypoglycemic reactions occur most frequently with the use of chlorpropamide (Diabinese), the longest acting
sulfonylurea.

If you experience a primary failure (on initial trial) or a secondary failure
(after a temporary period of effectiveness) on attempting control with a
sulfonylurea, you may need insulin to manage your diabetes successfully.

Insulin is used primarily to control the levels of blood sugar. It is not
required to prevent acidosis except under stressful conditions, such as
infections, trauma or surgery.

Type II diabetes is often well controlled with a single daily dose of an intermediate-acting insulin. Some individuals with a high degree of insulin
resistance may require unusually high doses of insulin to achieve satisfactory control.

Use of Insulins
1. Twenty percent of all diabetics require insulin for satisfactory control.
2. Available insulins differ in their times of peak action and duration of
   action. An understanding of these differences is necessary for planning
   an insulin schedule and adjusting it to control your individual pattern
   of blood-sugar fluctuations during each 24-hour day. The following
   chart illustrates the characteristics of the three principal types of insulin.

Type of insulin	Peak action (hours)	Duration (hours)	Hypoglycemia most likely to occur
Short-acting			
Regular	2–4	5–7	Before lunch
Semilente	2–8	12–16	Before lunch
Actrapid	2.5–5	8	Before lunch
Semitard	7	9	Early afternoon
Velosulin	2–5	8	Before lunch
Humulin R	2–5	6–8	Before lunch
Intermediate-acting			
Lente	8–12	18–28	Late afternoon
NPH	6–12	18–28	Late afternoon
Monotard	7–15	18–24	Late afternoon
Lentard	8–12	16–24	Late afternoon
Insulatard	4–12	16–24	Mid-afternoon
Humulin N	6–12	14–24	Late afternoon
Novolin N	4–12	18–24	Mid-afternoon

Long-acting

Protamine Zinc	14–24	24–36	During night—early morning
Ultralente	18–24	32–36	During night—early morning
Ultratard	10–28	24–36	During night—early morning

3. The peak action times and the duration of action vary greatly from person to person. Each individual will show variations of absorption from one injection site to another and from day to day. Insulin programs must be tailored to each person individually based on response to trials. All insulin schedules need adjustment from time to time.
4. Most insulin-dependent diabetics require from 20 to 60 units of insulin daily. If the requirement reaches 200 units/day, a marked degree of insulin resistance has developed. This is best treated with highly purified pork insulin or human insulin.
5. Most of the time satisfactory control can be achieved with an intermediate-acting insulin, or with the addition of a short-acting insulin. Regular insulin can be mixed with either Lente or NPH in the same syringe and given as a single injection. The mixture retains the short and intermediate characteristics of action.
6. Long-acting insulins are rarely necessary and are seldom used.
7. Hypoglycemia that occurs during the night (excessive insulin effect) causes a "rebound" hyperglycemia that is detected by blood- or urine sugar testing the next morning. This is known as the Somogyi effect. The proper adjustment is to reduce the dose of the long-acting insulin taken in the morning or the dose of the intermediate-acting insulin taken before the evening meal; this will prevent the nocturnal hypoglycemia that causes the confusing high blood or urine sugar on arising.
8. If a true allergy to insulin develops, or if the fatty tissue under the skin at the sites of insulin injection should disappear (lipoatrophy), change to highly purified pork or human insulin.
9. If insulin use is to be intermittent (as in some cases of type II diabetes), it is best to use human insulin to reduce the possibility of developing insulin antibodies that cause insulin resistance.
10. Insulin pumps using either Regular or Ultralente insulin have been developed for use in selected individuals. While they are capable of providing excellent control, their use is quite complex and demanding. They are suitable only for the highly motivated and educated individual who needs and is dedicated to achieving "tight control."

Use of Sulfonylureas (Oral Hypoglycemic Drugs)
1. These drugs are used only for the treatment of type II, NIDDM, in those whose diabetes is not adequately controlled by diet and exercise and who cannot or will not take insulin.
2. The best candidates for a trial of sulfonylureas
   - are over 50 years old.
   - are otherwise healthy.

- are not allergic to "sulfa" drugs.
- have no tendency to develop acidosis.
- have an insulin requirement of less than 30 units/day.
- prefer tablets by mouth to injections.

3. Sulfonylureas are not suitable for treating
   - type I, insulin-dependent diabetes.
   - the acutely ill diabetic with acidosis.
   - the diabetic with infection or with injury, or undergoing surgery.
   - the diabetic using long-term cortisonelike steroids.
   - the pregnant diabetic.
   - the diabetic whose blood sugar is over 300 mg.

4. Sulfonylureas should be used with caution in treating
   - the very old.
   - alcoholics.
   - those taking multiple drugs.
   - those with significantly impaired liver or kidney function.
   - those who comply poorly with recommendations.

5. Recommended dosage schedules

Short-acting	Duration	Doses/day
tolbutamide	6–12 hrs.	2–3
Intermediate-acting		
acetohexamide	12–24 hrs.	1–2
glipizide	18–30 hrs.	1–2
glyburide	10–30 hrs.	1–2
tolazamide	10–18 hrs.	1–2
Long-acting		
chlorpropamide	60 hrs.	1

6. All sulfonylureas can cause hypoglycemia. Because of its accumulative effects and long period of action, chlorpropamide requires the greatest caution in use; any hypoglycemic reaction is apt to be quite prolonged.

7. Sulfonylureas as a group have a high rate of primary failure (40%). A primary failure is an inability to control hyperglycemia after 3 months of continual treatment with adequate dosage. Secondary failures (25% to 30%) occur when a sulfonylurea drug loses its effectiveness after an initial period of demonstrated ability to control hyperglycemia.

8. During apparently successful long-term use of a sulfonylurea, it is prudent to periodically reduce the dosage and gradually withdraw the drug to determine if its continued use is justified. The success rate of adequate control by long-term use of sulfonylureas is no more than 20% to 30%.

9. There appears to be no general support for the concurrent use of sulfonylureas and insulin. If it is found that insulin is necessary for adequate control, the customary practice is to discontinue the sulfonylurea.

Ancillary Drug Treatment (as required)

Condition	Drug Treatment
For yeast infections of skin:	ciclopirox (Loprox) clotrimazole (Lotrimin) haloprogin (Halotex) miconazole (Micatin) nystatin (Mycostatin)
For yeast infections of the vagina:	clotrimazole (Gyne-Lotrimin, Mycelex-G) miconazole (Monistat)
For diabetic diarrhea:	diphenoxylate (Lomotil) loperamide (Imodium)
For peripheral neuritis:	carbamazepine (Tegretol) and amitriptyline (Elavil) concurrently
For neurogenic bladder:	bethanechol (Urecholine)
For high blood pressure:	see Profile of Hypertension in this section

Note: Drug selection, dosage and administration schedule must be determined by the physician for each patient individually.

EPILEPSY

Other Names: Seizure Disorders, Convulsive Disorders

Prevalence in USA: Approximately 2 million, 1% of the population.

Age Group: 24% of epileptics are under 18 years of age; 53% are 18 to 44 years; 18% are 45 to 64 years; 4% are 65 to 74 years; 1% is 75 years and older.

Male to Female Ratio: About equal.

Principal Features: True epilepsy is a chronic disorder characterized by recurring seizures lasting from a few seconds to several minutes and requiring specific medication for prevention and control. Sixty-six percent of epileptic patients require lifelong drug therapy. The principal types of epilepsy include:

Tonic-Clonic Seizures (Grand Mal): Sudden attacks that begin with an involuntary cry, followed by a loss of consciousness and falling, violent convulsive movements of the head, trunk and extremities, excessive salivation and sometimes loss of bladder and/or rectal control. The seizure lasts from 1 to 3 minutes. The individual awakens spontaneously, is dazed, confused and exhausted, and usually falls into a deep sleep that lasts several hours. The subject cannot remember the episode.

Absence Seizures (Petit Mal): These begin between 2 and 12 years of age; 90% cease by 20 years; 50% go on to develop tonic-clonic seizures by 20 years. The seizure consists of a sudden, momentary lapse of consciousness lasting several seconds (30 at the most), during which the subject has a blank stare and is oblivious of surroundings; there is no actual loss of consciousness, no fall and no convulsion; there may be a minor twitching of an eyelid or facial muscle, chewing movements or a jerk of a hand or arm. Such episodes may recur more than 100 times a day. Following each seizure, the subject resumes normal functioning as though nothing had happened; the attack is not remembered.

Complex Partial Seizures (Psychomotor or Temporal Lobe Epilepsy): This type comprises 40% of all epilepsies. It consists of sudden alterations of behavior that involve speech, hearing, memory and emotional response. Some episodes begin with an "aura" that may take the form of distorted vision, unpleasant odors, visual and auditory hallucinations and bizarre illusions; the subject may walk about aimlessly, talk irrationally, laugh, engage in purposeless and inappropriate actions, such as striking at walls in anger or fear. When the seizure ends, the subject is confused and does not recall what has happened.

Causes: The actual epileptic seizure is due to a sudden, abnormal and excessive electrical discharge within the brain. Normal electrical impulses of 80/second are suddenly increased to 500/second. In primary epilepsy the basic cause is unknown; there is usually a familial (genetic) predisposition. Secondary epilepsy can be a complication following head injuries, bacterial meningitis and malaria; it is often associated with cerebral palsy, mental retardation, brain tumors and cysts and hydrocephalus.

Drugs That Can Cause This Disorder: The following drugs have been reported to cause seizures or to aggravate existing epileptic disorders:

amphetamines
antihistamines
chloroquine
cimetidine (with large doses in the elderly)
cycloserine
isoniazid
metronidazole

monoamine oxidase inhibitors (MAOI's)
nalidixic acid
oral contraceptives
phenothiazines
tricyclic antidepressants
vincristine

Drugs Used to Treat This Disorder (in order of preference)
Generalized Tonic-Clonic Seizures (Grand Mal)
- phenytoin (Dilantin).
- phenobarbital (Luminal).
- carbamazepine (Tegretol).
- primidone (Mysoline).

Absence Seizures (Petit Mal)
- ethosuximide (Zarontin).
- valproic acid (Depakene).
- trimethadione (Tridione).
- clonazepam (Clonopin).

Complex Partial Seizures (Psychomotor, Temporal Lobe)
- carbamazepine (Tegretol).
- phenytoin (Dilantin).
- primidone (Mysoline).
- clonazepam (Clonopin).
- valproic acid (Depakene).

Goals of Drug Treatment

Complete prevention of seizures if possible (or marked reduction in frequency), with no (or minimal) adverse drug effects.

Restoration of ability to function independently.

Promotion of participation in school, employment and societal activities.

Drug Management

General Principles

Each individual who is subject to epilepsy experiences a pattern of seizures that is unique; the onset, frequency, severity and specific type (or types) of seizures are never exactly the same as those experienced by someone else.

The drugs used to control epilepsy are selected according to the specific type(s) of seizures the patient experiences.

Antiepileptic drugs are not curative; they are used to control seizures—to reduce their frequency and severity. Seizures should be prevented whenever possible; repeated, uncontrolled convulsions can cause significant brain damage.

When the drug of choice is used in adequate dosage to manage a correctly diagnosed type of epilepsy, seizures can be controlled completely in 60% of patients and substantially reduced in another 20%.

In every case a period of trial and error is necessary to find the most effective drug, the optimal dose and the correct timing of use.

Complete control of seizures with one drug is the ideal; this is possible in 85% of cases. If one drug does not give adequate control, a second drug may be added. The first drug may be continued or gradually withdrawn, depending upon individual response.

Dosage schedules are adjusted gradually to achieve the maximum of seizure control with the minimum of drug side-effects.

Because of the wide variation in drug absorption and elimination from person to person, the periodic measurement of drug levels in blood is necessary to determine the optimal dosage for each drug. An attempt is made to establish for each individual that drug level which will ensure freedom from seizures without toxic drug effects. Blood samples for measurement are usually taken just before the morning dose. (See Therapeutic Drug Monitoring in Section One.)

All antiepileptic drugs have toxic effects when taken in large doses; dosage adjustments are often necessary to prevent toxicity. However, the controllable risks of proper use do not justify withholding treatment in view of the much greater risks resulting from uncontrolled repeated seizures.

Birth defects are two to three times higher in children whose parents (father or mother) are using antiepileptic drugs, especially phenytoin, trimethadione and valproic acid. Consult your physician regarding the best course of action for you in managing your epilepsy during pregnancy.

Do not discontinue any antiepileptic drug suddenly unless advised to do so by your physician. Normally the dosage should be reduced gradually over a period of several weeks. Abrupt withdrawal can cause status epilepticus—a prolonged period of continual seizures without interruption.

Any consideration of discontinuing antiepileptic medications permanently should be made jointly with your physician. Such consideration can be made for absence seizures (petit mal) after a period of 2 to 3 years without a seizure. For other types of epilepsy, a period of 3 to 5 years is advisable. Seizures tend to return in 20% to 50% of cases after stopping medication. Any attempt to withdraw medication must be done very gradually over a period of several months.

Use of Phenytoin
1. Used to control all types of epilepsy except absence seizures.
2. A drug blood level within the therapeutic range correlates well with a decrease in seizure frequency and relative freedom from toxic effects.
3. Due to variation of absorbability among available products, it is advisable to stay with the same brand to gain and maintain control.
4. When the daily maintenance requirement has been established, it may be taken in a single dose.
5. Possible adverse effects include a measleslike rash within the first 2 weeks, excessive growth of hair (5%) and enlargement of the gums (30%).
6. Indications of early toxicity include rapid involuntary eye movements (nystagmus), dizziness, unsteadiness, lethargy and slurred speech.
7. If another drug is added for concurrent use, any significant interaction will occur within 6 weeks.

Use of Phenobarbital
1. Used to control all types of epilepsy except absence seizures.
2. Use with caution if liver or kidney function is impaired.
3. Should be taken twice a day with the largest dose at bedtime.
4. More sedative than phenytoin and carbamazepine, but relatively free of long-term adverse effects.
5. Indications of early toxicity include drowsiness, unsteadiness and impaired thinking.

Use of Primidone
1. Closely related to phenobarbital. Used to control all types of epilepsy except absence seizures.
2. Must be taken in divided doses because of its sedative effect.
3. Indications of early toxicity are the same of those for phenobarbital.

Use of Ethosuximide
1. Used to control absence seizures and some myoclonic seizures. About 75% effective in reducing the frequency of absence seizures when used in adequate dosage.
2. Indications of early toxicity include headache, drowsiness and dizziness.

Use of Valproic Acid
1. Used primarily to control both simple and complex absence seizures. Also used adjunctively to control all other types of epilepsy. It may control both absence and tonic-clonic seizures in the same individual.
2. Multiple doses are necessary to maintain 24-hour control.
3. Avoid use in presence of liver disease.
4. A possible side-effect is weight gain.
5. Monitor for indications of liver toxicity.
6. If used concurrently with other antiepileptic drugs, the periodic measurement of blood levels of all drugs being used is necessary to ensure adequate dosage and prevent toxicity.

Use of Carbamazepine
1. Used to control both tonic-clonic seizures and partial complex seizures (psychomotor epilepsy).
2. Should be taken with food to improve absorption.
3. Avoid use in presence of liver disease or impaired function.
4. Indications of early toxicity include double vision, blurred vision, dizziness, unsteadiness and tremor.
5. Routine, periodic, complete blood counts are mandatory to detect early bone marrow toxicity.

Ancillary Drug Treatment (as required)

Condition	*Drug Treatment*
For increased seizures before or after menstruation:	acetazolamide (Diamox)
For anxiety:	benzodiazepines (Tranxene, Valium, etc.)
For depression:	see Profile of Depression in this section

Note: Drug selection, dosage and administration schedule must be determined by the physician for each patient individually.

GLAUCOMA

Other Names: Primary Glaucoma, Secondary Glaucoma

Prevalence in USA: 1.7 million known, an estimated 1 million undiagnosed; 2% of the population over 40 years of age.

Age Group: Under 18 years—13,000; 18 to 44 years—124,000; 45 to 64 years—513,000; 65 to 74 years—534,000; 75 years and over—527,000.

Male to Female Ratio: Under 45 years—same incidence in men and women; 45 to 64 years—more common in men; 65 years and over—more common in women.

Principal Features: A chronic disorder characterized by abnormally high internal eye pressure that destroys the optic nerve and causes partial to complete loss of vision. Principal types include
Chronic Open-Angle (Simple, Wide-Angle) Glaucoma: The most common type, a primary glaucoma that is rare in children and young adults; usually begins after 30. The rise in intraocular pressure is gradual; the loss of vision is insidious and slowly progressive. Usually both eyes are affected. Characteristic symptoms include blurring of vision, frequent need for change of glasses, occasional headache, colored halos seen around electric lights and impaired visual adaptation to the dark.
Acute/Chronic Angle-Closure (Narrow-Angle, Closed-Angle) Glaucoma: A primary glaucoma that usually occurs after 60. The acute glaucoma attack begins in one eye; the rise in intraocular pressure is sudden and dramatic. Within a few hours the patient experiences severe headache, throbbing eye pain, blurred vision, halos around lights, tearing, swollen eyelids, nausea and vomiting. Initially the episode may be misdiagnosed as an acute abdominal disorder, such as gallbladder disease. Attacks of lesser severity can recur in chronic fashion.
Secondary Glaucoma: The rise in intraocular pressure is a consequence of a preexistent condition, such as infection (uveitis), eye tumor, enlarged cataract or long-term treatment with cortisonelike drugs. Headache, halos and blurred vision occur in proportion to the degree and duration of increased pressure.

Causes: Increased intraocular pressure is due to an imbalance between production and drainage of the liquid (aqueous humor) in the front portion of the eye; obstruction to normal drainage is the main mechanism. The primary types of glaucoma occur in individuals with hereditary predisposition, but specific initiating causes responsible for the rise in pressure are not known. Secondary types of glaucoma are associated with other eye disorders: uveitis, tumors, cataracts, hemorrhage, injury. "Steroid responders" develop increased pressure after 1 to 8 weeks of using cortisonelike steroids.

Drugs That Can Cause This Disorder: The following drugs do not cause true, permanent glaucoma, but they can increase intraocular pressure and thereby precipitate an attack of acute angle-closure glaucoma or aggravate chronic open-angle glaucoma:

amyl nitrite	nitroglycerin
atropine and atropinelike drugs	phenylephrine
cortisonelike drugs	tolazoline
epinephrine	tricyclic antidepressants
isosorbide dinitrate	

Drugs Used to Treat This Disorder

Eye Drops/Inserts (for Local Effects)
- carbachol (Carbacel, Isopto Carbachol).
- demecarium (Humorsol).
- dipivefrin (DPE, Propine).
- echothiopate (Phospholine).
- epinephrine (Epifrin, Epitrate, Glaucon, Lyophrin).
- phenylephrine (Neo-Synephrine, Ocusol).
- pilocarpine solution (Almocarpine, Isoptocarpine, etc.).
- pilocarpine inserts (Ocuserts Pilo-20, Pilo-40).
- timolol (Timoptic).

Internal Medications (for Systemic Effects)
- acetazolamide (Diamox).
- glycerine (Glyrol, Osmoglyn).

Goals of Drug Treatment

Prompt reduction of intraocular pressure in acute angle-closure glaucoma; stabilization of eye status in preparation for corrective eye surgery.

Gradual reduction and long-term normalization of intraocular pressure in chronic, simple, open-angle glaucoma.

Prevention of optic nerve damage; preservation of vision.

Drug Management

General Principles

Drug treatment cannot cure but can control glaucoma.

Factors that can increase intraocular pressure and reduce the effectiveness of drugs include emotional stress (anger, fear, worry); heavy physical exertion; straining with defecation; tight collars, belts and girdles; upper respiratory infections.

Periodic measurement of intraocular pressure is most advisable during long-term use of cortisonelike steroid drugs, especially eye drops and ointments.

Soft contact lens can act as a drug reservoir for pilocarpine (when administered in eye-drop solutions).

Some individuals cannot use pilocarpine Ocuserts successfully; some cannot retain them in the eye, and the loss may be unnoticed; some cannot tolerate the foreign-body sensation.

Pilocarpine is the pupil-constricting (miotic) drug of choice for use in the elderly. The stinging sensation felt on initial use usually disappears with continued application. Some blurring of distant vision is unavoidable.

Timolol (a beta-blocker) is as effective as pilocarpine in treating open-angle and secondary glaucoma; twice daily dosage (every 12 hours) is usually sufficient; it should be used very cautiously in those with asthma, slow heart rates or borderline congestive heart failure.

Epinephrine may be used concurrently with pilocarpine (or other miotic drugs) for greater effectiveness in reducing intraocular pressure; it is important that the pilocarpine be used first and be allowed to act for 5 minutes before using epinephrine. Avoid use in presence of high blood pressure (hypertension). Do not use discolored solutions of epinephrine.

Acetazolamide is usually reserved for glaucoma that is unresponsive to eye drops alone. Effectiveness is improved when both are used concurrently.

For Chronic Open-Angle Glaucoma

Eye drops: pilocarpine, timolol, carbachol, epinephrine, dipivefrin, demecarium.

Internal medications: acetazolamide.

Most cases are controlled by eye drops alone.

Treatment is started with the weakest strength; the most effective strength and dosage schedule are determined by trial and error.

Acetazolamide is not used routinely; it is added after an adequate trial of eye drops fails to maintain normal intraocular pressure.

For Acute Angle-Closure Glaucoma (Acute Attack)

Eye drops: pilocarpine, timolol.

Internal medications: glycerine and water mixture, acetazolamide.

The initial treatment is designed to lower intraocular pressure as rapidly as possible to prevent irreversible damage to the optic nerve. Eye drops and internal medications are used concurrently. The combination can reduce the pressure rapidly and abort the acute attack.

The ultimate treatment for this condition is surgical.

For Chronic, Recurrent Episodes of Subacute Angle-Closure Glaucoma

Eye drops: pilocarpine and timolol concurrently.

Internal medications: glycerine and water; acetazolamide is used only during the acute phase, not long-term.

The ultimate treatment is surgical.

For Secondary Glaucoma

Eye drops: atropine, cortisonelike steroids.

Internal medications: cortisonelike steroids, acetazolamide.

When appropriate, corrective treatment is directed at the primary eye disorder that is causing increased intraocular pressure.

For Cortisone-Induced Glaucoma

Discontinue all cortisonelike steroids if possible.

Eye drops: pilocarpine, timolol, demecarium.

Internal medications: acetazolamide.

Ancillary Drug Treatment (as required)

Condition	Drug Treatment
For itching, burning, redness of eyes:	naphazoline (Naphcon, Privine, Vasoclear) tetrahydralazine (Visine)

Note: Drug selection, dosage and administration schedule must be determined by the physician for each patient individually.

GOUT

Other Names: Gouty Arthritis, Podagra (gouty arthritis of the big toe), Hyperuricemia (abnormally high blood uric acid)

Prevalence in USA: Approximately 2.3 million, 2.8% of males in middle age. Hyperuricemia occurs in 5% to 10% of the population; 1% to 2% will have gout manifestations during a lifetime.

Age Group: Under 18 years—12,000; 18 to 44 years—316,000; 45 to 64 years—1.01 million; 65 to 74 years—494,000; 75 years and over—396,000.

Male to Female Ratio: Approximately 95% in men, 5% in women.

Principal Features: Gout consists of a group of related disorders having a single underlying feature—abnormally high blood levels of uric acid; this is referred to as hyperuricemia and implies a blood level of more than 7.0 mg of uric acid per 100 ml of blood. (The normal ranges generally recognized are 2.5 to 8.0 mg for men and 1.5 to 7.0 mg for women.) During the early years of primary (genetic) gout, hyperuricemia may exist without any symptoms to indicate its presence. During a lifetime, a small minority of these individuals will experience recurrent acute attacks of severe joint pain with tender swelling (usually one joint in an upper or lower limb), episodes of kidney stones, serious impairment of kidney function or the development of tophi—localized deposits of uric acid salts in the skin, on earlobes, on tendons and bones in and around joints (tophaceous gout).

Causes: Primary gout is due to an inherited defect in the metabolism of purines—end products of protein digestion. In approximately 10% of cases the defect results in an overproduction of uric acid; in 90% the defect is responsible for decreased excretion of uric acid by the kidneys. Either defect causes hyperuricemia. When tissue fluids cannot dissolve excessive levels of uric acid (due to saturation), uric acid crystals are deposited in joints (acute arthritis), kidneys (kidney damage and stone formation) and in soft tissue (tophi).

Drugs That Can Cause This Disorder: The following drugs can raise the blood level of uric acid and precipitate acute gouty arthritis in susceptible individuals:

acetazolamide	furosemide
alcohol	levodopa
antineoplastic drugs	nicotinic acid
aspirin (less than 2 grams/day)	pyrazinamide
ethacrynic acid	thiazide diuretics
ethambutol	triamterene

Drugs Used to Treat This Disorder
For Reducing Blood and Tissue Levels of Uric Acid
- allopurinol (Lopurin, Zyloprim).
- probenecid (Benemid).
- sulfinpyrazone (Anturane).

For Treating and Preventing Acute Attacks of Arthritis
- colchicine.
- fenoprofen (Nalfon).
- ibuprofen (Advil, Motrin, Nuprin, Rufen).
- indomethacin (Indocin).
- naproxen (Naprosyn).
- oxyphenbutazone (Oxalid).
- phenylbutazone (Azolid, Butazolidin).
- piroxicam (Feldene).
- prednisone (Deltasone, Meticorten, Orasone, etc.).
- sulindac (Clinoril).
- tolmetin (Tolectin).

Goals of Drug Treatment
Prompt relief of symptoms of acute attack of gouty arthritis.
Maintenance of blood uric acid level below 6 mg/100 ml. (Prevention of recurrent attacks of acute arthritis, kidney stone formation, kidney damage and tophi formation.)
Dissolution of existing tophi.

Drug Management
General Principles
Only 20% of individuals with hyperuricemia will develop manifestations of gout during their lifetime. At present there is no way of identifying those who will.
Gouty arthritis is the most responsive to treatment and the most easily controlled of all types of arthritis.
The patient and physician together should determine by trial and error which drug is most effective and acceptable for treating acute attacks of gouty arthritis.
After the acute attack of arthritis has subsided, minor symptoms may persist for 2 to 3 months. If maintenance treatment with antigout drugs is started, it is advisable to use low-dose colchicine concurrently to prevent recurrent flare-ups.

Measurement of the amount of uric acid in a 24-hour collection of urine can identify the overproducer of uric acid (greater than 800 mg) and the underexcretor (less than 800 mg). The overproducer is best treated with allopurinol; the underexcretor is best treated with probenecid or sulfinpyrazone.

Authorities differ on whether and when to initiate long-term treatment for hyperuricemia. Conservative opinion: initiate drug therapy only after 2 or more episodes of gouty arthritis or kidney stone within a year. Many first attacks are not followed by recurrent episodes. Withholding long-term treatment avoids the risks of adverse drug reactions. Aggressive opinion: initiate drug therapy after the first episode of gouty arthritis or kidney stone to prevent recurrent attacks and reduce the risks of kidney damage and tophi formation. Hyperuricemia is often present for 20 years or more before the first attack; bone, cartilage and kidney damage may already have occured. The risks of untreated hyperuricemia are thought to exceed the risks of long-term drug therapy. The prudent physician will consider the pros and cons of each case individually and make the decision jointly with the patient.

Once long-term treatment is started with allopurinol and/or probenecid or sulfinpyrazone, it should be maintained for life. Start-stop treatment has no lasting benefit and may precipitate acute attacks. Low-dose colchicine should be taken preventively until the uric acid blood level is stabilized below 6.0 mg/100ml and there have been no acute attacks for 6 to 12 months.

Acute attacks of gouty arthritis can be precipitated by injury, surgery, systemic infections and severe medical illnesses. Colchicine may be used preventively to minimize acute episodes of arthritis when such events occur.

Patients with kidney stones should use allopurinol to treat hyperuricemia; probenecid and sulfinpyrazone should be avoided because they increase the uric acid content of urine.

Do not take aspirin (or other salicylates) in doses of less than 2 grams while taking probenecid or sulfinpyrazone. It abolishes the effectiveness of these drugs and raises the blood level of uric acid.

Avoid fasting to lose weight; fasting can raise the blood level of uric acid. Treat obesity by long-term reduction of food intake and gradual loss of weight.

While taking antigout drugs on a regular basis, drink 2 to 3 quarts of liquids daily to ensure a copious flow of dilute urine.

Use of Allopurinol
1. Used to lower the blood level of uric acid by reducing its formation. Of no value in treating the acute attack, and should not be started until all symptoms of acute arthritis have subsided.
2. The drug of choice for individuals who
   - are overproducers of uric acid (more than 800 mg/24-hour urine excretion).
   - are over 60 years of age.
   - have impaired kidney function.

- are subject to kidney stones.
- have tophi formations.
- are allergic or overly sensitive to probenecid or sulfinpyrazone.
3. The total daily requirement may be taken in a single dose.
4. Once started, a commitment should be made to a lifetime of continual use.
5. May be combined with all other antigout drugs as appropriate for increased effectiveness.
6. Recommended for use prior to and during chemotherapy or irradiation therapy for selected cancers to counteract resulting hyperuricemia.
7. Serious toxicity is extremely rare.

Use of Colchicine
1. Used to treat acute attacks of gouty arthritis. It does not lower the blood level of uric acid.
2. For the quickest response and best results, treatment should be started as soon as possible after the onset of symptoms. If started within the first 12 hours, colchicine gives effective relief of acute arthritis in 90% of cases.
3. The long-term use of low-dose colchicine is very effective in preventing recurrent acute attacks of gouty arthritis.
4. Its use is recommended during the early months of maintenance therapy with allopurinol and/or probenecid or sulfinpyrazone to prevent flare-ups of acute arthritis.
5. Use with caution and reduce the dose in the presence of liver disease or impaired liver function.
6. Colchicine is destroyed by exposure to light. Be sure your supply is fresh and fully effective.

Use of Indomethacin (and Other Nonsteroidal Anti-inflammatory Drugs)
1. Now considered by many authorities to be the drug(s) of choice for treating acute attacks of gouty arthritis. They relieve pain and inflammation, but do not lower the blood level of uric acid.
2. When given promptly and in adequate dosage, these drugs usually provide relief within 6 to 12 hours and complete recovery in 3 days.
3. Take with food to prevent stomach irritation and indigestion.
4. Avoid in the presence of active peptic ulcer disease. Use with caution in hypertension and congestive heart failure.

Use of Phenylbutazone or Oxyphenbutazone
1. Used to provide prompt relief of acute gouty arthritis. It reduces pain and inflammation effectively, but does not lower the blood level of uric acid.
2. Because of its rare but very serious potential for causing bone marrow depression, this drug should never be used for long-term treatment. Treatment courses of no more than 5 to 7 days are advised.
3. This drug should not be used by the elderly (over 60 years of age).

Use of Prednisone (or Similar Cortisonelike Steroids)
1. Used to abort acute attacks of gouty arthritis. Relieves inflammation, swelling and pain, but does not lower the blood level of uric acid.

2. Should be used only after adequate trials of all other appropriate drugs have failed to relieve the acute attack.
3. "Rebound" attacks are common following withdrawal of steroid medications.
4. Not recommended for frequently repeated or long-term use.

Use of Probenecid or Sulfinpyrazone
1. Used to lower the blood level of uric acid by increasing its excretion in the urine. Of no value in treating the acute attack, and should not be started until acute arthritis has subsided.
2. Best suited for individuals who
   - are underexcretors of uric acid (less than 800 mg/24-hour urine excretion).
   - are under 60 years of age.
   - have good kidney function.
   - have no history of kidney stones.
3. Should not be used by those who
   - are overproducers of uric acid (more than 800 mg/24-hour urine excretion).
   - have impaired kidney function and low urine volume.
   - are subject to kidney stones.
4. Begin treatment with small doses to avoid precipitating an acute attack of arthritis.
5. Must be taken in 2 to 4 doses/day.
6. If the tolerance of either drug is limited, the two drugs can be taken concurrently in reduced dosage.
7. Ensure a high intake of liquids (up to 3 quarts daily). Effectiveness is improved by the concurrent use of sodium bicarbonate or potassium citrate.

Ancillary Drug Treatment (as required)

Condition	Drug Treatment
For mild pain:	acetaminophen (Tylenol, etc.) Do not use aspirin or other salicylates.
For severe pain:	codeine or meperidine (Demerol)
For diarrhea due to colchicine:	paregoric or loperimide (Imodium)
For high blood pressure:	see Profile of Hypertension in this section
For "secondary" gout due to chemotherapy for leukemia, lymphoma, multiple myeloma, polycythemia:	allopurinol (Zyloprim)

Note: Drug selection, dosage and administration schedule must be determined by the physician for each patient individually.

HYPERTENSION

Other Names: Arterial Hypertension, Essential Hypertension, Primary Hypertension, Secondary Hypertension

Prevalence in USA: 26.5 million—15% of adult white population; 25% of adult black population.

Age Group: Under 18 years—184,000; 18 to 44 years—5.6 million; 45 to 64 years—10.8 million; 65 to 74 years—6 million; 75 years and over—3.8 million.

Male to Female Ratio: Under 45 years—same incidence in men and women; 45 to 64 years—slightly more common in women; 65 years and over—more common in women (2 to 1).

Principal Features: During the early years of high blood pressure there are usually no symptoms. Brief periods of sudden elevation of blood presure above usual levels may cause throbbing headaches and/or dizziness. After years of untreated high blood pressure, manifestations of "target organ" disease include stroke (blood clot or hemorrhage in the brain), impaired vision (retinal hemorrhage and deterioration), heart attack (myocardial infarction), congestive heart failure and kidney failure (uremia).

Causes: In primary (essential) hypertension (95% of all hypertension), no specific cause is apparent. There is a definite hereditary predisposition; 80% of hypertensive individuals have a close relative with high blood pressure. In those who are genetically susceptible, obesity and high salt intake contribute significantly to the development of hypertension. Secondary hypertension (5% of all hypertension) is due to a demonstrable (and sometimes curable) cause: narrowing of the main artery to one or both kidneys, chronic kidney disease, adrenalin or renin producing tumors, coarctation of the aorta.

Drugs That Can Cause This Disorder: The following drugs (or drug combinations) can cause significant elevations of blood pressure:

amphetamines and related drugs
carbenoxolone
ephedrine
ergot preparations
licorice
oral contraceptives
phenylephrine

phenylpropanolamine
pseudoephedrine
tricyclic antidepressants taken
   concurrently with appetite
   suppressants, decongestants or
   antihistamines

Drugs Used to Treat This Disorder
Diuretics
- thiazides (see Drug Class, Section Four).
- chlorthalidone (Hygroton).
- quinethazone (Hydromox).
- metolazone (Diulo, Zaroxolyn).

- indapamide (Lozol).
- bumetanide (Bumex).
- furosemide (Lasix).
- *potassium-saving diuretics:* amiloride (Midamor); spironolactone (Aldactone); triamterene (Dyrenium).

Drugs Acting on the Sympathetic Nervous System
Beta-Adrenergic Blocking Drugs
- acebutolol (Sectral).
- atenolol (Tenormin).
- labetalol (Normodyne, Trandate).
- metoprolol (Lopressor).
- nadolol (Corgard).
- pindolol (Visken).
- propranolol (Inderal).
- timolol (Blocadren).

Alpha-Adrenergic Blocking Drugs
- prazosin (Minipres).

Centrally Acting Drugs (in the Brain)
- clonidine (Catapres).
- guanabenz (Wytensin).
- methyldopa (Aldomet).

Peripherally Acting Drugs (in Peripheral Blood Vessels)
- guanadrel (Hylorel).
- guanethidine (Ismelin).
- reserpine (Serpasil).

Direct Vasodilators
- hydralazine (Apresoline).
- minoxidil (Loniten).

Calcium Channel Blocking Drugs
- diltiazem (Cardizem).
- nifedipine (Procardia).
- verapamil (Calan, Isoptin).

Angiotensin Converting Enzyme (ACE) Inhibitors
- captopril (Capoten).
- enalapril (Vasotec).

Goals of Drug Treatment
Maintenance of blood pressure below 140/90, or as close as possible to this level with an acceptable program of drug therapy (minimal drug side-effects and expense).

Prevention or postponement of "target organ" disease in the brain, retina (eye), heart, major blood vessels and kidneys.

Drug Management
General Principles
Although hypertension is difficult to define precisely, blood pressure is considered to be abnormally high if the systolic level is 140 or above or the diastolic level is 90 or above.

Hypertension may be classified as follows:
  Diastolic pressure less than 85—normal
  Diastolic pressure of 85 to 89—high normal
  Diastolic pressure of 90 to 104—mild hypertension
  Diastolic pressure of 105 to 114—moderate hypertension
  Diastolic pressure of 115 or above—severe hypertension
  Systolic pressure less than 140—normal
  Systolic pressure of 140 to 159—borderline systolic hypertension
  Systolic pressure of 160 or above—systolic hypertension
Most men who develop primary hypertension will have a diastolic pressure
  of 90 or above by age 35, most women by age 40 to 45.
An adequate program of drug therapy for hypertension will postpone seri-
  ous disability and death for most hypertensive individuals.
The selection of antihypertensive drugs for initial treatment is based upon
  the range of the abnormally high pressures recorded on repeated measurements *and* the status of the "target organs" (brain, heart, kidneys
  and blood vessels) at the time hypertension is discovered.
One practical and effective approach to drug therapy for hypertension initiates treatment with a single drug and adds stronger drugs in stepwise
  fashion as needed to control blood pressure:

Step 1	begin treatment	either a diuretic or a beta-blocker drug.
Step 2	if necessary, add	clonidine, methyldopa or prazosin (or a diuretic or a beta-blocker if not used in Step 1)
Step 3	if necessary, add	hydralazine, a calcium channel blocker, or an ACE inhibitor
Step 4	if necessary, add	guanethidine or minoxidil

For most individuals, the initial drug treatment will normalize blood
  pressure within the first 2 months. Up to 60% of cases are controlled
  with a diuretic alone; 50% can be controlled with a beta-blocker
  alone. From 70% to 80% of all hypertensive individuals will achieve
  satisfactory blood pressure control by compliance with Step 1 or
  Step 2 drug therapy. The majority of the remainder can be controlled
  by Steps 3 and 4.
Tranquilizers and sedatives are not effective for lowering elevated blood
  pressure and should not be relied upon as primary treatment for hypertension.
Obtain a blood pressure measuring instrument (preferably an aneroid
  manometer, arm cuff and stethoscope) and ask your physician to teach
  you how to take your own blood pressure. Measurements of blood pressure made at home (or at work) are far more representative of your
  actual day-by-day pressures than are readings made in the physician's
  office. By taking your own blood pressure at home, at work and at varying times and under different circumstances, you can create a record
  that clearly reflects your response to the antihypertensive drugs prescribed for you.
Read the Drug Profiles (Section Three) of the drugs you are taking. If you

think you may be experiencing any of the side-effects or adverse effects listed in the Profile, discuss this with your physician so appropriate adjustments can be made. It is to your benefit to work along with your physician until a satisfactory selection of drugs is reached.

Avoid isometric exercises—body building, weight lifting, push-ups; these raise the blood pressure significantly. Consult your physician regarding the advisability of isotonic exercises—walking, bicycling, swimming.

Consumption of more than 2 ounces of alcohol daily can raise the blood pressure. One ounce of alcohol is present in 2 ounces of 100-proof whiskey, in 8 ounces of wine, or in 24 ounces of beer.

Five percent of oral contraceptive users will develop a diastolic blood pressure of over 90. If this occurs, the contraceptive pill should be discontinued for 6 months and the blood pressure monitored. Women with this sensitivity should use an alternative method of contraception.

The elderly individual with hypertension must approach antihypertensive drug therapy very cautiously. Goals of drug treatment are more liberal; reduction of pressures to 140–160/95–100 are usually adequate. This can usually be achieved with small doses of a diuretic. If a Step 2 drug is needed, methyldopa is better tolerated than the other choices. However, the response to all drugs must be observed closely. Drugs that cause emotional depression in the young individual can cause symptoms in the elderly that closely resemble senile dementia.

In type I diabetes, thiazides are well tolerated, but beta-blockers may mask the symptoms of hypoglycemia. In type II diabetes, thiazides are best avoided; small doses of furosemide or spironolactone are preferable. Beta-blockers can impair insulin release.

After blood pressure has been well controlled for a year, consideration may be given to a "step-down" reduction of both drug dosage and the number of drugs used. The blood pressure response to the gradual withdrawal of drugs must be monitored very carefully. A recent study showed that 28% of the group of hypertensives studied had normal blood pressure one year after discontinuing all antihypertensive medication. Your physician can determine if and when you meet the criteria for attempting to discontinue your program of drug treatment.

Treatment of Hypertension According to Severity

For Borderline Hypertension (120–160/90–94)
- Reduce excessive weight.
- Reduce salt intake moderately.
- Reduce stress in daily living.
- Avoid excessive consumption of alcohol.
- Stop smoking.
- Avoid isometric exercise.
- Increase isotonic exercise.
- Defer drug treatment for 3 to 6 months to determine effectiveness of above measures.

For Mild Hypertension (140–160/95–104) (80% of All Hypertensives)
- Urge all of the above measures.
- Begin Step 1 drug treatment: Use a single drug—currently a thia-

zide diuretic or a beta-blocker. Some authorities are now advocating a trial of a calcium channel blocker or an ACE inhibitor for initiating treatment.

For Moderate Hypertension (140–180/105–114)

- Begin with Step 2 drug treatment; it is not likely that a single drug will control this degree of hypertension.
- A diuretic will enhance the effectiveness of a beta-blocker, a calcium channel blocker, or a centrally acting drug.

For Severe Hypertension (160+/115+)

- Adequate control may require Step 3 or Step 4 drug treatment. When multiple drugs are used, smaller doses of individual drugs are often effective and better tolerated. A trial-and-error approach is often necessary to determine the most effective and acceptable combination of drugs.

For Isolated Systolic Hypertension (160+/85–90)

- This is usually found in the elderly. Cautious and conservative drug treatment is recommended for those under age 70.
- Calcium channel blocking drugs may be very effective for this type of hypertension.
- If a diuretic is used, avoid dehydration and potassium loss.
- If methyldopa is used, monitor for any tendency to depression or dementia.

Use of Diuretics

1. Used as Step 1 or Step 2 drugs, diuretics are most appropriate for treating hypertensives who are black or elderly, those with congestive heart failure or kidney failure and those who cannot use a beta-blocker drug.
2. A thiazide diuretic is the initial drug tried in the majority of cases. It is effective in a single dose taken in the morning.
3. While using thiazide diuretics, observe for loss of potassium (10% of users), increased blood level of uric acid (66% of users) and increased blood-sugar level.
4. Spironolactone and triamterene are as effective as thiazides in reducing blood pressure; they are used to prevent potassium loss.
5. The more potent diuretics furosemide and ethacrynic acid are no more effective than the thiazides for reducing blood pressure.
6. The most practical and reliable way to prevent a significant decline in the potassium blood level is to use a potassium-saving diuretic—amiloride, spironolactone or triamterene. The use of high-potassium foods is often unreliable. Compliance with the long-term use of oral potassium supplements is very poor.
7. It is advisable to discontinue the use of diuretics gradually to prevent fluid retention (edema) after withdrawal.

Use of Beta-Adrenergic Blocking Drugs

1. Used as Step 1 or Step 2 drugs, beta-blockers are most appropriate for treating hypertensives who are young, those who have an overactive heart (fast rate, palpitation, premature beats) and those with gout, migraine headaches and angina (coronary artery disease).

2. Avoid beta-blockers if you have asthma, emphysema or a history of heart block or congestive heart failure.
3. These drugs characteristically cause fatigue and lethargy. Propranolol and metoprolol can cause emotional depression.
4. When propranolol is used alone, 10% of users can experience an increase in blood pressure. It is advisable to use a diuretic prior to starting propranolol in sensitive individuals.
5. Avoid sudden discontinuation of beta-blockers, especially in the presence of coronary artery disease. Abrupt withdrawal can cause rapid heart rate, palpitation and intensification of angina; myocardial infarction has been reported.

Use of Labetalol (an Alpha- and Beta-adrenergic Blocker)
1. This drug may be effective when the beta-blockers have failed to control blood pressure.
2. Functions primarily as a vasodilator in the elderly, with no significant alteration of heart function.
3. Avoid in presence of asthma, emphysema, heart block and congestive heart failure.

Use of Clonidine
1. Characteristically causes drowsiness, fatigue and dry mouth. Is capable of causing depression.
2. Do not discontinue this drug abruptly; sudden withdrawal can cause a severe rebound hypertension with higher blood pressure than prior to treatment. Withdraw over 2 to 4 days.
3. After discontinuation of clonidine, delay the start of a beta-blocker drug for 48 hours.

Use of Methyldopa
1. Usually causes lethargy and fatigue at beginning of treatment; these often subside with continued use. Is also capable of causing depression.
2. This drug causes salt and water retention; a diuretic should be taken concurrently.
3. Discontinue this drug if any of the following develop: emotional depression, drug fever, breast enlargement, milk production, indications of liver toxicity (loss of appetite, nausea, jaundice).
4. Sudden discontinuation of this drug can cause agitation, insomnia, rapid heart rate and intensification of angina.

Use of Prazosin
1. In 10% of users, this drug can provoke an idiosyncratic reaction that results in a sudden extreme drop in blood pressure following the first dose. It is advisable to begin treatment with a bedtime dose and a warning to arise cautiously the next morning in anticipation of possible orthostatic hypotension (see Glossary).
2. This drug can cause fluid retention and can aggravate angina. It is best used in conjunction with a diuretic and a beta-blocker.
3. Do not use this drug concurrently with hydralazine or guanethidine because of the potential for additive postural hypotension.

4. A rapid loss of effectiveness can limit this drug's long-term usefulness.

Use of Hydralazine
1. This drug is rarely used alone. It can cause fluid retention and should be used concurrently with a diuretic.
2. This drug characteristically increases heart activity, which can be counteracted by the concurrent use of a beta-blocker drug.
3. Use cautiously in the presence of angina (coronary artery disease).
4. Monitor for possible development of a lupuslike drug reaction.

Use of Reserpine
1. Limit the daily dose to 0.25 mg or less.
2. Avoid completely if you have a history of depression.
3. This drug can cause salt and water retention; a diuretic should be used concurrently.
4. Do not use this drug concurrently with methyldopa; the combination can cause marked sedation, excessive dreaming and sexual impotence.
5. Observe for the following possible adverse effects: drowsiness, lethargy, depression (can be very insidious), nightmares, nasal congestion, acid indigestion (possible ulcer), diarrhea, impotence, parkinsonlike syndrome.

Use of Guanethidine
1. This is the most potent antihypertensive drug in general use. It is usually reserved to treat the most severe cases of hypertension and those that have been difficult to control.
2. It causes marked orthostatic hypotension. Users should avoid prolonged sitting (without moving the legs) and prolonged standing (without walking around); these are conducive to excessive drops in blood pressure and resultant fainting. Users should also arise cautiously in the morning to avoid fainting shortly after getting out of bed.
3. This drug causes salt and water retention and should be taken concurrently with a diuretic.
4. Tricyclic antidepressants can reduce this drug's antihypertensive effectiveness.

Use of Minoxidil
1. This drug is a potent, long-acting vasodilator. Its use is usually restricted to treating those whose blood pressure cannot be controlled by conventional treatment with other drugs.
2. It is generally used concurrently with a diuretic and a beta-blocker drug.
3. Observe for excessive growth of hair.

Use of Calcium Channel Blocking Drugs
1. These drugs are approved by the U.S. Food and Drug Administration only for use in the management of angina (coronary artery disease). However, they are effective antihypertensives and are being used as such by many physicians.
2. They may be used as Step 1, 2, or 3 drugs in the management of hypertension.

3. They are especially useful in treating the elderly individual with isolated systolic hypertension.
4. Use these drugs with caution if a beta-blocker drug is being used concurrently.
5. A dosage of 3 to 4 times daily is required.
6. Observe for fluid retention. Effectiveness is improved if a thiazide diuretic is taken concurrently.

Use of Angiotensin Converting Enzyme (ACE) Inhibitors
1. These may be used as Step 1, 2, 3, or 4 drugs in the management of hypertension.
2. To prevent an excessive drop in blood pressure, any diuretic in use should be discontinued 5 to 7 days before starting an ACE inhibitor. After the dose is stabilized, a diuretic may be resumed if necessary.
3. Captopril should be taken 1 hour before eating, 2 to 3 times daily, for maximal effectiveness. Enalapril may be taken once or twice daily without regard to eating.
4. Full effectiveness of these drugs may not be apparent until after several weeks of continual use.
5. These drugs may increase the blood potassium level. Do not use any commercial salt substitute (most of which contain potassium) without first consulting your physician.

Ancillary Drug Treatment (as required)

Condition	*Drug Treatment*
For thiazide-induced gout:	allopurinol (Zyloprim) probenecid (Benemid)
For drug-induced fluid retention:	hydrochlorothiazide (HydroDiuril, etc.)
For guanethidine-induced diarrhea:	diphenoxylate (Lomoti)
For tension headache:	acetaminophen (Tylenol, etc.)
For migraine headache (short-term use):	ibuprofen (Motrin, Advil, Nuprin) oxycodone (Percodan) Avoid ergotamine preparations.
For musculo-skeletal pain, arthritis (long-term use):	sulindac (Clinoril)

Note: Drug selection, dosage and administration schedule must be determined by the physician for each patient individually.

HYPOTHYROIDISM

Other Names: Hypometabolism, Myxedema, Primary Hypothyroidism, Secondary Hypothyroidism

Prevalence in USA: 1.9 million—0.8% of the general population; 1 in 5000 newborn infants has hypothyroidism (cretinism).

Age Group: Juvenile hypothyroidism: under 18 years—2% of total incidence. Adult hypothyroidism: percentage of total incidence by age: 18 to 44 years—34%; 45 to 64 years—40%; 65 years and over—24%.

Male to Female Ratio: More common in women—8 to 1.

Principal Features: Hypothyroidism spans a wide spectrum from very mild thyroid hormone deficiency (hypometabolism) with few nonspecific symptoms to severe deficiency (myxedema) that can be fatal if not treated adequately. The most common form of hypothyroidism is the mild to moderate hormone deficiency seen primarily in women age 20 to 65. The onset is usually insidious and the early symptoms are so vague that medical attention is rarely sought. With progression of the deficiency, the subject gradually becomes aware of lethargy, fatigability, intolerance of cold, weight gain (with no increased food intake), loss of hair, vague muscle and joint pains, and irregular menstruation. The skin may become dry and scaly, the face may appear puffy (fluid retention), the speech slows, the voice becomes hoarse and the pattern of activity becomes sluggish. Hypothyroidism in the elderly can cause mental changes, confusion, paranoia, depression and dementia.

Causes: Primary hypothyroidism can be due to (1) a congenital defect in thyroid gland development or function; (2) an "autoimmune" impairment of thyroid hormone production (45% of cases); (3) a lack of iodine in the food or water supply; or (4) intentional thyroid gland suppression by the administration of radioactive iodine or by surgical removal of thyroid tissue (35% of cases). Secondary hypothyroidism is due to inadequate stimulation of thyroid gland function from the hypothalamus (in the brain) or from the pituitary gland (the "master" gland that regulates most hormone-producing glands).

Drugs That Can Cause This Disorder: The following drugs can impair the normal production of thyroid hormones and induce varying degrees of hypothyroidism (see Drug Classes, Section Four):

amiodarone	methimazole
cyclophosphamide	pentazocine
disulfiram (?)	phenylbutazone
ethionamide	propylthiouracil
iodine compounds (iodides)	sulfonylurea antidiabetic drugs
lithium	

Drugs Used to Treat This Disorder
- synthetic thyroxine (T-4) (Synthroid, Levothroid).
- synthetic liothyronine (T-3) (Cytomel).
- synthetic liotrix (combinations of T-4 and T-3) (Euthroid, Thyrolar).
- thyroid extract (animal origin) (Dessicated thyroid Armour).
- thyroglobulin (animal origin) (Proloid).

Goals of Drug Treatment

Adequate replacement of thyroxine; restoration of normal blood levels of T-4, T-3 and the Thyroid Stimulating Hormone (TSH).

Relief of symptoms associated with deficiency of thyroid hormones (hypothyroidism, cretinism, myxedema).

Drug Management

General Principles

Primary hypothyroidism is diagnosed by finding the blood level of the principal thyroid hormone—thyroxine (T-4)—below the normal range and the blood level of the pituitary hormone—Thyroid Stimulating Hormone (TSH)—above the normal range.

Once the diagnosis of true primary hypothyroidism is established, treatment for life is generally thought to be necessary. However, periodic evaluation is advisable to determine the need for continual thyroid hormone replacement.

Individuals taking replacement thyroid hormones should be monitored every 6 to 12 months by measurements of T-4 and TSH along with evaluation of general well-being.

Until thyroid deficiency is adequately corrected, the subject may be overly sensitive to drugs that depress brain function—sedatives, tranquilizers, hypnotics, narcotic analgesics.

In treating hypothyroidism of infancy, avoid formula feedings that contain soybean extract; they can prevent the absorption of thyroxine and perpetuate cretinism.

Anxious, thin individuals usually require smaller doses of maintenance thyroxine than lethargic, obese individuals require. Significant reduction in weight (correction of obesity) is usually followed by a reduction in the daily requirement of maintenance thyroxine.

The use of thyroid hormones for weight reduction in the presence of normal thyroid function (no hormone deficiency) is unjustified and dangerous.

Hypothyroidism causes an increase in bone mass. Thyroid replacement therapy can result in a significant loss of bone (osteoporosis) in the lumbar vertebrae (spine). Consult your physician regarding the advisability of taking supplements of calcium and vitamin D during thyroid hormone replacement. (See Profile of Osteoporosis in this section.)

Use of Thyroxine

1. Hypothyroidism is best treated with a synthetic preparation of thyroxine (see Drug Profile, Section Three). This provides replacement that

approximates most closely the normal status of thyroid hormones in circulating blood.

2. Young, basically healthy individuals with hypothyroidism may take thyroxine in full dosage—1 microgram per pound of body weight daily. This usually achieves normal blood levels of T-4 and TSH.

3. Older individuals, with incipient or established heart disease, should initiate thyroxine treatment with small doses that can be increased gradually over 2 to 3 months. This reduces the risk of precipitating disturbances of heart function, such as angina and abnormal rhythm.

4. Thyroxine should be taken in the morning on an empty stomach to ensure maximal absorption and uniform effectiveness.

5. Cholestyramine and colestipol can prevent absorption of thyroxine and liothyronine; for best results, take thyroxine (and/or liothyronine) first (preferably in the morning, fasting), 2 to 3 hours before the first daily dose of either cholestyramine or colestipol.

6. Observe for possible seasonal variation in your response to thyroxine replacement therapy. Some individuals may need less in warm months and more in cold months. If the winter dose of thyroxine is somewhat excessive for summer requirements, you may develop nervousness, insomnia, headaches, intolerance of heat and loss of weight. Consult your physician if you think dosage adjustment is necessary.

7. Do not purchase thyroxine tablets in large quantities (such as 500 to 1000). Thyroxine products can lose up to 6% of their potency per year. It is advisable to obtain a 3 to 6 months' supply (100 to 200 tablets) to ensure full-strength medication.

Ancillary Drug Treatment (as required)

Condition	Drug Treatment
For anemia:	iron preparations
	vitamin B-12 (if appropriate for type of anemia)
For constipation:	docusate (Colace, Doxinate, etc.)
	docusate with casanthranol (Peri-Colace, etc.)
For muscle or joint ache/pain:	aspirin
	acetaminophen (Tylenol, Panadol, etc.)
	ibuprofen (Advil, Nuprin, etc.)

Note: Drug selection, dosage and administration schedule must be determined by the physician for each patient individually.

MENOPAUSE

Other Names: Menopausal Syndrome, Estrogen Withdrawal Syndrome, Female Climacteric, Change of Life

Prevalence in USA: 12.8 million women (candidates for menopause).

Age Group: 45 to 55 years; the mean age of natural menopause is 50 years.

Principal Features: The term "menopause" refers to the permanent cessation of menstruation. This occurs naturally in most women between 45 and 55 years of age. The characteristic indication of the "change"—altered menstrual pattern with eventual cessation of menstrual periods—usually lasts from 6 to 18 months. The majority of women (85%) experience some physical effects of progressive estrogen withdrawal: recurring hot flushes, episodic sweating, shrinkage of breast tissue, reduction of vaginal secretions and a variety of nervous and emotional symptoms—anxiety, depression, insomnia, headaches, dizziness, nausea. For approximately 25%, the symptoms are of sufficient intensity to warrant a trial of estrogen replacement therapy. Up to 35% of menopausal women experience hot flushes for 5 or more years.

Causes: Natural menopause occurs spontaneously to terminate reproductive capability. Therapeutic menopause follows surgical removal of the uterus or ovaries and irradiation or removal of the pituitary gland.

Drugs That Can Cause This Disorder: The following drugs can cause cessation of menstruation for varying periods of time, sometimes permanently: busulfan, chlorambucil, cyclophosphamide, mechlorethamine, oral contraceptives and vincristine. The antiestrogen drug tamoxifen, used for the treatment of breast cancer, can cause hot flushes, dizziness and menstrual irregularities typical of the menopausal syndrome.

Drugs Used to Treat This Disorder
"Natural-type" estrogens are preferred:
- conjugated estrogens (Genisis, Premarin).
- esterified estrogens (Evex, Menest).
- estradiol cypionate (Depo-Estradiol, injection).
- estradiol valerate (Delestrogen, injection).
- estriol (Hormonin, a mixture of estriol, estradiol, and estrone).
- piperazine estrone sulfate (Ogen).
- micronized 17-B estradiol (Estrace).
- transdermal estradiol skin patch (Estraderm-50 and 100).*

Goals of Drug Treatment
Reduction in the frequency and severity of hot flushes and night sweats with attendant insomnia.
Relief of nervous and emotional symptoms.

*Approval by FDA for marketing expected in late 1986.

Prevention or relief of atrophic changes of the vulva, vagina and urethra.
Prevention of thinning of the skin.
Prevention of osteoporosis (long-term treatment).

Drug Management
General Principles

It is now generally held that for the well-informed menopausal woman who has obvious symptoms of estrogen deficiency and does not have any contraindications to its use, the benefits of estrogen replacement therapy outweigh the possible risks. The use of estrogen is considered effective and safe when prescribed appropriately and monitored properly.

As each women reaches the menopausal years (45 to 55), she should assess her own status and perceived needs. Next she should familiarize herself with the benefits and possible risks of estrogen replacement therapy. (See the Drug Profile of Estrogen, Section Three.) If she thinks she needs medical guidance and/or treatment, she should discuss all aspects of her situation with her physician and share in the decision regarding the use of hormones.

A clear indication for the use of estrogen should exist. It should not be given routinely to the menopausal woman, but should be reserved to treat those with symptoms of estrogen deficiency. Estrogen does not retard the natural progression of general aging; it should not be used for the sole purpose of "preserving femininity."

Before estrogen therapy is started, appropriate examinations should be performed and due consideration given to the following possible contra-indications to the use of estrogen:

1. Pregnancy
2. History of deep venous thrombosis or pulmonary embolism
3. Present or previous cancer of the breast
4. Cancer of the uterus
5. Strong family history of breast or uterine cancer
6. Current liver disease or previous drug-induced jaundice
7. Chronic gallbladder disease, with or without stones
8. Abnormal elevation of blood fats (cholesterol, triglycerides, etc.)
9. History of porphyria
10. Large uterine fibroid tumors
11. Any estrogen-dependent tumor
12. Combination of obesity, varicose veins and cigarette smoking
13. Diabetes mellitus
14. Severe hypertension

In the young woman experiencing premature menopause (destruction or removal of both ovaries), the *long-term* use of estrogen replacement is justified, provided appropriate precautions are observed (see Guidelines below).

In the menopausal woman experiencing hot flushes and/or atrophic vaginitis, the *short-term* use of estrogen therapy is generally felt to be acceptable with appropriate supervision and guidance. Estrogen replacement therapy provides symptomatic relief; it is not a permanent cure for hot flushes.

Long-term estrogen therapy for *all* women after the menopause cannot be justified. Treatment must be carefully individualized (see Guidelines below).

It is generally recommended that estrogens be taken cyclically. The customary schedule is from the 1st through the 25th day of each month, with no estrogen during the remaining days of the month. After 6 to 12 months of continuous use, the estrogen dose should be gradually reduced over a period of 2 to 3 months and then discontinued to assess the individual's need for resumption of use.

The lowest effective daily dose of estrogen should be determined and maintained for the duration of the treatment.

Vaginal cream preparations of estrogen may be considered instead of orally administered estrogen if the only indication is atrophic vaginitis. However, it should be noted that these preparations allow rapid absorption of estrogen into the systemic circulation, and do not permit accurate control of dosage. They should be used intermittently and only as needed to correct the symptoms of atrophic vaginitis. (Note: The estrogen in vaginal creams can be absorbed through the skin of the penis and cause tenderness of the breast in men.)

The unnecessary prolongation of estrogen therapy should be avoided. It is advisable to use estrogens in the lowest effective dose and for only as long as necessary to relieve symptoms.

Guidelines for the Use of Estrogens in Specific Deficiency States

I. The young woman (under 45 years of age) with both ovaries and uterus removed:

1. Choice of estrogen: a conjugated "natural" estrogen (see list of estrogen preparations).
    The lowest effective dose should be used.*

2. Dosage schedule: once daily from the 1st through the 25th day of each month.
    Note: If the uterus is present, it is advisable to add a progestin (medroxyprogesterone), 4 to 10 mg daily during the last 7 to 10 days of the estrogen course.**

3. Duration of use: if well tolerated, until 50 years of age, when assessment of continued need is made individually.

4. Periodic examinations:
    Base-line mammogram (low-radiation-dose xeroradiography); mammogram should be repeated only as necessary to evaluate

---

*The lowest effective dose is determined by keeping a daily "flush count" to ascertain the lowest daily dose that will reduce the frequency and severity of flushes to an acceptable level.

**The use of a supplemental progestin during the last 7 to 10 days of estrogen administration is still controversial. A possible benefit is the reduced potential for uterine cancer; a possible risk is the increased potential for coronary artery disease; a possible inconvenience is withdrawal bleeding (induced menstruation). The risks of this form of long-term progestin therapy are not known.

possible breast tumor (American Cancer Society guideline).

Self-examination of breasts monthly.

Physician examination of breasts (and uterus if present) every 6 to 12 months.

Measurement of blood pressure.

II. The woman experiencing the "menopausal syndrome" of hot flushes and sweating (usually 45 to 55 years of age):

  A. Uterus not removed

    1. Choice of hormones and recommended dosage range:

Estrogen: conjugated equine estrogens—0.3 to 0.625 mg daily. (See list of alternative estrogen preparations.)

Progestin: medroxyprogesterone—5 to 10 mg daily.

The lowest effective dose of estrogen should be used.*

    2. Dosage schedule:

Estrogen: once daily from the 1st through the 25th day of each month.

Progestin: once daily during the last 7 to 10 days of the estrogen course.**

    3. Duration of use: 6 to 12 months, followed by gradual reduction of dose over a period of 2 to 3 months, and then discontinuation to assess the need for continued use. Treatment should be resumed only if symptoms require it. An attempt should be made to discontinue all hormones after 2 to 3 years of continual use, unless a clear need for continuation is apparent.

    4. Periodic examinations:

Base-line mammogram (low-radiation-dose xeroradiography).

Low-dose mammogram annually (over 50 years of age) during continuous use of estrogen (American Cancer Society guideline).

Self-examination of breasts monthly.

Physician examination of breasts every 6 to 12 months.

Cervical cytology and endometrial biopsy (aspiration curettage) annually.

Blood pressure measurement every 3 to 6 months.

Two-hour blood sugar assay annually.

  B. Uterus removed

    1. Choice of estrogen and dose: conjugated equine estrogens—0.3 to 0.625 mg daily.

The lowest effective dose should be used.*

    2. Dosage schedule: once daily from the 1st through the 25th day of each month.

    3. Duration of use: 6 to 12 months, followed by gradual reduction of

---

*The lowest effective dose is determined by keeping a daily "flush count" to ascertain the lowest daily dose that will reduce the frequency and severity of flushes to an acceptable level.

**The use of a supplemental progestin during the last 7 to 10 days of estrogen administration is still controversial. A possible benefit is the reduced potential for uterine cancer; a possible risk is the increased potential for coronary artery disease; a possible inconvenience is withdrawal bleeding (induced menstruation). The risks of this form of long-term progestin therapy are not known.

dose over a period of 2 to 3 months, and then discontinuation to assess the need for continued use. Treatment should be resumed only if symptoms require it. An attempt should be made to discontinue all hormones after 2 to 3 years of continual use.

4. Periodic examinations:

Base-line mammogram (low-radiation-dose xeroradiography).

Low-dose mammogram annually (over 50 years of age) during continuous use of estrogen (American Cancer Society guideline).

Self-examination of breasts monthly.

Physician examination of breasts every 6 to 12 months.

Blood pressure measurement every 3 to 6 months.

Two-hour blood sugar assay annually.

III. The woman in the "post-menopausal" period (usually over 55 years of age): treatment should be individualized as follows:

1. If there are no specific symptoms of estrogen deficiency (hot flushes or atrophic vaginitis), estrogen should not be given.

2. If specific symptoms of estrogen deficiency persist to a degree requiring subjective relief, the recommendations in category II apply. However, in addition to limiting courses of estrogen to 6 to 12 months followed by gradual withdrawal, dosage might be limited to 3 times weekly on a trial basis. Estrogen should be discontinued altogether as soon as possible. If only flushes persist beyond 60 years of age, all estrogen should be discontinued. Nonhormonal drugs such as clonidine, ergot preparations and certain sedatives may be substituted for the relief of hot flushes.

3. Although we do not yet have accurate and reliable predictive indicators, an attempt should be made to identify the woman who may be at high risk for the development of osteoporosis. The following features suggest the possibility of increased risk:

   (1) slender build, light-boned, white or Oriental race
   (2) a sedentary life style or restricted physical activity
   (3) a family history (mother or sister) of osteoporosis (reported by some investigators)
   (4) a low-sodium diet (also likely to be a low-calcium diet)
   (5) heavy smoking
   (6) excessive use of antacids that contain aluminum
   (7) long-term use of cortisone-related drugs
   (8) habitual use of carbonated beverages (reported by some investigators)
   (9) excessive consumption of alcohol
   (10) increased urinary excretion of calcium

   For the woman thought to be at increased risk for the development of osteoporosis, estrogen treatment should be started within 3 years after menstruation ceases. The following schedule of estrogen therapy may be recommended for prevention: conjugated equine estrogens—0.625 mg daily or 3 times weekly, for the first 3 weeks of each month. Periodic examinations as outlined in category II above should be performed. Estrogen replacement therapy may continue indefinitely, always with appropriate supervision.

In addition to the prudent use of estrogen, regular exercise and a daily intake of 1500 mg of calcium and 400 units of vitamin D are generally thought to be beneficial in slowing the development of osteoporosis.

Ancillary Drug Treatment (as required)

Condition	Drug Treatment
For anxiety and/or depression:	alprazolam (Xanax), for intermittent short-term use
For insomnia:	doxylamine (Unisom), available OTC
	diphenhydramine (Benadryl)
For headache:	aspirin
	acetaminophen (Tylenol, Panadol, etc.)
	ibuprofen (Advil, Nuprin, etc.)
For atrophic vaginitis and painful intercourse:	estrogen creams (Dienestrol, Estrace, Premarin)

Note: Drug selection, dosage and administration schedule must be determined by the physician for each patient individually.

OSTEOARTHRITIS

Other Names: Osteoarthrosis, Degenerative Arthritis, Degenerative Joint Disease, Hypertrophic Arthritis

Prevalence in USA: 16 million—8.7% of the adult population; 10% of the elderly population.

Age Group: 55 years and over.

Male to Female Ratio: Same incidence in men and women.

Principal Features: Osteoarthritis is the most common joint disease and the major cause of disability of our older population. It is an insidious, slowly progressive deterioration of the surface cartilage on the ends of bones where they come together to form joints. During the early phases of change, there are no symptoms. With progressive destruction of protective cartilage, bone surface becomes exposed and irritated; this results in pain, stiffness and muscle spasm. As the central area of cartilage is destroyed, new bone and cartilage begin to form on the edges of the joint (spur formation). These degenerative changes can start as early as the fourth decade of life; they usually begin to cause symptoms in sixth and seventh decades; by age 75, all individuals have some degree of osteoarthritis in one or more joints. The most commonly involved joints are: fingers, thumb, shoulders, hips, knees, base of the first toe, neck and lower (lumbar) spine. Progressive changes in the weight-bearing joints, principally the lower spine, hips and knees, eventually give rise to pain, deep ache and muscle spasm. Discomfort grows worse after prolonged activity that involves diseased joints.

Causes: There is no apparent initiating cause for primary osteoarthritis. The disorder does have a familial pattern, and it is thought that genetic bio-chemical defects in cartilage structure predispose some individuals to excessive "wear and tear" deterioration of vulnerable joints. Secondary osteoarthritis is due to congenital joint malformations, joint injuries and infections and other infrequent causes of bone and cartilage deteriora-tion.

Drugs That Can Cause This Disorder: Although some drugs are capable of causing joint aches and pains (e.g., barbiturates, "sulfa" drugs, oral con-traceptives, isoniazid, pyrazinamide), no drugs cause the bone and carti-lage destruction characteristic of osteoarthritis. Rarely the systemic (internal) use of cortisonelike steroid drugs can cause aseptic necrosis of bone (destruction without infection); this can initiate a secondary form of osteoarthritis.

Drugs Used to Treat This Disorder: There are no drugs that can prevent, halt the progression of or reverse the degenerative changes of osteoar-thritis. The following drugs are used to relieve pain, stiffness and mus-cle spasm.

Nonsteroidal Anti-inflammatory Drugs (NSAIDs)

Salicylates
- aspirin (Bufferin, Ascriptin, Cama, etc.).
- aspirin, enteric-coated (Easprin, Ecotrin, etc.).
- aspirin, zero-order-release (Zorpin).
- magnesium salicylate (Magan, Mobidin).
- choline magnesium salicylate (Trisilate).
- salsalate (Disalcid).
- diflunisal (Dolobid).
- sodium salicylate.

Indole derivatives
- indomethacin (Indocin).
- sulindac (Clinoril).
- tolmetin (Tolectin).

Propionic acid derivatives
- fenoprofen (Nalfon).
- ibuprofen (Motrin, Rufen, Advil, etc.).
- ketoprofen (Orudis).
- naproxen (Naprosyn).
- suprofen (Suprol).

Fenamic acid derivatives
- meclofenamate (Meclomen).
- mefenamic acid (Ponstel).

Oxicam derivatives
- piroxicam (Feldene).

Simple Analgesics
- acetaminophen (Tylenol, Panadol, etc.).
- propoxyphene (Darvon, etc.).
- codeine (Tylenol with codeine, etc.).
- hydrocodone (Vicodin, etc.).
- oxycodone (Percodan, Percocet, Tylox).

Muscle Relaxants
- carisoprodol (Soma).
- cyclobenzaprine (Flexeril).
- diazepam (Valium).
- methocarbamol (Robaxin).
- orphenadrine (Norflex).

Goals of Drug Treatment

Relief of pain and stiffness sufficient to permit continued activity, therapeutic exercise and physiotherapy.

Relief of associated anxiety and/or depression.

Drug Management

General Principles

Osteoarthritis is a chronic but slowly progressive disorder; although there is no curative treatment available, the symptoms are generally mild for long periods of time and can usually be relieved satisfactorily with available drugs.

Nonsteroidal anti-inflammatory drugs (NSAIDs) are the primary drugs of choice for managing osteoarthritis. Their principal actions are within the tissues of the diseased joint.

Simple analgesics, such as propoxyphene, codeine, oxycodone, etc., suppress pain perception in the brain; they are used to supplement the analgesic effects of NSAIDs.

Cortisonelike steroids by mouth should not be used in the management of osteoarthritis. They may be helpful when injected directly into osteoarthritis joints, sometimes providing prompt and lasting relief of pain and swelling. If effective, steroid injections may be repeated at intervals of 4 to 6 months for a limited number of times.

Symptomatic drug treatment will be more effective if it is supplemented by appropriate physiotherapy and the use of physical aids, such as canes, crutches, walkers, railings, etc.

Avoid prolonged and repeated overuse of diseased joints to (1) slow the progression of joint destruction and (2) minimize requirements for analgesic drugs.

Excessive body weight (obesity) can accelerate deterioration of weight-bearing joints. Prudent weight reduction programs are a most important part of treatment for osteoarthritis of the lower spine, hips and knees.

Use of Nonsteroidal Anti-inflammatory Drugs (NSAIDs)

1. These drugs are not thought to be able to favorably influence the natural course of osteoarthritis, but they can relieve pain and inflammation and thereby improve joint function and mobility.
2. Treatment is usually initiated with aspirin (lowest cost). Unfortunately, large doses (2 to 4 tablets of 325 mg each, 3 to 4 times daily) are often necessary to achieve satisfactory relief. The high blood levels required can cause ringing in the ears (tinnitus) and loss of hearing, especially in the elderly. Measurements of salicylate blood levels can be most helpful in establishing correct dosage. (See Therapeutic Drug Monitoring in Section One.)
3. Soluble aspirin preparations (regular aspirin, Bufferin, Ascriptin, etc.) often cause stomach ulceration and bleeding; they should be taken with food to minimize this effect.
4. The preferred forms of aspirin for continual use in large doses include (1) enteric-coated preparations and (2) zero-order-release tablets. (See list above.)
5. Salicylates other than aspirin can also be used. (See list above.) These cause significantly less stomach irritation; some are effective with twice daily dosage.
6. All NSAID aspirin substitutes are better tolerated than aspirin. However, they may share a cross-sensitivity in individuals who are allergic to aspirin and may induce asthmatic reactions.
7. An NSAID should be used on a regular schedule for a trial period of 3 to 4 weeks; if it is not effective, another one should be tried in sequence (selecting one from a different chemical group). An attempt is made to find the NSAID that provides the best relief with the fewest side-effects.
8. Authorities do not recommend the use of NSAIDs in combination with each other. A small dose of aspirin taken along with an NSAID may provide additional relief of pain.
9. NSAIDs have a potential for injuring the kidney and impairing kidney function. They should be used with caution in individuals over 50 years old, in those with hypertension, diabetes, congestive heart failure and especially in those taking diuretics.
10. NSAIDs can increase the effects of oral antidiabetic drugs (sulfonylureas) and anticoagulants. Dosage adjustments may be necessary.

Use of Narcoticlike Analgesics

1. In advanced cases of osteoarthritis, mild analgesics such as acetaminophen or propoxyphene may not provide adequate pain relief. Codeine, hydrocodone and oxycodone may be tried cautiously on an intermittent schedule to avoid tolerance and dependence.
2. The use of stronger narcotic (opioid) analgesics (morphine, meperidine, etc.) should be avoided completely. Their potential for causing depen-

dence (addiction) precludes repetitious, long-term use in chronically painful disorders like osteoarthritis.

Use of Muscle Relaxants

1. Muscle spasm prevents exercise and use of affected joints. The cautious use of muscle relaxants in conjunction with physiotherapy may be beneficial in preserving joint mobility and muscle strength.
2. Muscle relaxants are most useful in managing osteoarthritis of the lower spine with associated lumbo-sacral muscle spasm.

Ancillary Drug Treatment (as required)

Condition	*Drug Treatment*
For anxiety and/or mild depression:	alprazolam (Xanax), for intermittent, short-term use
For moderate or severe depression:	trazodone (Desyrel) (see Profile of Depression in this section)
For drug-induced constipation:	docusate with casanthranol (Peri-Colace)

Note: Drug selection, dosage and administration schedule must be determined by the physician for each patient individually.

OSTEOPOROSIS

Other Names: Osteopenia, Type I Postmenopausal or Spinal Osteoporosis (95% of all cases), Type II Senile Osteoporosis

Prevalence in USA: 15 to 20 million—approximately 25% of white women over 60 years of age have osteoporosis; 1.3 million fractures due to osteoporosis occur annually.

Age Group: Type I osteoporosis—50 to 65 years. Type II osteoporosis—65 years and over.

Male to Female Ratio: Much higher incidence in women: 8 to 1.

Principal Features: Osteoporosis is a major disorder of bone in the elderly, occurring most often in postmenopausal women. As ovarian function declines and estrogen is withdrawn, the natural loss of bone mass is accelerated. This eventually weakens bone structure and predisposes to fractures that can result from minimal trauma. Osteoporosis can be localized in a single bone (a leg immobilized in a cast), but it is usually more widely distributed, with most fractures occurring in the spine, wrist and hip. The basic defect is a relative increase in the rate of bone destruction without a compensating increase in the reformation of new bone. There are usually no symptoms prior to the occurrence of a spontaneous or traumatic fracture. A sudden compression fracture of a vertebra in the middle or lower section of the spine can result from such minor strains as bending, lifting or sneezing; it causes immediate pain and disability lasting several weeks. Gradual compression of the vertebrae (usually painless) causes loss of height and the development of a stooped, rounded back ("dowager's hump"). A spontaneous fracture of a hip (femur) can occur on arising from a chair or while walking. Untreated osteoporosis can cause a loss of 30% to 60% of bone mass.

Causes: Primary osteoporosis is a normal consequence of aging. A woman loses approximately 50% of bone mass, and a man approximately 25%, during a normal life span. Type I primary osteoporosis refers to the estrogen withdrawal syndrome following menopause. Type II primary osteoporosis occurs later as a feature of senility. Secondary osteoporosis refers to the bone loss that is associated with other diseases and disorders: hyperthyroidism, hyperparathyroidism, adrenal cortical hormone excess (Cushing's syndrome or drug-induced), multiple myeloma, diabetes, and alcoholism.

Drugs That Can Cause This Disorder
- Cortisonelike steroids, especially in immobilized women over 50 years of age receiving large doses.
- Heparin, when used in long-term therapy.
- Methotrexate, when used in prepubertal children for long-term therapy.

Drugs Used to Treat This Disorder
Estrogens ("Natural-type" Estrogens Are Preferred)
- conjugated estrogens (Genisis, Premarin).
- esterified estrogens (Evex, Menest).
- estradiol cypionate (Depo-Estradiol, injection).
- estradiol valerate (Delestrogen, injection).
- estriol (Hormonin, a mixture of estriol, estradiol and estrone).
- piperazine estrone sulfate (Ogen).
- micronized 17-B estadiol (Estrace).
- transdermal estradiol skin patch (Estraderm-50 and 100).*
Calcium Preparations
- calcium carbonate (40% calcium) (generic tablets, Alka-2, Biocal, Caltrate, OsCal-500, Tums).
- calcium gluconate (9% calcium) (generic tablets).
- calcium lactate (13% calcium) (generic tablets).
- dibasic calcium phosphate (31% calcium) (generic tablets).
Vitamin D Analogs
- calcifediol (Calderol).
- calcitriol (Rocaltrol).

*Approval by FDA for marketing expected in late 1986.

Other Drugs
- calcitonin (Calcimar).
- fluorides (investigational).

Goals of Drug Treatment

Primary prevention: early initiation of estrogen therapy—during or immediately after menopause—to prevent acceleration of natural bone loss.

Secondary prevention: initiation of estrogen therapy 3 or more years following menopause (after some degree of osteoporosis is present) to arrest or retard progressive bone loss.

Prevention of osteoporosis-related fractures.

Relief of pain and muscle spasm associated with fracture of osteoporotic bone.

Drug Management

General Principles

It is now firmly established that excessive bone loss (osteoporosis) following menopause can be prevented or significantly reduced by the timely administration of low-dose estrogen.

Accurate assessment of bone mass for the detection of osteoporosis can be made by quantitative CAT scan of vertebrae and by photon absorptiometry of wrist bones. However, these procedures are expensive and not generally available.

Currently it is not feasible to screen all postmenopausal women for osteoporosis. To identify those who may benefit from estrogen used preventively, the following "risk factors" characterize the candidates for postmenopausal osteoporosis:

1. slender build, light-boned, white or Oriental race
2. a sedentary life style or restricted physical activity
3. a family history of osteoporosis (grandmother, mother, aunt, sister)
4. a high-protein diet
5. a low-sodium diet (also likely to be a low-calcium diet)
6. lifelong avoidance of dairy products
7. heavy smoking
8. excessive use of antacids that contain aluminum
9. long-term use of cortisonelike steroid drugs
10. habitual use of carbonated beverages
11. excessive consumption of alcohol
12. increased urinary excretion of calcium

Thyroid replacement therapy (in appropriate dosage) may increase bone loss and predispose to the development of osteoporosis in the vertebrae of the lower spine. If you are taking a thyroid preparation to correct hypothyroidism, consult your physician regarding a possible need for calcium and vitamin D supplements to prevent potential bone loss.

Use of Estrogens

1. Estrogen increases the absorption of dietary calcium and reduces the rate of calcium loss from bone.

2. Estrogen does not substantially increase bone mass; it does not enhance restoration of bone following loss.
3. To be effective in preventing significant osteoporosis, estrogen therapy must begin within 3 years after menopause. Available evidence seems to indicate that continued protection against the development of osteoporosis requires ongoing use of estrogen—probably for life by those at risk.
4. Fifty percent of women are protected by 0.3 mg of conjugated estrogens daily; close to 100% are protected by 0.625 mg daily. Your physician can advise the dose most appropriate for you.
5. For detailed information regarding the use of estrogen, see the Profile of Menopause in this section and the Drug Profile of Estrogen in Section Three.

Use of Calcium Preparations
1. Calcium supplementation of the diet is appropriate for preventing or treating osteoporosis because the calcium content of the diet is usually less than the ongoing requirement for the maintenance of normal bone density. The average dietary intake of calcium by women is 500 to 600 mg daily. The daily requirement for the postmenopausal woman is 1500 to 2000 mg (all sources).
2. There is some evidence that calcium supplements (taken alone) may reduce the rate of bone loss and the incidence of fracture, but further proof is needed. Calcium is most effective when taken in conjunction with vitamin D and estrogen.
3. Supplemental calcium must not be taken in excessive doses. The recommended daily intake of calcium is approximately 1000 mg if taking estrogen and 1500 mg if not taking estrogen.
4. Excessive intake of supplemental calcium (more than 2000 mg daily) can cause abnormal increases in the blood and urine levels of calcium and predispose to kidney stone formation.
5. The most appropriate calcium preparations to use for supplementation are listed above.
6. Calcium supplements made from bone meal or mineral clay (dolomite, montmorillomite) may contain lead or other toxic metals and should be avoided.
7. Calcium supplements may be more effective if taken as a single late-evening dose to suppress the normal nocturnal rise in parathyroid hormone that increases bone loss.
8. Calcium may decrease the effects of aspirin (and other salicylates), calcium channel blocking drugs, iron and tetracyclines. Do not take calcium preparations within 2 hours of taking other drugs.

Use of Vitamin D Analogs
1. Elderly individuals with osteoporosis who have a normal life style are not likely to a have a vitamin D deficiency; they usually have an adequate supply from their diet and exposure to sunlight.
2. Shut-ins (those confined to home, nursing home or hospital) probably need a supplement of vitamin D. Currently recommended sources include Calderol and Rocaltrol.

3. When vitamin D is used, limit calcium intake to 600 to 700 mg daily to prevent excessive absorption and abnormally high calcium levels in blood and urine.

Use of Calcitonin (a Thyroid Hormone That Reduces Bone Loss)
1. Studies to date show that calcitonin in doses of 100 units daily can produce an increase in total body calcium (99% in bone) after 2 years of treatment. A favorable response was achieved in 70% of users.
2. Calcitonin is given by injection and is used in conjunction with calcium and vitamin D.
3. Studies using other dosage forms of calcitonin—oral, buccal (cheek), intranasal—are under way.

Use of Fluoride
1. The use of fluoride in the prevention and treatment of osteoporosis is still investigational. Directions for its optimal use have not been established.
2. A dose of 40 to 65 mg/day is required to stimulate bone formation. Adverse effects occur in over 30% of users; these include nausea, stomach pain, gastrointestinal bleeding, bone and joint pain and severe foot discomfort, often intense enought to preclude compliance with treatment.
3. Calcium must always be used concurrently with fluoride to avoid the development of osteomalacia (abnormal mineral composition of bone).

Ancillary Drug Treatment (as required)

Condition	*Drug Treatment*
For calcium-induced constipation:	docusate (Colace, etc.)
	docusate with casanthranol (Peri-Colace, etc.)
For fracture pain:	acetaminaphen with codeine (Tylenol with codeine)
	acetaminophen with propoxyphene (Darvocet-N 100)
	Avoid opiate analgesics stronger than codeine.
For muscle spasm:	diazepam (Valium)
For mild depression:	alprazolam (Xanax), for intermittent, short-term use
For marked depression:	trazodone (Desyrel)

Note: Drug selection, dosage and administration schedule must be determined by the physician for each patient individually.

PARKINSON'S DISEASE

Other Names: Paralysis Agitans, Parkinsonism, Parkinsonian Syndrome

Prevalence in USA: Approximately 1 million—50,000 new cases annually; 1% of the population over 50 years old.

Age Group: 10% of cases under 40 years old; 20% of cases 40 to 50 years old; 70% of cases 50 years old and over.

Male to Female Ratio: More common in men, 3 to 2.

Principal Features: Parkinson's disease is a slowly progressive, debilitating disorder of certain brain centers that contribute to the control and regulation of body movement. The earliest symptoms begin very insidiously; one arm or one leg (or the arm and leg on one side) will gradually develop a sense of weakness, retarded movement and stiffness. A fine tremor in a hand or foot will appear in 70% of cases; this occurs at rest and disappears with intentional use of the affected limb and while asleep. Symptoms may remain mild for years or they may progress steadily. Eventually the principal features of the disorder become generalized; the tremor spreads, most of the body musculature becomes rigid, the posture is stooped, movement is slow and jerky, the gait is shuffling and unsteady. Facial expression is lost; the voice grows weak and speech indistinct. Withdrawal and depression may occur as disability advances. Loss of mental acuity occurs in 30% of cases within 7 to 10 years. Currently available drug therapy can slow the progress of the disorder significantly for many, and life expectancy has been extended to equal the norms.

Causes: Primary Parkinson's disease is due to degeneration of the nerve cells in the brain that produce dopamine, one of the major nerve impulse transmitters. In most instances, the initiating cause of the cellular degeneration is unknown. Infrequently a virus infection of the brain (encephalitis) can initiate the degenerative process. Secondary parkinsonism can be caused by hardening of brain arteries, strokes, brain tumors, trauma, carbon monoxide or manganese poisoning and a few rare degenerative disorders of brain tissue.

Drugs That Can Cause This Disorder: The following drugs can block the action of dopamine and cause a form of secondary parkinsonism with features that are indistinguishable from primary Parkinson's disease: phenothiazines, haloperidol, reserpine, thiothixene, methyldopa, metoclopramide. (See respective Drug Profiles in Section Three or Drug Classes in Section Four.)

Drugs Used to Treat This Disorder
- levodopa (Dopar, Larodopa).
- levodopa + carbidopa (Sinemet).
- levodopa + bensarazide (Prolopa in Canada).

- amantadine (Symmetrel).
- anticholinergics (atropinelike drugs): benztropine (Cogentin), diphenhydramine (Benadryl), trihexyphenidyl (Artane).
- bromocriptine (Parlodel).
- deprenyl (or selegiline)—investigational.

Goals of Drug Treatment

Improvement of overall function and mobility.
Reduction of muscular rigidity and tremor.
Reversal of slowed movement.
Improvement of posture, balance, gait, speech and writing.

Drug Management

General Principles

The symptoms of Parkinson's disease are due to a relative increase in the effects of acetylcholine in the brain centers that regulate body movement. The exaggerated acetylcholine effects are the result of a reduced supply of dopamine (primary Parkinson's disease) or to a blocking of dopamine action (drug-induced parkinsonism).

Drugs used to manage parkinsonism utilize three distinct mechanisms of action: (1) anticholinergic drugs reduce the excessive effects of acetylcholine; (2) levodopa is converted to dopamine in the brain, increasing its supply to restore a balance closer to normal; (3) bromocriptine serves as a substitute for dopamine by stimulating its receptor cells directly. Amantadine is thought to have both anticholinergic and direct-stimulating effects.

Appropriate drugs, properly used, can improve function and mobility for significant periods of time; up to 50% of those treated have no major disabilities after 10 years of disease.

The optimal drug program—either one drug used alone or two or more used in combination—is that which provides satisfactory relief of symptoms or the most acceptable compromise between symptom relief and drug side-effects. (Complete relief of symptoms may not be possible.)

Drug selection and dosage schedules *must be carefully individualized*; adjustments will be necessary throughout the course of this disorder. Daily fluctuations in symptoms and drug responses occur in almost every individual and vary greatly from person to person. A "trial-and-error" process is unavoidable in determining the best drug(s) and the best dosage schedule. For the best treatment results, keep your physician informed regarding all aspects of your response to the drugs prescribed.

Combinations of several drugs taken in small doses are often more beneficial than a single drug taken in large doses.

Use of Levodopa

1. Only 25% of levodopa taken alone by mouth enters the brain. The large doses required to be effective often cause unacceptable side-effects. To prevent this, levodopa is combined with carbidopa; the combination (marketed as Sinemet) permits a 75% dosage reduction of levodopa.
2. Levodopa has been the drug of choice for managing primary parkin-

sonism for the past 15 years. Approximately 80% of users achieve 80% improvement in muscular rigidity and retarded movement.

3. Levodopa may be tried at any time during the course of this disorder. However, authorities differ in their opinions as to the best time to use levodopa. Some advise early use—within the first year of symptoms—to obtain the fullest benefit possible. Others advise later use to delay the onset of side-effects and adverse effects that develop with long-term use of levodopa.

4. Levodopa is more completely absorbed when taken on an empty stomach. However, it may be necessary to take it following food to prevent nausea. If so, avoid meat when possible; proteins can interfere with absorption of levodopa.

5. After a year or more of continual use of levodopa, 80% of users will develop abnormal involuntary movements (dyskinesias) of various muscle groups—jerks and twitches of the head and face or purposelike movement of the extremities. In 30% of the users these may be severe enough to interfere with normal functioning. They last for a few minutes to several hours and seem to coincide with the times of both high and low blood levels of levodopa.

6. Another 20% of users will experience "on-off' episodes—changes from relatively good function and mobility (drug effects "on") to marked loss of function and mobility (drug effects "off"). To minimize these periods of fluctuating effectiveness, levodopa may be taken in small doses every 1 to 3 hours throughout the day to maintain a more constant blood level.

7. Levodopa can cause a variety of mental disturbances: euphoria, hypomania, depression, confusion, nightmares, vivid hallucinations.

8. Levodopa should not be used concurrently with those antipsychotic drugs that block the action of dopamine; or with monoamine oxidase (MAO) inhibitors that increase the risk of a hypertensive crisis.

9. Some authorities advocate the use of "drug holidays" to reduce the toxic manifestations of levodopa. The very gradual withdrawal and reintroduction of the drug are essential to success.

Use of Amantadine

1. This drug probably releases dopamine from nerve cells and increases its availability. It may also seve as a dopamine substitute and stimulate receptor cells directly. It has anticholinergic effects that contribute to its effectiveness.

2. Amantadine may be tried first in all patients. It can produce a 15% to 25% improvement in 60% of users. A trial period of 1 week is usually adequate; if not beneficial or if mentality is adversely affected, discontinue use.

3. Amantadine may also be used in conjunction with anticholinergics and levodopa. It is usually well tolerated by the elderly.

4. This drug has a low incidence of side-effects. Ankle swelling and a reddish-blue mottling of the arms or legs may occur after 1 month to 1 year of use. These are not serious and are reversible.

5. Doses over 200 mg can cause excitement, increased tremor, jerkiness, insomnia and nightmares in sensitive individuals.

6. Amantadine may lose some of its effectiveness after 6 to 12 weeks of continual use.

Use of Anticholinergic Drugs

1. These atropinelike drugs are often used to initiate treatment when symptoms are mild. They can produce a 20% to 30% improvement by suppressing effects due to overactivity of acetylcholine: tremor, excessive salivation, rigidity and slow movement.

2. They may be used alone as long as symptoms remain mild. They may be combined with any of the other drugs used and at any stage of the disorder.

3. These drugs are not well tolerated by individuals over 70 years old. They can provoke latent glaucoma and can aggravate urinary retention in men with prostatism (see Glossary).

4. Unavoidable side-effects include blurring of near vision, dry mouth, constipation and urinary hesitancy. High doses may cause drowsiness, confusion, impaired memory, hallucinations and nightmares.

5. Following long-term use, these drugs must be discontinued very gradually to avoid a dangerous withdrawal syndrome.

Use of Bromocriptine

1. This drug may be used alone but is usually added to the treatment program at a later stage. It is the drug of choice for alleviating the abnormal involuntary movements associated with long-term levodopa use. It can also have a stabilizing effect when the "on-off" effects of levodopa therapy become apparent.

2. Bromocriptine is initiated with very small doses, and the dose is increased very slowly. Some individuals develop extreme hypotension (low blood pressure) with the first doses. It is advisable to try a test dose at bedtime for several days to determine individual blood pressure response.

3. This drug may not be effective in severe Parkinson's disease or in those with a poor response to levodopa.

4. High doses can cause acute personality changes, mood swings and other intolerable adverse effects; 40% of users discontinue this drug because of undesirable reactions.

5. This drug is an ergot derivative; it should be used with caution in the presence of angina, hypertension or any form of peripheral vascular disease.

Ancillary Drug Treatment (as required)

Condition	*Drug Treatment*
For levodopa-induced drowsiness:	methylphenidate (Ritalin)
For levodopa-induced nausea:	diphenidol (Vontrol)

Ancillary Drug Treatment (as required) *(continued)*

Condition	*Drug Treatment*
For action tremor:	propranolol (Inderal)
For muscle spasm and rigidity:	diazepam (Valium)
For nocturnal leg cramps:	quinine (Quinamm) at bedtime
For constipation:	docusate (Colace)
	docusate with casanthranol (Peri-Colace)
For insomnia:	chloral hydrate (Noctec, Somnos)
For ankle swelling:	hydrochlorothiazide (generic)
For depression:	amitriptyline (Elavil)
	desipramine (Norpramin)
	imipramine (Tofranil)

Note: Drug selection, dosage and administration schedule must be determined by the physician for each patient individually.

PEPTIC ULCER

Other Names: Peptic Ulcer Disease, Duodenal Ulcer, Gastric Ulcer

Prevalence in USA: 10% of the general population will have a symptomatic peptic ulcer sometime during life; 25% of men and 16% of women have scars of peptic ulcer disease on autopsy examination.

Age Group: Duodenal ulcer occurs most commonly between 25 and 40 years. Gastric ulcer occurs most commonly between 40 and 55 years. Of all ulcers, 1.9% occur under 18 years; 43% occur between 18 and 44 years; 36% occur between 45 and 64 years; 12.8% occur between 65 and 74 years; 6.3% occur at 75 years and over.

Male to Female Ratio: Duodenal ulcer: higher incidence in men—2 to 1. Gastric ulcer: same incidence in men and women.

Principal Features: Peptic ulcer disease refers to an intermittent disorder of the stomach and first portion of the small intestine (duodenum) that is characterized by the formation of ulcers in the lining of these organs. The tissues subject to ulceration are constantly bathed in digestive juices produced in the stomach; the principal components of these juices include hydrochloric acid and the digestive enzyme pepsin (hence "peptic" ulcer). Most individuals with peptic ulcer disease produce excessive amounts of acid and pepsin, which overwhelm the normal protection of the lining tissues and cause erosion (ulceration). The singular feature of an active duodenal ulcer is a gnawing or burning pain in the upper midabdomen that usually occurs between meals and in the early morning hours—when acid secretion is high. The pain is characteristically relieved by food or antacids. The pattern of pain-food-relief typifies active duodenal ulcer. Episodes of ulcer activation occur unpredictably, but are often more frequent and troublesome in the spring and fall of the year. By nature, peptic ulcer disease is a chronically recurrent disorder. The recurrence rate of duodenal ulcer is approximately 70% within 1 year and 90% within 2 years. Frequent recurrence predisposes to serious complications in 30% of ulcer patients, 10% to 15% will experience bleeding, 5% to 10% will suffer perforation of the duodenal wall and 5% will develop obstruction at the stomach outlet (pylorus) due to the extensive scarring that follows ulcer healing.

Causes: A predisposition to develop peptic ulcer disease appears to be hereditary. The primary initiating cause of ulceration is not known. Those individuals who produce excessive amounts of stomach acid and pepsin are often prone to the development of duodenal ulcer. Others with normal amounts of acid and pepsin develop ulceration because the protective mechanisms in the lining tissues are defective and inadequate. Certain states of physical stress (burns, trauma, surgery) can increase the incidence of peptic ulcer.

Drugs That Can Cause This Disorder: The following drugs can initiate ulceration of the stomach or duodenum in susceptible individuals or aggravate existing ulcers:

alcohol	cortisonelike steroids
aminophylline	phenylbutazone
aspirin and other nonsteroidal anti-inflammatory drugs	reserpine (?)

Drugs Used to Treat This Disorder
- antacids (Delcid, Maalox TC, Mylanta II, etc.).
- cimetidine (Tagamet).
- ranitidine (Zantac).
- sucralfate (Carafate).
- anticholinergic drugs (Darbid, Pro-Banthine, Robinul) for adjunctive use.

Goals of Drug Treatment
Short-term control of stomach acidity sufficient to relieve pain and promote ulcer healing.
Long-term control of stomach acidity to prevent ulcer recurrence.
Prevention of complications.

Drug Management
General Principles
Most cases of peptic ulcer disease can be managed successfully by appropriate drug therapy. A treatment program of 4 to 6 weeks will heal up to 90% of duodenal ulcers. Surgery is needed only for the management of ulcer complications: uncontrolled bleeding, perforation, obstruction, persistent pain.

The four principal drugs used to promote healing of duodenal ulcer are all equally effective when taken in adequate dosage for 4 to 6 weeks. However, some individuals may respond more favorably to 2 (or more) drugs used concurrently. In the treatment of gastric ulcer, antacids are less effective than cimetidine, ranitidine, or sucralfate.

Anticholinergic (atropinelike) drugs are used only when ulcer symptoms are not adequately controlled by antacids and/or cimetidine or ranitidine.

Tranquilizers and sedatives should not be used routinely but only as necessary to relieve significant anxiety and nervous tension that could possibly contribute to hyperacidity.

If possible, it is advisable to avoid cortisonelike steroid therapy in the presence of active peptic ulcer or in those individuals who are subject to recurrently active peptic ulcer disease. If steroid treatment is necessary, antacids and/or cimetidine (or ranitidine) should be used protectively.

The chronic use of aspirin (and substitute nonsteroidal anti-inflammatory drugs) increases the chance of developing active peptic ulcer.

Cigarette smoking doubles the chance of developing peptic ulcer disease; it also delays healing significantly.

Caffeine-containing beverages (coffee, tea, cola) can stimulate stomach acid production and aggravate an existing ulcer.

Alcohol (in excess) can aggravate gastric ulcer and increase the risk of bleeding.

Use of Antacids
1. These drugs are used to neutralize stomach acids and thereby (1) relieve pain, heartburn and acid indigestion; and (2) correct hyperacidity and promote ulcer healing.
2. The antacids of choice are composed of magnesium aluminum hydroxide (Delcid, Maalox TC, Mylanta II). The optimal treatment schedule is 1 ounce taken 1 hour and 3 hours after meals and at bedtime until free of pain for 2 weeks; then 1 hour after meals and at bedtime for an additional 4 weeks.
3. Avoid long-term use of aluminum hydroxide and magnesium trisilicate preparations; they may cause depletion of phosphate and increase the risk of osteomalacia (softening of bones).
4. Avoid calcium-containing antacids (Alka-2, Titralac, Tums); these stimulate secretion of gastrin, a stomach hormone that in turn stimulates production of hydrochloric acid and pepsin, referred to as rebound hyperacidity.
5. When practical, antacid liquids (suspensions) are more effective than tablets.
6. Antacids can interfere with the absorption of cimetidine (but not ranitidine), digoxin, iron, isoniazid and tetracyclines.

Use of Cimetidine or Ranitidine
1. Both of these drugs reduce the production of hydrochloric acid by blocking the stomach's response to stimulation by histamine. They promote healing of peptic ulcer in 70% to 80% of cases when taken for 4 to 6 weeks.

2. Treatment with cimetidine alone is a reasonable alternative to high-dose antacid therapy.
3. Cimetidine may cause confusion and unsteadiness in the elderly, especially those with impaired kidney function; infrequently it can cause breast enlargement and impotence in men; it increases the effects of warfarin when taken concurrently.
4. Ranitidine taken in a single dose at bedtime is as effective as other multidose drug regimens for healing peptic ulcer.
5. Ranitidine is less likely to cause confusion, unsteadiness, breast changes or altered sexual functions; in addition, it does not appear to be involved in any significant drug-drug interactions.
6. In the presence of liver disease or impaired liver function, avoid the concurrent use of ranitidine and acetaminophen to reduce the risk of liver toxicity.
7. Both cimetidine and ranitidine, taken once daily at bedtime, can reduce the recurrence rate (in 1 year) for duodenal ulcer from 70% to 10%, and for gastric ulcer from 56% to 20%.

Use of Sucralfate
1. This drug is used for short-term (8 weeks') treatment of active duodenal ulcer. It promotes ulcer healing by forming a dense coating over the ulcer that protects it from the erosive action of hydrochloric acid. Its effectiveness is comparable to antacids and histamine blockers (cimetidine and ranitidine) when used alone.
2. Sucralfate should not be used in conjunction with antacids or histamine blockers.
3. Food may impair the effectivemess of sucralfate. The recommended schedule is as follows:
   (1) If other drugs are being used concurrently, take these 1 hour before sucralfate.
   (2) Take sucralfate on an empty stomach, 1 hour before meals and at bedtime.
   (3) Food may be taken 1 hour after sucralfate.
4. This drug is very safe; it has no contraindications and minimal side-effects—constipation (2%).
5. It can interfere with the absorption of tetracyclines and phenytoin.

Ancillary Drug Treatment (as required)

Condition	*Drug Treatment*
For persistant nocturnal ulcer pain:	isopropamide (Combid, Darbid) taken at bedtime
For constipation:	docusate (Colace, etc.)
	docusate with casanthranol (Peri-Colace, etc.)
For anxiety or nervous tension:	diazepam (Valium)

Ancillary Drug Treatment (as required) *(continued)*

Condition	*Drug Treatment*
For headache, minor aches and pains:	acetaminophen (Tylenol, etc.) propoxyphene (Darvon) Avoid aspirin.

Note: Drug selection, dosage and administration schedule must be determined by the physician for each patient individually.

RHEUMATOID ARTHRITIS

Other Names: Atrophic Arthritis, Chronic Inflammatory Arthritis, Proliferative Arthritis

Prevalence in USA: Approximately 7 million—2% to 3% of the general population.

Age Group: Affects all ages—infancy to senescence. Usual onset is between 20 and 50 years. Mean age at onset is 30 to 40 years.

Male to Female Ratio: In 20-to-50-year age group—more common in women, 3 to 1. Over 50 years—same incidence in men and women.

Principal Features: Rheumatoid arthritis is a highly complex inflammatory disorder that can affect several systems of the body simultaneously. It is quite variable in its manifestations: it may last a few days or up to 50 years; it may affect a single joint or up to 60 joints; it may involve the skin, the eyes, the nervous system, the lungs, the heart and blood vessels and the spleen; it can be mild, moderately severe or life-threatening in its most virulent forms. It usually begins with fatigue, poor appetite, loss of weight, morning stiffness and joint pains. Initially the small joints of the hands, wrists and feet are affected; larger joints may be affected later. The painful and destructive disease of the joints is the major feature of this disorder. The disease process begins with a severe inflammation of the joint lining (synovial membrane). This is followed by the formation of thick granulation tissue that ultimately destroys joint cartilage, bone and adjacent ligaments. The affected joints are swollen, warm, tender, stiff and painful to use; after a sustained period of active disease, joint destruction results in irreversible deformity. All of the joints that are affected will show evidence of disease within the first 2 years. Ten percent of cases will have a spontaneous complete remission (recovery) within 6 to 24 months after the onset of symptoms.

Causes: A specific definitive cause for rheumatoid arthritis has not been established. However, there is evidence to support the theory that the disease process is initiated by a virus that infects the joints of individuals who are genetically susceptible because of a defective immune system.

Drugs That Can Cause This Disorder: There are no drugs that induce true rheumatoid arthritis. The following drugs may aggravate an active or latent arthritis: iron dextran, isoniazid and pyrazinamide (in combination), oral contraceptives (?).

Drugs Used to Treat This Disorder: There are no drugs that can cure rheumatoid arthritis. The drugs currently available for use in managing this form of arthritis fall into 2 groups: (1) those that relieve symptoms but do not alter the basic disease process—do not produce remission; (2) those that may retard or arrest the disease and initiate remission.

Drugs Used to Relieve Symptoms
Salicylates
- aspirin (Bufferin, Ascriptin, Cama, etc.).
- aspirin, enteric-coated (Easprin, Ecotrin, etc.).
- aspirin, zero-order-release (Zorprin).
- magnesium salicylate (Magan, Mobidin).
- choline magnesium salicylate (Trisilate).
- salsalate (Disalcid).
- diflunisal (Dolobid).
- sodium salicylate (Pabalate).

Other Nonsteroidal Anti-inflammatory Drugs (NSAIDs)
Indole derivatives:
- indomethacin (Indocin). ⚕
- sulindac (Clinoril).
- tolmetin (Tolectin).
Propionic acid derivatives:
- fenoprofen (Nalfon).
- ibuprofen (Motrin, Rufen). ⚕
- ketoprofen (Orudis).
- naproxen (Naprosyn). ⚕
- suprofen (Suprol).
Fenamic acid derivatives: meclofenamate (Meclomen)
Oxicam derivatives: piroxicam (Feldene)

Cortisonelike Steroid Drugs
- prednisone.
- triamcinolone (Aristocort).
- dexamethasone (Decadron).
- methylprednisolone (Medrol).

Immunosuppressive Drugs
- azathioprine (Imuran).
- chlorambucil (Leukeran).
- cyclophosphamide (Cytoxan).
- methotrexate (Mexate).

Drugs Used to Produce Remission
  Gold Preparations:
  • auranofin (Ridaura).
  • aurothioglucose (Solganal).
  • gold sodium thiomalate (Myochrysine).
  hydroxychloroquine (Plaquenil)
  penicillamine (Cuprimine, Depen)

Goals of Drug Treatment
  Relief of pain, tenderness and stiffness.
  Control of inflammation in joint tissues.
  Production of remission; arrest of active disease.
  Prevention of joint destruction; preservation of joint function.

Drug Management
General Principles
  Rheumatoid arthritis can be the most difficult of all arthritic disorders to
    control; in its more severe forms, it is the most damaging to joint tissues.
    Its course is usually intermittent to chronic. No cure is known.
  If the diagnosis is made early, and if adequate treatment is started
    promptly, severe crippling can often be prevented or minimized.
  Every case of rheumatoid arthritis is a unique, individual problem; suc-
    cessful management depends upon a treatment program that is carefully
    individualized.
  Many drugs are available to treat rheumatoid arthritis. None is curative,
    and none is effective in all cases. Drugs that control inflammation can
    provide symptomatic relief but do not modify the underlying disease
    process; they cannot induce a remission. Disease-altering drugs are used
    in an attempt to modify the actual disease process and thereby initiate a
    remission. If successful, maintenance drug treatment may be continued
    for months or years.
  Treatment is usually started with the safest and best tolerated drugs. There
    is marked individual variation in response to most drugs; this is very
    apparent with the use of the nonsteroidal anti-inflammatory drugs (aspi-
    rin substitutes). Trial-and-error experimentation is necessary to find the
    most effective and acceptable anti-inflammatory drug for each person.
  Drug treatment of rheumatoid arthritis often requires a combination of
    drugs. The more severe forms of this arthritis respond more favorably
    when a disease-modifying drug is added to an established program of
    salicylates or NSAIDs. (See drugs listed above).
Use of Salicylates
  1. Aspirin is often the first drug used to provide adequate anti-inflam-
     matory effects; it must be taken in large doses. A trial of salicylates is
     indicated in all cases of rheumatoid arthritis. (Avoid if there is a history
     of aspirin allergy, peptic ulcer disease, gastritis or gastrointestinal
     bleeding.)
  2. Aspirin preparations that are designed for absorption in the small intes-
     tine (instead of in the stomach) are preferred: Disalcid, Easprin, Eco-
     trin, Zorprin.

3. The measurement of salicylate blood levels is advisable to determine the optimal dose of the salicylate used and to avoid serious toxicity.

4. Warning symptoms of early salicylate toxicity are ringing in the ears (tinnitus) and loss of hearing. However, these may not occur in the very young or in the elderly.

5. Approximately 50% of patients cannot tolerate the large doses of aspirin required to achieve adequate anti-inflammatory effects. Other salicylates may be tried or a nonsteroidal anti-inflammatory drug may be substituted.

Use of Other Nonsteroidal Anti-inflammatory Drugs (NSAIDs)

1. These may be used as substitutes for aspirin by those who cannot tolerate (or should not take) salicylates; or they may be used to initiate treatment at the outset.

2. As a group, the NSAIDs are not superior to salicylates in anti-inflammatory effect, but they are generally better tolerated.

3. These drugs produce significant decrease in morning stiffness, improve comfort and function and may be more effective than aspirin for some.

4. Fenoprofen and naproxen are among the more active NSAIDs; a trial of 2 weeks will identify those who can respond favorably.

5. Response to NSAIDs is highly variable from person to person. If an NSAID from one chemical class proves to be ineffective or unacceptable, a drug from another class within the NSAID group should be tried. A trial of 2 weeks is usually adequate to determine effectiveness and tolerance. (See drugs listed above).

Use of Cortisonelike Steroid Drugs

1. Steroids are used infrequently and for short periods of time in both acute and chronic stages of rheumatoid arthritis. They are always added to existing drug programs as needed. Their use is justified, in small doses, to control acute "flares" of inflammation that prevent any degree of mobility in severly diseased joints.

2. Steroids provide a powerful anti-inflammatory effect, but they do not alter the underlying disease process or induce remission. They should be used to provide short-term comfort as necessary but not to abolish all symptoms.

3. Long-term maintenance use of steroids—even in small doses—must be avoided. Risks of excessive use include cataracts, osteoporosis, muscle wasting, atherosclerosis.

Use of Immunosuppressive Drugs

1. These highly toxic and hazardous drugs are used only when arthritis activity persists in spite of combined treatment with NSAIDs and disease-modifying agents. They are used in an attempt to prevent further joint destruction, deformity and disability.

2. Cyclophosphamide is the most effective drug of this group. Its use is reserved for patients with disabling systemic complications of rheumatoid arthritis.

3. Methotrexate is often the first choice of this group to try in the treatment of severe rheumatoid arthritis that has not responded to conventional therapy. In low dosage it can be very effective in approximately

50% of patients. Potential risks include severe depression of the bone marrow, liver damage, ulceration of the mouth and intestine and birth defects. Avoid alcohol and salicylates during methotrexate therapy.

Use of Gold Preparations
1. Based upon long experience with its use, gold is the standard disease-modifying drug for treating rheumatoid arthritis. It is often the first choice to add to an established program of NSAID therapy.
2. Gold is used only when arthritis cannot be controlled with safer drugs. A trial of 6 months or longer is necessary to determine its ability to induce remission. Approximately 50% of patients respond favorably.
3. Risks of gold therapy include dermatitis, kidney damage and blood cell and bone marrow toxicity. Treatment should be stopped immediately if any of the following develop: skin rash, mouth ulcers, fever, sore throat, abnormal bleeding or bruising.

Use of Hydroxychloroquine
1. This drug is used to treat mild or moderately severe rheumatoid arthritis. It can be very effective in some cases, relieving symptoms and retarding disease activity.
2. A trial of 6 months is necessary to determine this drug's ability to induce remission.
3. After 1 year of continual use, this drug can (rarely) damage eye structures and impair vision. Corneal deposits, retinal pigmentation and optic neuritis have been reported. The estimated incidence is 1 in 1000 to 1 in 2000 patients.
4. Other possible adverse drug effects include skin rash, abnormally low white blood cells and peripheral neuritis (see Glossary).
5. This drug can aggravate existing psoriasis.

Use of Penicillamine
1. This drug is an effective substitute for gold therapy when a disease-modifying drug is needed.
2. A trial of 6 to 12 months is necessary to determine its ability to induce remission.
3. For maximal effectiveness, this drug should be taken on an empty stomach.
4. This is a potent drug; it can cause the following adverse effects: dermatitis, kidney damage, blood cell and bone marrow toxicity, bronchiolitis (dry cough and shortness of breath) and a pattern of muscular weakness similar to myasthenia gravis.

Ancillary Drug Treatment (as required)

Condition	*Drug Treatment*
For additional analgesia:	propoxyphene (Darvon)
	hydrocodone (Vicodin) (for short-term, intermittent use only)
For night pain:	indomethacin (Indocin) (taken with food at bedtime)

Ancillary Drug Treatment (as required) *(continued)*

Condition	Drug Treatment
For anemia:	iron preparations
	folic acid (if appropriate for type of anemia)
For anxiety and tension:	diazepam (Valium)
For depression:	tricylic antidepressants (see Profile of Depression in this section)
For drug-induced peptic ulcer:	
	cimetidine (Tagamet) ⩒
	ranitidine (Zantac) (see Profile of Peptic Ulcer in this section)

Note: Drug selection, dosage and administration schedule must be determined by the physician for each patient individually.

SCHIZOPHRENIA

Other Names: Dementia Praecox

Prevalence in USA: Approximately 2.4 million—1% of the general population; 100,000 new cases annually.

Age Group: Onset most common between 16 and 25 years of age. Onset uncommon after 30 and rare after 40 years of age.

Male to Female Ratio: Equal incidence in men and women.

Principal Features: Schizophrenia refers to a group of disorders of the brain manifested by severe disturbances of the mind and personality. Cardinal features are abnormal thinking, behavior and mood; the schizophrenic pattern is characterized by misinterpretation of reality, withdrawal, delusions, hallucinations (usually auditory), bizarre or regressive behavior. It usually begins early in life, may be mild and transient in nature or may develop into a psychosis of major dimension that is intermittent or chronic for life. The first group—referred to as schizophreniform—experiences one episode of varying severity (often in response to stress), responds well to treatment and has no relapse after treatment is stopped. The second group—classical chronic schizophrenia—experiences recurrent episodes of disabling symptoms that require long-term antipsychotic drug therapy for control. Most of this group will relapse if maintenance treatment is stopped. A variety of subtypes are identified according to their dominant features: delusions of persecution and grandeur (paranoid type); primitive mentality, markedly disorganized thought and behavior (hebephrenic type); withdrawn, negativistic, uncommunicative, apathetic behavior pattern (catatonic); disorganized thinking, delusions, hallucinations accompanied by either mania or depression (schizo-affective); insidious loss of motivation and ambition, avoidance of interpersonal relationships (simple type); mixed or indefinite symptom complex (undifferentiated type). Though the presentations may vary according to type, the same group of antipsychotic drugs is used to treat all types without distinction.

Causes: The fundamental cause of schizophrenia is unknown. No anatomical or biochemical abnormality of the brain has been identified. Studies suggest that a genetic predisposition is necessary for the development of schizophrenia, rendering the subject vulnerable to disturbances of neurochemical transmission of nerve impulses or to alterations of brain circuitry. Effective antipsychotic drugs block dopamine receptors in certain brain cells; this suggests that increased dopamine activity is somehow responsible for the schizophrenic syndrome.

Drugs That Can Cause This Disorder: The following drugs may aggravate existing schizophrenia or produce schizophrenialike symptoms in normal individuals:

albuterol
alcohol (intoxication)
amantadine
amphetamines (abuse)
anticonvulsants
apomorphine
atropinelike drugs
bromides
bromocriptine
cimetidine
cocaine

cortisonelike steroids
digitalis
disopyramide
disulfiram (toxicity)
indomethacin
isoniazid
levodopa
methyldopa
propranolol
tocainide
triazolam

Drugs Used to Treat This Disorder

Phenothiazines
Aliphatic type:
  • chlorpromazine (Thorazine)
Piperidine type:
  • thioridazine (Mellaril)
  • mesoridazine (Serentil)
Piperazine type:
  • perphenazine (Trilafon)
  • trifluoperazine (Stelazine)
  • fluphenazine (Prolixin, Permitil)
Thioxanthenes
  • thiothixene (Navane).
Butyrophenones
  • haloperidol (Haldol).
Dibenzoxazepines
  • loxapine (Loxitane).

Dihydroindolones
- molindone (Moban).

Goals of Drug Treatment

Good control of symptoms with the lowest possible dose of antipsychotic drug.

Determination of the most effective drug and dosage schedule for each individual: intermittent dosage (as needed) versus continual long-term dosage.

Prevention of relapse (recurrent psychotic episode).

Improvement of capacity to function in society as normally as possible.

Drug Management

General Principles

The primary management of schizophrenia is based upon the rational use of antipsychotic drugs. Psychotherapy and drug therapy are considered to be complementary; psychotherapy can improve the patient's social adjustment; drug therapy can control disabling symptoms and make the situation somewhat manageable. Drug therapy is not curative.

If appropriate drug treatment is started early, 30% to 50% of patients will have a satisfactory remission; another 30% will improve sufficiently to live outside of a hospital. Drug therapy can abolish delusions, hallucinations, hyperactivity and combative behavior. Approximately 10% to 20% of patients do not respond to any drugs currently available.

The initial treatment of an acute psychotic episode consists of a course of carefully selected antipsychotic drugs taken for 6 to 12 months. Many individuals will respond favorably to one drug and not at all to another. History of previous drug use and response can be very helpful in selecting a drug for the management of recurrent episodes.

Current practice is to attempt withdrawal of antipsychotic drugs from all patients who have had a good response to drug treatment during their first episode of schizophrenia. This allows identification of those who will have a self-limited type of schizophrenia (schizophreniform disorder) and will do well without maintenance drug therapy. From 15% to 30% of patients will recover spontaneously following the initial episode and drug withdrawal. Antipsychotic drugs should be discontinued gradually over a period of 1 to 2 weeks.

The majority of schizophrenic patients will require continual drug therapy for long periods of time—possibly for life. Many will relapse rapidly and severely after drugs are discontinued. The nature of the drug maintenance program is determined by the type and frequency of continuing psychotic symptoms and the pattern of relapses experienced by each individual. When the patient complies well, maintenance drug therapy is successful in 85% of cases.

The principal action of antipsychotic drugs is to block dopamine receptors in the brain. By blocking dopamine action in the mesolimbic system, the drugs control the abnormal manifestations of schizophrenia; by blocking dopamine action in the nigrostriatal system, the drugs cause parkinsonism (and related adverse effects). Thus parkinsonism is now recognized as an *unavoidable* side-effect of most antipsychotic drugs. It is usually very responsive to the anticholinergic drugs used to treat Parkinson's disease, but not to levodopa. (See Profile of Parkinson's Disease in this section.)

It is generally recommended that antiparkinsonism drugs *not* be used routinely while taking antipsychotic drugs. Reasons given are: (1) antiparkinsonism drugs can produce toxic brain syndromes; (2) they can interfere with the effectiveness of antipsychotic drugs; (3) they may increase the risk of developing tardive dyskinesia.

Tardive dyskinesia (see Glossary) is one of the most serious adverse effects of long-term antipsychotic drug use. The reported incidence ranges from 3% after 1 year of medication to 21% after 7 years of medication. It appears to occur more frequently in elderly women.

"Drug holidays" of 4 to 6 weeks without medication are being used by some physicians treating chronic schizophrenia to reduce the risk of developing tardive dyskinesia. Among those who have been on maintenance therapy for 1 year without relapsing, 66% will not relapse within 6 months after stopping medication. For this group of patients, a "drug holiday" is feasible and possibly beneficial.

Antipsychotic drugs usually improve behavior. However, excessively high doses can cause a toxic state that worsens behavior. Drug response and tolerance vary greatly from person to person and must be monitored carefully in each individual.

Patients with schizo-affective disorders will probably require an antipsychotic drug and an additional drug for the affective component; this could be either lithium or an antidepressant.

Lithium may aggravate the neurological complications of antipsychotic drug therapy. The concurrent use of these two drugs requires caution and careful monitoring.

Use of Phenothiazines

1. Because of its numerous side-effects, chlorpromazine (the first phenothiazine) is used less frequently.
2. Because of its relatively greater sedative effects, thioridazine is favored for treatment of acute psychotic episodes. It causes parkinsonism (and possibly tardive dyskinesia) less frequently.
3. Fluphenazine is less sedating but is thought to have a higher risk for causing parkinsonism and tardive dyskinesia.
4. Trifluoperazine is thought to be preferable for the elderly schizophrenic because it has less sedative and atropinelike side-effects.

Use of Thiothixene

1. This antipsychotic drug is thought to be more effective for the retarded and regressed schizophrenic.
2. Because of its mild antidepressant effect, this drug is preferred for the schizo-affective patient who has features of depression.
3. This drug has less sedative and atropinelike side-effects, but a higher risk for causing parkinsonism.

Use of Haloperidol
1. This drug is reported to be effective in patients who are not responsive to chlorpromazine.
2. It can control aggressive behavior without causing significant sedation.
3. Although it has a relatively high potential for causing parkinsonism (and related effects), it is useful in the elderly because it is less sedating and has fewer atropinelike side-effects.

Use of Loxapine
1. This drug is especially useful in treating the paranoid schizophrenic.
2. It is less sedating than chlorpromazine and equal to haloperidol in effectiveness.

Use of Molindone
1. This is the only antipsychotic drug that appears to contribute to weight loss; many antipsychotic drugs tend to promote weight gain.
2. This drug is as effective as other major antipsychotics and is less sedating than many.

Ancillary Drug Treatment (as required)

Condition	*Drug Treatment*
For anxiety:	buspirone (Buspar)
For depression:	see Profile of Depression in this section
For insomnia:	chloral hydrate (Noctec, etc.)
	temazepam (Restoril)
	triazolam (Halcion)
For constipation:	docusate (Colace, etc.)
	docusate with casanthranol (Peri-Colace)
For parkinsonism:	benztropine (Cogentin)
	trihexyphenidyl (Artane)
For akathisia (marked restlessness):	propranolol (Inderal)
	diphenhydramine (Benadryl)

Note: Drug selection, dosage and administration schedule must be determined by the physician for each patient individually.

ULCERATIVE COLITIS

Other Names: Idiopathic Proctocolitis, Inflammatory Bowel Disease

Prevalence in USA: 1 million (includes 100,000 children); 15,000 new cases annually.

Age Group: Peak incidence occurs between 19 and 49 years of age; 75% of cases develop before the age of 40.

Male to Female Ratio: Same incidence in men and women.

Principal Features: Ulcerative colitis is a chronically recurrent disorder of the colon (large intestine) and rectum characterized by inflammation and ulceration. Its course follows a pattern of frequent spontaneous remissions and recurrences without apparent cause. It may be associated with disease in other organs of the body, notably the skin, joints, eye, liver and blood vessels, making it a multiple system disorder. The principle symptoms of the diseased colon are abdominal cramping and bloody diarrhea; associated symptoms include fatigue, weakness, occasional low-grade fever, weight loss, anemia and dehydration. The more severe forms of ulcerative colitis can be very difficult to control.

Causes: The basic cause of ulcerative colitis is not known. Theories of possible causes include infection, environmental toxins, psychological stress, sensitivities to foods and "autoimmunity"—a disorder of the immune system that results in the selective destruction of body tissues. There is some evidence that indicates a familial pattern, suggesting a hereditary susceptibility to a causative agent.

Drugs That Can Cause This Disorder: No drugs initiate true ulcerative colitis. However, the following anti-infective drugs can cause pseudomembranous colitis, a disorder that closely resembles an acute attack of ulcerative colitis:

amoxicillin
ampicillin
cephalosporins
chloramphenicol
clindamycin
lincomycin

penicillin
tetracycline
trimethoprim and
  sulfamethoxsazole in
  combination

Drugs Used to Treat This Disorder
sulfasalazine (Azulfidine)
Cortisonelike Steroids:
  • prednisone, prednisolone (generic).
  • hydrocortisone enemas (Cortenema).
  • methylprednisolone enema (Medrol Enpak).
Antidiarrheals
  • diphenoxylate (Lomotil).
  • loperamide (Imodium).
Antispasmodics
  • dicyclomine (Bentyl).
  • propantheline (Pro-Banthine).

Goals of Drug Treatment
Control of pain and diarrhea.
Prompt control of acute attacks; surppression of inflammation and ulceration.
Induction of a remission.
Prevention of recurrence of acute attacks.

Drug Management

General Principles

The majority (up to 90%) of cases of active ulcerative colitis respond well to medical treatment or have a spontaneous remission. Approximately 20% have a prolonged remission after the first acute attack.

Studies indicate that 55% of individuals who experience ulcerative colitis remain in remission at any given time during the course of the disorder. To minimize the risks of long-term drug use, the smallest dose of maintenance drugs (azulfidine and steroids) that prevents recurrence should be determined.

It is essential that every recurrence of acute colitis (relapse) be treated promptly and vigorously. Chronically active ulcerative colitis predisposes to a higher than normal incidence of cancer of the colon and rectum. Estimates are 3% after the first 10 years of disease, increasing to 20% per decade thereafter. Everyone subject to ulcerative colitis should have a thorough examination of the colon and rectum annually regardless of the status of the disorder.

Antidiarrheal drugs should be used with extreme caution. Excessive use can induce a paralysis of colon activity and increase the risk of developing toxic megacolon—a massive distention of the colon with air; perforation constitutes a surgical emergency.

Iron preparations for anemia should not be taken during a period of acute inflammation or active ulceration. Withhold iron therapy until a remission is established.

Use of Sulfasalazine

1. This effective and reliable drug is used to treat acute attacks of active colitis and to prevent relapse during periods of remission.
2. It is used concurrently with cortisonelike steroids during acute attacks to control inflammation and ulceration and to induce remission.
3. During the quiescent phase of colitis, it is used in small doses (up to 2 grams/day) for the long-term maintenance of remission. It may be taken indefinitely.
4. This drug is best taken with or following food to reduce stomach irritation.
5. The long-term use of this drug can impair folic acid absorption and may cause a folic acid deficiency. Consult your physician regarding the need for a supplement.
6. During long-term use, it is advisable to monitor blood cell counts to detect the development of anemia or abnormally low white blood cells.

Use of Cortisonelike Steroids

1. These drugs are the mainstay of treatment for acute, active ulcerative colitis. They can induce remission in 70% to 80% of cases.
2. Steroids should be used when there are obvious symptoms of disease activity: diarrhea, bloody stools, nocturnal bowel movements, anemia, weight loss, etc. They are also of value in treating the systemic manifestations of this disorder: dermatitis, arthritis, iritis, etc.
3. To ensure prompt and adequate control of acute inflammation, initial dosage should be high. Response usually occurs within 10 to 14 days.

4. After a remission has been induced, steroid dosage is reduced to a minimum that will stabilize the colon and prevent relapse. The long-term maintenance use of steroids is controversial. If individual circumstances warrant the continual use of low-dose steroids, it is preferable to use alternate-day dosage—a single morning dose every 48 hours. This is effective in preventing recurrence for some patients and it carries a lower risk of causing adverse effects.

5. When the inflammation and ulceration are limited to the rectum, steroids can be administered in the form of enemas, foams and suppositories for local application. This minimizes systemic effects.

6. The long-term use of steroids (even in small doses) can cause significant adverse effects:
   - susceptibility to infection.
   - mineral and water imbalance.
   - reduced tolerance for sugar, potential for diabetes.
   - cataracts.
   - hypertension.
   - acne, excessive hair growth.
   - muscle wasting.
   - mental disturbances.
   - osteoporosis.
   - peptic ulcer activation.
   - retarded growth in children.

Ancillary Drug Treatment (as required)

Condition	*Drug Treatment*
For abdominal cramps:	dicyclomine (Bentyl) propantheline (Pro-Banthine) Use these sparingly.
For diarrhea:	diphenoxylate (Lomotil) loperamide (Imodium) Use these sparingly.
For anxiety:	buspirone (Buspar), nonsedating diazepam (Valium), sedating
For depression:	see Profile of Depression in this section
For anemia:	iron preparations (not during acute stage of colitis) folic acid (if appropriate for type of anemia)

Note: Drug selection, dosage and administration schedule must be determined by the physician for each patient individually.

SECTION THREE

DRUG PROFILES

NOTE

The designation [CD] following the brand names of any drugs in these Profiles indicates a combination drug (a drug product with more than one active ingredient).

ACEBUTOLOL
(a se BYU toh lohl)

Introduced: 1973

Class: Antihypertensive, Heart Rhythm Regulator, Beta-Adrenergic Blocker

Prescription: USA: Yes

Controlled Drug: USA: No

Available as Generic: No

Brand Names: Sectral

BENEFITS versus RISKS

Possible Benefits	*Possible Risks*
ANTIHYPERTENSIVE in mild to moderate high blood pressure	CONGESTIVE HEART FAILURE in advanced heart disease
	Worsening of angina in coronary heart disease (abrupt withdrawal)
	Masking of low blood sugar (hypoglycemia) in drug-treated diabetes

---

> **Principal Uses**

As a Single Drug Product: The treatment of mild to moderately severe high blood pressure. May be used alone or concurrently with other antihypertensive drugs, such as diuretics. Also used to prevent premature ventricular heartbeats.

How This Drug Works: By blocking certain actions of the sympathetic nervous system, this drug

- reduces the rate and contraction force of the heart, thus lowering the ejection pressure of the blood leaving the heart.
- reduces the degree of contraction of blood vessel walls, resulting in their relaxation and expansion and consequent lowering of the blood pressure.
- prolongs the conduction time of nerve impulses through the heart, of benefit in the management of certain heart rhythm disorders.

Available Dosage Forms and Strengths
Capsules — 200 mg, 400 mg

> **Usual Adult Dosage Range:** Initially 400 mg daily, either as a single dose in the morning or as 200 mg taken morning and evening (12 hours apart). The usual maintenance dose is 400 to 800 mg/24 hrs. The total dose should not exceed 1200 mg/24 hrs, given as 600 mg twice daily. **Note: Actual dosage and administration schedule must be determined by the physician for each patient individually.**

> **Dosing Instructions:** May be taken without regard to eating. Capsule may be opened for administration. Do not discontinue this drug abruptly.

Usual Duration of Use: Continual use on a regular schedule for 10 to 14 days is usually necessary to determine this drug's effectiveness in lowering the blood pressure or abolishing premature heartbeats. The long-term use of this drug will be determined by the course of your blood pressure over time and your response to the overall treatment program (weight reduction, salt restriction, smoking cessation, etc.).

▷ **This Drug Should Not Be Taken If**
- you have had an allergic reaction to it previously.
- you have congestive heart failure.
- you have an abnormally slow heart rate or a serious form of heart block.
- you are taking, or have taken within the past 14 days, any monoamine oxidase (MAO) inhibitor drug (see Drug Class, Section Four).

▷ **Inform Your Physician Before Taking This Drug If**
- you have had an adverse reaction to any "beta-blocker" drug in the past (see Drug Class, Section Four).
- you have a history of serious heart disease, with or without episodes of heart failure.
- you have a history of hay fever (allergic rhinitis), asthma, chronic bronchitis or emphysema.
- you have a history of overactive thyroid function (hyperthyroidism).
- you have a history of low blood sugar (hypoglycemia).
- you have impaired liver or kidney function.
- you have diabetes or myasthenia gravis.
- you are currently taking any form of digitalis, quinidine or reserpine, or any "calcium-blocker" drug (see Drug Class, Section Four).
- you plan to have surgery under general anesthesia in the near future.

Possible Side-Effects   (natural, expected and unavoidable drug actions)
Lethargy and fatigability (11%), cold extremities (0.2%), slow heart rate, lightheadedness in upright position (see orthostatic hypotension in Glossary).

▷ **Possible Adverse Effects**   (unusual, unexpected and infrequent reactions)
If any of the following develop, consult your physician promptly.
Mild Adverse Effects
Allergic Reactions: Skin rash, itching.
Headache, dizziness, insomnia, abnormal dreams.
Indigestion, nausea, constipation, diarrhea.
Joint and muscle discomfort, fluid retention (edema).
Serious Adverse Effects
Mental depression (2%), anxiety, impotence (2%).
Chest pain, shortness of breath, precipitation of congestive heart failure.
Induction of bronchial asthma (in asthmatic individuals).

CAUTION
1. *Do not discontinue this drug suddenly* without the knowledge and guidance of your physician. Carry a notation on your person that you are taking this drug.

2. Consult your physician or pharmacist before using nasal decongestants usually present in over-the-counter cold preparations and nose drops. These can cause sudden increases in blood pressure when taken concurrently with beta-blocker drugs.
3. Report the development of any tendency to emotional depression.

Precautions for Use

By Infants and Children: Safety and effectiveness for use by those under 12 years of age have not been established. However, if this drug is used, observe for the development of low blood sugar (hypoglycemia) during periods of reduced food intake.

By Those over 60 Years of Age: Proceed *cautiously* with all antihypertensive drugs. Unacceptably high blood pressure should be reduced without creating the risks associated with excessively low blood pressure. Start treatment with small doses, and monitor the blood pressure response frequently. Sudden, rapid and excessive reduction of blood pressure can predispose to stroke or heart attack. Total daily dosage should not exceed 800 mg. Observe for dizziness, unsteadiness, tendency to fall, confusion, hallucinations, depression or urinary frequency.

▷ **Advisability of Use During Pregnancy**

Pregnancy Category: B (tentative). See Pregnancy Code inside back cover.

Animal studies: No significant increase in birth defects found in rats or rabbits.

Human studies: Information from adequate studies in pregnant women is not available.

Use this drug only if clearly needed. Ask physician for guidance.

Advisability of Use if Breast-Feeding

Presence of this drug in breast milk: Yes.

Avoid drug or refrain from nursing.

Habit-Forming Potential: None.

Effects of Overdosage: Weakness, slow pulse, low blood pressure, fainting, cold and sweaty skin, congestive heart failure, possible coma and convulsions.

Possible Effects of Long-Term Use: Reduced heart reserve and eventual heart failure in susceptible individuals with advanced heart disease.

Suggested Periodic Examinations While Taking This Drug   (at physician's discretion)

Measurements of blood pressure, evaluation of heart function.

▷ **While Taking This Drug, Observe the Following**

Foods: No restrictions. Avoid excessive salt intake.

Beverages: No restrictions. May be taken with milk.

▷ *Alcohol*: Use with caution until the combined effect has been determined. Alcohol may exaggerate this drug's ability to lower the blood pressure and may increase its mild sedative effect.

Tobacco Smoking: Nicotine may reduce this drug's effectiveness in treating high blood pressure. In addition, high doses of this drug may potentiate the constriction of the bronchial tubes caused by regular smoking.

▷ *Other Drugs*

Acebutolol may *increase* the effects of

- other antihypertensive drugs and cause excessive lowering of the blood pressure. Dosage adjustments may be necessary.
- reserpine (Ser-Ap-Es, etc.) and cause sedation, depression, slowing of the heart rate and lowering of the blood pressure.

Acebutolol *taken concurrently* with

- clonidine (Catapres) requires close monitoring for rebound high blood pressure if clonidine is withdrawn while acebutolol is still being taken.
- insulin requires close monitoring to avoid undetected hypoglycemia (see Glossary).

The following drugs may *decrease* the effects of acebutolol

- indomethacin (Indocin), and possibly other "aspirin substitutes," may impair acebutolol's antihypertensive effect.

▷ *Driving, Hazardous Activities*: Use caution until the full extent of drowsiness, lethargy and blood pressure change have been determined.

Aviation Note: The use of this drug *is a disqualification* for piloting. Consult a designated Aviation Medical Examiner.

Exposure to Sun: No restrictions.

Exposure to Heat: Caution advised. Hot environments can lower the blood pressure and exaggerate the effects of this drug.

Exposure to Cold: Caution advised. Cold environments can enhance the circulatory deficiency in the extremities that may occur with this drug. The elderly should take precautions to prevent hypothermia (see Glossary).

Heavy Exercise or Exertion: It is advisable to avoid exertion that produces lightheadedness, excessive fatigue or muscle cramping. The use of this drug may intensify the hypertensive response to isometric exercise.

Occurrence of Unrelated Illness: The fever that accompanies systemic infections can lower the blood pressure and require adjustment of dosage. Illnesses that cause nausea or vomiting may interrupt the regular dosage schedule. Ask your physician for guidance.

Discontinuation: It is advisable to avoid sudden discontinuation of this drug in all situations. If possible, gradual reduction of dose over a period of 2 to 3 weeks is recommended. Ask your physician for specific guidance.

ACETAMINOPHEN
(a set a MEE noh fen)

Other Names: APAP, Paracetamol

Introduced: 1893

Class: Mild Analgesic and Antipyretic

Prescription: No

Controlled Drug: No

Available as Generic: Yes

Brand Names: Anacin-3, Anacin-3 with Codeine [CD], ✤Apo-Acetaminophen, Arthralgen [CD], Aspirin-Free Excedrin [CD], ✤Atasol, ✤Atasol-8 [CD], Bromo-Seltzer [CD], ✤Campain, CoTylenol Children's Liquid Cold Formula [CD], CoTylenol Tablets [CD], Darvocet-N [CD], Datril, Demerol-APAP [CD], Empracet with Codeine [CD], Excedrin [CD], ✤Exdol, ✤Exdol-8, -15, -30 [CD], Fioricet [CD], Hycomine Compound [CD], Panadol, Parafon Forte [CD], Percocet [CD], Percogesic [CD], Phenaphen, Phenaphen with Codeine [CD], ✤Robigesic, ✤Rounox, ✤Rounox with Codeine [CD], Sine-Aid [CD], SK-APAP with Codeine [CD], SK-65 APAP [CD], St. Joseph Aspirin-Free, Talacen [CD], Tapar, Tempra, Trigesic [CD], Tylenol, Tylenol with Codeine [CD], Tylox [CD], Valadol, Vanquish [CD], Vicodin [CD], Wygesic [CD]

BENEFITS versus RISKS

Possible Benefits	*Possible Risks*
EFFECTIVE RELIEF OF MILD TO MODERATE PAIN REDUCTION OF FEVER	Rare anemia, liver or kidney damage (with prolonged or excessive use)

> **Principal Uses**

As a *Single Drug Product*: To relieve mild to moderate pain from any cause, and to reduce high fever. It is often used instead of aspirin for these purposes.

As a *Combination Drug Product* [CD]: Often combined with other analgesics to enhance pain relief. Also combined with antihistamines and decongestants to relieve the discomfort of respiratory tract infections; and with muscle relaxants to augment the relief of discomfort associated with muscle spasm.

How This Drug Works: It reduces the tissue concentrations of prostaglandins, chemicals involved in the production of pain and inflammation.

Available Dosage Forms and Strengths

Capsules — 325 mg, 500 mg
Elixir — 120 mg, 160 mg, 325 mg per teaspoonful (5 ml)
Liquid — 160 mg, 167 mg per teaspoonful (5 ml)
Solution — 100 mg per ml, 120 mg per 2.5 ml
Suppositories — 120 mg, 125 mg, 325 mg, 650 mg
Tablets — 160 mg, 325 mg, 500 mg, 650 mg
Chewable tablets — 80 mg, 120 mg

> **Usual Adult Dosage Range:**   325 to 650 mg/4 hrs as needed, or 1000 mg (1 gram)/4 to 6 hrs (not to exceed 4 times/24 hrs). **Note: For long-term use, actual dosage and administration schedule must be determined by the physician for each patient individually.**

> **Dosing Instructions:**   May be taken on empty stomach or with food or milk. Capsule may be opened for administration.

Usual Duration of Use: Continual use (at above dosage) should not exceed 10 days at a time. For long-term use under physician supervision, the daily dosage should not exceed 2600 mg/24 hrs.

▷ **This Drug Should Not Be Taken If**
- you have had an allergic reaction to any dosage form of it previously.

▷ **Inform Your Physician Before Taking This Drug If**
- you have impaired liver or kidney function.
- you are currently taking any anticoagulant drug ("blood thinner").

Possible Side-Effects   (natural, expected and unavoidable drug actions)
Drowsiness (in sensitive individuals).

▷ **Possible Adverse Effects**   (unusual, unexpected and infrequent reactions)
If any of the following develop, consult your physician promptly
Mild Adverse Effects
Allergic Reactions: Skin rash, hives (rare).
Impaired thinking and concentration.
Serious Adverse Effects
Allergic Reactions: Swelling of the vocal cords, difficult breathing, anaphylactic reaction (see Glossary). Hemolytic anemia (see Glossary).
Fever, sore throat (abnormally low white blood cells).
Abnormal bleeding or bruising (reduced blood platelets, see Glossary).
Decreased urine volume, bloody urine (kidney damage).
Jaundice (liver damage).

CAUTION
1. If you have bronchial asthma and you are also allergic to aspirin, use this drug with caution until your sensitivity to it has been determined.
2. If you are taking an oral anticoagulant drug ("blood thinner"), high-dose acetaminophen may alter your response to it and increase the risk of abnormal bleeding. Ask physician for guidance.
3. Avoid the long-term use of this drug concurrently with aspirin or aspirin substitutes. This combination, especially in high doses, can increase the risk of kidney damage.

Precautions for Use
By Infants and Children: Dosage is based upon age; ask physician for guidance if in doubt. Do not exceed 5 doses/24 hrs. Continual use should not exceed 5 days at a time without physician guidance.
By Those over 60 Years of Age: Do not exceed a total dose of 2600 mg/24 hrs. Prolonged use in excessive doses can cause anemia, liver damage with jaundice and kidney damage.

▷ **Advisability of Use During Pregnancy**
Pregnancy Category: B (tentative). See Pregnancy Code inside back cover.
Animal studies: No birth defects due to this drug.
Human studies: Adequate information not available.

Advisability of Use if Breast-Feeding
Presence of this drug in breast milk: Yes.
No adverse effects on nursing infants reported.

Habit-Forming Potential: None.

Effects of Overdosage: Nausea, vomiting, stomach pain, drowsiness, stupor, convulsions, coma, jaundice (in 2 to 5 days after large overdose).

Possible Effects of Long-Term Use: Formation of abnormal hemoglobin (methemoglobin). Development of anemia.

Suggested Periodic Examinations While Taking This Drug (at physician's discretion)
None required for short-term use.
During long-term use, examination for abnormal hemoglobin, anemia, reduced white blood cells or platelets, liver and kidney function.

▷ **While Taking This Drug, Observe the Following**
Foods: No restrictions.
Beverages: No restrictions. May be taken with milk or juices.
▷ *Alcohol*: No interactions expected.
Tobacco Smoking: No interactions expected.
▷ *Other Drugs*
Acetaminophen may *increase* the effects of
• oral anticoagulants if the acetaminophen is taken continually in daily doses of 2000 mg or more.
The following drug may *increase* the effects of acetaminophen
• diflunisal (Dolobid) may increase the risk of acetaminophen toxicity.
▷ *Driving, Hazardous Activities*: Usually no restrictions. Be alert to the rare occurrence of drowsiness and/or impaired thinking, and restrict activities accordingly.
Aviation Note: Usually no restrictions. However, it is advisable to observe for the possible occurrence of drowsiness or impaired thinking and to restrict activities accordingly.
Exposure to Sun: No restrictions.

ACETAZOLAMIDE
(a set a ZOHL a mide)

Introduced: 1953

Class: Antiglaucoma, Diuretic, Sulfonamides

Prescription: USA: Yes
Canada: Yes

Controlled Drug: USA: No
Canada: No

Available as Generic: USA: Yes
Canada: No

Brand Names: ✟Acetazolam, ✟Apo-Acetazolamide, Diamox, Diamox Sequles

```
┌─────────────────────────────────────────────────────────────┐
│                    BENEFITS versus RISKS                     │
│                                                              │
│      Possible Benefits              Possible Risks           │
│   REDUCTION OF INTERNAL EYE     Acidosis with long-term use  │
│     PRESSURE in selected cases of  Increased risk of kidney stone│
│     glaucoma                    Rare bone marrow, liver or kidney│
│   CONTROL OF ABSENCE (PETIT        injury                    │
│     MAL) SEIZURES                                            │
│   TREATMENT OF PERIODIC                                      │
│     PARALYSIS                                                │
└─────────────────────────────────────────────────────────────┘
```

▷ **Principal Uses**

As a Single Drug Product: Primarily to treat certain types of glaucoma. Also used with other anticonvulsant drugs to manage petit mal epilepsy. Used less frequently to treat familial periodic paralysis and to prevent altitude sickness.

How This Drug Works: By inhibiting the action of the enzyme carbonic anhydrase, it decreases the formation of fluid (the aqueous humor) in the eye and increases the volume of urine.

Available Dosage Forms and Strengths

Capsules, Prolonged-action — 500 mg
Tablets — 125 mg, 250 mg

▷ **Usual Adult Dosage Range:** For glaucoma: 250 to 1000 mg/24 hrs, in 2 or 3 doses. For epilepsy: 250 to 1000 mg/24 hrs. As a diuretic: 250 to 375 mg/24 hrs, in one morning dose. **Note: Actual dosage and administration schedule must be determined by the physician for each patient individually.**

▷ **Dosing Instructions:** Best taken with food or milk to prevent stomach irritation. Tablet may be crushed. Diamox Sequels may be opened, but do not chew or crush contents for administration.

Usual Duration of Use: Treatment of glaucoma and epilepsy require long-term use. If taken to control seizures, do not stop this drug abruptly.

▷ **This Drug Should Not Be Taken If**
  • you have had an allergic reaction to any dosage form of it previously.
  • you have serious liver or kidney disease.
  • you have Addison's disease.

▷ **Inform Your Physician Before Taking This Drug If**
  • you have had an allergic reaction to any "sulfa" drug in the past.
  • you have gout or lupus erythematosus.

Possible Side-Effects (natural, expected and unavoidable drug actions)
Drowsiness, temporary nearsightedness.

▷ **Possible Adverse Effects** (unusual, unexpected and infrequent reactions)
If any of the following develop, consult your physician promptly.

Mild Adverse Effects
Allergic Reactions: Skin rash, hives, drug fever.
Reduced appetite, indigestion, nausea.
Fatigue; weakness; dizziness; tingling of face, arms or legs.

Serious Adverse Effects
Allergic Reactions: Hemolytic anemia (see Glossary), spontaneous bruising (reduced blood platelets, see Glossary).
Bone marrow depression (see Glossary)—fatigue, weakness, fever, sore throat, abnormal bleeding or bruising.
Hepatitis with jaundice (see Glossary)—yellow eyes and skin, dark-colored urine, light-colored stools.

▷ **Adverse Effects That May Mimic Natural Diseases or Disorders**
Toxic liver reaction may suggest viral hepatitis.
Lupus erythematosuslike syndrome.

Natural Diseases or Disorders That May Be Activated by This Drug
Gout, acidosis secondary to chronic obstructive lung disease—asthma, bronchitis, emphysema.

CAUTION
1. Observe for possible loss of drug effectiveness when used as a diuretic or to control seizures.
2. Emotional depression may occur and not be recognized as an adverse effect of this drug.
3. This drug may cause an excessive loss of potassium from the body. Consult your physician regarding the need for a high-potassium diet or potassium supplements.

Precautions for Use
By Infants and Children: Excessive dosage may cause drowsiness and numbness of the face and extremities. Not recommended for use as a diuretic in children.
By Those over 60 Years of Age: Do not exceed recommended doses. Increased dosage may cause excessive loss of sodium and potassium, with resultant weakness, confusion, numbness in the extremities and nausea. If taking a digitalis preparation (digitoxin, digoxin), consult your physician regarding the need for a high-potassium diet or potassium supplements.

▷ **Advisability of Use During Pregnancy**
Pregnancy Category: C (tentative). See Pregnancy Code inside back cover.
Animal studies: Limb and skeletal defects reported in mice and rats.
Human studies: Information from adequate studies in pregnant women is not available.
Avoid completely during the first 3 months and during labor and delivery.

Advisability of Use if Breast-Feeding
Presence of this drug in breast milk: Probable.
Diuretic effect of drug may temporarily impair milk production. Monitor nursing infant closely and discontinue drug or nursing if adverse effects develop.

Habit-Forming Potential: None.

Effects of Overdosage: Drowsiness, numbness and tingling, thirst, nausea, vomiting, confusion, excitement, convulsions, coma.

Possible Effects of Long-Term Use: The development of low blood potassium and/or acidosis.

Suggested Periodic Examinations While Taking This Drug (at physician's discretion)

Complete blood cell counts, measurements of blood sodium, potassium and uric acid levels, liver and kidney function tests.

▷ **While Taking This Drug, Observe the Following**

Foods: Consult your physician regarding the advisability of eating a high-potassium diet. See Section Six for the Table of High Potassium Foods.

Beverages: No restrictions. May be taken with milk.

▷   *Alcohol*: Use with caution until the combined effect has been determined. Alcohol may impair the anticonvulsant effect of this drug and reduce its control of seizures.

Tobacco Smoking: No interactions expected.

▷   *Other Drugs*

Acetazolamide may *increase* the effects of
  • quinidine
Acetazolamide may *decrease* the effects of
  • lithium

▷   *Driving, Hazardous Activities*: Usually no restrictions. Be alert to the possible occurrence of drowsiness or dizziness.

Aviation Note: The use of this drug *may be a disqualification* for piloting. Consult a designated Aviation Medical Examiner.

Exposure to Sun: No restrictions.

ACYCLOVIR
(ay SI kloh ver)

Introduced: 1979

Class: Antiviral

Prescription: USA: Yes
    Canada: Yes

Controlled Drug: USA: No
    Canada: No

Available as Generic: No

Brand Names: Zovirax

BENEFITS versus RISKS	
Possible Benefits	*Possible Risks*
HASTENED RECOVERY FROM INITIAL EPISODE OF GENITAL HERPES	Nausea, vomiting, diarrhea (8% in long-term use)
PREVENTION OF RECURRENCE OF GENITAL HERPES	Nervousness, depression (less than 3%)
	Joint and muscle pain (3%)

▷ **Principal Uses**

As a Single Drug Product: Treatment of initial episodes and prevention of recurrent episodes of genital herpes in selected individuals.

How This Drug Works: By inhibiting DNA replication of the herpes simplex virus, this drug arrests the multiplication and spread of the infecting virus and thus reduces the severity and duration of the herpes infection.

Available Dosage Forms and Strengths

Capsules — 200 mg

Ointment — 5%

▷ **Usual Adult Dosage Range:** For initial episode of genital herpes—200 mg/4 hrs for a total of 5 capsules daily for 10 consecutive days (total dose of 50 capsules). For intermittent recurrence—200 mg/4 hrs for a total of 5 capsules daily for 5 consecutive days (total dose of 25 capsules). Begin treatment at the earliest indication of recurrence. For prevention of frequent recurrence—200 mg taken 3 to 5 times daily for up to 6 months. For the ointment form—cover all infected areas every 3 hours for a total of 6 times daily for 7 consecutive days. Begin treatment at the earliest indication of infection. **Note: Actual dosage and administration schedule must be determined by the physician for each patient individually.**

▷ **Dosing Instructions:** May be taken without regard to eating. Capsule may be opened for administration. Take the full course of the exact dose prescribed. Use a finger cot or rubber glove to apply the ointment.

Usual Duration of Use: Continual use on a regular schedule for 10 days is usually necessary to determine this drug's effectiveness in reducing the severity and duration of the initial infection. Continual use for 4 to 6 months may be necessary to prevent frequent recurrence of herpes eruptions.

▷ **This Drug Should Not Be Taken If**
- you have had an allergic reaction to any dosage form of it previously.

▷ **Inform Your Physician Before Taking This Drug If**
- you have impaired liver or kidney function.
- you are taking any other drugs at this time.

Possible Side-Effects (natural, expected and unavoidable drug actions)

With use of capsules—none. With use of ointment—mild pain, burning or stinging at site of application (28%).

▷ **Possible Adverse Effects** (unusual, unexpected and infrequent reactions)
If any of the following develop, consult your physician promptly.
Mild Adverse Effects
Allergic Reactions: Skin rash.
Headache, dizziness, nervousness, insomnia, depression, fatigue.
Nausea, vomiting, diarrhea.
Joint pains, muscle cramps, altered menstruation.
Acne, hair loss.

Serious Adverse Effects
Superficial thrombophlebitis, enlarged lymph glands.

CAUTION
1. This drug does not eliminate all herpes virus and is not a permanent cure. Observe for possible recurrence and resume treatment at the earliest indication of active infection.
2. Avoid sexual intercourse while herpes blisters and inflammation are visible.
3. Do not exceed the prescribed dosage.
4. Inform physician if the frequency and severity of recurrent infections do not improve.

Precautions for Use
By Infants and Children: Safety and effectiveness for use by those under 12 years of age have not been established.
By Those over 60 Years of Age: Avoid dehydration. Drink 2 to 3 quarts of liquids daily.

▷ **Advisability of Use During Pregnancy**
Pregnancy Category: C (tentative). See Pregnancy Code inside back cover.
Animal studies: No birth defects found in mouse, rat or rabbit studies.
Human studies: Information from adequate studies in pregnant women is not available.
Avoid use if possible. Use only if clearly needed.

Advisability of Use if Breast-Feeding
Presence of this drug in breast milk: Unknown.
Avoid drug or refrain from nursing.

Habit-Forming Potential: None.

Effects of Overdosage: Possible impairment of kidney function.

Possible Effects of Long-Term Use: Development of strains of herpes virus that are resistant to this drug.

Suggested Periodic Examinations While Taking This Drug (at physician's discretion)
Kidney function tests.

▷ **While Taking This Drug, Observe the Following**
Foods: No restrictions.
Beverages: No restrictions. May be taken with milk. Drink 2 to 3 quarts of liquids daily.
▷ *Alcohol*: Use caution until the combined effects have been determined. Dizziness or fatigue may be accentuated.
Tobacco Smoking: No interactions expected.
▷ *Other Drugs*
The following drugs may *increase* the effects of acyclovir
• probenecid (Benemid) may delay its elimination.

▷ *Driving, Hazardous Activities*: Use caution if dizziness or fatigue occurs.
  Aviation Note: The use of this drug *may be a disqualification* for piloting.
  Consult a designated Aviation Medical Examiner.
  Exposure to Sun: No restrictions.

ALBUTEROL
(al BYU ter ohl)

Other Names: Salbutamol

Introduced: 1968   **Class:** Antiasthmatic, Bronchodilator

Prescription: USA: Yes   **Controlled Drug:** USA: No
     Canada: Yes   Canada: No

Available as Generic: No

Brand Names: Proventil Inhaler, Proventil Tablets, Ventolin Inhaler, Ventolin Tablets

BENEFITS versus RISKS	
Possible Benefits	*Possible Risks*
VERY EFFECTIVE RELIEF OF BRONCHOSPASM	Increased blood pressure Fine hand tremor Irregular heart rhythm (with excessive use)

▷ **Principal Uses**
  As a Single Drug Product: To relieve acute bronchial asthma and to reduce the frequency and severity of chronic, recurrent asthmatic attacks.

How This Drug Works: It is thought that by increasing the production of cyclic AMP, this drug relaxes constricted bronchial muscles to relieve asthmatic wheezing.

Available Dosage Forms and Strengths
  Aerosol — 90 mcg per actuation
  Syrup — 2 mg/5 ml teaspoonful
  Tablets — 2 mg, 4 mg

▷ **Usual Adult Dosage Range:** Inhaler—1 to 2 inhalations (90 to 180 mcg) up to 4 times daily, every 4 to 6 hours. Tablets—2 to 4 mg 3 to 4 times daily, every 4 to 6 hours. **Do not exceed** 8 inhalations (720 mcg)/24 hrs, or 32 mg (tablet form)/24 hrs. **Note: Actual dosage and administration schedule must be determined by the physician for each patient individually.**

▷ **Dosing Instructions:** May be taken on empty stomach or with food or milk. Tablet may be crushed. For inhaler, follow the written instructions carefully. Do not overuse.

Usual Duration of Use: According to individual requirements. Do not use beyond the time necessary to terminate episodes of asthma.

▷ **This Drug Should Not Be Taken If**
- you have had an allergic reaction to any dosage form of it previously.
- you currently have an irregular heart rhythm.
- you are taking, or have taken within the past 2 weeks, any monoamine oxidase (MAO) inhibitor drug (see Drug Class, Section Four).

▷ **Inform Your Physician Before Taking This Drug If**
- you have any type of heart or circulatory disorder, especially high blood pressure or coronary heart disease.
- you have diabetes.
- you are taking any form of digitalis or any stimulant drug.

Possible Side-Effects   (natural, expected and unavoidable drug actions)
Aerosol—dryness or irritation of mouth or throat, altered taste. Tablet—nervousness, palpitation.

▷ **Possible Adverse Effects**   (unusual, unexpected and infrequent reactions)
If any of the following develop, consult your physician promptly.
Mild Adverse Effects
Headache (7%), dizziness (2%), restlessness, insomnia, fine tremor of hands (20%).
Nausea (2%), heartburn, vomiting.
Leg cramps (3%), flushing of skin.
Serious Adverse Effects
Rapid or irregular heart rhythm, increased blood pressure, difficult urination.

Natural Diseases or Disorders That May Be Activated By This Drug
Latent coronary artery disease, diabetes or high blood pressure.

CAUTION
1. Concurrent use of this drug by inhalation with beclomethasone aerosol (Beclovent, Vanceril) may increase the risk of toxicity due to fluorocarbon propellants. It is advisable to use albuterol aerosol 20 to 30 minutes *before* beclomethasone aerosol. This will reduce the risk of toxicity and will enhance the penetration of beclomethasone.
2. The excessive or prolonged use of this drug by inhalation can reduce its effectiveness and cause serious heart rhythm disturbances, including cardiac arrest.

Precautions for Use
By Infants and Children: Safety and effectiveness of use in children under 12 years of age have not been established.
By Those over 60 Years of Age: Avoid excessive and continual use. If acute asthma is not relieved promptly, other drugs will have to be tried. Observe for the development of nervousness, palpitations, irregular heart rhythm and muscle tremors.

▷ **Advisability of Use During Pregnancy**
 Pregnancy Category: C (tentative). See Pregnancy Code inside back cover.
  Animal studies: Cleft palate reported in mice.
  Human studies: Information from adequate studies in pregnant women is
   not available.
  Avoid use during first 3 months if possible.

Advisability of Use if Breast-Feeding
 Presence of this drug in breast milk: Unknown.
 Avoid drug or refrain from nursing.

Habit-Forming Potential: None.

Effects of Overdosage: Nervousness, palpitation, rapid heart rate, sweating,
  headache, tremor, vomiting, chest pain.

Possible Effects of Long-Term Use: Loss of effectiveness.

Suggested Periodic Examinations While Taking This Drug (at physician's
  discretion)
 Blood pressure measurements, evaluation of heart status.

▷ **While Taking This Drug, Observe the Following**
 Foods: No restrictions.
 Beverages: Avoid excessive use of caffeine-containing beverages—coffee, tea,
  cola, chocolate.
▷ *Alcohol*: No interactions expected.
 Tobacco Smoking: No interactions expected.
▷ *Other Drugs*
  Albuterol *taken concurrently* with
  • monoamine oxidase (MAO) inhibitor drugs may cause excessive increase
   in blood pressure and undesirable heart stimulation.
▷ *Driving, Hazardous Activities*: Use caution if excessive nervousness or dizzi-
   ness occurs.
 Aviation Note: The use of this drug *is a disqualification* for piloting. Consult a
  designated Aviation Medical Examiner.
 Exposure to Sun: No restrictions.
 Heavy Exercise or Exertion: Use caution. Excessive exercise can induce
  asthma in sensitive individuals.

ALLOPURINOL
(al oh PURE i nohl)

Introduced: 1963

Class: Antigout

Prescription: USA: Yes
 Canada: Yes

Controlled Drug: USA: No
 Canada: No

Available as Generic: USA: Yes
 Canada: No

Brand Names: ❦Alloprin, ❦Apo-Allopurinol, Lopurin, ❦Novopurol, ❦Puri-
nol, ❦Roucol, Zyloprim

BENEFITS versus RISKS

Possible Benefits	*Possible Risks*
EFFECTIVE CONTROL OF GOUT CONTROL OF HIGH BLOOD URIC ACID due to polycythemia, leukemia, cancer and chemotherapy	Increased frequency of acute gout initially Peripheral neuritis Allergic reactions in skin, blood vessels and liver Bone marrow depression (questionable)

▷ **Principal Uses**

As a Single Drug Product: Used primarily in the long-term management of gout to *prevent* episodes of acute gout. (It does not relieve the symptoms of acute gout attacks.) Also used to prevent abnormally high blood levels of uric acid in individuals who have recurrent uric acid kidney stones, and in those receiving chemotherapy or radiation therapy for cancer.

How This Drug Works: By inhibiting the action of the tissue enzyme xanthine oxidase, this drug decreases the conversion of purines (protein nutrients) to uric acid.

Available Dosage Forms and Strengths

Tablets — 100 mg, 300 mg (and 200 mg in Canada)

▷ **Usual Adult Dosage Range:**   Initially 100 mg/24 hrs. Increase by 100 mg/24 hrs at intervals of 1 week until uric acid blood level is 6 mg/dl or less. Usual dose is 200 to 300 mg/24 hrs for mild gout, and 400 to 600 mg/24 hrs for moderate to severe gout. Daily doses of 300 mg or less may be taken as a single dose. Doses exceeding 300 mg daily should be divided into 2 or 3 equal portions; for the high uric acid levels associated with cancer, 600 to 800 mg/24 hrs, divided into 3 equal portions. **Note: Actual dosage and administration schedule must be determined by the physician for each patient individually.**

▷ **Dosing Instructions:**   Best taken with food or milk to reduce stomach irritation. Tablet may be crushed. Drink 2 to 3 quarts of liquids daily.

Usual Duration of Use: According to individual requirements. Blood uric acid levels usually begin to decrease in 48 to 72 hours and may reach a normal range in 1 to 3 weeks. Regular use for several months may be required to prevent attacks of acute gout. Continual use for many years may be necessary for adequate control.

▷ **This Drug Should Not Be Taken If**
- you have had an allergic reaction to any dosage form of it previously.
- you are experiencing an acute attack of gout at the present time.

▷ **Inform Your Physician Before Taking This Drug If**
- you have a personal or family history of hemochromatosis.
- you have a history of liver or kidney disease.
- you have had a blood cell or bone marrow disorder.
- you have any type of convulsive disorder (epilepsy).

Possible Side-Effects   (natural, expected and unavoidable drug actions)
An increase in the frequency and severity of episodes of acute gout may occur during the first several weeks of drug use. Consult your physician regarding the need for other drugs during this period.

▷ **Possible Adverse Effects**   (unusual, unexpected and infrequent reactions)
If any of the following develop, consult your physician promptly.
Mild Adverse Effects
Allergic Reactions: Skin rash, hives, itching, drug fever.
Headache, dizziness, drowsiness.
Nausea, vomiting, diarrhea, stomach cramps.
Loss of scalp hair.
Serious Adverse Effects
Allergic Reactions: Severe skin reactions, high fever, chills, joint pains, swollen glands, kidney damage.
Hepatitis with or without jaundice (see Glossary)—yellow eyes and skin, dark-colored urine, light-colored stools.
Bone marrow depression (see Glossary)—questionable.
Seizures, peripheral neuritis.
Macular eye damage, cataract formation—questionable.

▷ **Adverse Effects That May Mimic Natural Diseases or Disorders**
Toxic liver reaction may suggest viral hepatitis.
Severe skin reactions may resemble the Stevens-Johnson syndrome (erythema multiforme).

CAUTION
1. During the early weeks of treatment, the frequency of acute attacks of gout may increase. These subside with continuation of treatment.
2. This drug will not relieve the symptoms of acute gout. It should not be started during the presence of acute gout symptoms.
3. Vitamin C in doses of 2 grams or more daily may acidify the urine and increase the risk of kidney stone formation during the use of allopurinol.
4. The concurrent use of thiazide diuretics (see Drug Class, Section Four) is reported to cause a possible allergic-type kidney damage. Avoid this drug combination.

Precautions for Use
By Infants and Children: Monitor closely for allergic skin reactions and blood cell disorders. This drug may increase the toxicity of azathioprine (Imuran) or mercaptopurine (Purinethol) in children receiving chemotherapy for cancer.

By Those over 60 Years of Age: The natural decline in kidney function makes it advisable to use smaller initial and maintenance doses of this drug.

▷ **Advisability of Use During Pregnancy**
Pregnancy Category: C (tentative). See Pregnancy Code inside back cover.
Animal studies: Results are conflicting and inconclusive.
Human studies: Information from adequate studies in pregnant women is not available.
Avoid use of drug during the first 3 months.

Advisability of Use if Breast-Feeding
Presence of this drug in breast milk: Unknown.
Avoid drug or refrain from nursing.

Habit-Forming Potential: None.

Effects of Overdosage: Nausea, vomiting or diarrhea may occur as a result of individual sensitivity. No serious toxic effects expected.

Possible Effects of Long-Term Use: None identified.

Suggested Periodic Examinations While Taking This Drug   (at physician's discretion)
Blood uric acid levels, complete blood cell counts, liver and kidney function tests. If appropriate, eye examinations for possible cataract formation or macular damage. A cause-and-effect relationship (see Glossary) between this drug and eye changes has not been established.

▷ **While Taking This Drug, Observe the Following**
Foods: Follow physician's advice regarding the need for a low-purine diet.
Beverages: No restrictions. May be taken with milk.
▷ *Alcohol*: No interactions expected.
Tobacco Smoking: No interactions expected.
▷ *Other Drugs*
Allopurinol may *increase* the effects of
• azathioprine (Imuran) and mercaptopurine (Purinethol), making it necessary to reduce their dosages.
• oral anticoagulants (see Drug Class, Section Four) in *some* individuals.
• theophylline (aminophylline, Elixophyllin, Theo-Dur, etc.)
Allopurinol *taken concurrently* with
• ampicillin may increase the incidence of skin rash.
▷ *Driving, Hazardous Activities*: Drowsiness may occur in some individuals. Determine sensitivity before engaging in hazardous activities.
Aviation Note: The use of this drug *may be a disqualification* for piloting. Consult a designated Aviation Medical Examiner.
Exposure to Sun: No restrictions.

✕ ALPRAZOLAM
(al PRAY zoh lam)

Introduced: 1973

Class: Mild Tranquilizer, Benzodiazepines

Prescription: USA: Yes
Canada: Yes

Controlled Drug: USA: C-IV*
Canada: No

Available as Generic: No

Brand Names: Xanax

BENEFITS versus RISKS

Possible Benefits	*Possible Risks*
RELIEF OF ANXIETY AND NERVOUS TENSION in 75% of users	Habit-forming potential with prolonged use
Wide margin of safety with therapeutic doses	Minor impairment of mental functions with therapeutic doses

---

▷ **Principal Uses**

As a Single Drug Product: Used primarily as a mild tranquilizer for the short-term relief of mild to moderate anxiety and nervous tension.

How This Drug Works: It is thought that this drug produces a calming effect by enhancing the action of the nerve transmitter gamma-aminobutyric acid (GABA), which in turn blocks the arousal of higher brain centers.

Available Dosage Forms and Strengths

Tablets — 0.25 mg, 0.5 mg, 1 mg

▷ **Usual Adult Dosage Range:** 0.25 mg to 0.5 mg 3 times daily. The maximal dose is 4 mg/24 hrs, taken in divided doses. **Note: Actual dosage and administration schedule must be determined by the physician for each patient individually.**

▷ **Dosing Instructions:** May be taken on empty stomach or with food or milk. Tablet may be crushed for administration. Do not discontinue this drug abruptly if taken for more than 4 weeks.

Usual Duration of Use: Several days to several weeks. Avoid prolonged and uninterrupted use. Continual use should not exceed 8 weeks without evaluation by your physician.

▷ **This Drug Should Not Be Taken If**
- you have had an allergic reaction to it previously.
- you are pregnant (first 3 months).
- you have acute narrow-angle glaucoma.
- you have myasthenia gravis.

*See Schedules of Controlled Drugs inside back cover.

▷ **Inform Your Physician Before Taking This Drug If**
- you are allergic to other benzodiazepine drugs (see Drug Class, Section Four).
- you are pregnant (last 6 months) or planning pregnancy.
- you are breast-feeding.
- you have a history of depression or serious mental illness (psychosis).
- you have a history of alcoholism or drug abuse.
- you have impaired liver or kidney function.
- you have open-angle glaucoma.
- you have a seizure disorder (epilepsy).
- you have severe chronic lung disease.

Possible Side-Effects   (natural, expected and unavoidable drug actions)
Drowsiness, lightheadedness.

▷ **Possible Adverse Effects**   (unusual, unexpected and infrequent reactions)
If any of the following develop, consult your physician promptly.
Mild Adverse Effects
Allergic Reactions: Skin rash, hives.
Headache, dizziness, fatigue, blurred vision, dry mouth.
Nausea, vomiting, constipation.
Serious Adverse Effects
Confusion, hallucinations, depression, unexpected excitement, agitation (paradoxical reaction).

CAUTION
1. This drug should not be discontinued abruptly if it has been taken continually for more than 4 weeks.
2. The concurrent use of some over-the-counter drug products that contain antihistamines (allergy and cold preparations, sleep aids) can cause excessive sedation in sensitive individuals.

Precautions for Use
By Infants and Children: Safety and effectiveness for use by those under 18 years of age have not been established.
By Those over 60 Years of Age: The starting dose should be 0.25 mg 2 or 3 times daily. Monitor for excessive drowsiness, dizziness, unsteadiness and incoordination (possible low blood pressure).

▷ **Advisability of Use During Pregnancy**
Pregnancy Category: D (tentative). See Pregnancy Code inside back cover.
Animal studies: Diazepam (a closely related benzodiazepine) can cause cleft palate in mice and skeletal defects in rats. No information available for alprazolam.
Human studies: Some studies suggest a possible association between the use of diazepam and defects such as cleft lip and heart deformities. Information from adequate studies on the use of alprazolam in pregnant women is not available.
Avoid use during entire pregnancy if possible.

Advisability of Use if Breast-Feeding
　　Presence of this drug in breast milk: Probably yes.
　　Avoid drug or refrain from nursing.

Habit-Forming Potential:　This drug can produce psychological and/or physical dependence (see Glossary) if used in large doses for an extended period of time.

Effects of Overdosage:　Marked drowsiness, weakness, feeling of drunkenness, staggering gait, tremor, stupor progressing to deep sleep or coma.

Possible Effects of Long-Term Use:　Psychological and/or physical dependence.

Suggested Periodic Examinations While Taking This Drug　(at physician's discretion)
　　None required for short-term use.

▷　**While Taking This Drug, Observe the Following**
　　Foods: No restrictions.
　　Beverages: Avoid excessive intake of caffeine-containing beverages: coffee, tea, cola. This drug may be taken with milk.
▷　*Alcohol*: Use with extreme caution and in very small amounts until the combined effect is determined. Alcohol may increase the sedative effects of alprazolam. Alprazolam may increase the intoxicating effects of alcohol. Avoid alcohol completely—throughout the day and night—if you find it necessary to drive or to engage in *any* hazardous activity.
　　Tobacco Smoking: Heavy smoking may reduce the calming action of alprazolam.
　　Marijuana Smoking
　　　Occasional (once or twice weekly): Mild increase in the sedative effect of this drug.
　　　Daily: Marked increase in the sedative effect of this drug.
▷　*Other Drugs*
　　Alprazolam may *increase* the effects of
　　• digoxin (Lanoxin), and cause digoxin toxicity.
　　Alprazolam may *decrease* the effects of
　　• levodopa (Sinemet, etc.), and reduce its effectiveness in treating Parkinson's disease.
　　The following drugs may *increase* the effects of alprazolam
　　• cimetidine (Tagamet).
　　• disulfiram (Antabuse).
　　• isoniazid (INH, Rifamate, etc.).
　　• oral contraceptives.
　　• valproic acid (Depakene).
　　The following drugs may *decrease* the effects of alprazolam
　　• rifampin (Rimactane, etc.).
　　• theophylline (aminophylline, Theo-Dur, etc.).
▷　*Driving, Hazardous Activities*: This drug can impair mental alertness, judgment, physical coordination and reaction time. Avoid hazardous activities accordingly.

Aviation Note: The use of this drug *is a disqualification* for piloting. Consult a designated Aviation Medical Examiner.

Exposure to Sun: No restrictions.

Discontinuation: If it has been necessary to use this drug for an extended period of time, do not discontinue it abruptly. Reduce dose gradually at the rate of 1 mg every 3 days.

ALUMINUM HYDROXIDE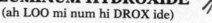
(ah LOO mi num hi DROX ide)

Other Names: Antacid

Introduced: 1936   **Class:** Antacids

Prescription: USA: No   **Controlled Drug:** USA: No
    Canada: No   Canada: No

Available as Generic: Yes

Brand Names: Algicon [CD], ALternaGEL, Aludrox [CD], ✿Alu-Tab, Amphojel, ✿Amphojel Plus [CD], ✿Amphojel 500 [CD], Camalox [CD], Creamalin [CD], Delcid [CD], Di-Gel Liquid [CD], Di-Gel Tablets [CD], ✿Diovol [CD], ✿Diovol Ex [CD], Gaviscon [CD], Gelusil Preparations [CD], Kolantyl [CD], Maalox Preparations [CD], Mylanta Preparations [CD], ✿Neutralca-S [CD], Rolaids [CD], ✿Univol Suspension [CD], ✿Univol Tablets [CD], WinGel [CD]

BENEFITS versus RISKS

Possible Benefits	*Possible Risks*
EFFECTIVE NEUTRALIZATION OF STOMACH ACIDS (Short-term)	CONSTIPATION
EFFECTIVE RELIEF OF HEARTBURN, SOUR STOMACH AND ACID INDIGESTION	

▷ **Principal Uses**

As a Single Drug Product: Used primarily to provide symptomatic relief in the treatment of peptic ulcer disease, gastritis, esophagitis, hiatal hernia and conditions associated with the production of excessive stomach acid.

As a Combination Drug Product [CD]: Antacids of different chemical composition are often combined to reduce unwanted side-effects of each other. For example, the constipating effects of aluminum hydroxide can correct the laxative effects of magnesium antacids—hence their frequent combination in popular antacid products. Antacids are sometimes combined with drugs that cause stomach irritation, such as aspirin and related compounds, to make such drugs less irritating.

How This Drug Works: By neutralizing some of the hydrochloric acid in the stomach, this drug reduces the degree of acidity and thus lessens the irritating effect of digestive juices on inflamed or ulcerated tissues. By reducing the action of the digestive enzyme pepsin, this drug is thought to create a more favorable environment for the healing of peptic ulcer.

Available Dosage Forms and Strengths

Capsules — 475 mg, 500 mg
Oral suspensions — 320 mg, 600 mg per teaspoonful (5 ml)
Tablets — 300 mg, 600 mg
Chewable tablets — 500 mg

▷ **Usual Adult Dosage Range:** 300 to 600 mg 3 to 6 times daily. Total dose should not exceed 3600 mg/24 hrs. **Note: For long-term use, actual dosage and administration schedule must be determined by the physician for each patient individually.**

▷ **Dosing Instructions:** Best taken between meals and at bedtime. When used on a regular basis for continuous effect, it is most effective when taken 1 hour after eating. May be followed by a sip of water. Tablet may be crushed and capsule opened for administration.

Usual Duration of Use: Continuous use on a regular schedule should not exceed 2 weeks without your physician's guidance.

▷ **This Drug Should Not Be Taken If**
• you have a known allergy or sensitivity to any of its components.

▷ **Inform Your Physician Before Taking This Drug If**
• you have chronic constipation.
• you are taking any form of tetracycline antibiotic.

Possible Side-Effects (natural, expected and unavoidable drug actions)
Constipation.

▷ **Possible Adverse Effects** (unusual, unexpected and infrequent reactions)
If any of the following develop, consult your physician promptly.
Mild Adverse Effects
Nausea, vomiting.
Serious Adverse Effects
Aluminum hydroxide taken in large doses and with inadequate fluids can cause intestinal obstruction.

CAUTION
1. Do not take *any antacid* regularly for more than 2 weeks without your physician's guidance.
2. If symptoms requiring the use of antacids persist, consult your physician for definitive diagnosis and appropriate treatment.
3. If frequent and continual use of antacids is necessary, it is advisable to use aluminum and/or magnesium preparations; they are less absorbable than calcium and sodium antacids.
4. Do not exceed the maximal daily dose stated on the product label.

5. Do not swallow chewable tablets and wafers whole. These preparations must be thoroughly sucked or chewed before swallowing, and preferably followed by a small amount of water or milk. Antacid tablets designed for chewing can cause intestinal obstruction if swallowed whole.
6. Shake all liquid preparations of antacids well before measuring the dose.

Precautions for Use
By Infants and Children: Ask physician for guidance.

By Those over 60 Years of Age: If you develop constipation with the use of this antacid, consult your physician or pharmacist for guidance. Do not allow this condition to go uncorrected.

▷ **Advisability of Use During Pregnancy**
Pregnancy Category: B (tentative). See Pregnancy Code inside back cover.
Animal studies: No birth defects found in chicken and rat studies.
Human studies: Information from adequate studies in pregnant women is not available. Some studies indicate the possibility of fetal damage from antacids containing *magnesium*. Read the label on the antacid product carefully to determine its exact composition. Ask physician for guidance regarding the use of aluminum antacid preparations.

Advisability of Use if Breast-Feeding
Presence of this drug in breast milk: Unknown.
Avoid drug or refrain from nursing. Ask physician for guidance.

Habit-Forming Potential: None.

Effects of Overdosage: Nausea, vomiting, constipation.

Possible Effects of Long-Term Use: Decreased levels of blood phosphates resulting in loss of calcium and phosphate from bone with weakening of bone structure (osteomalacia).

Suggested Periodic Examinations While Taking This Drug   (at physician's discretion)
Measurements of blood calcium and phosphorus levels (with long-term use).

▷ **While Taking This Drug, Observe the Following**
Foods: Follow the diet prescribed by your physican. Maintain regular intake of high-phosphate foods such as meats, poultry, fish, eggs, dairy products and cereals.

Beverages: No restrictions. Tablets may be taken with milk.

▷ *Alcohol*: No interactions expected. However, alcoholic beverages may increase stomach acidity and thus increase antacid requirements.

Tobacco Smoking: No interactions expected. However, nicotine may increase stomach acidity and thus increase antacid requirements.

▷ *Other Drugs*
Aluminum Hydroxide may *decrease* the effects of
• beta-adrenergic blocking drugs (see Drug Class, Section Four).
• chloroquine (Aralen).

- diflunisal (Dolobid).
- digoxin (Lanoxin).
- iron preparations.
- penicillamine (Cuprimine, Depen).
- phenothiazines (Thorazine, etc., see Drug Class, Section Four).
- sodium polystyrene sulfonate (Kayexalate).
- tetracyclines (see Drug Class, Section Four).

▷ *Driving, Hazardous Activities*: No precautions or restrictions.
Aviation Note: No restrictions.
Exposure to Sun: No restrictions.

AMILORIDE
(a MIL oh ride)

Introduced: 1967

Prescription: USA: Yes
         Canada: Yes

Available as Generic: No

Brand Names: Midamor, ♣Moduret [CD], Moduretic [CD]

Class: Diuretic

Controlled Drug: USA: No
         Canada: No

BENEFITS versus RISKS	
Possible Benefits	*Possible Risks*
EFFECTIVE DIURETIC WITHOUT LOSS OF POTASSIUM	ABNORMALLY HIGH BLOOD POTASSIUM with excessive use Rare bone marrow depression

---

▷ **Principal Uses**
As a Single Drug Product: To eliminate excessive fluid retention (edema).
As a Combination Drug Product [CD]: It is combined with other diuretics of the thiazide class primarily to prevent the loss of potassium from the body.

How This Drug Works: It is thought that this drug promotes the loss of sodium and water from the body and the retention of potassium by altering the enzyme systems of the kidney that control the formation of urine.

Available Dosage Forms and Strengths
Tablets — 5 mg

▷ **Usual Adult Dosage Range:**   Initially 5 mg once daily, preferably in the morning. May increase up to 15 mg daily as needed and tolerated. Should not exceed 20 mg/24 hrs. **Note: Actual dosage and administration schedule must be determined by the physician for each patient individually.**

▷ **Dosing Instructions:**   Preferably taken on arising, with the stomach empty. For best results, withhold food for 4 hours. May be taken with food if necessary to reduce stomach irritation. Tablet may be crushed for administration.

Usual Duration of Use: As needed for elimination of edema or maintenance of normal blood pressure. Intermittent or alternate-day use is recommended to minimize imbalance of sodium and potassium.

▷ **This Drug Should Not Be Taken If**
- you have had an allergic reaction to any dosage form of it previously.
- your blood potassium level is above the normal range.
- your kidneys are not producing urine.

▷ **Inform Your Physician Before Taking This Drug If**
- you have diabetes or glaucoma.
- you have a history of kidney disease or impaired kidney function.
- you are taking any other diuretic, blood pressure drug, any form of digitalis or lithium.

Possible Side-Effects   (natural, expected and unavoidable drug actions)
Abnormally high blood potassium level (10% of users), abnormally low blood sodium level, dehydration, constipation.

▷ **Possible Adverse Effects**   (unusual, unexpected and infrequent reactions)
If any of the following develop, consult your physician promptly.
Mild Adverse Effects
Allergic Reactions: Skin rash, itching.
Headache, dizziness, weakness, fatigue, numbness and tingling.
Dry mouth, nausea, vomiting, stomach pains, diarrhea.
Loss of scalp hair.
Serious Adverse Effects
Idiosyncratic Reactions: Joint and muscle pains.
Excessively high blood potassium level—marked fatigue and weakness, confusion, numbness and tingling of lips and extremities, slow and irregular heartbeats.
Increased internal eye pressure (of concern in glaucoma).
Mental depression, visual disturbances, ringing in ears, tremors.
Decreased sexual interest and performance.
Aplastic anemia (see Glossary)—unusual fatigue or weakness, fever, sore throat, abnormal bleeding or bruising.

▷ **Adverse Effects That May Mimic Natural Diseases or Disorders**
Nervousness, confusion and/or depression may resemble spontaneous mental disorder.

Natural Diseases or Disorders That May Be Activated by This Drug
Preexisting peptic ulcer, latent glaucoma.

CAUTION
1. Do not take potassium supplements, and do not increase your intake of high-potassium foods.
2. If taking any form of digitalis, report as directed for periodic measurements of your blood potassium level.

3. Do not discontinue this drug abruptly unless directed to do so by your physician.

Precautions for Use

By Infants and Children: Safety and effectiveness for use by those under 12 years of age have not been established.

By Those over 60 Years of Age: The natural decline in kidney function may predispose to excessive retention of potassium in the body. It is advisable to limit use of this drug to periods of 2 to 3 weeks if possible. Overdosage and extended use can cause excessive loss of body water, increased viscosity of the blood and an increased tendency to abnormal blood clotting (thrombosis, heart attack, stroke).

▷ **Advisability of Use During Pregnancy**

Pregnancy Category: B (tentative). See Pregnancy Code inside back cover.

Animal studies: No birth defects reported.

Human studies: Information from adequate studies in pregnant women is not available.

Advisability of Use if Breast-Feeding

Presence of this drug in breast milk: Unknown, but probably present.

This drug may suppress milk production.

Avoid drug if possible. If use is necessary, monitor nursing infant closely and discontinue drug or nursing if adverse effects develop.

Habit-Forming Potential: None.

Effects of Overdosage: Thirst, drowsiness, fatigue, weakness, nausea, vomiting, confusion, numbness and tingling of face and extremities, irregular heart rhythm, shortness of breath.

Suggested Periodic Examinations While Taking This Drug   (at physician's discretion)

Complete blood cell counts; measurements of blood levels of sodium, potassium and chloride; kidney function tests; and assessment of water balance (state of hydration).

▷ **While Taking This Drug, Observe the Following**

Foods: No restrictions. Avoid excessive restriction of salt.

Avoid excessive amounts of high-potassium foods.

Beverages: No restrictions. May be taken with milk.

▷ *Alcohol*: Use with caution until the combined effect has been determined. Alcohol can exaggerate the blood-pressure-lowering effect of this drug and cause orthostatic hypotension (see Glossary).

Tobacco Smoking: No interactions expected.

▷ *Other Drugs*

Amiloride may *increase* the effects of

• other blood-pressure-lowering drugs. Dosage adjustments may be necessary.

Amiloride may *decrease* the effects of

• digoxin (Lanoxin, etc.), and reduce its effectiveness in treating heart failure.

Amiloride *taken concurrently* with
- spironolactone (Aldactone, Aldactazide) or triamterene (Dyrenium, Dyazide) may cause excessive (dangerous) increase in blood potassium levels. Avoid the concurrent use of these drugs.
- lithium may cause lithium accumulation to toxic levels.

▷ *Driving, Hazardous Activities*: This drug may cause drowsiness, dizziness and orthostatic hypotension in sensitive individuals. If these drug effects occur, avoid hazardous activities.

Aviation Note: The use of this drug *may be a disqualification* for piloting. Consult a designated Aviation Medical Examiner.

Exposure to Sun: No restrictions.

Exposure to Heat: Caution advised. Excessive perspiration can cause water, sodium and potassium imbalance. Hot environments can cause lowering of blood pressure.

Occurrence of Unrelated Illness: Consult your physician if you contract an illness that causes vomiting or diarrhea.

Discontinuation: With high dosage or prolonged use, withdraw this drug gradually. Sudden withdrawal can cause excessive loss of potassium from the body.

AMITRIPTYLINE
(a mee TRIP ti leen)

Introduced: 1961

Class: Antidepressant

Prescription: USA: Yes
Canada: Yes

Controlled Drug: USA: No
Canada: No

Available as Generic: Yes

Brand Names: Amitril, ♣Apo-Amitriptyline, Elavil, Endep, Etrafon [CD], Etrafon-A [CD], Etrafon-Forte [CD], ♣Levate, Limbitrol [CD], ♣Meravil, ♣Novotriptyn, SK-Amitriptyline, Triavil [CD]

BENEFITS versus RISKS

Possible Benefits	*Possible Risks*
EFFECTIVE RELIEF OF ENDOGENOUS DEPRESSION in 60% to 75% of users	ADVERSE BEHAVIORAL EFFECTS: Confusion, disorientation, hallucinations CONVERSION OF DEPRESSION TO MANIA in manic-depressive disorders Irregular heart rhythms Rare blood cell abnormalities

---

▷ **Principal Uses**

As a Single Drug Product: To relieve the symptoms associated with spontaneous (endogenous) depression, and to initiate the restoration of normal mood. This drug should be used only when a diagnosis of a true, primary depression of significant degree has been established. It should not be used to treat the symptoms of mild and transient (reactive) depression that may be associated with many life situations in the absence of a bona fide affective illness.

As a Combination Drug Product [CD]: This drug is available in combination with chlordiazepoxide, a mild tranquilizer of the benzodiazepine class. This combination is used to relieve anxiety that may accompany depression. This drug is also available in combination with perphenazine, a strong tranquilizer of the phenothiazine class. This combination is used to relieve severe agitation that may accompany depression.

How This Drug Works: It is thought that this drug relieves depression by slowly restoring to normal levels certain constituents of brain tissue (norepinephrine and serotonin) that transmit nerve impulses.

Available Dosage Forms and Strengths
Tablets — 10 mg, 25 mg, 50 mg, 75 mg, 100 mg, 150 mg

▷ **Usual Adult Dosage Range:**   Initially 25 mg 2 to 4 times daily. Dose may be increased cautiously as needed and tolerated by 10 to 25 mg daily at intervals of 1 week. Usual maintenance dose is 50 to 100 mg/24 hrs. Total dose should not exceed 150 mg/24 hrs. When the optimal requirement is determined, it may be taken at bedtime as one dose. **Note: Actual dosage and administration schedule must be determined by the physician for each patient individually.**

▷ **Dosing Instructions:**   May be taken without regard to meals. Tablet may be crushed for administration.

Usual Duration of Use: Some benefit may be apparent within 1 to 2 weeks, but adequate response may require continuous use for 4 to 6 weeks or longer. Long-term use should not exceed 6 months without evaluation regarding the need for continuation of the drug.

▷ **This Drug Should Not Be Taken If**
- you are allergic to any of the drugs bearing the brand names listed above.
- you are taking or have taken within the past 14 days any monoamine oxidase (MAO) inhibitor drug (see Drug Class, Section Four).
- you are recovering from a recent heart attack.
- you have narrow-angle glaucoma.

▷ **Inform Your Physician Before Taking This Drug If**
- you are allergic or sensitive to any other tricyclic antidepressant (see Drug Class, Section Four).
- you have a history of any of the following: diabetes, epilepsy, glaucoma, heart disease, prostate gland enlargement or overactive thyroid function.
- you plan to have surgery under general anesthesia in the near future.

Possible Side-Effects   (natural, expected and unavoidable drug actions)
Drowsiness, blurred vision, dry mouth, constipation, impaired urination.

▷ **Possible Adverse Effects**   (unusual, unexpected and infrequent reactions)
If any of the following develop, consult your physician promptly.
Mild Adverse Effects
Allergic Reactions: Skin rash, hives, swelling of face or tongue, drug fever (see Glossary).
Headache, dizziness, weakness, fainting, unsteady gait, tremors.
Peculiar taste, irritation of tongue or mouth, nausea, indigestion.
Breast enlargement, milk formation, swelling of testicles.
Fluctuation of blood sugar levels.
Serious Adverse Effects
Allergic Reactions: Hepatitis, with or without jaundice (see Glossary).
Confusion, hallucinations, agitation, restlessness, nightmares.
Heart palpitation and irregular rhythm.
Bone marrow depression (see Glossary)—fatigue, weakness, fever, sore throat, abnormal bleeding or bruising.
Peripheral neuritis (see Glossary)—numbness, tingling, pain, loss of strength in arms and legs.
Parkinson-like disorders (see Glossary)—usually mild and infrequent; more likely to occur in the elderly.

▷ **Adverse Effects That May Mimic Natural Diseases or Disorders**
Liver toxicity may suggest viral hepatitis.

Natural Diseases or Disorders That May Be Activated by This Drug
Latent diabetes, epilepsy, glaucoma, impaired urination due to prostate gland enlargement.

CAUTION
1. Dosage must be adjusted for each person individually. Report for follow-up evaluation and laboratory tests as directed by your physician.
2. It is advisable to withhold this drug if electroconvulsive therapy (ECT, "shock" treatment) is to be used to treat your depression.

Precautions for Use
By Infants and Children: Safety and effectiveness for use by those under 12 years of age have not been established.
By Those over 60 Years of Age: During the first 2 weeks of treatment, observe for the development of confusion, agitation, forgetfulness, disorientation, delusions and hallucinations. Reduction of dosage or discontinuation may be necessary. Unsteadiness may predispose to falling and injury. This drug can increase the degree of impaired urination associated with prostate gland enlargement (prostatism).

▷ **Advisability of Use During Pregnancy**
Pregnancy Category: C (tentative). See Pregnancy Code inside back cover.
Animal studies: Skull deformities reported in rabbits.

Human studies: No defects reported in 21 exposures. Information from adequate studies in pregnant women is not available.

Avoid use of drug during first 3 months.

Advisability of Use if Breast-Feeding

Presence of this drug in breast milk: Yes, in small amounts.

Monitor nursing infant closely and discontinue drug or nursing if adverse effects develop.

Habit-Forming Potential: Psychological or physical dependence is rare and unexpected.

Effects of Overdosage: Confusion, hallucinations, marked drowsiness, heart palpitations, dilated pupils, tremors, stupor, deep sleep, coma, convulsions.

Suggested Periodic Examinations While Taking This Drug   (at physician's discretion)

Complete blood cell counts, liver function tests, serial blood pressure readings and electrocardiograms.

▷ **While Taking This Drug, Observe the Following**

Foods: No restrictions. This drug may increase the appetite and cause excessive weight gain.

Beverages: No restrictions. May be taken with milk.

▷   *Alcohol*: Avoid completely. This drug can markedly increase the intoxicating effects of alcohol and accentuate its depressant action on brain function.

Tobacco Smoking: May hasten the elimination of this drug. Higher doses may be necessary.

▷   *Other Drugs*

Amitriptyline may *increase* the effects of

• atropinelike drugs (see Drug Class, Section Four).

Amitriptyline may *decrease* the effects of

• clonidine (Catapres).

• guanethidine (Ismelin).

Amitriptyline *taken concurrently* with

• monoamine oxidase (MAO) inhibitor drugs may cause high fever, delirium and convulsions (see Drug Class, Section Four).

• thyroid preparations may impair heart rhythm and function.

Ask physician for guidance regarding adjustment of thyroid dose.

▷   *Driving, Hazardous Activities*: This drug may impair mental alertness, judgment, physical coordination and reaction time. Avoid hazardous activities.

Aviation Note: The use of this drug *is a disqualification* for piloting. Consult a designated Aviation Medical Examiner.

Exposure to Sun: Use caution until sensitivity to sun has been determined. This drug may cause photosensitivity (see Glossary).

Exposure to Heat: This drug can inhibit sweating and impair the body's adaptation to hot environments, increasing the risk of heat stroke. Avoid saunas.

Exposure to Cold: The elderly should use caution and avoid conditions conducive to hypothermia (see Glossary).

Discontinuation: It is advisable to discontinue this drug gradually. Abrupt withdrawal after long-term use can cause headache, malaise and nausea.

AMOXAPINE
(a MOX a peen)

Introduced: 1970

Prescription: USA: Yes
Canada: Yes

Available as Generic: No

Brand Names: Asendin

Class: Antidepressant

Controlled Drug: USA: No
Canada: No

BENEFITS versus RISKS

Possible Benefits	*Possible Risks*
EFFECTIVE RELIEF OF PRIMARY DEPRESSIONS: Endogenous, neurotic, reactive Well tolerated by most persons	ADVERSE BEHAVIORAL EFFECTS: Confusion, delusions, disorientation, hallucinations CONVERSION OF DEPRESSION TO MANIA in manic-depressive disorders Rare blood cell abnormalities

---

▷ **Principal Uses**

As a Single Drug Product: To provide symptomatic relief in all types of depression, and to initiate the restoration of normal mood.

How This Drug Works: It is thought that by increasing the availability of certain nerve impulse transmitters (norepinephrine and serotonin) in brain tissue, this drug relieves the symptoms associated with depression.

Available Dosage Forms and Strengths

Tablets — 25 mg, 50 mg, 100 mg, 150 mg

▷ **Usual Adult Dosage Range:**   Initially 50 mg 3 times daily. Dose may be increased cautiously on the third day as needed and tolerated to 100 mg 3 times daily. Usual maintenance dose is 200 to 300 mg/24 hrs. Total dosage should not exceed 400 mg/24 hrs. When determined, the optimal requirement may be taken at bedtime as one dose, not to exceed 300 mg. **Note: Actual dosage and administration schedule must be determined by the physician for each patient individually.**

▷ **Dosing Instructions:**   May be taken without regard to meals. Tablet may be crushed for administration.

Usual Duration of Use: Benefit may be apparent within 4 to 7 days in some individuals, but continual use on a regular schedule for 2 to 3 weeks is usually necessary to determine this drug's effectiveness. Long-term use should not exceed 6 months without evaluation regarding the need for continuation.

▷ **This Drug Should Not Be Taken If**
- you have had an allergic reaction to it previously.
- you are taking or have taken within the past 14 days any monoamine oxidase (MAO) inhibitor drug (see Drug Class, Section Four).
- you are recovering from a recent heart attack.

▷ **Inform Your Physician Before Taking This Drug If**
- you are allergic or overly sensitive to other antidepressant drugs.
- you have a history of any of the following: diabetes, epilepsy, glaucoma, heart disease, paranoia, prostate gland enlargement, schizophrenia or overactive thyroid function.
- you plan to have surgery under general anesthesia in the near future.

Possible Side-Effects   (natural, expected and unavoidable drug actions)
Drowsiness, blurred vision, dry mouth, constipation, impaired urination.

▷ **Possible Adverse Effects**   (unusual, unexpected and infrequent reactions)
If any of the following develop, consult your physician promptly.
Mild Adverse Effects
Allergic Reactions: Skin rash, hives, swellings, drug fever (see Glossary).
Insomnia, nervousness, palpitations, dizziness, unsteadiness, tremors, fainting.
Peculiar taste, indigestion, nausea, vomiting.
Altered libido, breast enlargement, milk formation.
Serious Adverse Effects
Behavioral effects: anxiety, confusion, excitement, disorientation, hallucinations, delusions.
Aggravation of paranoid psychosis and schizophrenia.
Aggravation of epilepsy (seizures).
Altered menstrual pattern, impotence.
Parkinson-like disorders (see Glossary).
Peripheral neuritis (see Glossary)—numbness, tingling, pain, loss of strength in arms and legs.
Reduced white blood cell count—fever, sore throat.

Natural Diseases or Disorders That May Be Activated by This Drug
Latent epilepsy, glaucoma, prostatism.

CAUTION
1. The dosage of this drug must be adjusted carefully for each person individually. This requires observation of symptom improvement and, in some instances, the measurement of drug levels in the blood.
2. Observe for early indications of toxicity: confusion, agitation, rapid heartbeat.
3. It is advisable to withhold this drug if electroconvulsive therapy (ECT, "shock" treatment) is to be used.

Precautions for Use

By Infants and Children: Safety and effectiveness for use by those under 16 years of age have not been established.

By Those over 60 Years of Age: During the first 2 weeks of treatment, observe for the development of confusion, restlessness, agitation, forgetfulness, disorientation, delusions and hallucinations. Reduction of dosage or discontinuation may be necessary. Observe for unsteadiness that may predispose to falling and injury. This drug can increase the degree of impaired urination associated with prostate gland enlargement (prostatism). It is advisable to take the total dose at bedtime to reduce the risk of postural hypotension (see Glossary).

▷ **Advisability of Use During Pregnancy**

Pregnancy Category: C (tentative). See Pregnancy Code inside back cover.

Animal studies: Reveal toxic effects on the embryo in rats and rabbits but no birth defects in the newborn.

Human studies: Information from adequate studies in pregnant women is not available.

Avoid drug during first 3 months.

Advisability of Use if Breast-Feeding

Presence of this drug in breast milk: Yes, in small amounts.

Monitor nursing infant closely and discontinue drug or nursing if adverse effects develop.

Habit-Forming Potential: None.

Effects of Overdosage: Confusion, hallucinations, marked drowsiness, tremors, dilated pupils, cold skin, stupor, coma, convulsions, rapid heartbeat, low blood pressure.

Suggested Periodic Examinations While Taking This Drug   (at physician's discretion)

Complete blood cell counts, serial blood pressure readings and electrocardiograms.

▷ **While Taking This Drug, Observe the Following**

Foods: No restrictions. Drug may increase appetite and cause excessive weight gain.

Beverages: No restrictions. May be taken with milk.

▷   *Alcohol*: Avoid completely. This drug can markedly increase the intoxicating effects of alcohol and accentuate its depressant action on brain function.

Tobacco Smoking: May hasten the elimination of this drug. Higher doses may be necessary.

▷   *Other Drugs*

Amoxapine may *increase* the effects of

• atropinelike drugs (see Drug Class, Section Four).

Amoxapine may *decrease* the effects of

• clonidine (Catapres).

• guanethidine (Ismelin).

Amoxapine *taken concurrently* with
- monoamine oxidase (MAO) inhibitor drugs may cause high fever, delirium and convulsions (see Drug Class, Section Four).
- thyroid preparations may impair heart rhythm and function. Ask physician for guidance regarding adjustment of thyroid dose.

▷ *Driving, Hazardous Activities*: This drug may impair mental alertness, judgment, physical coordination and reaction time. Avoid hazardous activities.

Aviation Note: The use of this drug *is a disqualification* for piloting. Consult a designated Aviation Medical Examiner.

Exposure to Sun: Use caution until sensitivity to sun has been determined. This drug may cause photosensitivity (see Glossary).

Exposure to Heat: This drug can inhibit sweating and impair the body's adaptation to hot environments, increasing the risk of heat stroke. Avoid saunas.

Exposure to Cold: The elderly should use caution and avoid conditions conducive to hypothermia (see Glossary).

Discontinuation: It is advisable to discontinue this drug gradually. Abrupt withdrawal after long-term use can cause headache, malaise and nausea.

AMOXICILLIN
(a mox i SIL in)

Introduced: 1969

Class: Antibiotic, Penicillins

Prescription: USA: Yes
    Canada: Yes

Controlled Drug: USA: No
    Canada: No

Available as Generic: USA: Yes
    Canada: No

Brand Names: Amoxil, Augmentin [CD], ✚Clavulin, Larotid, ✚Novamoxin, Polymox, Sumox, Trimox, Utimox, Wymox

---

BENEFITS versus RISKS

Possible Benefits	*Possible Risks*
EFFECTIVE TREATMENT OF INFECTIONS due to susceptible microorganisms	ALLERGIC REACTIONS, mild to severe, in 3% of the general population and 15% of allergic individuals Superinfections (yeast) Drug-induced colitis

---

▷ **Principal Uses**

As a Single Drug Product: To treat certain infections of the skin and soft tissues; of the ear, nose and throat; and of the genitourinary tract, including gonorrhea.

How This Drug Works: This drug destroys susceptible infecting bacteria by interfering with their ability to produce new protective cell walls as they multiply and grow.

Available Dosage Forms and Strengths

Capsules — 250 mg, 500 mg
Chewable tablets — 125 mg, 250 mg
Oral suspension — 125 mg, 250 mg per teaspoonful (5 ml)
Pediatric drops — 50 mg per ml

▷ **Usual Adult Dosage Range:**   250 to 500 mg/8 hrs. The usual maximal dose is 4500 mg/24 hrs. **Note: Actual dosage and administration schedule must be determined by the physician for each patient individually.**

▷ **Dosing Instructions:**   May be taken on an empty stomach or with food, milk, fruit juice, ginger ale or other cold drinks. Capsule may be opened for administration.

Usual Duration of Use: For all streptococcal infections—not less than 10 consecutive days (without interruption) to reduce the possibility of developing rheumatic fever or glomerulonephritis. For all other infections—as long as necessary to eradicate the infection.

▷ **This Drug Should Not Be Taken If**
- you have had an allergic reaction to any dosage form of it previously.
- you are certain you are allergic to *any* form of penicillin.

▷ **Inform Your Physician Before Taking This Drug If**
- you suspect you may be allergic to penicillin or you have a history of a previous "reaction" to penicillin.
- you are allergic to cephalosporin antibiotics (Ancef, Ceporan, Ceporex, Kafocin, Keflex, Keflin, Kefzol, Loridine).
- you are allergic by nature (hay fever, asthma, hives, eczema).

Possible Side-Effects   (natural, expected and unavoidable drug actions)
Superinfections (see Glossary), often due to yeast organisms.

▷ **Possible Adverse Effects**   (unusual, unexpected and infrequent reactions)
If any of the following develop, consult your physician promptly.
Mild Adverse Effects
Allergic Reactions: Skin rashes, hives, itching.
Irritations of mouth and tongue, "black tongue," nausea, vomiting, mild diarrhea, dizziness (rare).
Serious Adverse Effects
Allergic Reactions: Anaphylactic reaction (see Glossary), severe skin reactions, drug fever, swollen painful joints, sore throat, abnormal bleeding or bruising.

CAUTION
1. Take the exact dose and the full course prescribed.
2. This drug should not be used concurrently with antibiotics like erythromycin or tetracycline.

Precautions for Use

By Infants and Children: A generalized rash occurs in approximately 90% of individuals who take this drug during an episode of infectious mononucleosis. This drug may cause diarrhea, which sometimes necessitates discontinuation.

By Those over 60 Years of Age: Natural changes in the skin may predispose to prolonged itching reactions in the genital and anal regions. Report such reactions promptly.

▷ **Advisability of Use During Pregnancy**

Pregnancy Category: B (tentative). See Pregnancy Code inside back cover.
Animal studies: No information available.
Human studies: Information from adequate studies in pregnant women indicates no increased risk of birth defects in 3546 pregnancies exposed to penicillin derivatives.
Ask physician for guidance.

Advisability of Use if Breast-Feeding

Presence of this drug in breast milk: Probably yes.
The nursing infant may be sensitized to penicillin.
Avoid drug if possible or refrain from nursing.

Habit-Forming Potential: None.

Effects of Overdosage: Possible nausea, vomiting and/or diarrhea.

Possible Effects of Long-Term Use: Superinfections, often due to yeast organisms.

Suggested Periodic Examinations While Taking This Drug   (at physician's discretion)
Complete blood cell counts.

▷ **While Taking This Drug, Observe the Following**

Foods: No restrictions.
Beverages: No restrictions. May be taken with milk, fruit juices or carbonated drinks.

▷ *Alcohol*: No interactions expected.

Tobacco Smoking: No interactions expected.

▷ *Other Drugs*

Amoxicillin may *decrease* the effects of
• oral contraceptives in some women, and impair their effectiveness in preventing pregnancy.
The following drugs may *decrease* the effects of amoxicillin
• antacids reduce the absorption of amoxicillin.
• chloramphenicol (Chloromycetin).
• erythromycin (Erythrocin, E-Mycin, etc.).
• tetracyclines (Achromycin, Declomycin, Minocin, etc.). (See Drug Class, Section Four.)

▷ *Driving, Hazardous Activities*: Usually no restrictions. Be alert to the rare occurrence of dizziness and/or nausea, and restrict activities accordingly.

Aviation Note: The use of this drug *may be a disqualification* for piloting. Consult a designated Aviation Medical Examiner.

Exposure to Sun: No restrictions.

Special Storage Instructions: Oral suspension and pediatric drops should be refrigerated.

Observe the Following Expiration Times: Do not take the oral suspension or drops of this drug if older than 7 days when kept at room temperature or 14 days when kept refrigerated.

AMPICILLIN
(am pi SIL in)

Introduced: 1961

Prescription: USA: Yes
Canada: Yes

Class: Antibiotic, Penicillins

Controlled Drug: USA: No
Canada: No

Available as Generic: Yes

Brand Names: Amcill, ✦Ampicin, ✦Ampilean, ✦Novo-Ampicillin, Omnipen, ✦Penbritin, Polycillin, Polycillin-PRB [CD], Principen, SK-Ampicillin, Supen, Totacillin

---

BENEFITS versus RISKS

Possible Benefits	*Possible Risks*
EFFECTIVE TREATMENT OF INFECTIONS due to susceptible microorganisms	ALLERGIC REACTIONS, mild to severe, in 3% of the general population and 15% of allergic individuals Superinfections (yeast) Drug-induced colitis

---

▷ **Principal Uses**

As a Single Drug Product: To treat certain infections of the skin and soft tissues, of the respiratory tract, of the gastrointestinal tract, and of the genitourinary tract (including gonorrhea in females). Also used to treat certain types of septicemia and meningitis.

As a Combination Drug Product [CD]: May be combined with probenecid (Benemid) to delay the elimination of ampicillin by the kidney and thereby increase its level in the blood. This combination drug is designed primarily for the treatment of gonorrhea in males and females.

How This Drug Works: This drug destroys susceptible infecting bacteria by interfering with their ability to produce new protective cell walls as they multiply and grow.

Available Dosage Forms and Strengths
Capsules — 250 mg, 500 mg

Oral suspension — 125 mg, 250 mg, 500 mg per teaspoonful (5 ml)
Pediatric drops — 100 mg per ml

▷ **Usual Adult Dosage Range:** 250 to 500 mg/6 hrs. The usual maximal dose is 6000 mg/24 hrs. **Note: Actual dosage and administration schedule must be determined by the physician for each patient individually.**

▷ **Dosing Instructions:** Best taken on an empty stomach, 1 hour before or 2 hours after eating. Capsule may be opened for administration.

Usual Duration of Use: For all streptococcal infections—not less than 10 consecutive days (without interruption) to reduce the possibility of developing rheumatic fever or glomerulonephritis. For all other infections—as long as necessary to eradicate the infection.

▷ **This Drug Should Not Be Taken If**
• you have had an allergic reaction to any dosage form of it previously.
• you are certain you are allergic to *any* form of penicillin.

▷ **Inform Your Physician Before Taking This Drug If**
• you suspect you may be allergic to penicillin or you have a history of a previous "reaction" to penicillin.
• you are allergic to cephalosporin antibiotics (Ancef, Ceporan, Ceporex, Kafocin, Keflex, Keflin, Kefzol, Loridine).
• you are allergic by nature (hay fever, asthma, hives, eczema).

Possible Side-Effects (natural, expected and unavoidable drug actions)
Superinfections (see Glossary), often due to yeast organisms.

▷ **Possible Adverse Effects** (unusual, unexpected and infrequent reactions)
If any of the following develop, consult your physician promptly.
Mild Adverse Effects
Allergic Reactions: Skin rashes, hives, itching.
Irritations of mouth and tongue, "black tongue," nausea, vomiting, mild diarrhea, dizziness (rare).
Serious Adverse Effects
Allergic Reactions: Anaphylactic reaction (see Glossary), severe skin reactions, drug fever, swollen painful joints, sore throat, abnormal bleeding or bruising.

CAUTION
1. Take the exact dose and the full course prescribed.
2. This drug should not be used concurrently with antibiotics like erythromycin or tetracycline.

Precautions for Use
By Infants and Children: A generalized rash occurs in approximately 90% of individuals who take this drug during an episode of infectious mononucleosis. This drug may cause diarrhea, which sometimes necessitates discontinuation.
By Those over 60 Years of Age: Natural changes in the skin may predispose to

prolonged itching reactions in the genital and anal regions. Report such reactions promptly.

▷ **Advisability of Use During Pregnancy**
Pregnancy Category: B (tentative). See Pregnancy Code inside back cover.
Animal studies: No birth defects due to this drug found in mice or rats.
Human studies: Information from adequate studies in pregnant women indicates no increased risk of birth defects in 3546 pregnancies exposed to penicillin derivatives.
Ask physician for guidance.

Advisability of Use if Breast-Feeding
Presence of this drug in breast milk: Yes, in small amounts.
The nursing infant may be sensitized to penicillin.
Avoid drug if possible or refrain from nursing.

Habit-Forming Potential: None.

Effects of Overdosage: Possible nausea, vomiting and/or diarrhea.

Possible Effects of Long-Term Use: Superinfections, often due to yeast organisms.

Suggested Periodic Examinations While Taking This Drug   (at physician's discretion)
Complete blood cell counts.

▷ **While Taking This Drug, Observe the Following**
Foods: No restrictions.
Beverages: No restrictions. May be taken with milk.
▷   *Alcohol*: No interactions expected.
Tobacco Smoking: No interactions expected.
▷   *Other Drugs*
Ampicillin may *decrease* the effects of
• oral contraceptives in some women, and impair their effectiveness in preventing pregnancy.
The following drugs may *decrease* the effects of ampicillin
• antacids reduce the absorption of amoxicillin.
• chloramphenicol (Chloromycetin).
• erythromycin (Erythrocin, E-Mycin, etc.).
• tetracyclines (Achromycin, Declomycin, Minocin, etc.). (See Drug Class, Section Four.)
▷   *Driving, Hazardous Activities*: Usually no restrictions. Be alert to the rare occurrence of dizziness and/or nausea, and restrict activities accordingly.
Aviation Note: The use of this drug *may be a disqualification* for piloting. Consult a designated Aviation Medical Examiner.
Exposure to Sun: No restrictions.
Special Storage Instructions: Oral suspension and pediatric drops should be refrigerated.
Observe the Following Expiration Times: Do not take the oral suspension or drops of this drug if older than 7 days when kept at room temperature or 14 days when kept refrigerated.

ASPIRIN*
(AS pir in)

Other Names: ASA, Acetylsalicylic Acid

Introduced: 1899

Class: Mild Analgesic, Anti-inflammatory, Antipyretic, Salicylates

Prescription: USA: No   Canada: No

Controlled Drug: USA: No   Canada: No

Available as Generic: Yes

Brand Names: A.S.A., Aspergum, ✤Aspirin*, Aspirjen, Jr., ✤Astrin, Bayer Aspirin, Bayer Timed Release Aspirin, Easprin, Ecotrin Preparations, Empirin, ✤Entrophen, Excedrin, Measurin, ✤Novasen, ✤Sal-Adult, ✤Sal-Infant, Stanback Max-Extra Strength, St. Joseph Children's Aspirin, ✤Supasa, ✤Triaphen-10

OTC Preparations Containing Aspirin: Alka-Seltzer Plus [CD], Alka-Seltzer Effervescent Pain Reliever and Antacid [CD], Anacin [CD], Anacin Maximum Strength [CD], Ascriptin [CD], Ascriptin A/D [CD], Bufferin [CD], Bufferin, Arthritis Strength [CD], Bufferin, Extra Strength [CD], Cama Arthritis Pain Reliever [CD], Cope [CD], 4-Way Cold Tablets [CD], Midol Caplets [CD], Midol Maximum Strength Caplets [CD], Stanback Analgesic Powders [CD], Synalgos [CD], Vanquish [CD]

BENEFITS versus RISKS

Possible Benefits	*Possible Risks*
EFFECTIVE RELIEF OF MILD TO MODERATE PAIN and INFLAMMATION	Stomach irritation, bleeding, and/or ulceration
REDUCTION OF FEVER	Hearing loss
PREVENTION OF BLOOD CLOTS (as in heart attack, phlebitis and stroke)	Decreased numbers of white blood cells and platelets
	Hemolytic anemia

▷ **Principal Uses**

As a Single Drug Product: To relieve mild to moderate pain from any cause, to provide symptomatic relief in conditions characterized by inflammation and to reduce high fever. A major use is to treat musculoskeletal disorders, especially acute and chronic arthritis. It is also used selectively in low dosage to prevent platelet embolism to the brain (in men) and to reduce the risk of thromboembolism in patients recovering from a recent heart attack, in those with artificial heart valves and in those undergoing hip surgery. (See Blood Platelets in the Glossary.)

*In the United States *aspirin* is an official generic designation. In Canada *Aspirin* is the Registered Trade Mark of the Bayer Company Division of Sterling Drug Limited.

As a Combination Drug Product [CD]: Frequently combined with other mild or strong analgesic drugs to enhance pain relief. Also combined with antihistamines and decongestants in many cold preparations to relieve the headache and general discomfort that often accompany respiratory infections.

How This Drug Works: Aspirin reduces the tissue concentrations of prostaglandins, chemicals involved in the production of inflammation and pain. By modifying the temperature-regulating center in the brain, dilating blood vessels in the skin, and increasing sweating, aspirin hastens the loss of body heat and reduces fever. By preventing the production of thromboxane in blood platelets, aspirin inhibits the aggregation of platelets and the initiation of blood clots.

Available Dosage Forms and Strengths

                Capsules — 325 mg, 500 mg

           Gum tablets — 227.5 mg

        Suppositories — 60 mg, 130 mg, 195 mg, 300 mg, 325 mg, 600 mg, 650 mg, 1.2 g

                Tablets — 65 mg, 81 mg, 325 mg, 487.5 mg, 500 mg, 650 mg

      Tablets, chewable — 81 mg

   Tablets, enteric-coated — 325 mg, 487.5 mg, 500 mg, 650 mg, 975 mg

 Tablets, prolonged-action — 650 mg, 800 mg

▷ **Usual Adult Dosage Range:**   For pain or fever—325 to 650 mg/4 hrs as needed. For arthritis (and related conditions)—3600 to 5400 mg daily in divided doses. For the prevention of blood clots—80 to 150 mg/24 to 48 hrs. **Note: For long-term use, actual dosage and administration schedule must be determined by the physician for each patient individually.**

▷ **Dosing Instructions:**   Take with food, milk, or a full glass of water to reduce stomach irritation. Regular tablets may be crushed and capsules opened for administration. Enteric-coated tablets, prolonged-action tablets, A.S.A. Enseals, Cama tablets and Ecotrin tablets should not be crushed.

Usual Duration of Use: Short-term use is recommended—3 to 5 days. Daily use should not exceed 10 days without physician supervision. Continual use on a regular schedule for 1 week is usually necessary to determine this drug's effectiveness in relieving the symptoms of chronic arthritis.

▷ **This Drug Should Not Be Taken If**
- you have had an allergic reaction or unfavorable response to any form of aspirin previously.
- you have any type of bleeding disorder (such as hemophilia).
- you have active peptic ulcer disease.
- it has an odor resembling vinegar. This is due to the presence of acetic acid and indicates the decomposition of aspirin.

▷ **Inform Your Physician Before Taking This Drug If**
- you are taking any anticoagulant drug.

- you are taking oral antidiabetic drugs.
- you have a history of peptic ulcer disease or gout.
- you have lupus erythematosus.
- you are pregnant or planning pregnancy.
- you plan to have surgery of any kind in the near future.

Possible Side-Effects   (natural, expected and unavoidable drug actions)
Mild drowsiness in sensitive individuals.

▷ **Possible Adverse Effects**   (unusual, unexpected and infrequent reactions)
If any of the following develop, consult your physician promptly.
Mild Adverse Effects
Allergic Reactions: Skin rash, hives, nasal discharge (resembling hay fever), nasal polyps.
Stomach irritation, heartburn, nausea, vomiting, constipation.
Serious Adverse Effects
Allergic Reactions: Acute anaphylactic reaction (see Glossary), asthma, unusual bruising due to allergic destruction of blood platelets (see Glossary).
Idiosyncratic Reactions: Hemolytic anemia (see Glossary).
Erosion of stomach lining, with silent bleeding.
Activation of peptic ulcer, with or without hemorrhage.
Bone marrow depression (see Glossary)—fatigue, weakness, fever, sore throat, abnormal bleeding or bruising.
Hepatitis with jaundice (see Glossary)—yellow skin and eyes, dark-colored urine, light-colored stool (very rare).
Kidney damage, if used in large doses or for a prolonged period of time.

▷ **Adverse Effects That May Mimic Natural Diseases or Disorders**
Liver damage may suggest viral hepatitis.

CAUTION
1. It is most important to understand that aspirin is a drug. While it is one of our most useful drugs, we have an unrealistic sense of safety and unconcern regarding its action within the body and its potential for adverse effects.
2. In order to know if you are taking aspirin, make it a point to learn the contents of all drugs you take—those prescribed by your physician and those you purchase over-the-counter (OTC) without prescription.
3. Limit the dose of aspirin to no more than 3 tablets (975 mg) at one time, allow at least 4 hours between doses and take no more than 10 tablets (3250 mg) in 24 hours without physician supervision.
4. Remember that aspirin can
   - cause new illnesses.
   - complicate existing illnesses.
   - complicate pregnancy.
   - complicate surgery.
   - interact unfavorably with other drugs.
5. When your physician asks "Are you taking any drugs?" the answer is

yes if you are taking aspirin. This also applies to *any* nonprescription drug you may be taking. (See OTC drugs in the Glossary.)

Precautions for Use

By Infants and Children: Reye syndrome (brain and liver damage in children, often fatal) can follow flu or chicken pox in children and teenagers. While the exact cause and nature of the syndrome are not known, some reports suggest that the use of aspirin by children with flu or chicken pox can increase the risk of developing this complication. Consult your physician before giving aspirin to a child or teenager with chicken pox, flu or similar infection.

Usual dosage schedule for children:

Up to 2 years of age—consult physician.

2 to 4 years of age—160 mg/4 hrs, up to 5 doses/24 hrs.

4 to 6 years of age—240 mg/4 hrs, up to 5 doses/24 hrs.

6 to 9 years of age—320 mg/4 hrs, up to 5 doses/24 hrs.

9 to 11 years of age—400 mg/4 hrs, up to 5 doses/24 hrs.

11 to 12 years of age—480 mg/4 hrs, up to 5 doses/24 hrs.

Do not exceed 5 days of continual use without consulting your physician.

Give all doses with food, milk or a full glass of water.

By Those over 60 Years of Age: The natural decline in kidney function can reduce your tolerance for aspirin. Observe for indications of excessive dosage: nervous irritabilty, confusion, ringing in the ears, deafness, loss of appetite, nausea and stomach irritation. Aspirin can cause excessive bleeding from the stomach in sensitive individuals. This can occur as "silent" bleeding of small amounts over an extended period of time, resulting in anemia. In addition, sudden hemorrhage can occur, even without a history of stomach ulcer. Observe stools for gray to black discoloration—an indication of stomach bleeding.

▷ **Advisability of Use During Pregnancy**

Pregnancy Category: B (tentative). See Pregnancy Code inside back cover.

Animal studies: Significant birth defects due to this drug have been reported.

Human studies: Information from studies in pregnant women indicates no increased risk of birth defects in 32,164 pregnancies exposed to aspirin. However, studies show that the regular use of salicylates during pregnancy is often detrimental to the health of the mother and to the welfare of the infant. Excessive use of salicylate drugs can cause anemia, hemorrhage before and after delivery and an increased incidence of stillbirths. It is advisable to limit the use of aspirin during pregnancy to small doses and for brief periods of time, and to avoid aspirin altogether during the last 3 months.

Advisability of Use if Breast-Feeding

Presence of this drug in breast milk: Yes.

Avoid drug or refrain from nursing.

Habit-Forming Potential: Use of this drug in large doses for a prolonged period of time may cause a form of psychological dependence (see Glossary).

Effects of Overdosage: Stomach distress, nausea, vomiting, ringing in the ears, dizziness, impaired hearing, sweating, stupor, fever, deep and rapid breathing, muscular twitching, delirium, hallucinations, convulsions.

Possible Effects of Long-Term Use
A form of psychological dependence (see Glossary).
Anemia due to chronic blood loss from erosion of stomach lining.
The development of stomach ulcer.
The development of "aspirin allergy"—nasal discharge, nasal polyps, asthma.
Kidney damage.
Excessive prolongation of bleeding time, of major importance in the event of injury or surgery.

Suggested Periodic Examinations While Taking This Drug (at physician's discretion)
Complete blood cell counts.
Kidney function tests and urine analyses.
Liver function tests.

▷ **While Taking This Drug, Observe the Following**
Foods: No restrictions.
Nutritional Support: If supplementing the diet with vitamin C, take no more than the recommended daily allowance. Do not take large doses of vitamin C while taking aspirin on a regular basis.
Beverages: No restrictions. May be taken with milk.
▷ *Alcohol*: No interactions expected. However, the concurrent use of alcohol and aspirin may significantly increase the possibility of erosion and ulceration of the stomach lining and may result in bleeding.
Tobacco Smoking: No interactions expected.
▷ *Other Drugs*
Aspirin may *increase* the effects of
- oral anticoagulants, and cause abnormal bleeding. Dosage adjustment is often necessary.
- oral antidiabetic drugs and insulin, and cause hypoglycemia (see Glossary). Dosage adjustment is often necessary.
- heparin, and cause abnormal bleeding.
- methotrexate, and increase its toxic effects.
- valproic acid (Depakene).
Aspirin may *decrease* the effects of
- beta-adrenergic blocking drugs (see Drug Class, Section Four).
- captopril (Capoten).
- probenecid (Benemid), and reduce its effectiveness in the treatment of gout—with aspirin doses of less than 2 grams/24 hrs.
- spironolactone (Aldactone), and reduce its diuretic effect.

- sulfinpyrazone (Anturane), and reduce its effectiveness in the treatment of gout—with aspirin doses of less than 2 grams/24 hrs.

The following drugs may *increase* the effects of aspirin

- acetazolamide (Diamox).
- para-aminobenzoic acid (Pabalate).
- vitamin C, taken as ascorbic acid and in large doses, may acidify the urine in some individuals and cause aspirin accumulation and toxicity.

The following drugs may *decrease* the effects of aspirin

- antacids, in regular continual use.
- cortisonelike drugs (see Drug Class, Section Four).
- urinary alkalizers (sodium bicarbonate, sodium citrate).

▷ *Driving, Hazardous Activities*: No restrictions or precautions.

Aviation Note: Usually no restrictions. However, it is advisable to observe for the possible occurrence of mild drowsiness and to restrict activities accordingly.

Exposure to Sun: No restrictions.

Discontinuation: The use of aspirin should be discontinued completely at least 1 week before surgery of any kind.

ATENOLOL
(a TEN oh lohl)

Introduced: 1973

Class: Antihypertensive, Beta-Adrenergic Blocker

Prescription: USA: Yes
Canada: Yes

Controlled Drug: USA: No
Canada: No

Available as Generic: No

Brand Names: Tenoretic [CD], Tenormin

BENEFITS versus RISKS	
Possible Benefits	*Possible Risks*
EFFECTIVE, WELL-TOLERATED ANTIHYPERTENSIVE in mild to moderate high blood pressure	CONGESTIVE HEART FAILURE in advanced heart disease Worsening of angina in coronary heart disease (abrupt withdrawal) Masking of low blood sugar (hypoglycemia) in drug-treated diabetes Provocation of bronchial asthma (with high doses)

▷ **Principal Uses**

As a Single Drug Product: The treatment of mild to moderately severe high blood pressure. May be used alone or concurrently with other antihypertensive drugs, such as diuretics.

How This Drug Works: By blocking certain actions of the sympathetic nervous system, this drug
- reduces the rate and contraction force of the heart, thus lowering the ejection pressure of the blood leaving the heart.
- reduces the degree of contraction of blood vessel walls, resulting in their relaxation and expansion and consequent lowering of blood pressure.

Available Dosage Forms and Strengths
Tablets — 50 mg, 100 mg

▷ **Usual Adult Dosage Range:**   Initially 50 mg once daily. Dose may be increased gradually at intervals of 7 to 10 days as needed and tolerated up to 100 mg/24 hrs. The usual maintenance dose is 50 to 100 mg/24 hrs. The total dose should not exceed 100 mg/24 hrs. **Note: Actual dosage and administration schedule must be determined by the physician for each patient individually.**

▷ **Dosing Instructions:**   May be taken without regard to eating. Tablet may be crushed for administration. Do not discontinue this drug abruptly.

Usual Duration of Use: Continual use on a regular schedule for 10 to 14 days is usually necessary to determine this drug's effectiveness in lowering blood pressure. The long-term use of this drug will be determined by the course of your blood pressure over time and your response to the overall treatment program (weight reduction, salt restriction, smoking cessation, etc.)

▷ **This Drug Should Not Be Taken If**
- you have had an allergic reaction to it previously.
- you have congestive heart failure.
- you have an abnormally slow heart rate or a serious form of heart block.
- you are taking, or have taken within the past 14 days, any monoamine oxidase (MAO) inhibitor drug (see Drug Class, Section Four).

▷ **Inform Your Physician Before Taking This Drug If**
- you have had an adverse reaction to any "beta-blocker" drug in the past (see Drug Class, Section Four).
- you have a history of serious heart disease, with or without episodes of heart failure.
- you have a history of hay fever (allergic rhinitis), asthma, chronic bronchitis or emphysema.
- you have a history of overactive thyroid function (hyperthyroidism).
- you have a history of low blood sugar (hypoglycemia).
- you have impaired liver or kidney function.
- you have diabetes or myasthenia gravis.

- you are currently taking any form of digitalis, quinidine or reserpine, or any "calcium-blocker" drug (see Drug Class, Section Four).
- you plan to have surgery under general anesthesia in the near future.

Possible Side-Effects   (natural, expected and unavoidable drug actions)

Lethargy, fatigability, cold extremities, slow heart rate, lightheadedness in upright position (see orthostatic hypotension in Glossary).

▷ **Possible Adverse Effects**   (unusual, unexpected and infrequent reactions)

If any of the following develop, consult your physician promptly.

Mild Adverse Effects

Allergic Reactions: Skin rash, itching.

Headache, dizziness, drowsiness, abnormal dreams.

Indigestion, nausea, diarrhea.

Joint and muscle discomfort, fluid retention (edema).

Serious Adverse Effects

Mental depression, anxiety, impotence.

Chest pain, shortness of breath, precipitation of congestive heart failure.

Induction of bronchial asthma (in asthmatic individuals).

CAUTION

1. *Do not discontinue this drug suddenly* without the knowledge and guidance of your physician. Carry a notation on your person that you are taking this drug.
2. Consult your physician or pharmacist before using nasal decongestants usually present in over-the-counter cold preparations and nose drops. These can cause sudden increases in blood pressure when taken concurrently with beta-blocker drugs.
3. Report the development of any tendency to emotional depression.

Precautions for Use

By Infants and Children: Safety and effectiveness for use by those under 12 years of age have not been established. However, if this drug is used, observe for the development of low blood sugar (hypoglycemia) during periods of reduced food intake.

By Those over 60 Years of Age: Proceed *cautiously* with all antihypertensive drugs. Unacceptably high blood pressure should be reduced without creating the risks associated with excessively low blood pressure. Start treatment with small doses, and monitor the blood pressure response frequently. Sudden, rapid and excessive reduction of blood pressure can predispose to stroke or heart attack. Total daily dosage should not exceed 100 mg. Observe for dizziness, unsteadiness, tendency to fall, confusion, hallucinations, depression or urinary frequency.

▷ **Advisability of Use During Pregnancy**

Pregnancy Category: C (tentative). See Pregnancy Code inside back cover.

Animal studies: Increased resorptions of embryo and fetus reported in rats, but no birth defects.

Human studies: Information from adequate studies in pregnant women is not available.

Avoid use of drug during the first 3 months if possible. Avoid use during labor and delivery because of the possible effects on the newborn infant.

Advisability of Use if Breast-Feeding
Presence of this drug in breast milk: Yes.
Avoid drug if possible. If drug is necessary, observe nursing infant for slow heart rate and indications of low blood sugar.

Habit-Forming Potential: None.

Effects of Overdosage: Weakness, slow pulse, low blood pressure, fainting, cold and sweaty skin, congestive heart failure, possible coma and convulsions.

Possible Effects of Long-Term Use: Reduced heart reserve and eventual heart failure in susceptible individuals with advanced heart disease.

Suggested Periodic Examinations While Taking This Drug   (at physician's discretion)
Measurements of blood pressure, evaluation of heart function.

▷ **While Taking This Drug, Observe the Following**
Foods: No restrictions. Avoid excessive salt intake.
Beverages: No restrictions. May be taken with milk.
▷   *Alcohol*: Use with caution until the combined effect has been determined. Alcohol may exaggerate this drug's ability to lower blood pressure and may increase its mild sedative effect.
Tobacco Smoking: Nicotine may reduce this drug's effectiveness in treating high blood pressure. In addition, high doses of this drug may potentiate the constriction of the bronchial tubes caused by regular smoking.
▷   *Other Drugs*
Atenolol may *increase* the effects of
- other antihypertensive drugs and cause excessive lowering of blood pressure. Dosage adjustments may be necessary.
- reserpine (Ser-Ap-Es, etc.) and cause sedation, depression, slowing of heart rate and lowering of blood pressure.
Atenolol *taken concurrently* with
- clonidine (Catapres) requires close monitoring for rebound high blood pressure if clonidine is withdrawn while atenolol is still being taken.
- insulin requires close monitoring to avoid undetected hypoglycemia (see Glossary).
The following drugs may *decrease* the effects of atenolol
- indomethacin (Indocin), and possibly other "aspirin substitutes," may impair atenolol's antihypertensive effect.
▷   *Driving, Hazardous Activities*: Use caution until the full extent of drowsiness, lethargy, and blood pressure change has been determined.
Aviation Note: The use of this drug *is a disqualification* for piloting. Consult a designated Aviation Medical Examiner.
Exposure to Sun: No restrictions.
Exposure to Heat: Caution advised. Hot environments can lower blood pressure and exaggerate the effects of this drug.

Exposure to Cold: Caution advised. Cold environments can enhance the circulatory deficiency in the extremities that may occur with this drug. The elderly should take precautions to prevent hypothermia (see Glossary).

Heavy Exercise or Exertion: It is advisable to avoid exertion that produces lightheadedness, excessive fatigue, or muscle cramping. The use of this drug may intensify the hypertensive response to isometric exercise.

Occurrence of Unrelated Illness: The fever that accompanies systemic infections can lower blood pressure and require adjustment of dosage. Illnesses that cause nausea or vomiting may interrupt the regular dosage schedule. Ask your physician for guidance.

Discontinuation: It is advisable to avoid sudden discontinuation of this drug in all situations. If possible, gradual reduction of dose over a period of 2 to 3 weeks is recommended. Ask your physician for specific guidance.

ATROPINE*
(A troh peen)

Other Names: Belladonna Alkaloids, Hyoscyamine, Scopolamine

Introduced: 1831

Class: Antispasmodic, Atropine-like Drugs, Anticholinergics

Prescription: USA: Yes
Canada: No

Controlled Drug: USA: No
Canada: No

Available as Generic: Yes

Brand Names: Barbidonna [CD], Belladenal [CD], Belladenal-S [CD], ♣Belladenal Spacetabs [CD], Bellergal [CD], Bellergal-S [CD], ♣Bellergal Spacetabs [CD], Butibel [CD], Chardonna-2 [CD], Donnagel [CD], ♣Donnagel w/Neomycin [CD], Donnagel-PG [CD], Donnatal [CD], Donnazyme [CD], Isopto Atropine, Kinesed [CD], Lomotil [CD], ♣SMP Atropine, Urised [CD],

---

BENEFITS versus RISKS

Possible Benefits	*Possible Risks*
EFFECTIVE ANTISPASMODIC ACTION in spastic disorders of the stomach and intestine	Increased internal eye pressure (important in glaucoma) Constipation (may be quite marked) Urinary retention (in predisposed persons)

▷ **Principal Uses**

As a Single Drug Product: Used primarily for its antispasmodic effect in the

---

*Atropine, hyoscyamine, and scopolamine are the principal belladonna alkaloids. The characteristics of atropine are representative of the group.

treatment of spastic disorders of the digestive tract and lower urinary tract.

As a Combination Drug Product [CD]: Frequently combined with mild sedatives (especially barbiturates) to utilize their calming effects in the management of functional disorders associated with anxiety and nervous tension. The combination of a mild tranquilizer and an antispasmodic medication is more effective than either drug used alone.

How This Drug Works: By blocking the action of the chemical (acetylcholine) that transmits impulses at parasympathetic nerve endings, this drug prevents stimulation of muscular contraction and glandular secrection within the organs involved. This results in reduced overall activity, including the prevention or relief of muscle spasm.

Available Dosage Forms and Strengths

          Injection — 0.05 mg, 0.1 mg, 0.3 mg, 0.4 mg, 0.5 mg, 1 mg, 1.2 mg, all per ml

          Tablets — 0.4 mg

    Tablets, soluble — 0.3 mg, 0.4 mg, 0.6 mg

▷ **Usual Adult Dosage Range:** 0.3 to 1.2 mg/4 to 6 hrs. **Note: Actual dosage and administration schedule must be determined by the physician for each patient individually.**

▷ **Dosing Instructions:** For maximal absorption and effect, this drug should be taken 30 to 60 minutes before eating. Regular tablets may be crushed and regular capsules may be opened for administration. Prolonged-action and sustained-release dosage forms should be taken whole (neither crushed nor opened).

Usual Duration of Use: Continual use on a regular schedule for 2 to 5 days is usually necessary to determine this drug's effectiveness in relieving the symptoms of spastic disorders of the digestive system. Limit use to the relief of symptoms as necessary. Ask physician for guidance regarding long-term use.

▷ **This Drug Should Not Be Taken If**
- you have had an allergic reaction or unfavorable response to any atropine or belladonna preparation in the past.
- your stomach cannot empty properly into the intestine (pyloric obstruction).
- you are unable to empty the urinary bladder completely.
- you have glaucoma (narrow-angle type).
- you have severe ulcerative colitis.

▷ **Inform Your Physician Before Taking This Drug If**
- you have glaucoma (open-angle type).
- you have angina or coronary heart disease.
- you have chronic bronchitis.
- you have a hiatal hernia or peptic ulcer disease.
- you have enlargement of the prostate gland.

- you have myasthenia gravis.
- you plan to have surgery under general anesthesia in the near future.

Possible Side-Effects   (natural, expected and unavoidable drug actions)
Blurring of near vision (impairment of focus), dryness of mouth and throat, constipation, hesitancy in urination.

▷ **Possible Adverse Effects**   (unusual, unexpected and infrequent reactions)
If any of the following develop, consult your physician promptly.
Mild Adverse Effects
Allergic Reactions: Skin rash, hives.
Lightheadedness, dizziness, unsteadiness.
Dilation of pupils, causing sensitivity to light.
Flushing and dryness of skin, reduced sweating.
Serious Adverse Effects
Allergic Reactions: Severe skin reactions—exfoliative dermatitis.
Idiosyncratic Reactions: Paradoxical excitement, nervousness, confusion, delirium.
Increased internal eye pressure, development of glaucoma in susceptible individuals.

Natural Diseases or Disorders That May Be Activated by This Drug
Latent glaucoma (narrow-angle type), latent myasthenia gravis.

CAUTION
1. Use cautiously in the presence of asthma and chronic bronchitis. This drug can thicken bronchial secretions and promote retention of mucous plugs.
2. Many over-the-counter medications (see OTC Drugs in the Glossary) for allergies, colds and coughs contain antihistamines that can augment this drug's drying effects. Ask your physician or pharmacist for guidance before using such preparations.

Precautions for Use
By Infants and Children: Children are particularly vulnerable to atropine toxicity. Start with low doses and increase cautiously as needed and tolerated. Observe for idiosyncratic reactions consisting of flushing, high fever, agitation, rapid pulse and breathing. Children with Down's syndrome or brain damage are more susceptible to this type of reaction.
By Those over 60 Years of Age: Observe for agitation, confusion, loss of short-term memory, disorientation, visual and auditory hallucinations, delirium. This drug can increase the degree of impaired urination associated with prostate gland enlargement (prostatism).

▷ **Advisability of Use During Pregnancy**
Pregnancy Category: C (tentative). See Pregnancy Code inside back cover.
Animal studies: Birth defects reported in mouse studies.
Human studies: No increase in birth defects reported in 1198 exposures to this drug. Information from adequate studies in pregnant women is not available.
Avoid drug completely during first 3 months.

Advisability of Use if Breast-Feeding
Presence of this drug in breast milk: Yes, in very small amounts.
Monitor nursing infant closely and discontinue drug or nursing if adverse effects develop.

Habit-Forming Potential: None.

Effects of Overdosage: Dilated pupils, blurring of near vision, dryness of mouth and throat, heart palpitation, impaired urination, high fever, hot skin, excitement, confusion, hallucinations, delirium, convulsions, coma.

Possible Effects of Long-Term Use: Chronic constipation, severe enough to result in fecal impaction. (Constipation should be treated promptly with effective laxatives.)

Suggested Periodic Examinations While Taking This Drug   (at physician's discretion)
Measurement of internal eye pressure to detect any significant increase that could indicate developing glaucoma.

▷ **While Taking This Drug, Observe the Following**
Foods: Avoid constipating foods, such as cheeses. Follow the diet prescribed by your physician.
Beverages: Avoid large amounts of tea (may be constipating).
▷ *Alcohol*: No interactions expected.
Tobacco Smoking: No interactions expected.
▷ *Other Drugs*
Atropine may *increase* the effects of
• all other drugs having atropinelike actions (see Drug Class, Section Four).
Atropine may *decrease* the effects of
• haloperidol (Haldol), and reduce its effectiveness.
• phenothiazines (Thorazine, etc.), and reduce their effectiveness.
• pilocarpine eye drops, and reduce their effectiveness in lowering internal eye pressure in the treatment of glaucoma.
▷ *Driving, Hazardous Activities*: This drug may cause drowsiness, dizziness or blurred vision. Avoid hazardous activities if these drug effects occur.
Aviation Note: The use of this drug *is a disqualification* for piloting. Consult a designated Aviation Medical Examiner.
Exposure to Sun: No restrictions.
Exposure to Heat: Use extreme caution. The use of this drug in hot environments may significantly increase the risk of heat stroke.
Heavy Exercise or Exertion: Use caution in warm or hot environments. This drug may impair normal perspiration (heat loss) and interfere with the regulation of body temperature.
Discontinuation: Avoid prolonged and unnecessary use of this drug. When symptoms have been controlled for an adequate period of time, and discontinuation appears possible, reduce the dose gradually over a period of several days.

AURANOFIN
(aw RAY noh fin)

Introduced: 1976

Prescription: USA: Yes
Canada: Yes

Available as Generic: No

Brand Names: Ridaura

Class: Antiarthritic, Gold
Compounds

Controlled Drug: USA: No
Canada: No

BENEFITS versus RISKS

Possible Benefits	*Possible Risks*
REDUCTION OF JOINT PAIN, TENDERNESS AND SWELLING in active, severe RHEUMATOID ARTHRITIS Medication effective when taken by mouth	SIGNIFICANTLY REDUCED LEVELS OF RED AND WHITE BLOOD CELLS AND BLOOD PLATELETS (1 to 3%) LIVER DAMAGE WITH JAUNDICE (less than 0.1%) Diarrhea (47%), ulcerative colitis (less than 0.1%) Skin rash (24%) Mouth sores (13%)

▷ **Principal Uses**

As a Single Drug Product: Used *only* for the treatment of adults with active, severe rheumatoid arthritis who have had an inadequate and disappointing response to aspirin, aspirin substitutes and other antiarthritic drugs and treatment programs. It is usually added to a well-established program of antiarthritic drugs of the aspirin-substitute class.

How This Drug Works: Its method of action is unknown. It suppresses but does not cure arthritis and associated synovitis.

Available Dosage Forms and Strengths

Capsules — 3 mg

▷ **Usual Adult Dosage Range:** 6 mg daily, taken either as one dose every 24 hours or as two doses of 3 mg each every 12 hours. If response is inadequate after 6 months of regular continual use, the dose may be increased to 9 mg daily, taken as 3 doses of 3 mg each. If response remains inadequate after 3 months of 9 mg daily, this drug should be discontinued. **Note: Actual dosage and administration schedule must be determined by the physician for each patient individually.**

▷ **Dosing Instructions:** Take with or following food to reduce stomach irritation. Take the capsule whole with milk or a full glass of water.

Usual Duration of Use: Continual use on a regular schedule for 3 to 4 months is usually necessary to determine this drug's effectiveness in reducing the joint pain, tenderness and swelling associated with rheumatoid arthritis. The extent of long-term use will be determined by the degree of benefit and the pattern of adverse effects experienced by the individual patient.

▷ **This Drug Should Not Be Taken If**
  - you have had an allergic reaction or serious adverse effect from previous use of gold.
  - you have active ulcerative colitis.
  - you have a current blood cell or bone marrow disorder.
  - you have active liver or kidney disease.
  - you are pregnant or breast-feeding.
  - you are taking penicillamine or antimalarial drugs for your arthritis.

▷ **Inform Your Physician Before Taking This Drug If**
  - you are allergic by nature, or have a history of allergic reactions to drugs.
  - you have diabetes.
  - you have a history of heart disease, high blood pressure, circulatory disorders, liver or kidney disease, or ulcerative colitis.
  - you are taking any other drugs at this time.
  - you are planning pregnancy in the near future.

Possible Side-Effects   (natural, expected and unavoidable drug actions)
Metallic taste.

▷ **Possible Adverse Effects**   (unusual, unexpected and infrequent reactions)
  If any of the following develop, consult your physician promptly.
  Mild Adverse Effects
  Allergic Reactions: Itching, skin rash.
  Sores in mouth and throat and on tongue, loss of appetite, nausea, vomiting, stomach cramps, diarrhea.
  Headache, partial or complete hair loss.
  Serious Adverse Effects
  Allergic Reactions: Severe skin reactions, exfoliative dermatitis.
  Fever, cough, shortness of breath, drug-induced pneumonia and lung damage.
  Liver damage with jaundice, ulcerative colitis.
  Kidney damage.
  Blood cell and bone marrow toxicity—fatigue, weakness, sore throat, abnormal bleeding or bruising.
  Peripheral neuritis—pain, numbness, weakness of arms and legs.

Possible Delayed Adverse Effects
  Adverse effects from gold may occur many months after treatment has been discontinued. This is due to accumulation of gold in body tissues and its slow elimination. Report any indications of possible toxicity to your physician promptly.

▷ **Adverse Effects That May Mimic Natural Diseases or Disorders**
  Fever, cough and chest discomfort may suggest respiratory tract infections such as bronchitis or pneumonia.
  Liver damage may suggest viral hepatitis.

CAUTION
1. Periodic examinations (blood and urine tests) are mandatory during the use of this drug. Keep all appointments as directed by your physician.
2. Inform your physician promptly of any indications of possible toxic reactions. If there is a delay in reaching your physician, discontinue this drug until you obtain medical guidance.

Precautions for Use
By Infants and Children: Safety and effectiveness for use by those under 12 years of age have not been established.

By Those over 60 Years of Age: Tolerance to gold usually decreases with advancing age. Use small doses initially and observe closely for indications of adverse effects.

▷ **Advisability of Use During Pregnancy**
Pregnancy Category: C (tentative). See Pregnancy Code inside back cover.

Animal studies: Rabbit studies revealed an increase in resorptions, abortions and birth defects.

Human studies: Information from adequate studies in pregnant women is not available.

The manufacturer does not recommend the use of this drug during pregnancy.

Advisability of Use if Breast-Feeding
Presence of this drug in breast milk: Yes.
Avoid drug or refrain from nursing.

Habit-Forming Potential: None.

Effects of Overdosage: Nausea, vomiting, diarrhea, confusion, delirium, peripheral neuritis.

Suggested Periodic Examinations While Taking This Drug   (at physician's discretion)
Complete blood cell counts, urine analyses, liver and kidney function tests.

▷ **While Taking This Drug, Observe the Following**
Foods: No restrictions.
Beverages: No restrictions. May be taken with milk.
▷   *Alcohol*: Use caution until the combined effects have been determined. Alcohol may intensify the irritant effect of this drug on the gastrointestinal tract.
Tobacco Smoking: No interactions expected.
▷   *Other Drugs*
Auranofin may *increase* the effects of
• phenytoin (Dilantin), by increasing its blood level. Monitor closely for indications of phenytoin toxicity.
▷   *Driving, Hazardous Activities*: Usually no restrictions.

Aviation Note: The use of this drug *may be a disqualification* for piloting. Consult a designated Aviation Medical Examiner.

Exposure to Sun: Use caution. This drug may cause photosensitivity (see Glossary). Avoid sun and sun lamps if a drug-induced rash occurs.

AZATADINE
(a ZA ta deen)

Introduced: 1977

Prescription: USA: Yes
  Canada: Yes

Available as Generic: No

Brand Names: Optimine, Trinalin Repetabs [CD]

Class: Antihistamines

Controlled Drug: USA: No
  Canada: No

BENEFITS versus RISKS

Possible Benefits	*Possible Risks*
EFFECTIVE RELIEF OF ALLERGIC RHINITIS AND ALLERGIC SKIN DISORDERS	Mild sedation Atropinelike effects Rare blood cell disorders: hemolytic anemia, abnormally low white blood cells and platelets

---

▷ **Principal Uses**

As a Single Drug Product: Used primarily to provide symptomatic relief in allergic and related disorders: seasonal and perennial allergic rhinitis (hay fever), allergic conjunctivitis, and vasomotor rhinitis; also in hives and localized swellings (angioedema) of allergic origin.

As a Combination Drug Product [CD]: This drug is combined with a decongestant drug to enhance its ability to reduce tissue swelling and secretions in allergic and infectious disorders of the upper respiratory tract— hay fever, head colds and sinusitis.

How This Drug Works: Antihistamines reduce the intensity of the allergic response by blocking the action of histamine after it has been released from sensitized tissue cells in the eyes, nose and skin.

Available Dosage Forms and Strengths
  Tablets — 1 mg

▷ **Usual Adult Dosage Range:** 1 to 2 mg/12 hrs as needed (twice daily). **Note: Actual dosage and administration schedule must be determined by the physician for each patient individually.**

▷ **Dosing Instructions:**   Take with food or milk to prevent stomach irritation. The prolonged-action (combination) tablet should be swallowed whole (not crushed or chewed).

Usual Duration of Use: Continual use on a regular schedule for 2 to 3 days is usually necessary to determine this drug's effectiveness in relieving the symptoms of allergic rhinitis and dermatosis. It may be necessary to take this drug throughout the entire pollen season, depending upon individual sensitivity. However, antihistamines should not be taken continually (without interruption) for long-term use. Limit their use to periods that require symptomatic relief.

▷ **This Drug Should Not Be Taken If**
- you have had an allergic reaction to any dosage form of it previously.
- you are currently undergoing allergy skin tests.
- you are taking, or have taken within the past 14 days, any monoamine oxidase (MAO) inhibitor drug (see Drug Class, Section Four).

▷ **Inform Your Physician Before Taking This Drug If**
- you have had any allergic reactions or unfavorable responses to the previous use of antihistamines.
- you have glaucoma (narrow-angle type) or asthma.
- you have difficulty emptying the urinary bladder, especially if due to prostate gland enlargement.
- you are taking an anticoagulant at this time.
- you plan to have surgery under general anesthesia in the near future.

Possible Side-Effects   (natural, expected and unavoidable drug actions)
Drowsiness; sense of weakness; blurred vision; dryness of the nose, mouth and throat; impaired urination.

▷ **Possible Adverse Effects**   (unusual, unexpected and infrequent reactions)
If any of the following develop, consult your physician promptly.
Mild Adverse Effects
Allergic Reactions: Skin rash.
Headache, nervous agitation, dizziness, confusion.
Reduced tolerance for contact lenses.
Thickening of bronchial secretions in asthma or bronchitis.
Indigestion, nausea, vomiting.
Serious Adverse Effects
Hemolytic anemia (see Glossary).
Abnormally low white blood cells—fever, sore throat, infections.
Abnormally low blood platelets—abnormal bleeding or bruising.

CAUTION
1. Discontinue this drug 4 days before diagnostic skin testing procedures in order to prevent false negative test results.
2. Do not use this drug if you have active bronchial asthma, bronchitis or pneumonia. It can thicken bronchial mucus and make it more difficult to remove (by absorption or coughing).

Precautions for Use

By Infants and Children: Safety and effectiveness for use by those under 12 years of age have not been established.

By Those over 60 Years of Age: You may be more susceptible to the development of drowsiness, dizziness, and unsteadiness, and to impairment of thinking, judgment and memory. This drug can increase the degree of impaired urination associated with prostate gland enlargement (prostatism).

▷ **Advisability of Use During Pregnancy**

Pregnancy Category: B (tentative). See Pregnancy Code inside back cover.

Animal studies: Reproduction studies in rats and rabbits revealed no increase in birth defects.

Human studies: Information from adequate studies in pregnant women is not available.

Avoid this drug during the last 3 months because of the potential risk for serious adverse effects on the newborn infant.

Advisability of Use if Breast-Feeding

Presence of this drug in breast milk: Unknown.

Avoid drug or refrain from nursing.

Habit-Forming Potential: None.

Effects of Overdosage: Drowsiness; unsteadiness; faintness; marked dryness of mouth, nose and throat; flushing of face; shortness of breath; hallucinations; convulsions.

Possible Effects of Long-Term Use: Tardive dyskinesia (see Glossary) has been reported in association with the long-term use of several widely used antihistamines. It is advisable to avoid the prolonged, continual use of antihistamines without interruption.

Suggested Periodic Examinations While Taking This Drug   (at physician's discretion)

Complete blood cell counts.

▷ **While Taking This Drug, Observe the Following**

Foods: No restrictions.

Beverages: No restrictions. May be taken with milk.

▷   *Alcohol*: Use with extreme caution until the combined effects have been determined. The combination of antihistamine and alcohol can produce rapid and marked sedation.

Tobacco Smoking: No interactions expected.

▷   *Other Drugs*

Azatadine may *increase* the effects of

- all sedatives, sleep-inducing drugs, tranquilizers, analgesics, and narcotic drugs, and produce oversedation.

Azatadine may *decrease* the effects of

- oral anticoagulants (Warfarin, etc.), by hastening their elimination from the body. Consult physician regarding prothrombin time testing and dosage adjustment.

The following drugs may *increase* the effects of azatadine

- monoamine oxidase (MAO) inhibitor drugs (see Drug Class, Section Four) may prolong the action of antihistamines.

▷ *Driving, Hazardous Activities*: This drug can impair mental alertness, judgment, coordination and reaction time. Avoid hazardous activities until the full sedative effects have been determined.

Aviation Note: The use of this drug *may be a disqualification* for piloting. Consult a designated Aviation Medical Examiner.

Exposure to Sun: Use caution. This drug may cause photosensitivity in some individuals (see Glossary).

AZATHIOPRINE
(ay za THI oh preen)

Introduced: 1965

Class: Antiarthritic, Immunosuppressive

Prescription: USA: Yes
Canada: Yes

Controlled Drug: USA: No
Canada: No

Available as Generic: No

Brand Names: Imuran

BENEFITS versus RISKS

Possible Benefits	*Possible Risks*
REDUCTION OF JOINT PAIN, TENDERNESS AND SWELLING in active, severe RHEUMATOID ARTHRITIS (66% of users) PREVENTION OF REJECTION IN ORGAN TRANSPLANTATION	UNACCEPTABLE ADVERSE EFFECTS IN 15% OF USERS REDUCED LEVELS OF WHITE BLOOD CELLS (28% in rheumatoid arthritis 50% in kidney transplants) REDUCED LEVELS OF RED BLOOD CELLS AND PLATELETS LIVER DAMAGE WITH JAUNDICE (less than 1%) POSSIBLE INCREASED RISK OF MALIGNANCY (3%)

▷ **Principal Uses**

As a Single Drug Product: Used primarily as an immunosuppressant to prevent rejection in organ transplantation (mainly kidney transplants). Also used to manage active, severe rheumatoid arthritis (in adults) that has failed to respond adequately to conventional treatment. Progression of the arthritic process may be slowed or even stopped. Lesser uses include treatment of lupus erythematosus, ulcerative colitis, chronic active hepatitis and other "autoimmune" disorders.

How This Drug Works: Not fully known. It is thought that by impairing purine metabolism, blocking production of DNA and RNA, and inhibiting cell multiplication, this drug suppresses the immune reaction that is responsible for such "autoimmune" disorders as rheumatoid arthritis, lupus erythematosus, etc.

Available Dosage Forms and Strengths
   Tablets — 50 mg

▷ **Usual Adult Dosage Range:**   As immunosuppressant—3 to 5 mg/ kilogram of body weight daily, 1 to 3 days before transplantation surgery; for postoperative maintenance—1 to 2 mg/kilogram of body weight daily. As antiarthritic—1 mg/kilogram of body weight daily for 6 to 8 weeks; increase dose by 0.5 mg/kilogram of body weight every 4 weeks as needed and tolerated. Maximal daily dose is 2.5 mg/kilogram of body weight. Total dose may be taken once daily or divided into 2 equal doses taken 12 hours apart. **Note: Actual dosage and administration schedule must be determined by the physician for each patient individually.**

▷ **Dosing Instructions:**   Take with or following food to reduce stomach irritation. Tablet may be crushed for administration.

Usual Duration of Use: Continual use on a regular schedule for 12 weeks is usually necessary to determine this drug's effectiveness in favorably modifying the course of rheumatoid arthritis. This drug has been used successfully for periods of up to 11 years.

▷ **This Drug Should Not Be Taken If**
   • you have had an allergic reaction to it previously.
   • you are pregnant, and this drug is prescribed to treat rheumatoid arthritis.
   • you have an active blood cell or bone marrow disorder.
   • you are taking, or have recently taken, any form of chlorambucil (Leukeran), cyclophosphamide (Cytoxan) or melphalan (Alkeran).

▷ **Inform Your Physician Before Taking This Drug If**
   • you have any kind of active infection.
   • you have any form of cancer.
   • you have gout or are taking allopurinol (Zyloprim).
   • you have a history of blood cell or bone marrow disorders.
   • you have impaired liver or kidney function.
   • you are taking any form of gold, penicillamine or an antimalarial drug for arthritis.
   • you plan pregnancy in the near future.

Possible Side-Effects   (natural, expected and unavoidable drug actions)
   Development of infection (2.4%).

▷ **Possible Adverse Effects**   (unusual, unexpected and infrequent reactions)
   If any of the following develop, consult your physician promptly.

Mild Adverse Effects
Allergic Reactions: Skin rash (2%).
Loss of appetite, nausea, vomiting, diarrhea (19%).
Sores on lips and in mouth.
Serious Adverse Effects
Allergic Reactions: Drug fever (see Glossary), joint and muscle pain. Pancreatitis—severe stomach pain with nausea and vomiting (0.18%).
Bone marrow depression (see Glossary)—fatigue, weakness, fever, sore throat, abnormal bleeding or bruising.
Liver damage—yellow eyes and skin, dark-colored urine, light-colored stools (0.37%). (See Hepatitis and Jaundice in Glossary).
Drug-induced pneumonia—cough, shortness of breath.
Development of cancer—skin cancer, reticulum-cell sarcoma, lymphoma, leukemia (3.3%).

Possible Delayed Adverse Effects
Bone marrow depression may become apparent many weeks after discontinuing this drug.

▷ **Adverse Effects That May Mimic Natural Diseases or Disorders**
Liver damage may suggest viral hepatitis.

CAUTION
1. Report promptly any indications of a developing infection—fever, chills, lip or mouth sores, etc.
2. Inform your physician promptly if you become pregnant.
3. Periodic blood counts are mandatory for the safe use of this drug. Report for examinations as directed.

Precautions for Use
By Infants and Children: Safety and effectiveness for use by those under 12 years of age have not been established.
By Those over 60 Years of Age: To reduce the risk of possible toxic reactions, the minimal effective dose should be determined and maintained.

▷ **Advisability of Use During Pregnancy**
Pregnancy Category: D (tentative). See Pregnancy Code inside back cover.
Animal studies: Birth defects reported in rodent studies.
Human studies: Two incidents of birth defects reported.
Information from adequate studies in pregnant women is not available.
Avoid completely during entire pregnancy if possible.

Advisability of Use if Breast-Feeding
Presence of this drug in breast milk: Unknown.
Avoid drug or refrain from nursing.

Habit-Forming Potential: None.

Effects of Overdosage: Immediate—nausea, vomiting, diarrhea.
Delayed—lowered white blood cell and platelet counts.

Possible Effects of Long-Term Use: Susceptibility to infection, bone marrow depression, development of malignancies.

Suggested Periodic Examinations While Taking This Drug (at physician's discretion)

Complete blood cell counts, liver function tests.

▷ **While Taking This Drug, Observe the Following**

Foods: No restrictions.

Beverages: No restrictions. May be taken with milk.

▷ *Alcohol*: No interactions expected.

Tobacco Smoking: No interactions expected.

▷ *Other Drugs*

Azathioprine may *decrease* the effects of
- oral anticoagulants (warfarin, etc.), and make it necessary to increase their dosage.
- certain muscle relaxants (gallamine, pancuronium, tubocurarine), and make it necessary to increase their dosage.

The following drugs may *increase* the effects of azathioprine
- allopurinol (Zyloprim) may increase its activity and toxicity and make it necessary to reduce its dosage.

▷ *Driving, Hazardous Activities*: No restrictions.

Aviation Note: The use of this drug *may be a disqualification* for piloting. Consult a designated Aviation Medical Examiner.

Exposure to Sun: No restrictions.

Discontinuation: If possible, do not discontinue this drug suddenly. A gradual reduction in dosage is preferable. Consult your physician for a withdrawal schedule.

BACAMPICILLIN
(bak am pi SIL in)

Introduced: 1979

Prescription: USA: Yes
Canada: Yes

Class: Antibiotic, Penicillins

Controlled Drug: USA: No
Canada: No

Available as Generic: No

Brand Names: ✤Penglobe, Spectrobid

BENEFITS versus RISKS

Possible Benefits	*Possible Risks*
EFFECTIVE TREATMENT OF INFECTIONS due to susceptible microorganisms	ALLERGIC REACTIONS, mild to severe, in 3% of the general population and 15% of allergic individuals Superinfections (yeast) Drug-induced colitis

---

▷ **Principal Uses**

As a Single Drug Product: To treat certain infections of the skin and skin structures, of the upper and lower respiratory tract, and of the genito-urinary tract, including gonorrhea.

How This Drug Works: During its absorption from the gastrointestinal tract, bacampicillin is converted to ampicillin. The unique chemical modification that characterizes bacampicillin permits its more rapid and complete absorption than ampicillin. When given in equivalent doses, bacampicillin provides peak blood levels that are 3 times higher than the levels provided by unmodified ampicillin. Thus bacampicillin can be effective when given every 12 hours; ampicillin requires a dosage schedule of every 6 hours. (See the Drug Profile of ampicillin.)

Available Dosage Forms and Strengths
Oral suspension — 125 mg per teaspoonful (5 ml)
        Tablets — 400 mg

▷ **Usual Adult Dosage Range:**   400 to 800 mg/12 hrs. **Note: Actual dosage and administration schedule must be determined by the physician for each patient individually.**

▷ **Dosing Instructions:**   Tablets may be taken without regard to eating. The oral suspension should be taken on an empty stomach, 1 hour before or 2 hours after eating. The tablet may be crushed for administration.

Usual Duration of Use: Continual use on a regular schedule for 5 to 7 days is usually necessary to determine this drug's effectiveness in eradicating the infection. Treatment is usually continued for 2 to 3 days after all indications of infection are gone. Treatment for all streptococcal infections should be for no less than 10 consecutive days (without interruption) to reduce the possibility of developing rheumatic fever or glomerulonephritis.

▷ **While Taking This Drug, Observe the Following**
▷   *Other Drugs*
    Bacampicillin *taken concurrently* with
    • allopurinol (Zyloprim) substantially increases the incidence of skin rash.
    • disulfiram (Antabuse) can cause a disulfiramlike reaction (see Glossary). Avoid the concurrent use of these 2 drugs.
    The following drugs may *decrease* the effects of bacampicillin
    • chloramphenicol (Chloromycetin).
    • erythromycins (E-Mycin, Erythrocin, etc.).
    • sulfonamides ("Sulfa" drugs, see Drug Class, Section Four).
    • tetracyclines (see Drug Class, Section Four).

Note: The information categories provided in this Profile are appropriate for bacampicillin. For specific information that is normally found in those categories that have been omitted from this Profile, the reader is referred to the Drug Profile of ampicillin.

BECLOMETHASONE
(be kloh METH a sohn)

Introduced: 1976

Prescription: USA: Yes
Canada: Yes

Available as Generic: No

Class: Antiallergic, Antiasthmatic,
Cortisone-like Drugs

Controlled Drug: USA: No
Canada: No

Brand Names: Beclovent Inhaler, ✤Beclovent Rotacaps, ✤Beconase, Beconase Nasal Inhaler, Vancenase Nasal Inhaler, Vanceril Inhaler

---

BENEFITS versus RISKS

Possible Benefits	*Possible Risks*
EFFECTIVE RELIEF OF ALLERGIC RHINITIS	FUNGUS INFECTIONS OF THE MOUTH AND THROAT
EFFECTIVE CONTROL OF SEVERE, CHRONIC ASTHMA	Localized areas of "allergic" pneumonia

---

> **Principal Uses**
>> *As a Single Drug Product*: Used primarily to treat bronchial asthma in those individuals who do not respond to bronchodilators and who require cortisonelike drugs for asthma control. This inhalation dosage form is significantly more advantageous than cortisone taken by mouth (swallowed) or by injection in that it works locally on the tissues of the respiratory tract and does not require absorption and systemic distribution. This prevents the more serious adverse effects that usually result from the long-term use of cortisone taken for systemic effects.

How This Drug Works: Not established. One possibility is that by increasing the amount of cyclic AMP in appropriate tissues, this drug may thereby increase the concentration of epinephrine, which is an effective bronchodilator and antiasthmatic. Additional benefit may be due to the drug's ability to reduce local inflammation in the lining tissues of the respiratory tract.

Available Dosage Forms and Strengths
Nasal inhaler — 16.8 grams (200 doses of 42 mcg each)
Oral inhaler — 16.8 grams (200 doses of 42 mcg each)

> **Usual Adult Dosage Range:** Nasal inhaler—1 inhalation (42 mcg) 2 to 4 times daily. Oral inhaler—2 inhalations (84 mcg) 3 or 4 times daily. For severe asthma—12 to 16 inhalations daily. The maximal daily dose should not exceed 20 inhalations. **Note: Actual dosage and administration schedule must be determined by the physician for each patient individually.**

> **Dosing Instructions:** May be used as needed without regard to eating. Rinse the mouth and throat (gargle) with water thoroughly after each inhalation.

Usual Duration of Use: Continual use on a regular schedule for 1 to 4 weeks is usually necessary to determine this drug's effectiveness in relieving severe, chronic allergic rhinitis and in controlling severe, chronic asthma. Long-term use requires the supervision and guidance of the physician.

▷ **This Drug Should Not Be Taken If**
- you have had an allergic reaction to any of the drugs bearing the brand names listed above.
- you are experiencing severe acute asthma or status asthmaticus that requires more intense treatment for prompt relief.
- your asthma can be controlled by bronchodilators and other antiasthmatic drugs that are not related to cortisone.
- your asthma requires cortisonelike drugs infrequently for control.
- you have a form of nonallergic bronchitis with asthmatic features.

▷ **Inform Your Physician Before Taking This Drug If**
- you are now taking or have recently taken any cortisone-related drug (including ACTH by injection) for any reason (see Drug Class, Section Four).
- you have a history of tuberculosis of the lungs.
- you have chronic bronchitis or bronchiectasis.
- you think you may have an active infection of any kind, especially a respiratory infection.

Possible Side-Effects   (natural, expected and unavoidable drug actions)
Fungus infections (thrush) of the mouth and throat.

▷ **Possible Adverse Effects**   (unusual, unexpected and infrequent reactions)
If any of the following develop, consult your physician promptly.
Mild Adverse Effects
Allergic Reactions: Skin rash (rare).
Dryness of mouth, hoarseness, sore throat.
Serious Adverse Effects
Allergic Reactions: Localized areas of "allergic" pneumonitis (lung inflammation).
Bronchospasm, asthmatic wheezing (rare).

Natural Diseases or Disorders That May Be Activated by This Drug
Cortisone-related drugs that have systemic effects can impair immunity and lead to reactivation of "healed" or quiescent tuberculosis of the lungs. Individuals with a history of tuberculosis must be observed closely during use of this drug by inhalation.

CAUTION
1. This drug does not act primarily as a brochodilator and should not be relied upon for the immediate relief of acute asthma.
2. If you were using any cortisone-related drugs for treatment of your asthma *before* transferring to this inhaler drug, it may be necessary to resume the former cortisone-related drug if you experience injury or infection of any kind, or if you require surgery. Be sure to notify your

attending physician of your prior use of cortisone-related drugs taken either by mouth or by injection.

3. If you experience a return of severe asthma while using this drug, notify your physician immediately so that additional supportive treatment with cortisone-related drugs by mouth or injection can be provided as needed.

4. It is advisable to carry a card of personal identification with a notation (if applicable) that you have used cortisone-related drugs within the past year. During periods of stress it may be necessary to resume cortisone treatment in adequate dosage.

5. An interval of approximately 5 to 10 minutes should separate the inhalation of bronchodilators such as epinephrine, isoetharine, or isoproterenol (which should be used first) and the inhalation of this drug. This sequence will permit greater penetration of beclomethasone into the bronchial tubes. The delay between inhalations will also reduce the possibility of adverse effects from the propellants used in the two inhalers.

Precautions for Use

By Infants and Children: Safety and effectiveness for use of the nasal inhaler by those under 12 years of age have not been established. Safety and effectiveness for use of the oral inhaler by those under 6 years of age have not been established. The maximal daily dose in children 6 to 12 years of age should not exceed 10 inhalations.

By Those over 60 Years of Age: Individuals with bronchiectasis should be observed closely for the development of lung infections.

▷ **Advisability of Use During Pregnancy**

Pregnancy Category: C (tentative). See Pregnancy Code inside back cover.

Animal studies: Mouse, rat and rabbit studies reveal significant birth defects due to this drug.

Human studies: Information from adequate studies in pregnant women is not available.

Avoid drug during the first 3 months. Use infrequently and only as clearly needed during the last 6 months.

Advisability of Use if Breast-Feeding

Presence of this drug in breast milk: Probably yes.

Avoid drug or refrain from nursing.

Habit-Forming Potential: With recommended dosage, a state of functional dependence (see Glossary) is not likely to develop.

Effects of Overdosage: Indications of cortisone excess (due to systemic absorption)—fluid retention, flushing of the face, stomach irritation, nervousness.

Suggested Periodic Examinations While Taking This Drug (at physician's discretion)

Inspection of nose, mouth and throat for evidence of fungus infection.

Assessment of the status of adrenal function in individuals who have used cortisone-related drugs over an extended period of time prior to using this drug.

X-ray examination of the lungs of individuals with a prior history of tuberculosis.

▷ **While Taking This Drug, Observe the Following**

Foods: No specific restrictions beyond those advised by your physician.

Beverages: No specific restrictions.

▷ *Alcohol*: No interactions expected.

Tobacco Smoking: No interactions expected. However, smoking can affect the condition under treatment and reduce the effectiveness of this drug. Follow your physician's advice.

▷ *Other Drugs*

The following drugs may *increase* the effects of beclomethasone

• inhalant bronchodilators—epinephrine, isoetharine, isoproterenol.

• oral bronchodilators—aminophylline, ephedrine, terbutaline, theophylline, etc.

▷ *Driving, Hazardous Activities*: No restrictions.

Aviation Note: The use of this drug and the disorder for which this drug is prescribed *may be disqualifications* for piloting. Consult a designated Aviation Medical Examiner.

Exposure to Sun: No restrictions.

Occurrence of Unrelated Illness: Acute infections, serious injuries, and surgical procedures can create an urgent need for the administration of additional supportive cortisone-related drugs given by mouth and/or injection. Notify your physician immediately in the event of new illness or injury of any kind.

Discontinuation: If the regular use of this drug has made it possible to reduce or discontinue maintenance doses of cortisonelike drugs by mouth, *do not* discontinue this drug abruptly. If you find it necessary to discontinue this drug for any reason, consult your physician promptly. It may be necessary to resume cortisone preparations and to institute other measures for satisfactory management.

Special Storage Instructions

Store at room temperature. Avoid exposure to temperatures above 120 degrees F (49 degrees C). Do not store or use this inhaler near heat or open flame. Protect from light.

BENZTROPINE
(BENZ troh peen)

Introduced: 1954

Class: Antiparkinsonism, Atropinelike Drugs

Prescription: USA: Yes
Canada: No

Controlled Drug: USA: No
Canada: No

Available as Generic: No

Brand Names: 🍁Apo-Benztropine, 🍁Bensylate, Cogentin, 🍁PMS Benztropine

---

BENEFITS versus RISKS

Possible Benefits	*Possible Risks*
PARTIAL RELIEF OF SYMPTOMS OF PARKINSON'S DISEASE	Atropinelike side-effects: blurred vision, dry mouth, constipation, impaired urination

---

▷ **Principal Uses**

As a Single Drug Product: Used adjunctively in the management of all types of parkinsonism to relieve the characteristic rigidity, tremor and sluggish movement. Should it fail to provide adequate relief, it may be supplemented with more potent drugs such as levodopa and bromocriptine. This drug is also used to control the parkinsonian reactions that can result from the use of certain antipsychotic drugs, such as the phenothiazines and related compounds.

How This Drug Works: By restoring a more normal balance of the chemical activities responsible for the transmission of nerve impulses within the basal ganglia of the brain, this drug relieves the symptoms of parkinsonism.

Available Dosage Forms and Strengths
Injection — 1 mg/ml
Tablets — 0.5 mg, 1 mg, 2 mg

▷ **Usual Adult Dosage Range:** For Parkinson's disease—0.5 to 2 mg daily, taken in a single dose at bedtime. For drug-induced parkinsonian reactions—1 to 4 mg daily, either in a single dose or in 2 to 3 divided doses. The total daily dose should not exceed 6 mg. **Note: Actual dosage and administration schedule must be determined by the physician for each patient individually.**

▷ **Dosing Instructions:** May be taken with or following food to reduce stomach irritation. Tablet may be crushed for administration.

Usual Duration of Use: Continual use on a regular schedule for 2 to 4 weeks is usually necessary to determine this drug's effectiveness in relieving the symptoms of parkinsonism and to determine the optimal dosage schedule. Long-term use (months to years) requires physician supervision and guidance.

▷ **This Drug Should Not Be Taken If**
- you have had an allergic reaction to any dosage form of it previously.
- it is prescribed for a child under 3 years of age.

▷ **Inform Your Physician Before Taking This Drug If**
- you have experienced an unfavorable reaction to atropine or atropinelike drugs in the past.
- you have glaucoma or myasthenia gravis.

- you have heart disease or high blood pressure.
- you have a history of liver or kidney disease.
- you have difficulty emptying the urinary bladder, especially if due to an enlarged prostate gland.
- you are taking, or have taken within the past 2 weeks, any monoamine oxidase (MAO) inhibitor drug (see Drug Class, Section Four).

Possible Side-Effects   (natural, expected and unavoidable drug actions)
Nervousness, blurring of vision, dryness of mouth, constipation, impaired urination. (These often subside as drug use continues.)

▷ **Possible Adverse Effects**   (unusual, unexpected and infrequent reactions)
If any of the following develop, consult your physician promptly.
Mild Adverse Effects
Allergic Reactions: Skin rashes.
Headache, dizziness, drowsiness, muscle cramps.
Indigestion, nausea, vomiting.
Serious Adverse Effects
Idiosyncratic Reactions: Abnormal behavior, confusion, delusions, halluci-nations, agitation.

Natural Diseases or Disorders That May Be Activated by This Drug
Latent glaucoma, latent myasthenia gravis.

CAUTION
1. Many over-the-counter (OTC) medications for allergies, colds and coughs contain drugs that can interact unfavorably with this drug. Ask your physician or pharmacist for guidance before using such prepara-tions.
2. This drug may aggravate tardive dyskinesia (see Glossary). Ask physi-cian for guidance.

Precautions for Use
By Infants and Children: Safety and effectiveness for use by those under 3 years of age have not been established. Children are especially suscepti-ble to the atropinelike effects of this drug.
By Those over 60 Years of Age: Small doses are advisable until your response has been determined. You may be more susceptible to the development of impaired thinking, confusion, nightmares, hallucinations, increased internal eye pressure (glaucoma) and impaired urination associated with prostate gland enlargement (prostatism).

▷ **Advisability of Use During Pregnancy**
Pregnancy Category: C (tentative). See Pregnancy Code inside back cover.
Animal studies: No data available.
Human studies: Information from adequate studies in pregnant women is not available.
Avoid use if possible, especially close to delivery. This drug can impair the proper functioning of the infant's intestinal tract following birth.

Advisability of Use if Breast-Feeding
Presence of this drug in breast milk: Unknown.
Avoid drug or refrain from nursing.

Habit-Forming Potential: None with recommended doses. At higher doses it may cause euphoria and hallucinations, creating a potential for abuse.

Effects of Overdosage: Weakness; drowsiness; stupor; impaired vision; rapid pulse; excitement; confusion; hallucinations; dry, hot skin; skin rash; dilated pupils.

Possible Effects of Long-Term Use: Increased internal eye pressure—possible glaucoma, especially in the elderly.

Suggested Periodic Examinations While Taking This Drug (at physician's discretion)
Measurement of internal eye pressure at regular intervals.

▷ **While Taking This Drug, Observe the Following**
Foods: No restrictions.
Beverages: No restrictions.
▷ *Alcohol*: Use caution until the combined effects have been determined. Alcohol may increase the sedative effects of this drug.
Tobacco Smoking: No interactions expected.
▷ *Other Drugs*
Benztropine may *decrease* the effects of
• haloperidol (Haldol), and reduce its effectiveness.
• phenothiazines (Thorazine, etc.), and reduce their effectiveness.
The following drugs may *increase* the effects of benztropine
• antihistamines may add to the dryness of mouth and throat.
• tricyclic antidepressants (Elavil, etc.) may add to the effects on the eye and further increase internal eye pressure (dangerous in glaucoma).
• monoamine oxidase (MAO) inhibitor drugs may intensify all effects of this drug (see Drug Class, Section Four).
▷ *Driving, Hazardous Activities*: Drowsiness and dizziness may occur in sensitive individuals. Avoid hazardous activities until full effects and tolerance have been determined.
Aviation Note: The use of this drug *is a disqualification* for piloting. Consult a designated Aviation Medical Examiner.
Exposure to Sun: No restrictions.
Exposure to Heat: Use caution. This drug may reduce sweating, cause an increase in body temperature, and contribute to the development of heat stroke.
Heavy Exercise or Exertion: Use caution. Avoid in hot environments.
Discontinuation: Do not discontinue this drug abruptly. Ask physician for guidance in reducing the dose gradually.

BITOLTEROL
(bi TOHL ter ohl)

Introduced: 1985

Class: Antiasthmatic, Bronchodilator

Prescription: Yes

Controlled Drug: No

Available as Generic: No

Brand Names: Tornalate

BENEFITS versus RISKS	
Possible Benefits	*Possible Risks*
EFFECTIVE PREVENTION AND RELIEF OF ASTHMA for 5 to 8 hours	Fine hand tremor (14%) Nervousness (5%) Throat irritation (5%) Irregular heart rhythm (with excessive use)

▷ **Principal Uses**

As a Single Drug Product: To relieve acute bronchial asthma and to reduce the frequency and severity of chronic, recurrent asthmatic attacks.

How This Drug Works: It is thought that by increasing the production of cyclic AMP, this drug relaxes constricted bronchial muscles to relieve asthmatic wheezing.

Available Dosage Forms and Strengths

Aerosol inhaler — 15 ml (300 inhalations of 0.37 mg each)

▷ **Usual Adult Dosage Range:**   For acute bronchospasm—2 inhalations at intervals of 1 to 3 minutes, followed by a third inhalation in 3 to 4 minutes if needed. For prevention of bronchospasm—2 inhalations/8 hrs. **Note: Actual dosage and administration schedule must be determined by the physician for each patient individually.**

▷ **Dosing Instructions:**   May be used without regard to eating. Follow the written directions for use carefully. Do not overuse.

Usual Duration of Use: According to individual requirements. Do not use beyond the time necessary to terminate episodes of acute asthma. Ask physician for guidance regarding duration of use for prevention of asthma attacks.

▷ **This Drug Should Not Be Taken If**
- you have had an allergic reaction to it previously.
- you currently have an irregular heart rhythm.

- you are taking, or have taken within the past 2 weeks, any monoamine oxidase (MAO) inhibitor drug (see Drug Class, Section Four).

▷ **Inform Your Physician Before Taking This Drug If**
- you have any type of heart or circulatory disorder, especially high blood pressure or coronary heart disease.
- you have diabetes, epilepsy or an overactive thyroid gland.
- you are taking any form of digitalis or any stimulant drug.

Possible Side-Effects   (natural, expected and unavoidable drug actions)
Dryness or irritation of mouth or throat (5%).

▷ **Possible Adverse Effects**   (unusual, unexpected and infrequent reactions)
If any of the following develop, consult your physician promptly.
Mild Adverse Effects
Headache (4%), dizziness (3%), nervousness (5%), insomnia (less than 1%), fine tremor of hands (14%).
Nausea (3%), indigestion.
Serious Adverse Effects
Rapid or irregular heart rhythm or increased blood pressure can occur with excessive use.

Natural Diseases or Disorders That May Be Activated by This Drug
Latent coronary artery disease, diabetes or high blood pressure.

CAUTION
1. Concurrent use of this drug by inhalation with beclomethasone aerosol (Beclovent, Vanceril) may increase the risk of toxicity due to fluorocarbon propellants. It is advisable to use bitolterol aerosol 20 to 30 minutes *before* beclomethasone aerosol. This will reduce the risk of toxicity and will enhance the penetration of beclomethasone.
2. The excessive or prolonged use of this drug by inhalation can reduce its effectiveness and cause serious heart rhythm disturbances.

Precautions for Use
By Infants and Children: Safety and effectiveness for use by children under 12 years of age have not been established.
By Those over 60 Years of Age: Avoid excessive and continual use. If acute asthma is not relieved promptly, other drugs will have to be tried. Observe for the development of nervousness, palpitations, irregular heart rhythm and muscle tremors.

▷ **Advisability of Use During Pregnancy**
Pregnancy Category: C (tentative). See Pregnancy Code inside back cover.
Animal studies: Cleft palate reported in mice.
Human studies: Information from adequate studies in pregnant women is not available.
Avoid use during first 3 months if possible.

Advisability of Use if Breast-Feeding
Presence of this drug in breast milk: Unknown.
Avoid drug or refrain from nursing.

Habit-Forming Potential: None.

Effects of Overdosage: Nervousness, palpitation, rapid heart rate, sweating, headache, tremor, vomiting, chest pain.

Possible Effects of Long-Term Use: Loss of effectiveness.

Suggested Periodic Examinations While Taking This Drug (at physician's discretion)
Blood pressure measurements, evaluation of heart status.

▷ **While Taking This Drug, Observe the Following**
Foods: No restrictions.
Beverages: Avoid excessive use of caffeine-containing beverages—coffee, tea, cola, chocolate.
▷ *Alcohol*: No interactions expected.
Tobacco Smoking: No interactions expected.
▷ *Other Drugs*
Bitolterol *taken concurrently* with
• monoamine oxidase (MAO) inhibitor drugs (see Drug Class, Section Four) may cause excessive increase in blood pressure and undesirable heart stimulation.
▷ *Driving, Hazardous Activities*: Use caution if excessive nervousness or dizziness occurs.
Aviation Note: The use of this drug *is a disqualification* for piloting. Consult a designated Aviation Medical Examiner.
Exposure to Sun: No restrictions.
Heavy Exercise or Exertion: Use caution. Excessive exercise can induce asthma in sensitive individuals.

BROMOCRIPTINE
(broh moh KRIP teen)

Introduced: 1975

Class: Antiparkinsonism, Dopamine Agonist, Ergot Derivative

Prescription: USA: Yes
Canada: Yes

Controlled Drug: USA: No
Canada: No

Available as Generic: No

Brand Names: Parlodel

BENEFITS versus RISKS

Possible Benefits	*Possible Risks*
PARTIAL RELIEF OF SYMPTOMS OF PARKINSON'S DISEASE	ABNORMAL INVOLUNTARY MOVEMENTS AND ALTERED
PREVENTION OF LACTATION following childbirth	BEHAVIOR IN 20% to 35% of users taking high doses
CORRECTION OF INFERTILITY AND ABSENT MENSTRUATION in women with high prolactin levels	Raynaud's phenomenon (see Glossary) in 30 to 60% of users taking high doses

---

▷ **Principal Uses**

As a Single Drug Product: This drug is used primarily to

1. Treat the manifestations of Parkinson's disease. It may be used as the initial drug in treating those with early-stage symptoms. More often it is used in conjunction with levodopa when it is found that levodopa is losing its effectiveness, or the patient cannot tolerate the adverse effects of levodopa and dosage adjustment or withdrawal is necessary.
2. Suppress the production of milk and thereby prevent the breast congestion and engorgement that normally follow childbirth.
3. Treat those disorders that are due to excessive production of prolactin by the pituitary gland: absence of menstruation, infertility, and inappropriate production of milk.

How This Drug Works: By directly stimulating the dopamine receptor sites in the corpus striatum of the brain, this drug helps to offset the deficiency of dopamine that is responsible for the rigidity, tremor, and sluggish movement characteristic of Parkinson's disease. By inhibiting the production of the hormone prolactin by the anterior pituitary gland, this drug

- reduces the amount of prolactin in the blood to below the level required to stimulate the breast glands to produce milk.
- reduces abnormally high levels of prolactin in the blood, restoring it to normal levels that permit menstrual regularity and fertility.

Available Dosage Forms and Strengths

Capsules — 5 mg
Tablets — 2.5 mg

▷ **Usual Adult Dosage Range:** For Parkinson's disease—initially 1.25 to 2.5 mg once daily; for maintenance, 2.5 to 100 mg daily in divided doses. Increase dose by no more than 2.5 to 5 mg on alternate days. Do not exceed 300 mg daily. For suppression of lactation—2.5 mg 2 times a day for 14 days; may extend to 21 days if needed. For absent menstruation and infertility—initially 1.25 to 2.5 mg daily; for maintenance, 2.5 mg 2 or 3 times a day. **Note: Actual dosage and administration schedule must be determined by the physician for each patient individually.**

▷ **Dosing Instructions:**   Take with food or milk to reduce stomach irritation. Capsule may be opened and tablet may be crushed for administration.

Usual Duration of Use: Continual use on a regular schedule for 3 to 4 months is usually necessary to determine this drug's effectiveness in controlling the symptoms of Parkinson's disease. Treatment for 4 to 12 weeks restores fertility and normal menstruation in most women; however, treatment may be necessary for 6 to 12 months. Long-term use (up to 3 years or more) must be under physician supervision and guidance.

▷ **This Drug Should Not Be Taken If**
- you have had an allergic reaction to it previously.
- you have had a serious adverse effect from any ergot preparation in the past.
- you have severe coronary artery disease or peripheral vascular disease.
- you are pregnant.

▷ **Inform Your Physician Before Taking This Drug If**
- you have constitutionally low blood pressure.
- you are taking any antihypertensive drugs or phenothiazines (see Drug Classes, Section Four).
- you have any degree of coronary artery disease, especially with a history of a "heart attack" (myocardial infarction).
- you have a history of heart rhythm abnormalities.
- you have impaired liver function.
- you have a seizure disorder (epilepsy).

Possible Side-Effects   (natural, expected and unavoidable drug actions)
Fatigue, lethargy, lightheadedness in upright position (see orthostatic hypotension in Glossary).

▷ **Possible Adverse Effects**   (unusual, unexpected and infrequent reactions)
If any of the following develop, consult your physician promptly.
Mild Adverse Effects
Allergic Reactions: Skin rash.
Headache, drowsiness, dizziness, fainting, nervousness, nightmares.
Nasal congestion, dry mouth, loss of appetite, nausea, vomiting, stomach cramps, constipation, diarrhea.
Serious Adverse Effects
Abnormal involuntary movements, confusion, hallucinations, incoordination, visual disturbances, depression, seizures.
Swelling of feet and ankles (edema). Loss of urinary bladder control, inability to empty bladder.
Indications of "ergotism": numbness and tingling of fingers, cold hands and feet, muscle cramps of legs and feet.
Vomiting blood, bloody or black stools (gastrointestinal bleeding).

▷ **Adverse Effects That May Mimic Natural Diseases or Disorders**
Effects on mental function and behavior may resemble psychotic disorders.

Natural Diseases or Disorders That May Be Activated by This Drug
Coronary artery disease with anginal syndrome. Raynaud's syndrome.

CAUTION
1. During treatment of parkinsonism, avoid excessive and hurried activity as improvement occurs; this will reduce the risk of falls and injury.
2. The neurological and psychiatric disturbances due to this drug may last for 2 to 6 weeks after stopping it.
3. During treatment to reduce the blood level of prolactin and restore normal menstruation and fertility, it is mandatory that you use a barrier method of contraception to prevent pregnancy. Oral contraceptives should not be used while taking bromocriptine.
4. If pregnancy occurs, notify your physician immediately.

Precautions for Use
By Infants and Children: Safety and effectiveness for use by those under 15 years of age have not been established.
By Those over 60 Years of Age: Your initial test dose should be 1.25 mg. Observe closely for any tendency to lightheadedness or faintness on attempting to stand after this first dose. You may be more susceptible to the development of impaired thinking, confusion, agitation, nightmares, hallucinations, nausea or vomiting. Close monitoring and careful dosage adjustments are mandatory.

▷ **Advisability of Use During Pregnancy**
Pregnancy Category: X (tentative). See Pregnancy Code inside back cover.
Animal studies: Rabbit studies reveal an increase in cleft lip.
Human studies: Serious birth defects have been reported in infants whose mothers took this drug during early pregnancy. Because the incidence of these defects (3.3%) does not exceed that reported for the general population, a cause-and-effect relationship is uncertain. Information from adequate studies in pregnant women is not available.
Pending further studies, it is recommended that this drug not be taken during the entire pregnancy.

Advisability of Use if Breast-Feeding
This drug prevents the production of milk and makes nursing impossible.

Habit-Forming Potential: None.

Effects of Overdosage: Weakness, low blood pressure, nausea, vomiting, diarrhea, confusion, agitation, hallucinations, loss of consciousness.

Possible Effects of Long-Term Use: Drug-induced changes in the lung tissue, thickening of the pleura and pleural effusion (fluid formation within the chest cage). These effects appear to be reversible after discontinuation of the drug.

Suggested Periodic Examinations While Taking This Drug   (at physician's discretion)
Blood pressure measurements; CAT scan of the pituitary gland for enlarge-

ment due to tumor; pregnancy test; blood tests for anemia; evaluation of heart, lung and liver functions.

▷ **While Taking This Drug, Observe the Following**
Foods: No restrictions.
Beverages: No restrictions. May be taken with milk.
▷   *Alcohol*: Use caution until the combined effects have been determined. Alcohol can exaggerate the blood-pressure-lowering effects and sedative effects of this drug.
▷   *Other Drugs*
Bromocriptine *taken concurrently* with
• antihypertensive drugs (and other drugs that can lower blood pressure) requires careful monitoring for excessive drops in pressure. Dosage adjustments may be necessary.
The following drugs may *decrease* the effects of bromocriptine
• phenothiazines (see Drug Class, Section Four).
Theoretically, bromocriptine and phenothiazines have opposite effects on the utilization of dopamine in the brain. It is probably best to avoid the concurrent use of these drugs until the results of further studies are available.
▷   *Driving, Hazardous Activities*: Be alert to the possible occurrence of orthostatic hypotension, dizziness, drowsiness or impaired coordination.
Aviation Note: Parkinsonism *is a disqualification* for piloting. The use of this drug otherwise *may be a disqualification* for piloting. Consult a designated Aviation Medical Examiner.
Exposure to Sun: No restrictions.

BROMPHENIRAMINE
(brohm fen IR a meen)

Introduced: 1957   **Class:** Antihistamines

Prescription: USA: Varies   **Controlled Drug:** USA: No
Canada: No   Canada: No

Available as Generic: USA: Yes
Canada: No

Brand Names: Dimetane, Dimetane Cough Syrup [CD], Dimetane Deconges-tant Elixir [CD], Dimetane Decongestant Tablets [CD], ✦Dimetane Expectorant [CD], ✦Dimetane Expectorant-C [CD], ✦Dimetane Expec-torant-DC [CD], Dimetane Extentabs, Dimetane-Ten, Dimetapp Prepara-tions [CD], ✦Dimetapp-A Preparations [CD], ✦Dimetapp w/Codeine [CD], ✦Dimetapp-DM [CD], ✦Dimetapp Infant Drops [CD], Disophrol Preparations [CD], Drixoral Preparations [CD], Veltane

---

BENEFITS versus RISKS

Possible Benefits	*Possible Risks*
EFFECTIVE RELIEF OF ALLERGIC RHINITIS AND ALLERGIC SKIN DISORDERS	Mild sedation (23%) Atropinelike effects Rare blood cell disorders: abnormally low white blood cells and platelets

---

▷ **Principal Uses**

As a Single Drug Product: Used primarily to provide symptomatic relief in allergic and related disorders: seasonal and perennial allergic rhinitis (hay fever), allergic conjunctivitis and vasomotor rhinitis; also in hives and localized swellings (angioedema) of allergic origin.

As a Combination Drug Product [CD]: This drug is combined with a decongestant drug to enhance its ability to reduce tissue swelling and secretions in allergic and infectious disorders of the upper respiratory tract—hay fever, head colds and sinusitis. It is also combined with decongestants, expectorants and codeine to increase their effectiveness in the symptomatic treatment of allergic and infectious disorders of the lower respiratory tract, often with associated coughing.

How This Drug Works: Antihistamines reduce the intensity of the allergic response by blocking the action of histamine after it has been released from sensitized tissue cells in the eyes, nose, respiratory passages and skin.

Available Dosage Forms and Strengths
Elixir — 2 mg per teaspoonful (5 ml)
Injection — 10 mg per ml
Tablets — 4 mg
Tablets, prolonged-action — 8 mg, 12 mg

▷ **Usual Adult Dosage Range:** 4 mg/4 to 6 hrs, or 8 to 12 mg (prolonged-action form)/12 hrs. Total daily dosage should not exceed 24 mg. **Note: Actual dosage and administration schedule must be determined by the physician for each patient individually.**

▷ **Dosing Instructions:** Take with food or milk to prevent stomach irritation. The prolonged-action forms should be swallowed whole (not crushed or chewed).

Usual Duration of Use: Continual use on a regular schedule for 2 to 3 days is usually necessary to determine this drug's effectiveness in relieving the symptoms of allergic rhinitis and dermatosis. It may be necessary to take this drug throughout the entire pollen season, depending upon individual sensitivity. However, antihistamines should not be taken continually (without interruption) for long-term use. Limit their use to periods that require symptomatic relief.

▷ **This Drug Should Not Be Taken If**
- you have had an allergic reaction to any dosage form of it previously.

- you are currently undergoing allergy skin tests.
- you are taking, or have taken within the past 14 days, any monoamine oxidase (MAO) inhibitor drug (see Drug Class, Section Four).

▷ **Inform Your Physician Before Taking This Drug If**
- you have had any allergic reactions or unfavorable responses to the previous use of antihistamines.
- you have glaucoma (narrow-angle type) or asthma.
- you have epilepsy or a seizure disorder.
- you have difficulty emptying the urinary bladder, especially if due to prostate gland enlargement.
- you plan to have surgery under general anesthesia in the near future.

Possible Side-Effects   (natural, expected and unavoidable drug actions)
Drowsiness; sense of weakness; blurred vision; dryness of the nose, mouth and throat; impaired urination.

▷ **Possible Adverse Effects**   (unusual, unexpected and infrequent reactions)
If any of the following develop, consult your physician promptly.
Mild Adverse Effects
Allergic Reactions: Skin rash.
Headache, nervous agitation, dizziness, confusion, tremor, blurred or double vision, ringing in ears.
Reduced tolerance for contact lenses.
Thickening of bronchial secretions in asthma or bronchitis.
Indigestion, nausea, vomiting, diarrhea.
Serious Adverse Effects
Hemolytic anemia (see Glossary).
Abnormally low white blood cells—fever, sore throat, infections.
Abnormally low blood platelets—abnormal bleeding or bruising.

Natural Diseases or Disorders That May Be Activated by This Drug
Latent epilepsy, glaucoma, prostatism (see Glossary).

CAUTION
1. Discontinue this drug 4 days before diagnostic skin testing procedures in order to prevent false negative test results.
2. Do not use this drug if you have active bronchial asthma, bronchitis or pneumonia. It can thicken bronchial mucus and make it more difficult to remove (by absorption or coughing).

Precautions for Use
By Infants and Children: This drug should not be used in premature or full-term newborn infants. Doses for children should be small. The young child is especially sensitive to the effects of antihistamines on the brain and nervous system.
By Those over 60 Years of Age: You may be more susceptible to the development of drowsiness, dizziness, and unsteadiness, and to impairment of thinking, judgment and memory. This drug can increase the degree of impaired urination associated with prostate gland enlargement (prostatism). The sedative effects of antihistamines in the elderly can cause a

syndrome of underactivity that may be misinterpreted as senility or emotional depression.

▷ **Advisability of Use During Pregnancy**
Pregnancy Category: C (tentative). See Pregnancy Code inside back cover.
Animal studies: No information available.
Human studies: Information from adequate studies in pregnant women is not available. Birth defects have been reported in 10 infants whose mothers used this drug during the first 3 months of pregnancy.
Avoid this drug during the first 3 months, and the last 3 months because of the potential risk for serious adverse effects on the newborn infant.

Advisability of Use if Breast-Feeding
Presence of this drug in breast milk: Yes, in small amounts. Avoid drug or refrain from nursing.

Habit-Forming Potential: None.

Effects of Overdosage: Drowsiness; unsteadiness; faintness; marked dryness of mouth, nose and throat; flushing of face; shortness of breath; hallucinations; convulsions; stupor progressing to coma.

Possible Effects of Long-Term Use: Tardive dyskinesia (see Glossary) has been reported in association with the long-term use of several widely used antihistamines. It is advisable to avoid the prolonged, continual use of antihistamines without interruption.

Suggested Periodic Examinations While Taking This Drug (at physician's discretion)
Complete blood cell counts.

▷ **While Taking This Drug, Observe the Following**
Foods: No restrictions.
Beverages: No restrictions. May be taken with milk.
▷ *Alcohol*: Use with extreme caution until the combined effects have been determined. The combination of antihistamine and alcohol can produce rapid and marked sedation.
Tobacco Smoking: No interactions expected.
▷ *Other Drugs*
Brompheniramine may *increase* the effects of
• all sedatives, sleep-inducing drugs, tranquilizers, analgesics and narcotic drugs, and produce oversedation.
The following drugs may *increase* the effects of brompheniramine
• monoamine oxidase (MAO) inhibitor drugs (see Drug Class, Section Four) may prolong the action of antihistamines.
▷ *Driving, Hazardous Activities*: This drug can impair mental alertness, judgment, coordination and reaction time. Avoid hazardous activities until the full sedative effects have been determined.
Aviation Note: The use of this drug *is a disqualification* for piloting. Consult a designated Aviation Medical Examiner.
Exposure to Sun: Use caution. Some drugs of this class can cause photosensitivity (see Glossary).

BUMETANIDE
(byu MET a nide)

Introduced: 1983

Prescription: USA: Yes

Available as Generic: No

Brand Names: Bumex

Class: Diuretic

Controlled Drug: USA: No

BENEFITS versus RISKS

Possible Benefits	*Possible Risks*
POTENT, EFFECTIVE DIURETIC BY MOUTH OR INJECTION	ABNORMALLY LOW BLOOD POTASSIUM with excessive use Impaired sexual function

---

▷ **Principal Uses**

As a Single Drug Product: To relieve edema (fluid retention) associated with congestive heart failure, liver disease or kidney disease.

How This Drug Works: By increasing the elimination of salt and water from the body (through increased urine production), this drug reduces the volume of fluid in the blood and body tissues and lowers the sodium content throughout the body.

Available Dosage Forms and Strengths

Injection — 0.25 mg/ml (2 ml ampules; 2 ml, 4 ml, 10 ml vials)

Tablets — 0.5 mg, 1 mg

▷ **Usual Adult Dosage Range:** 0.5 to 2 mg daily, usually taken in the morning as a single dose. If needed, an additional second or third dose may be taken later in the day at 4- to 5-hour intervals. The total daily dose should not exceed 10 mg. Alternate-day dosage (taken every other day) may be adequate for some individuals. **Note: Actual dosage and administration schedule must be determined by the physician for each patient individually.**

▷ **Dosing Instructions:** May be taken with or following food to reduce stomach irritation. Tablet may be crushed for administration.

Usual Duration of Use: Continual use on a regular schedule for 2 to 3 days is usually necessary to determine this drug's effectiveness in relieving edema. After maximal benefit has been achieved, intermittent use will reduce the risk of sodium, potassium and water imbalance. Long-term use requires the supervision and guidance of the physician.

▷ **This Drug Should Not Be Taken If**
- you have had an allergic reaction to either dosage form previously.
- your kidneys are unable to produce urine.

▷ **Inform Your Physician Before Taking This Drug If**
- you are allergic to any form of "sulfa" drug.

- you are pregnant or planning pregnancy.
- you have impaired liver or kidney function.
- you have diabetes or a tendency to diabetes.
- you have a history of gout.
- you have impaired hearing.
- you are taking any form of cortisone, digitalis, oral antidiabetic drugs, insulin, probenecid (Benemid), indomethacin (Indocin), lithium or drugs for high blood pressure.
- you plan to have surgery under general anesthesia in the near future.

Possible Side-Effects   (natural, expected and unavoidable drug actions)
Light-headedness on arising from sitting or lying position (see orthostatic hypotension in Glossary).
Increase in level of blood sugar, affecting control of diabetes.
Increase in level of blood uric acid, affecting control of gout.
Decrease in levels of blood potassium and sodium, resulting in muscle weakness and cramping.

▷ **Possible Adverse Effects**   (unusual, unexpected and infrequent reactions)
If any of the following develop, consult your physician promptly.
Mild Adverse Effects
Allergic Reactions: Skin rashes, hives, itching.
Headache, dizziness, vertigo, fatigue, weakness, sweating, earache.
Nausea, vomiting, stomach pain, diarrhea.
Breast nipple tenderness, joint and muscle pains.
Serious Adverse Effects
Impaired hearing, precipitation of liver coma (in preexisting liver disease), reduced sexual potency, premature ejaculation.

Natural Diseases or Disorders That May Be Activated by This Drug
Latent diabetes, gout.

CAUTION
1. Do not exceed recommended doses. Increased dosage can cause excessive excretion of water, sodium and potassium, with resultant loss of appetite, nausea, weakness, confusion and profound drop in blood pressure (circulatory collapse).
2. If you are also taking a digitalis preparation (digitoxin, digoxin), ensure an adequate intake of high-potassium foods to prevent potassium deficiency—a potential cause of digitalis toxicity.
3. If you are being treated for cirrhosis of the liver, do not increase your dose without consulting your physician. Excessive dosage can alter blood chemistry significantly and induce liver coma.

Precautions for Use
By Infants and Children: Safety and effectiveness for use by those under 18 years of age have not been established.
By Those over 60 Years of Age: Small doses are advisable until your individual response has been determined. You may be more susceptible to the development of impaired thinking, orthostatic hypotension, potassium loss and elevation of blood sugar. Overdosage and prolonged use of this

drug can cause excessive loss of body water, thickening of the blood, and an increased tendency of the blood to clot, predisposing to stroke, heart attack or thrombophlebitis.

▷ **Advisability of Use During Pregnancy**
Pregnancy Category: C (tentative). See Pregnancy Code inside back cover.
Animal studies: High-dose studies in rats and rabbits reveal defects in bone development.
Human studies: Information from adequate studies in pregnant women is not available.
This drug should not be used during pregnancy unless a very serious complication of pregnancy occurs for which this drug is significantly beneficial.

Advisability of Use if Breast-Feeding
Presence of this drug in breast milk: Unknown.
Avoid drug or refrain from nursing.

Habit-Forming Potential: None.

Effects of Overdosage: Weakness, lethargy, dizziness, confusion, nausea, vomiting, muscle cramps, thirst, drowsiness progressing to deep sleep or coma, weak and rapid pulse.

Possible Effects of Long-Term Use: Impaired balance of water, salt, and potassium in blood and body tissues. Dehydration with resultant increase in blood viscosity and potential for abnormal clotting. Development of diabetes in predisposed individuals.

Suggested Periodic Examinations While Taking This Drug (at physician's discretion)
Complete blood cell counts; measurements of blood levels of sodium, potassium, chloride, sugar, uric acid; liver and kidney function tests.

▷ **While Taking This Drug, Observe the Following**
Foods: Consult your physician regarding the advisability of eating a high-potassium diet. See Section Six for the Table of High Potassium Foods. Follow your physician's instructions regarding the use of salt.
Beverages: No restrictions unless directed by your physician. May be taken with milk.
▷ *Alcohol*: Use with caution until the combined effect has been determined. Alcohol can exaggerate the blood-pressure-lowering effect of this drug and cause orthostatic hypotension (see Glossary).
Tobacco Smoking: No interactions expected. Follow your physician's advice regarding smoking.
▷ *Other Drugs*
Bumetanide may *increase* the effects of
• antihypertensive drugs. Careful adjustment of dosages is necessary to prevent excessive lowering of the blood pressure.
Bumetanide *taken concurrently* with
• aminoglycoside antibiotics (amikacin, gentamicin, kanamycin, neomy-

cin, streptomycin, tobramycin, viomycin) may increase the risk of hearing loss.

- cortisone-related drugs may cause excessive loss of potassium from the body.
- digitalis-related drugs requires very careful monitoring and dosage adjustments to prevent serious disturbances of heart rhythm.
- lithium may increase the risk of lithium toxicity.

The following drugs may *decrease* the effects of bumetanide

- indomethacin (Indocin) may reduce its diuretic effect.

▷ *Driving, Hazardous Activities*: Use caution until the possible occurrence of dizziness, weakness or orthostatic hypotension (see Glossary) has been determined.

Aviation Note: The use of this drug *may be a disqualification* for piloting. Consult a designated Aviation Medical Examiner.

Exposure to Sun: No restrictions.

Occurrence of Unrelated Illness: Illnesses that cause vomiting or diarrhea can produce a serious imbalance of important body chemistry. Report such illnesses promptly.

Discontinuation: It may be advisable to discontinue this drug 5 to 7 days before major surgery. Consult your physician, surgeon, or anesthesiologist for guidance regarding dosage reduction or withdrawal.

BUSPIRONE
(byu SPI rohn)

Introduced: 1979

Prescription: USA: Yes

Available as Generic: No

Brand Names: Buspar

Class: Mild Tranquilizer

Controlled Drug: USA: No

BENEFITS versus RISKS

Possible Benefits	*Possible Risks*
EFFECTIVE RELIEF OF MILD TO MODERATE ANXIETY without significant sedation or risk of dependence	Mild dizziness, faintness or headache (uncommon) Rare restlessness, tremor and rigidity (with high doses)

▷ **Principal Uses**

As a Single Drug Product: Used to relieve anxiety and nervous tension states of mild to moderate severity. Because of its lack of significant sedative effects and of abuse potential, it is particularly useful in the elderly, the alcoholic and the addiction-prone individual.

How This Drug Works: Not completely established. This drug is thought to be a "mid-brain modulator" with effects on dopamine, norepinephrine and serotonin transmission activities. Its exact method of action is not understood.

Available Dosage Forms and Strengths
Tablets — 5 mg, 10 mg

▷ **Usual Adult Dosage Range:**   20 to 30 mg/day, in divided doses. Initially, 5 mg three times/day; if needed, increase dose by 5 to 10 mg/day every 3 to 4 days, with individual doses every 6 to 8 hours. The total daily dose should not exceed 60 mg. **Note: Actual dosage and administration schedule must be determined by the physician for each patient individually.**

▷ **Dosing Instructions:**   May be taken without regard to food. The tablet may be crushed for administration.

Usual Duration of Use: Continual use on a regular schedule for 7 to 10 days is usually necessary to determine this drug's effectiveness in relieving anxiety and nervous tension. Use intermittently and only as necessary; avoid prolonged and uninterrupted use.

▷ **This Drug Should Not Be Taken If**
   • you have had an allergic reaction to it previously.

▷ **Inform Your Physician Before Taking This Drug If**
   • you are taking other drugs that affect the function of the brain and nervous system: tranquilizers, sedatives, hypnotics, analgesics, narcotics, antidepressants, antipsychotic drugs, anticonvulsants or drugs for parkinsonism.
   • you have impaired liver or kidney function.

Possible Side-Effects   (natural, expected and unavoidable drug actions)
Infrequent and mild drowsiness (less than with benzodiazepines), lethargy, fatigue.

▷ **Possible Adverse Effects**   (unusual, unexpected and infrequent reactions)
If any of the following develop, consult your physician promptly.
Mild Adverse Effects
Headache, dizziness, faintness, excitement, nausea.
Serious Adverse Effects
Depression (3%). With high doses: restlessness, rigidity, tremors.

CAUTION
Although this drug is reported to have no significant (or very mild) sedative effects and no potential for causing dependence, it should be used with caution and only when clearly needed. It has not been used by large numbers of people for long periods of time; some unexpected side-effects or adverse effects may become apparent after general use for several years.

Precautions for Use
By Infants and Children: Safety and effectiveness for use by those under 18 years of age have not been established.
By Those over 60 Years of Age: This drug should be tolerated much better

than benzodiazepines and barbiturates when used by this age group. Observe for some possible increase in dizziness and/or weakness; use caution to avoid falls.

> **Advisability of Use During Pregnancy**
Pregnancy Category: B (tentative). See Pregnancy Code inside back cover.
Animal studies: No birth defects found in rat and rabbit studies.
Human studies: Information from adequate studies in pregnant women is not available.
Use this drug during pregnancy only when clearly needed. Until more experience has been gained from wider use, it is advisable to avoid this drug during the first 3 months of pregnancy.

Advisability of Use if Breast-Feeding
Presence of this drug in breast milk: Unknown; probably yes.
Avoid drug or refrain from nursing.

Habit-Forming Potential: None demonstrated in premarketing trials.

Effects of Overdosage: No experience reported. Probable effects would be increased dizziness, weakness and lethargy.

Possible Effects of Long-Term Use: None reported.

Suggested Periodic Examinations While Taking This Drug (at physician's discretion)
None required or recommended at the time of this writing.

▷ **While Taking This Drug, Observe the Following**
Foods: No restrictions.
Beverages: No restrictions.
▷ *Alcohol*: No interactions expected.
Tobacco Smoking: No interactions expected.
▷ *Other Drugs*: No significant drug interactions have been reported at the time of this writing.
▷ *Driving, Hazardous Activities*: This drug may cause dizziness, faintness or fatigue. Restrict activities as necessary.
Aviation Note: The use of this drug *may be a disqualification* for piloting. Consult a designated Aviation Medical Examiner.
Exposure to Sun: No restrictions.

BUTALBITAL
(byu TAL bi tal)

Introduced: 1954

Class: Mild Sedative, Hypnotic, Barbiturates

Prescription: USA: Yes
Canada: Yes

Controlled Drug: USA: C-III*
Canada: C

*See Schedules of Controlled Drugs inside back cover.

Available as Generic: No

Brand Names: Axotal [CD], Fioricet [CD], Fiorinal [CD], ✦Fiorinal-C1/4, C1/2 [CD], Fiorinal w/Codeine [CD]

```
┌─────────────────────────────────────────────────────────────────────┐
│                      BENEFITS versus RISKS                            │
│                                                                       │
│        Possible Benefits                  Possible Risks              │
│    RELIEF OF ANXIETY AND          HABIT-FORMING POTENTIAL             │
│       NERVOUS TENSION                WITH EXCESSIVE USE               │
│                                   Minor impairment of mental          │
│                                     functions with usual doses        │
│                                   Allergic skin rashes and hepatitis  │
│                                   Rare blood cell changes:            │
│                                     abnormally low white blood cells  │
│                                     and blood platelets               │
└─────────────────────────────────────────────────────────────────────┘
```

▷ **Principal Uses**

As a Single Drug Product: This barbiturate, with short to intermediate duration of action, is a mild sedative that is infrequently used alone to relieve anxiety and nervous tension.

As a Combination Drug Product [CD]: This drug is used primarily in combination with aspirin, caffeine and codeine to treat headaches associated with nervous tension. Because of the significant emotional component in the perception of pain, the addition of a mild sedative to a mixture of analgesics renders the combination more effective in relieving pain.

How This Drug Works: Not completely established. It is thought that this drug relieves nervous tension by reducing the amount of available norepinephrine, one of the chemicals responsible for nerve impulse transmission in the brain.

Available Dosage Forms and Strengths

Capsules — 50 mg (in combination), 120 mg

Tablets — 50 mg (in combination), 120 mg

▷ **Usual Adult Dosage Range:**   50 mg (in combination capsule or tablet)/4 hrs as needed. Total daily dose should not exceed 6 capsules or tablets. **Note: Actual dosage and administration schedule must be determined by the physician for each patient individually.**

▷ **Dosing Instructions:**   Take with food or milk to prevent stomach irritation. The tablet may be crushed or the capsule opened for administration.

Usual Duration of Use: For short-term use only. Take only as needed to abort or relieve tension headaches. Avoid prolonged and uninterrupted use.

▷ **This Drug Should Not Be Taken If**
- you have had an allergic reaction to any dosage form of it previously.
- you have a history of porphyria.

> **Inform Your Physician Before Taking This Drug If**
>   - you are allergic or overly sensitive to any barbiturate drug.
>   - you are taking any other sedative drugs, tranquilizers, antihistamines or pain relievers.
>   - you have epilepsy.
>   - you have a history of liver or kidney disease.
>   - you plan to have surgery under general anesthesia in the near future.

Possible Side-Effects   (natural, expected and unavoidable drug actions)
Drowsiness, lethargy and sense of mental and physical sluggishness as "hangover" effect.

> **Possible Adverse Effects**   (unusual, unexpected and infrequent reactions)
> **If any of the following develop, consult your physician promptly.**
> *Mild Adverse Effects*
> Allergic Reactions: Skin rash; hives; localized swellings of eyelids, face or lips; drug fever (see Glossary).
> Headache, dizziness.
> Nausea, vomiting, diarrhea.
> *Serious Adverse Effects*
> Allergic Reactions: Drug-induced hepatitis, with or without jaundice (see Glossary).
> Idiosyncratic Reactions: Paradoxical excitement and delirium (rather than sedation). This is more likely to occur in the presence of pain and in the elderly.
> Abnormally low white blood cells—infection, fever, sore throat.
> Abnormally low blood platelets—abnormal bleeding or bruising.

> **Adverse Effects That May Mimic Natural Diseases or Disorders**
> Drug-induced jaundice may suggest viral hepatitis.

Natural Diseases or Disorders That May Be Activated by This Drug
Acute intermittent porphyria.

CAUTION
This drug is most commonly used in combination with caffeine and/or aspirin. For complete information, be sure to read the Profiles of these two drugs.

Precautions for Use
By Infants and Children: Observe for possible paradoxical excitement and hyperactivity. Barbiturates should not be given to the hyperkinetic child.
By Those over 60 Years of Age: Small doses are advisable until tolerance has been determined. The elderly or debilitated may experience agitation, excitement, confusion and delirium with standard doses. This drug may also cause excessive lowering of body temperature (hypothermia). Keep dosage to a minimum during cold weather; dress warmly.

> **Advisability of Use During Pregnancy**
> *Pregnancy Category*: C (tentative). See Pregnancy Code inside back cover.
> Animal studies: No information available.

Human studies: Information from adequate studies in pregnant women is not available.

Avoid the frequent use of this drug during the last 2 months because of the potential risk of adverse effects on the newborn infant.

Advisability of Use if Breast-Feeding

Presence of this drug in breast milk: Probably yes.

Avoid drug or refrain from nursing.

Habit-Forming Potential: If used for an extended period of time, this drug can cause both psychological and physical dependence (see Glossary).

Effects of Overdosage: Behavior similar to alcoholic intoxication: confusion, slurred speech, incoordination, staggering gait, drowsiness, deepening sleep, coma.

Possible Effects of Long-Term Use: Psychological and/or physical dependence. If dose is excessive, a form of chronic intoxication can occur: headache, impaired vision, slurred speech and depression.

Suggested Periodic Examinations While Taking This Drug   (at physician's discretion)

With frequent or continual use, complete blood cell counts and liver function tests are desirable.

▷ **While Taking This Drug, Observe the Following**

Foods: No restrictions.

Beverages: No restrictions.

▷   *Alcohol*: Avoid completely. Alcohol can increase greatly the sedative and depressant actions of this drug on brain function.

Tobacco Smoking: No interactions expected.

▷   *Other Drugs*

Butalbital may *increase* the effects of

- other sedatives, hypnotics, tranquilizers, antihistamines and pain relievers, and cause oversedation. Ask your physician for guidance regarding dosage adjustments.

Butalbital may *decrease* the effects of

- oral anticoagulants of the coumarin drug class. Ask physician for guidance regarding prothrombin time testing and adjustment of the anticoagulant dose.
- beta-blocker drugs (see Drug Class, Section Four).
- oral contraceptives (see Drug Profile, Section Three).
- cortisonelike drugs (see Drug Class, Section Four).
- doxycycline (Vibramycin, etc.).
- griseofulvin (Fulvicin, Grisactin, etc.).
- phenmetrazine (Preludin).
- quinidine (Quinaglute, Quinidex, etc.).
- theophylline (Bronkotabs, Quibron, Theo-Dur, etc.).

Butalbital *taken concurrently* with

- anticonvulsants may cause a change in the pattern of epileptic seizures.

Dosage adjustments may be necessary to achieve a balance of drug actions that will give the best protection from seizures.

▷ *Driving, Hazardous Activities*: This drug can cause drowsiness and can impair mental alertness, judgment, physical coordination and reaction time. Avoid hazardous activities until its full sedative effects have been determined.

Aviation Note: The use of this drug *is a disqualification* for piloting. Consult a designated Aviation Medical Examiner.

Exposure to Sun: Use caution until sensitivity has been determined. Some barbiturates can cause photosensitivity (see Glossary).

Discontinuation: If it has been necessary to use this drug for an extended period of time, do not discontinue it abruptly. Ask physician for guidance during gradual withdrawal. It may also be necessary to adjust the doses of other drugs taken concurrently with it.

CAFFEINE
(KAF een)

Introduced: 4700 B.C. (tea)

Class: Stimulant, Xanthines

Prescription: USA: No
Canada: No

Controlled Drug: USA: No
Canada: No

Available as Generic: Yes

Brand Names: Anacin [CD], Cafergot [CD], Cafergot-PB [CD], Fioricet [CD], Fiorinal [CD], Fiorinal with Codeine [CD], Hycomine Compound [CD], NoDoz, Norgesic [CD], Norgesic Forte [CD], Synalgos-DC [CD], Wigraine [CD]

BENEFITS versus RISKS

Possible Benefits	*Possible Risks*
RELIEF OF DROWSINESS AND FATIGUE	Nervousness, insomnia
	Irritability
RELIEF OF MIGRAINE AND RELATED HEADACHES (in combination drugs)	Impaired thinking
	Stomach irritation, heartburn, ulcer

▷ **Principal Uses**

As a Single Drug Product: This stimulant of brain activity is used primarily to prolong wakefulness and delay the onset of sleep.

As a Combination Drug Product [CD]: This drug is used most commonly in combination with ergotamine to treat vascular headaches, such as migraine and cluster headaches. Caffeine increases the absorption of ergotamine and renders it more effective.

How This Drug Works: By increasing the energy level of the chemical systems responsible for nerve tissue activity, this drug induces wakefulness and improves alertness and mental acuity. By constricting the walls of blood vessels, this drug corrects the excessive expansion (dilation) responsible for the pain of vascular headache.

Available Dosage Forms and Strengths
Capsules — 100 mg, 250 mg
Capsules, prolonged action — 200 mg, 250 mg
Tablets — 65 mg, 100 mg

▷ **Usual Adult Dosage Range:**   100 to 200 mg/4 hrs, as needed. Prolonged-action forms: 200 to 250 mg/6 hrs, as needed. **Note: For frequent or long-term use, actual dosage and administration schedule must be determined by the physician for each patient individually.**

▷ **Dosing Instructions:**   If necessary, take with food or milk to prevent stomach irritation. The prolonged-action forms should be taken whole (not crushed or chewed). Do not take within 6 hours of retiring.

Usual Duration of Use: Short-term use advised. Avoid frequent or prolonged use without physician supervision.

▷ **This Drug Should Not Be Taken If**
- you have had an allergic reaction to any dosage form of it previously.
- you have severe heart disease.
- you have an active peptic ulcer.

▷ **Inform Your Physician Before Taking This Drug If**
- you have serious disturbances of heart rhythm.
- you have a history of peptic ulcer disease.
- you are subject to hypoglycemia.
- you have epilepsy.

Possible Side-Effects   (natural, expected and unavoidable drug actions)
Nervousness, insomnia, increased urine output. (Nature and degree of side-effects depend upon the size of the dose and the susceptibility of the individual.)

▷ **Possible Adverse Effects**   (unusual, unexpected and infrequent reactions)
If any of the following develop, consult your physician promptly.
Mild Adverse Effects
Headache, irritability, light-headedness, feeling of drunkenness, impaired thinking and concentration.
Rapid, forceful heart action; palpitation.
Indigestion, stomach irritation, heartburn, nausea.
Serious Adverse Effects
Development of peptic ulcer (in susceptible individuals).

CAUTION
1. Do not exceed 250 mg/dose or 500 mg/24 hours.
2. Caffeine in excessive amounts can provoke migraine headache in susceptible individuals.

Precautions for Use

By Infants and Children: Use not recommended.

By Those over 60 Years of Age: Tolerance for caffeine often decreases after 60. You may be more susceptible to caffeine-induced nervousness, irritability, impaired thinking, tremor, insomnia, disturbed heart rhythm and acid indigestion.

▷ **Advisability of Use During Pregnancy**

Pregnancy Category: C (tentative). See Pregnancy Code inside back cover.

Animal studies: Significant birth defects are attributed to this drug.

Human studies: Information from studies in pregnant women indicates no increased birth defects in 12,696 exposures to this drug.

Avoid during first 3 months if possible.

It is advisable to limit coffee consumption to 3 cups daily during pregnancy.

Advisability of Use if Breast-Feeding

Presence of this drug in breast milk: Yes, in small amounts.

Monitor nursing infant closely and discontinue drug or nursing if adverse effects develop.

Habit-Forming Potential: Varying degrees of tolerance and psychological dependence (see Glossary) may occur with prolonged use.

Effects of Overdosage: Nervousness, restlessness, insomnia (followed by depression in some individuals), tremor, sweating, ringing in ears, spots before eyes, heart palpitation, diarrhea, excitement, delirium, hallucinations, seizures.

Possible Effects of Long-Term Use: Development of tolerance and psychological dependence; stomach irritation (gastritis), peptic ulcer.

Suggested Periodic Examinations While Taking This Drug (at physician's discretion)

None.

▷ **While Taking This Drug, Observe the Following**

Foods: No restrictions. Note: Chocolate contains 5 to 10 mg of caffeine per ounce.

Beverages: Keep in mind that caffeine beverages (coffee, tea, cola) will add to the total intake of caffeine taken in medicinal form. Avoid possible overdosage. The approximate caffeine content of popular beverages is as follows:

Regular coffee (average cup) 100—150 mg

Instant coffee (average cup) 80—100 mg

Coffee-grain blends (average cup) 14—37 mg

Decaffeinated coffee (average cup) 3—5 mg

Tea (average cup) 60—75 mg

Regular cola (6 ounces) 36 mg

Diet cola (6 ounces) 18 mg

Cocoa (6 ounces) 10 mg

▷ *Alcohol*: No interactions expected.

Tobacco Smoking: Consult physician regarding possible adverse effects of combined nicotine and caffeine. Smoking can hasten the elimination of caffeine and shorten its period of effectiveness.

▷ *Other Drugs*

Caffeine may *decrease* the effects of
- sedatives, tranquilizers, hypnotics and pain relievers.

The following drugs may *increase* the effects of caffeine
- cimetidine (Tagamet).
- oral contraceptives.

▷ *Driving, Hazardous Activities*: No restrictions.

Aviation Note: No restrictions.

Exposure to Sun: No restrictions.

Discontinuation: Sudden discontinuation of this drug after extended use can produce a "caffeine-withdrawal" headache. This is readily relieved by coffee or caffeine in medicinal form.

CALCIUM CARBONATE
(KAL see um KAR boh nayt)

Other Names: Antacid

Introduced: 1825   **Class:** Antacid, Calcium Supplements

Prescription: USA: No   **Controlled Drug:** USA: No
Canada: No   Canada: No

Available as Generic: Yes

Brand Names: Alka-2, Alkets [CD], BioCal, Bisodol Tablets [CD], Cal.Sup, Caltrate 600, Camalox [CD], Dicarbosil, Gustalac, Marblen [CD], ✤Os-Cal, Os-Cal 250 [CD], Os-Cal 500, Ratio [CD], Titralac, Tums

BENEFITS versus RISKS	
Possible Benefits	*Possible Risks*
EFFECTIVE RELIEF OF ACID INDIGESTION CORRECTION OF CALCIUM DEFICIENCY	Constipation Predisposition to calcified kidney stones and kidney damage (excessive use)

▷ **Principal Uses**

As a Single Drug Product: Used primarily to (1) relieve acid indigestion, heartburn and sour stomach, and (2) supplement the diet to meet the body's requirements for calcium in the formation and maintenance of normal bone. Used primarily in children to prevent or treat rickets, and in adults to prevent or treat osteoporosis or osteomalacia.

As a Combination Drug Product [CD]: Often combined with other antacids to enhance the product's ability to neutralize stomach acids. Also combined with vitamin D, which increases the intestinal absorption of calcium. Also available in combination with the entire spectrum of essential vitamins and minerals.

How This Drug Works: By neutralizing some of the hydrochloric acid in the stomach and by reducing the action of the digestive enzyme pepsin, antacids lessen the irritant effect of digestive juices on inflamed tissues and create a more favorable environment for the healing of peptic ulcers.

Available Dosage Forms and Strengths
    Chewing gum — 500 mg
Chewable tablets — 330 mg, 350 mg, 420 mg, 500 mg
        Tablets — 650 mg, 1250 mg
    Suspension — 1 gram per teaspoonful (5 ml)

▷ **Usual Adult Dosage Range:** (1) As antacid: 500 mg to 2 grams after meals and at bedtime, or as needed. Total daily dosage should not exceed 8 grams. (2) As supplement, the recommended daily dietary allowances are as follows:
Infants up to 6 months of age: 360 mg.
Infants 6 months to 1 year of age: 540 mg.
Children 1 to 10 years of age: 800 mg.
Males 11 to 18 years of age: 1200 mg.
Males 19 years of age and older: 800 mg.
Females 11 to 18 years of age: 1200 mg. Females 19 to 50 years of age: 800 mg.
Females after 50 years of age (postmenopausal): 1500 mg.
During pregnancy: 1200 mg.
While breast-feeding: 1200 mg.
Note: For long-term use, actual dosage and administration schedule must be determined by the physician for each patient individually.

▷ **Dosing Instructions:** As antacid for treatment of peptic ulcer disease, take 1 to 3 hours after meals and at bedtime. As supplement, take 1 to 2 hours after meals. Chewable tablets should be chewed thoroughly before swallowing. Shake suspension well before measuring dose. Do not take within 2 hours of other oral medications.

Usual Duration of Use: If used for the treatment of peptic ulcer disease, continual use on a regular schedule is recommended for 4 to 6 weeks after all symptoms of ulcer activity have disappeared. Long-term use, as antacid or supplement, should be under physician supervision.

▷ **This Drug Should Not Be Taken If**
  • your calcium blood level is abnormally high.
  • you have severe kidney disease.
  • you have calcified kidney stones.
  • you are immobilized for an extended period of time.

▷ **Inform Your Physician Before Taking This Drug If**
  • you have a history of kidney stones or impaired kidney function.
  • you have any form of heart disease.

- you have sarcoidosis.
- you have deficient or absent stomach acid.
- you are prone to constipation.
- you are taking any other oral medications at this time, especially thiazide diuretics, quinidine or tetracycline.

Possible Side-Effects   (natural, expected and unavoidable drug actions)
Constipation (may be severe with large doses).

▷ **Possible Adverse Effects**   (unusual, unexpected and infrequent reactions)
If any of the following develop, consult your physician promptly.
Mild Adverse Effects
Chalky taste in mouth, belching, intestinal gas.
Serious Adverse Effects
With normal dosage—none.
With excessive dosage—abnormally high level of blood calcium: headache, fatigue, weakness, loss of appetite, nausea, vomiting.

CAUTION
1. Calcium can interfere with the absorption of many drugs. Do not take any other oral medication within 2 hours of a dose of calcium carbonate.
2. Avoid large doses of vitamin D while taking any form of calcium. Ask physician for guidance regarding vitamin D dosage.

Precautions for Use
By Infants and Children: May cause constipation with frequent or chronic use. Limit use to short-term schedules.
By Those over 60 Years of Age: This drug should be avoided because of its potential for raising the blood calcium level and predisposing to kidney stones and impairment of kidney function.

▷ **Advisability of Use During Pregnancy**
Pregnancy Category: C (tentative). See Pregnancy Code inside back cover.
Animal studies: No information available.
Human studies: Information from adequate studies in pregnant women is not available.
This drug is considered safe for use during the last 6 months of pregnancy in doses not to exceed 1200 mg daily. The calcium content of the diet must be considered.

Advisability of Use if Breast-Feeding
Presence of this drug in breast milk: Calcium is a normal constituent of breast milk. This drug does not increase the calcium content of milk to any significant degree, but does prevent deficiency.

Habit-Forming Potential: None.

Effects of Overdosage: Headache, fatigue, weakness, nervousness, muscle twitching, stomach pain, nausea, vomiting, constipation, mental disturbance, delirium, coma.

Possible Effects of Long-Term Use: Development of calcium-containing kidney stones.

Suggested Periodic Examinations While Taking This Drug (at physician's discretion)
Measurement of blood calcium levels (chronic use).

▷ **While Taking This Drug, Observe the Following**
Foods: Avoid frequent and excessive intake of spinach, rhubarb, bran and whole grain cereals; these can interfere with the absorption of calcium.
Beverages: Avoid large quantities of milk while taking calcium.
▷ *Alcohol*: No interactions.
Tobacco Smoking: No interactions.
▷ *Other Drugs*
Calcium may *increase* the effects of
- quinidine by delaying its elimination.
Calcium may *decrease* the effects of
- iron preparations.
- salicylates (aspirin, etc.).
- tetracyclines.
Calcium *taken concurrently* with
- thiazide diuretics (see Drug Class, Section Four) may cause abnormally high blood levels of calcium.
▷ *Driving, Hazardous Activities*: No restrictions.

CAPTOPRIL
(KAP toh pril)

Introduced: 1979

Class: Antihypertensive, ACE Inhibitor

Prescription: USA: Yes
Canada: Yes

Controlled Drug: USA: No
Canada: No

Available as Generic: No

Brand Names: Capoten, Capozide [CD]

BENEFITS versus RISKS	
Possible Benefits	*Possible Risks*
EFFECTIVE CONTROL OF MILD TO SEVERE HIGH BLOOD PRESSURE USEFUL ADJUNCTIVE TREATMENT FOR CONGESTIVE HEART FAILURE	Rash, itching, fever (10%) Lost or altered taste (7%) Impaired white blood cell production (0.3%) Bone marrow depression (rare) Kidney damage (rare) Liver damage (rare)

▷ **Principal Uses**

As a Single Drug Product: Used primarily to treat all degrees of high blood pressure. Mild to moderate high blood pressure usually responds to low doses; severe high blood pressure requires higher doses, with greater risk of serious adverse effects. Also used to treat selected cases of advanced heart failure that have not responded to conventional treatment with digitalis and diuretics.

How This Drug Works: Not completely known. It is thought that by blocking certain enzyme systems that influence arterial function, this drug contributes to the relaxation of arterial walls throughout the body and thus lowers the resistance to blood flow that causes high blood pressure. This, in turn, reduces the workload of the heart and improves its performance.

Available Dosage Forms and Strengths
Tablets — 12.5 mg, 25 mg, 50 mg, 100 mg

▷ **Usual Adult Dosage Range:**   Initially 12.5 to 25 mg 2 or 3 times daily for 2 weeks. If necessary, dose may be increased to 50 mg 3 times daily. Usual maintenance dose is 50 to 100 mg 3 times daily. Total daily dose should not exceed 450 mg. **Note: Actual dosage and administration schedule must be determined by the physician for each patient individually.**

▷ **Dosing Instructions:**   Take on empty stomach, 1 hour before meals, at same time each day. Tablet may be crushed for administration.

Usual Duration of Use: Continual use on a regular schedule for several weeks is usually necessary to determine this drug's effectiveness in controlling high blood pressure. The proper treatment of high blood pressure usually requires the long-term use of effective medications. Consult your physician before stopping this drug.

▷ **This Drug Should Not Be Taken If**
  • you have had an allergic reaction to it previously.
  • you currently have a blood cell or bone marrow disorder.
  • you have active liver disease.
  • you have an abnormally high level of blood potassium.

▷ **Inform Your Physician Before Taking This Drug If**
  • you have a history of kidney disease or impaired kidney function.
  • you have scleroderma or systemic lupus erythematosus.
  • you have any form of heart disease.
  • you have diabetes.
  • you are taking any of the following drugs: other antihypertensives, diuretics, nitrates, allopurinol (Zyloprim), Indocin or potassium supplements.
  • you plan to have surgery under general anesthesia in the near future.

Possible Side-Effects   (natural, expected and unavoidable drug actions)
Dizziness, light-headedness, fainting (excessive drop in blood pressure).

▷ **Possible Adverse Effects**   (unusual, unexpected and infrequent reactions)
   If any of the following develop, consult your physician promptly.
   Mild Adverse Effects
      Allergic Reactions: Skin rash; swelling of face, hands or feet; fever.
      Lost or altered taste, mouth or tongue sores.
      Rapid heart rate, palpitation.
   Serious Adverse Effects
      Bone marrow depression—fatigue, weakness, fever, sore throat, abnormal
         bleeding or bruising.
      Kidney damage—water retention (edema).
      Liver damage—with or without jaundice.

CAUTION
   1. If possible, it is advisable to discontinue all other antihypertensive
       drugs (especially diuretics) for 1 week before starting captopril.
   2. **Report promptly** any indications of infection (fever, sore throat), and
       any indications of water retention (weight gain, puffiness, swollen feet
       or ankles).
   3. Do not use a salt substitute without your physician's knowledge and
       approval. (Many salt substitutes contain potassium.)
   4. It is advisable to obtain blood cell counts and urine analyses **before**
       starting this drug.

Precautions for Use
   By Infants and Children: Safety and effectiveness for use by those in this age
      group have not been established.
   By Those over 60 Years of Age: Small doses are advisable until tolerance has
      been determined. Sudden and excessive lowering of blood pressure can
      predispose to stroke or heart attack in those with impaired brain circula-
      tion or coronary artery heart disease.

▷ **Advisability of Use During Pregnancy**
   Pregnancy Category: C (tentative). See Pregnancy Code inside back cover.
      Animal studies: No birth defects found in rat, rabbit or hamster studies.
      Human studies: Information from adequate studies in pregnant women is
         not available.
      Avoid during first 3 months if possible.

Advisability of Use if Breast-Feeding
   Presence of this drug in breast milk: Yes, in small amounts.
   Monitor nursing infant closely and discontinue drug or nursing if adverse
      effects develop.

Habit-Forming Potential: None.

Effects of Overdosage: Excessive drop in blood pressure—light-headedness,
   dizziness, fainting.

Possible Effects of Long-Term Use: Gradual increase in blood potassium level.

Suggested Periodic Examinations While Taking This Drug   (at physician's
   discretion)
   Before starting drug: Complete blood cell counts; urine analysis with mea-

surement of protein content, blood potassium level. During use of drug: Blood cell counts every 2 weeks during the first 3 months of treatment, then periodically for duration of use. Urine protein measurements every month during the first 9 months of treatment, then periodically for duration of use. Periodic measurements of blood potassium.

▷ **While Taking This Drug, Observe the Following**
Foods: Consult physician regarding salt intake.
Nutritional Support: **Do not take** potassium supplements unless directed by your physician.
Beverages: No restrictions. May be taken with milk.
▷ *Alcohol*: Use caution until combined effect has been determined. Alcohol may enhance the blood-pressure-lowering effect of this drug.
Tobacco Smoking: No interactions expected.
▷ *Other Drugs*
Captopril *taken concurrently* with
• potassium preparations (K-Lyte, Slow-K, etc.) may cause increased blood levels of potassium with risk of serious heart rhythm disturbances.
• potassium-sparing diuretics: amiloride (Moduretic), spironolactone (Aldactazide), triamterene (Dyazide) may cause increased blood levels of potassium with risk of serious heart rhythm disturbances.
The following drugs may *decrease* the effects of captopril
• indomethacin (Indocin).
• salicylates (aspirin, etc.).
▷ *Driving, Hazardous Activities*: Usually no restrictions. Be aware of possible drops in blood pressure with resultant dizziness or faintness.
Aviation Note: The use of this drug **may be a disqualification** for piloting. Consult a designated Aviation Medical Examiner.
Exposure to Sun: Caution advised. This drug can cause photosensitivity.
Exposure to Heat: Caution advised. Avoid excessive perspiring with resultant loss of body water and drop in blood pressure.
Occurrence of Unrelated Illness: Report promptly any disorder that causes nausea, vomiting or diarrhea. Fluid and chemical imbalances must be corrected as soon as possible.

CARBAMAZEPINE ✗
(kar ba MAZ e peen)

Introduced: 1962

Class: Anticonvulsant, Antineuralgic

Prescription: USA: Yes
Canada: Yes

Controlled Drug: USA: No
Canada: No

Available as Generic: No

Brand Names: ♣Apo-Carbamazepine, ♣Mazepine, Tegretol

BENEFITS versus RISKS

Possible Benefits	*Possible Risks*

RELIEF OF PAIN IN
  TRIGEMINAL NEURALGIA
EFFECTIVE CONTROL OF
  CERTAIN TYPES OF EPILEPTIC
  SEIZURES
Relief of pain in some rare forms of
  neuralgia

RARE BONE MARROW
  DEPRESSION (reduced
  formation of all blood cells)
Liver damage with jaundice

▷ **Principal Uses**

As a Single Drug Product: This drug is used primarily in the management of two uncommon but serious disorders: (1) for relief of pain in true trigeminal neuralgia (tic douloureux) and glossopharyngeal neuralgia; (2) for control of several types of epilepsy, namely grand mal, psychomotor or temporal lobe, and mixed seizure patterns. Because of its potential for serious toxic effects, precise diagnosis and careful management are mandatory for its proper use.

How This Drug Works: Not completely known. It is thought that by reducing the transmission of impulses at certain nerve terminals, this drug relieves or reduces pain (of trigeminal neuralgia) and also reduces the excitability of certain nerve fibers in the brain and thereby inhibits the repetitious spread of electrical impulses along nerve pathways. This action may prevent seizures altogether or reduce their frequency and severity.

Available Dosage Forms and Strengths

Tablets — 200 mg
Tablets, chewable — 100 mg

▷ **Usual Adult Dosage Range:** Initially 200 mg/12 hrs. Dose may be increased by 200 mg/24 hrs as needed and tolerated. Total daily dosage should not exceed 1200 mg. **Note: Actual dosage and administration schedule must be determined by the physician for each patient individually.**

▷ **Dosing Instructions:** Take at same time each day, with or following food to reduce stomach irritation. Tablet may be crushed for administration.

Usual Duration of Use: Continual use on a regular schedule for 3 months is usually necessary to determine this drug's effectiveness in relieving the pain of trigeminal neuralgia. Longer periods, with dosage adjustment, may be required to determine its ability to control epileptic seizures. Careful evaluation of each individual's tolerance and response should be made every 3 months during long-term treatment.

▷ **This Drug Should Not Be Taken If**
  • you have had an allergic reaction to it previously.
  • you have active liver disease.

- you currently have a blood cell or bone marrow disorder.
- you are currently taking, or have taken within the past 14 days, any monoamine oxidase (MAO) inhibitor drug (see Drug Class, Section Four).

▷ **Inform Your Physician Before Taking This Drug If**
- you have had an allergic reaction to any tricyclic antidepressant drug (see Drug Class, Section Four).
- you have taken this drug in the past.
- you have a history of any kind of blood cell or bone marrow disorder, especially one due to a drug.
- you have a history of liver or kidney disease.
- you have had serious mental depression or other mental disorder.
- you have had thrombophlebitis.
- you have high blood pressure, heart disease or glaucoma.
- you take more than 2 alcoholic drinks a day.

Possible Side-Effects   (natural, expected and unavoidable drug actions)
Dry mouth and throat, constipation, impaired urination.

▷ **Possible Adverse Effects**   (unusual, unexpected and infrequent reactions)
If any of the following develop, consult your physician promptly.
Mild Adverse Effects
Allergic Reactions: Skin rash, hives, itching, drug fever.
Headache, dizziness, drowsiness, unsteadiness, fatigue, blurred vision, confusion.
Exaggerated hearing, ringing in ears.
Loss of appetite, nausea, vomiting, indigestion, diarrhea.
Water retention (edema), frequent urination, impaired sexual function.
Changes in skin pigmentation, hair loss.
Aching of muscles and joints, leg cramps.
Serious Adverse Effects
Allergic Reactions: Severe dermatitis with peeling of skin, irritation of mouth and tongue, swelling of lymph glands.
Bone marrow depression (see Glossary)—fatigue, weakness, fever, sore throat, abnormal bleeding or bruising.
Liver damage with jaundice (see Glossary)—yellow eyes and skin, dark-colored urine, light-colored stools.
Kidney damage—reduced urine volume, uremic poisoning.
Mental depression and agitation.
Double vision, visual hallucinations, speech disturbances, peripheral neuritis (see Glossary).
Thrombophlebitis.

▷ **Adverse Effects That May Mimic Natural Diseases or Disorders**
Liver reactions may suggest viral hepatitis.

Natural Diseases or Disorders That May Be Activated by This Drug
Latent psychosis, systemic lupus erythematosus.

CAUTION
1. Because this drug can cause serious adverse effects, it should be used only after a trial of less hazardous drugs has been ineffective.
2. *Before* the first dose is taken, pretreatment blood cell counts, liver function tests and kidney function tests should be performed.
3. Careful periodic testing for early indications of blood cell or bone marrow toxicity is *mandatory*.
4. During periods of spontaneous remission from trigeminal neuralgia, this drug *should not be used* to prevent recurrence.
5. If used to control epileptic seizures, *do not discontinue this drug suddenly*.

Precautions for Use
By Infants and Children: Because of the high frequency of adverse effects (up to 25%), careful testing of blood cell production, liver function and kidney function must be performed regularly. This drug can reduce the effectiveness of other anticonvulsant drugs. Blood levels of all anticonvulsant drugs should be monitored when this drug is added to the treatment program.

By Those over 60 Years of Age: This drug can cause confusion and agitation. Observe for the possible aggravation of glaucoma, coronary artery disease (angina) or prostatism (see Glossary).

▷ **Advisability of Use During Pregnancy**
Pregnancy Category: C (tentative). See Pregnancy Code inside back cover.
Animal studies: Rat studies reveal significant birth defects.
Human studies: Information from adequate studies in pregnant women is not available.
Avoid completely during the first 3 months. Use during the last 6 months only if clearly needed.

Advisability of Use if Breast-Feeding
Presence of this drug in breast milk: Yes.
Avoid drug or refrain from nursing.

Habit-Forming Potential: None.

Effects of Overdosage: Dizziness, unsteadiness, drowsiness, disorientation, tremor, involuntary movements, nausea, vomiting, flushed skin, dilated pupils, stupor progressing to coma.

Possible Effects of Long-Term Use: Water retention (edema), impaired liver function, possible liver damage with jaundice.

Suggested Periodic Examinations While Taking This Drug   (at physician's discretion)
Complete blood cell counts weekly during the first 3 months of treatment, and monthly thereafter until the drug is discontinued. Liver and kidney function tests. Complete eye examinations.

▷ **While Taking This Drug, Observe the Following**
Foods: No restrictions.

Beverages: No restrictions. May be taken with milk.

▷ *Alcohol*: Use caution until the combined effect has been determined. This drug may increase the sedative effect of alcohol.

Tobacco Smoking: No interactions expected.

▷ *Other Drugs*

Carbamazepine may *increase* the effects of
- sedatives, tranquilizers, hypnotics, narcotics, and enhance their sedative effects.

Carbamazepine may *decrease* the effects of
- doxycycline (Doxy-II, Vibramycin, etc.).
- warfarin (Coumadin, Panwarfin, etc.).

Carbamazepine *taken concurrently* with
- lithium may cause serious neurological disturbances: confusion, drowsiness, weakness, unsteadiness, tremors, muscle twitching.
- monoamine oxidase (MAO) inhibitor drugs (see Drug Class, Section Four) may cause severe toxic reactions.

The following drugs may *increase* the effects of carbamazepine
- erythromycin (E.E.S., E-Mycin, etc.).
- isoniazid (INH).
- propoxyphene (Darvon, Darvocet, etc.).
- troleandomycin (Tao).

▷ *Driving, Hazardous Activities*: This drug can cause dizziness and drowsiness. Adjust activities accordingly.

Aviation Note: The use of this drug *is a disqualification* for piloting. Consult a designated Aviation Medical Examiner.

Exposure to Sun: This drug can cause photosensitivity (see Glossary). Use caution until sensitivity to sun has been determined.

Heavy Exercise or Exertion: Use caution if you have coronary artery disease. This drug can intensify angina and reduce tolerance for physical activity.

Occurrence of Unrelated Illness: Because of this drug's potential for serious adverse effects, it is mandatory that you inform each physician and dentist you consult that you are taking carbamazepine.

Discontinuation: If used to treat trigeminal neuralgia, attempt should be made every 3 months to reduce the maintenance dose or to discontinue this drug altogether. If used to control epilepsy, this drug *must not be discontinued abruptly*.

CARBENICILLIN
(kar ben i SIL in)

Introduced: 1964   **Class:** Antibiotic, Penicillins

Prescription: USA: Yes   **Controlled Drug:** USA: No
Canada: Yes   Canada: No

Available as Generic: No

Brand Names: Geocillin, Geopen, ✤Geopen Oral, Pyopen

+---+
| **BENEFITS versus RISKS** |
| |
| *Possible Benefits*   *Possible Risks* |
| EFFECTIVE TREATMENT OF   ALLERGIC REACTIONS, mild to|
| INFECTIONS due to susceptible   severe |
| microorganisms   Superinfections (yeast) |
| Drug-induced colitis |
| Rare blood cell disorders |
+---+

▷ **Principal Uses**

As a Single Drug Product: Oral tablets are used to treat certain infections of the urinary tract and prostate gland. Injections are used to treat a wider variety of more serious infections.

How This Drug Works: This drug destroys susceptible infecting bacteria by interfering with their ability to produce new protective cell walls as they multiply and grow.

Available Dosage Forms and Strengths

Injections — Vials of 1 gram, 2 grams, 5 grams
Tablets, film-coated — 382 mg

▷ **Usual Adult Dosage Range:**   382 to 764 mg/6 hrs (4 doses/24 hrs). **Note: Actual dosage and administration schedule must be determined by the physician for each patient individually.**

▷ **Dosing Instructions:**   Take on an empty stomach, 1 hour before or 2 hours after eating, at same times each day. Tablet may be crushed for administration, but drug has a bitter taste.

Usual Duration of Use: For urinary tract infections—10 days. For prostate gland infections—2 to 4 weeks. Recurrent and chronic infections require longer periods of treatment.

▷ **This Drug Should Not Be Taken If**

• you have had an allergic reaction to any dosage form of it previously.
• you are certain you are allergic to *any* form of penicillin.

▷ **Inform Your Physician Before Taking This Drug If**

• you suspect you may be allergic to penicillin or you have a history of a previous "reaction" to penicillin.
• you are allergic to cephalosporin antibiotics (Ancef, Ceporan, Ceporex, Kafocin, Keflex, Keflin, Kefzol, Loridine).
• you are allergic by nature—hay fever, asthma, hives, eczema.
• you have a history of a bleeding disorder, kidney disease, regional enteritis or ulcerative colitis.

Possible Side-Effects   (natural, expected and unavoidable drug actions)
Superinfections (see Glossary), often due to yeast organisms.

▷ **Possible Adverse Effects**   (unusual, unexpected and infrequent reactions)
If any of the following develop, consult your physician promptly.

Mild Adverse Effects
Allergic Reactions: Skin rashes, hives, itching.
Irritations of mouth and tongue, unpleasant taste, nausea, vomiting, mild diarrhea.

Serious Adverse Effects
Allergic Reactions: Anaphylactic reaction (see Glossary), severe skin reactions, drug fever, swollen painful joints, sore throat, abnormal bleeding or bruising.
Hemolytic anemia (see Glossary).
Pseudomembranous colitis—severe diarrhea.

CAUTION
1. Take the exact dose and the full course prescribed.
2. This drug should not be used concurrently with antibiotics like erythromycin or tetracycline.

Precautions for Use
By Infants and Children: Safety and effectiveness for use by those under 12 years of age have not been established.

By Those over 60 Years of Age: It is advisable to evaluate kidney function before and during use of this drug to determine the need for dosage adjustment. Natural changes in the skin may predispose to prolonged itching reactions in the genital and anal regions. Report such reactions promptly.

▷ Advisability of Use During Pregnancy
Pregnancy Category: B (tentative). See Pregnancy Code inside back cover.
Animal studies: No information available.
Human studies: Information from adequate studies in pregnant women indicates no increased risk of birth defects in 3546 pregnancies exposed to penicillin derivatives.
Ask physician for guidance.

Advisability of Use if Breast-Feeding
Presence of this drug in breast milk: Probably yes.
The nursing infant may be sensitized to penicillin.
Avoid drug if possible or refrain from nursing.

Habit-Forming Potential: None.

Effects of Overdosage: Possible nausea, vomiting and/or diarrhea.

Possible Effects of Long-Term Use: Superinfections, often due to yeast organisms.

Suggested Periodic Examinations While Taking This Drug   (at physician's discretion)
Complete blood cell counts. Liver and kidney function tests with long-term use.

▷ While Taking This Drug, Observe the Following
Foods: No restrictions.
Beverages: No restrictions.

▷   *Alcohol*: No interactions expected.
    Tobacco Smoking: No interactions expected.
▷   *Other Drugs*
        Carbenicillin may *decrease* the effects of
        • oral contraceptives in some women, and impair their effectiveness in
            preventing pregnancy.
        The following drugs may *decrease* the effects of carbenicillin
        • antacids may reduce the absorption of carbenicillin.
        • chloramphenicol (Chloromycetin).
        • erythromycin (Erythrocin, E-Mycin, etc.).
        • tetracyclines (Achromycin, Declomycin, Minocin, etc.). (See Drug Class,
            Section Four.)
▷   *Driving, Hazardous Activities*: Usually no restrictions.
    Aviation Note: The use of this drug *may be a disqualification* for piloting.
        Consult a designated Aviation Medical Examiner.
    Exposure to Sun: No restrictions.

CEFACLOR
(SEF a klor)

Introduced: 1979

Prescription: USA: Yes
    Canada: Yes

Available as Generic: No

Brand Names: Ceclor

Class: Antibiotic, Cephalosporins

Controlled Drug: USA: No
    Canada: No

BENEFITS versus RISKS

Possible Benefits	*Possible Risks*
EFFECTIVE TREATMENT OF INFECTIONS due to susceptible microorganisms	ALLERGIC REACTIONS mild to severe (up to 5% of general population, up to 16% of those allergic to penicillin) Drug-induced colitis (rare) Superinfections (see Glossary)

▷ **Principal Uses**
    As a Single Drug Product: To treat certain infections of the skin and skin
        structures, the upper and lower respiratory tract (including middle ear
        infections and "strep" throat) and certain infections of the urinary tract.

How This Drug Works: This drug destroys susceptible infecting bacteria by
        interfering with their ability to produce new protective cell walls as they
        multiply and grow.

Available Dosage Forms and Strengths
        Capsules — 250 mg, 500 mg
        Oral Suspension — 125 mg, 250 mg per teaspoonful (5 ml)

▷ **Usual Adult Dosage Range:**   250 to 500 mg/8 hrs. Total daily dose should not exceed 4 grams. **Note: Actual dosage and administration schedule must be determined by the physician for each patient individually.**

▷ **Dosing Instructions:**   May be taken on an empty stomach or with food if stomach irritation occurs. Capsule may be opened for administration. Shake suspension well before measuring dose. Take the full course prescribed.

Usual Duration of Use: Continual use on a regular schedule for 3 to 5 days is usually necessary to determine this drug's effectiveness in controlling the infection under treatment. Response varies with the nature of the infection. Total treatment time will vary from 1 to 4 weeks. Certain infections require that this drug be taken for 10 consecutive days to prevent the development of rheumatic fever. Follow your physician's instructions regarding duration of use.

▷ **This Drug Should Not Be Taken If**
- you are allergic to any cephalosporin antibiotic (see Drug Class, Section Four).

▷ **Inform Your Physician Before Taking This Drug If**
- you have a history of allergy to any form of penicillin (see Drug Class, Section Four).
- you have a history of regional enteritis or ulcerative colitis.
- you have impaired kidney function.

Possible Side-Effects   (natural, expected and unavoidable drug actions)
Superinfections (see Glossary).

▷ **Possible Adverse Effects**   (unusual, unexpected and infrequent reactions)
If any of the following develop, consult your physician promptly.
Mild Adverse Effects
Allergic Reactions: Skin rash, itching, hives.
Nausea and vomiting (1 in 90), mild diarrhea (1 in 70), sore mouth or tongue.
Serious Adverse Effects
Allergic Reactions: Drug fever (see Glossary), joint aches and pains, anaphylactic reaction (see Glossary).
Idiosyncratic Reactions: Minor and temporary changes in white blood cell counts and liver function tests (infrequent).
Genital itching (may represent a fungus superinfection).
Severe diarrhea, possibly indicating a drug-induced form of colitis (rare).

▷ **Adverse Effects That May Mimic Natural Diseases or Disorders**
Skin rash and fever may resemble measles.

CAUTION
In the management of diabetes it should be noted that this drug can cause a false positive test result for urine sugar when using Clinitest tablets, Benedict's solution or Fehling's solution, but not with Tes-Tape.

Precautions for Use
By Infants and Children: Not recommended for use in infants less than 1 month old. The maximal dose in children should not exceed 1 gram/24 hrs.
By Those over 60 Years of Age: Dosage must be carefully individualized and based upon evaluation of kidney function. Natural changes in the skin may predispose to severe and prolonged itching reactions in the genital and anal regions. Such reactions should be reported promptly.

▷ **Advisability of Use During Pregnancy**
Pregnancy Category: B (tentative). See Pregnancy Code inside back cover.
Animal studies: No birth defects reported.
Human studies: Information from adequate studies in pregnant women is not available.
Generally considered to be safe. Ask physician for guidance.

Advisability of Use if Breast-Feeding
Presence of this drug in breast milk: Yes, in small amounts.
Avoid drug or refrain from nursing.

Habit-Forming Potential: None.

Effects of Overdosage: Nausea, vomiting, stomach cramps and/or diarrhea.

Possible Effects of Long-Term Use: Superinfections (see Glossary).

Suggested Periodic Examinations While Taking This Drug   (at physician's discretion)
Complete blood cell counts.

▷ **While Taking This Drug, Observe the Following**
Foods: No restrictions.
Beverages: No restrictions. May be taken with milk.
▷ *Alcohol*: No interactions expected.
Tobacco Smoking: No interactions expected.
▷ *Other Drugs*
Cefaclor *taken concurrently* with
• probenecid (Benemid) will slow the elimination of cefaclor, resulting in higher blood levels and prolonged effect.
▷ *Driving, Hazardous Activities*: Usually no restrictions.
Aviation Note: The use of this drug *may be a disqualification* for piloting. Consult a designated Aviation Medical Examiner.

Exposure to Sun: No restrictions.
Special Storage Instructions: Oral suspension should be refrigerated.
Observe the Following Expiration Times: Do not take the oral suspension of
  this drug if it is older than 14 days.

CEFADROXIL
(sef a DROX il)

Introduced: 1977

Prescription: USA: Yes
  Canada: Yes

Available as Generic: No

Brand Names: Duricef, Ultracef

Class: Antibiotic, Cephalosporins

Controlled Drug: USA: No
  Canada: No

BENEFITS versus RISKS

Possible Benefits	*Possible Risks*
EFFECTIVE TREATMENT OF INFECTIONS due to susceptible microorganisms	ALLERGIC REACTIONS mild to severe (up to 5% of general population, up to 16% of those allergic to penicillin) Drug-induced colitis (rare) Superinfections (see Glossary)

▷ **Principal Uses**

  As a Single Drug Product: To treat certain infections of the skin and skin
    structures, the upper respiratory tract (including tonsillitis and "strep"
    throat) and certain infections of the urinary tract.

How This Drug Works: This drug destroys susceptible infecting bacteria by
  interfering with their ability to produce new protective cell walls as they
  multiply and grow.

Available Dosage Forms and Strengths
    Capsules — 500 mg
    Oral Suspension — 125 mg, 250 mg, 500 mg per teaspoonful (5 ml)
    Tablets — 1000 mg (1 gram)

▷ **Usual Adult Dosage Range:** Skin infections—500 mg/12 hrs, or 1 gram daily.
  "Strep" throat—500 mg/12 hrs for 10 days. Urinary tract infections—500
  mg to 1 gram/12 hrs, or 1 to 2 grams daily. Total daily dosage should not
  exceed 6 grams. **Note: Actual dosage and administration schedule must
  be determined by the physician for each patient individually.**

▷ **Dosing Instructions:** May be taken on an empty stomach or with food if stomach irritation occurs. Capsule may be opened for administration. Shake
  suspension well before measuring dose. Take the full course prescribed.

Usual Duration of Use: Continual use on a regular schedule for 3 to 5 days is usually necessary to determine this drug's effectiveness in controlling the infection under treatment. Response varies with the nature of the infection. Total treatment time will vary from 1 to 4 weeks. Certain infections require that this drug be taken for 10 consecutive days to prevent the development of rheumatic fever. Follow your physician's instructions regarding duration of use.

▷ **This Drug Should Not Be Taken If**
- you are allergic to any cephalosporin antibiotic (see Drug Class, Section Four).

▷ **Inform Your Physician Before Taking This Drug If**
- you have a history of allergy to any form of penicillin (see Drug Class, Section Four).
- you have a history of regional enteritis or ulcerative colitis.
- you have impaired kidney function.

Possible Side-Effects   (natural, expected and unavoidable drug actions)
Superinfections (see Glossary).

▷ **Possible Adverse Effects**   (unusual, unexpected and infrequent reactions)
If any of the following develop, consult your physician promptly.
Mild Adverse Effects
Allergic Reactions: Skin rash, itching, hives, localized swellings.
Headache, drowsiness, dizziness.
Indigestion, stomach cramping, nausea, vomiting, mild diarrhea, sore mouth or tongue.
Serious Adverse Effects
Allergic Reactions: Drug fever (see Glossary), joint aches and pains, anaphylactic reaction (see Glossary).
Idiosyncratic Reactions: Minor and temporary changes in white blood cell counts and liver function tests (infrequent).
Genital itching (may represent a fungus superinfection).
Severe diarrhea, possibly indicating a drug-induced form of colitis (rare).

▷ **Adverse Effects That May Mimic Natural Diseases or Disorders**
Skin rash and fever may resemble measles.

CAUTION
In the management of diabetes it should be noted that this drug can cause a false positive test result for urine sugar when using Clinitest tablets, Benedict's solution or Fehling's solution, but not with Tes-Tape.

Precautions for Use
By Infants and Children: Dosage is based upon weight, and must be determined by the physician for each individual. Follow your physician's instructions exactly.
By Those over 60 Years of Age: Dosage must be carefully individualized and based upon evaluation of kidney function. Natural changes in the skin

may predispose to severe and prolonged itching reactions in the genital and anal regions. Such reactions should be reported promptly.

▷ **Advisability of Use During Pregnancy**
Pregnancy Category: B (tentative). See Pregnancy Code inside back cover.
Animal studies: No birth defects reported.
Human studies: Information from adequate studies in pregnant women is not available.
Generally considered to be safe. Ask physician for guidance.

Advisability of Use if Breast-Feeding
Presence of this drug in breast milk: Yes, in small amounts.
Avoid drug or refrain from nursing.

Habit-Forming Potential: None.

Effects of Overdosage: Nausea, vomiting, stomach cramps and/or diarrhea.

Possible Effects of Long-Term Use: Superinfections (see Glossary).

Suggested Periodic Examinations While Taking This Drug (at physician's discretion)
Complete blood cell counts. Liver and kidney function tests.

▷ **While Taking This Drug, Observe the Following**
Foods: No restrictions.
Beverages: No restrictions. May be taken with milk.
▷ *Alcohol*: No interactions expected.
Tobacco Smoking: No interactions expected.
▷ *Other Drugs*
Cefadroxil *taken concurrently* with
• probenecid (Benemid) will slow the elimination of cefadroxil, resulting in higher blood levels and prolonged effect.
▷ *Driving, Hazardous Activities*: Usually no restrictions. If drowsiness or dizziness occurs, restrict activities accordingly.
Aviation Note: The use of this drug *may be a disqualification* for piloting. Consult a designated Aviation Medical Examiner.
Exposure to Sun: No restrictions.
Special Storage Instructions: Oral suspension should be refrigerated.
Observe the Following Expiration Times: Do not take the oral suspension of this drug if it is older than 14 days.

CEPHALEXIN ✒
(sef a LEX in)

Introduced: 1969	**Class:** Antibiotic, Cephalosporins
Prescription: USA: Yes	**Controlled Drug:** USA: No
Canada: Yes	Canada: No
Available as Generic: No	

Brand Names: ✦Ceporex, Keflex, ✦Novolexin

BENEFITS versus RISKS

Possible Benefits	*Possible Risks*
EFFECTIVE TREATMENT OF INFECTIONS due to susceptible microorganisms	ALLERGIC REACTIONS mild to severe (up to 5% of general population, up to 16% of those allergic to penicillin)
	Drug-induced colitis (rare)
	Superinfections (see Glossary)

▷ **Principal Uses**

   As a Single Drug Product: To treat certain infections of the skin and skin structures, the upper respiratory tract (including middle ear infections and "strep" throat), the genitourinary tract and certain infections involving bones and joints.

How This Drug Works: This drug destroys susceptible infecting bacteria by interfering with their ability to produce new protective cell walls as they multiply and grow.

Available Dosage Forms and Strengths

                    Capsules — 250 mg, 500 mg
            Oral Suspension — 125 mg, 250 mg per teaspoonful (5 ml)
   Pediatric Oral Suspension — 100 mg/ml
                    Tablets — 1000 mg (1 gram)

▷ **Usual Adult Dosage Range:** 250 to 500 mg/6 hrs. Total daily dose should not exceed 4 grams. **Note: Actual dosage and administration schedule must be determined by the physician for each patient individually.**

▷ **Dosing Instructions:** May be taken on an empty stomach or with food if stomach irritation occurs. Capsule may be opened and tablet may be crushed for administration. Shake suspension well before measuring dose. Take the full course prescribed.

Usual Duration of Use: Continual use on a regular schedule for 3 to 5 days is usually necessary to determine this drug's effectiveness in controlling the infection under treatment. Response varies with the nature of the infection. Total treatment time will vary from 1 to 4 weeks. Certain infections require that this drug be taken for 10 consecutive days to prevent the development of rheumatic fever. Follow your physician's instructions regarding duration of use.

▷ **This Drug Should Not Be Taken If**
   • you are allergic to any cephalosporin antibiotic (see Drug Class, Section Four).

▷ **Inform Your Physician Before Taking This Drug If**
   • you have a history of allergy to any form of penicillin (see Drug Class, Section Four).

- you have a history of regional enteritis or ulcerative colitis.
- you have impaired kidney function.

Possible Side-Effects   (natural, expected and unavoidable drug actions)
Superinfections (see Glossary).

▷ **Possible Adverse Effects**   (unusual, unexpected and infrequent reactions)
If any of the following develop, consult your physician promptly.
Mild Adverse Effects
Allergic Reactions: Skin rash (0.8%), itching, hives (0.3%).
Headache, drowsiness, dizziness.
Irritation of mouth or tongue, indigestion, stomach cramping, nausea, vomiting (1.8%), diarrhea (1.1%).
Serious Adverse Effects
Allergic Reactions: Drug fever (see Glossary), joint aches and pains, anaphylactic reaction (see Glossary).
Idiosyncratic Reactions: Minor and temporary changes in white blood cell counts and liver function tests (infrequent).
Genital itching (may represent a fungus superinfection).
Severe diarrhea, possibly indicating a drug-induced form of colitis (rare).

▷ **Adverse Effects That May Mimic Natural Diseases or Disorders**
Skin rash and fever may resemble measles.

CAUTION
1. In the management of diabetes it should be noted that this drug can cause a false positive test result for urine sugar when using Clinitest tablets, Benedict's solution or Fehling's solution, but not with Tes-Tape.
2. Do not use this drug concurrently with other antibiotics such as erythromycin or tetracyclines.

Precautions for Use
By Infants and Children: Not recommended for use in infants less than 1 year old. Monitor allergic children closely for evidence of developing allergy to this drug.
By Those over 60 Years of Age: Dosage must be carefully individualized and based upon evaluation of kidney function. Natural changes in the skin may predispose to severe and prolonged itching reactions in the genital and anal regions. Such reactions should be reported promptly.

▷ **Advisability of Use During Pregnancy**
Pregnancy Category: B (tentative). See Pregnancy Code inside back cover.
Animal studies: No birth defects reported.
Human studies: Information from adequate studies in pregnant women is not available.
Generally considered to be safe. Ask physician for guidance.

Advisability of Use if Breast-Feeding
Presence of this drug in breast milk: Yes, in small amounts.
Avoid drug or refrain from nursing.

Habit-Forming Potential: None.

Effects of Overdosage: Nausea, vomiting, stomach cramps and/or diarrhea.

Possible Effects of Long-Term Use: Superinfections (see Glossary).

Suggested Periodic Examinations While Taking This Drug (at physician's discretion)
Complete blood cell counts. Liver and kidney function tests.

▷ **While Taking This Drug, Observe the Following**
Foods: No restrictions.
Beverages: No restrictions. May be taken with milk.
▷ *Alcohol*: No interactions expected.
Tobacco Smoking: No interactions expected.
▷ *Other Drugs*
Cephalexin *taken concurrently* with
• probenecid (Benemid) will slow the elimination of cephalexin, resulting in higher blood levels and prolonged effect.
▷ *Driving, Hazardous Activities*: Usually no restrictions. Use caution if drowsiness or dizziness occurs.
Aviation Note: The use of this drug *may be a disqualification* for piloting. Consult a designated Aviation Medical Examiner.
Exposure to Sun: No restrictions.
Special Storage Instructions: Oral suspension should be refrigerated.
Observe the Following Expiration Times: Do not take the oral suspension of this drug if it is older than 14 days.

CHLORAL HYDRATE
(klor al HI drayt)

Introduced: 1832

Prescription: USA: Yes
Canada: Yes

Available as Generic: Yes

Class: Sedative, Hypnotic

Controlled Drug: USA: C-IV*
Canada: No

Brand Names: Aquachloral Supprettes, Noctec, ♣Novochlorhydrate, SK-Chloral Hydrate

BENEFITS versus RISKS	
Possible Benefits	*Possible Risks*
EFFECTIVE HYPNOTIC for short-term use (2 weeks)	DRUG DEPENDENCE with prolonged use
Effective daytime sedative for intermittent use	Severe allergic skin reactions
	Paradoxical excitement, delirium, psychotic behavior (infrequent)

*See Schedules of Controlled Drugs inside back cover.

▷ **Principal Uses**

   As a Single Drug Product: Used primarily as a bedtime sedative in sufficient dosage to induce sleep. It is the drug of choice for use in the elderly because it produces less "hangover" effect and is less likely to cause the confusion so commonly seen with use of barbiturates.

   How This Drug Works: Not completely known. It is converted into an alcohol, which is thought to have a sedative effect on the wake-sleep centers of the brain.

   Available Dosage Forms and Strengths
           Capsules — 250 mg, 500 mg
              Elixir — 500 mg per teaspoonful (5 ml)
      Suppositories — 324 mg, 500 mg, 648 mg
              Syrup — 250 mg, 500 mg per teaspoonful (5 ml)

▷ **Usual Adult Dosage Range:**   As sedative—250 mg 3 times daily. As hypnotic—500 to 1000 mg, 15 to 30 minutes before bedtime. Total daily dosage should not exceed 2000 mg (2 grams). **Note: Actual dosage and administration schedule must be determined by the physician for each patient individually.**

▷ **Dosing Instructions:**   Take capsules whole (unopened) with a full glass of water, fruit juice or ginger ale to prevent stomach irritation. Mix the elixir or syrup in 1/2 glass of water, fruit juice or ginger ale. Daytime doses are best taken after meals.

   Usual Duration of Use: As sedative, use intermittently and not on a regular basis. As hypnotic, limit use to periods of 7 to 10 days. Avoid continual and prolonged use. Duration of use should not exceed 14 days without drug-free periods of several days, and reappraisal of continued need.

▷ **This Drug Should Not Be Taken If**
   • you have had an allergic or unfavorable reaction to it previously.
   • you have severely impaired liver or kidney function.
   • you have severe heart disease.
   • you have active gastritis or peptic ulcer disease.
   • you have a history of intermittent porphyria.

▷ **Inform Your Physician Before Taking This Drug If**
   • you have a history of heart disease or peptic ulcer disease.
   • you are taking other sedatives, hypnotics, tranquilizers or narcotic drugs of any kind.
   • you plan to have surgery under general anesthesia in the near future.

   Possible Side-Effects   (natural, expected and unavoidable drug actions)
   Light-headedness in upright position, unsteadiness, weakness.
   "Hangover" effect following nighttime use as hypnotic.

▷ **Possible Adverse Effects**   (unusual, unexpected and infrequent reactions)
   If any of the following develop, consult your physician promptly.

459 — 8310

Health One

Ophthalmology

Mild Adverse Effects
   Allergic Reactions: Skin rashes, hives, conjunctivitis.
   Dizziness, confusion, hallucinations, nightmares.
   Unpleasant taste, stomach irritation, nausea, vomiting, diarrhea.
Serious Adverse Effects
   Allergic Reactions: Severe forms of dermatitis.
   Idiosyncratic Reactions: Sleepwalking, delirium, disorientation, paranoid
      behavior.
   Double vision, temporary blindness.
   Reduced formation of white blood cells.

Possible Delayed Adverse Effects
   Allergic skin reactions may occur up to 10 days following the last dose.

▷ **Adverse Effects That May Mimic Natural Diseases or Disorders**
   Paradoxical excitement or delirium may suggest latent psychosis.

Natural Diseases or Disorders That May Be Activated by This Drug
   Intermittent porphyria.

CAUTION
   1. Use with caution in the presence of bronchial asthma. Avoid high and
      frequent doses.
   2. Take all doses well diluted with water, milk, fruit juice or ginger ale to
      prevent stomach irritation.

Precautions for Use
   By Infants and Children: Avoid concurrent use with other drugs that have a
      sedative effect. Use very cautiously in asthmatic children.
   By Those over 60 Years of Age: Small doses are advisable until your individ-
      ual response has been determined. You may be more susceptible to the
      development of "hangover" effect, dizziness, confused thinking,
      impaired memory, unsteadiness, loss of bladder control or constipa-
      tion.

▷ **Advisability of Use During Pregnancy**
   Pregnancy Category: C (tentative). See Pregnancy Code inside back cover.
      Animal studies: No information available.
      Human studies: Information from adequate studies in pregnant women is
         not available.
      Use this drug only if clearly needed. Continual use during pregnancy can
         cause withdrawal symptoms in the newborn infant.

Advisability of Use if Breast-Feeding
   Presence of this drug in breast milk: Yes.
   Monitor nursing infant closely and discontinue drug or nursing if adverse
      effects develop.

Habit-Forming Potential: This drug can cause psychological and/or physical
   dependence (see Glossary). Avoid large doses and continual use.

Effects of Overdosage: Marked drowsiness, confusion, incoordination, slurred speech, staggering gait, weakness, vomiting, stupor, deep sleep.

Possible Effects of Long-Term Use: Psychological and/or physical dependence, toxic psychosis, liver and kidney damage.

Suggested Periodic Examinations While Taking This Drug (at physician's discretion)
Complete blood cell counts, liver and kidney function tests.

▷ **While Taking This Drug, Observe the Following**
Foods: No restrictions.
Beverages: No restrictions. May be taken with milk.
▷ *Alcohol*: Avoid completely for at least 6 hours before taking this drug. Alcohol can greatly increase the sedative and depressant actions of this drug on brain function.
Tobacco Smoking: No interactions expected.
Marijuana Smoking: Increased drowsiness, impaired mental and physical performance.
▷ *Other Drugs*
Chloral hydrate may *increase* the effects of
• oral anticoagulants (Coumadin, etc.), and cause abnormal bleeding or hemorrhage. Consult physician regarding prothrombin time testing and dosage adjustment.
▷ *Driving, Hazardous Activities*: This drug can impair mental alertness, judgment, physical coordination and reaction time. Avoid hazardous activities until all sensation of drowsiness has disappeared.
Aviation Note: The use of this drug *is a disqualification* for piloting. Consult a designated Aviation Medical Examiner.
Exposure to Sun: No restrictions.
Discontinuation: If this drug has been used continually over an extended period of time, it should be discontinued gradually under physician supervision.

CHLORAMPHENICOL
(klor am FEN i kohl)

Introduced: 1947

Class: Antibiotic

Prescription: USA: Yes
Canada: Yes

Controlled Drug: USA: No
Canada: No

Available as Generic: USA: Yes
Canada: No

Brand Names: Antibiopto, Chloromycetin, Chloroptic, Econochlor, ✤Fenicol, ✤Isopto Fenicol, ✤Minims, Mychel, ✤Nova-Phenicol, ✤Novochlorocap, Ophthochlor, Pentamycetin

---

BENEFITS versus RISKS

Possible Benefits	*Possible Risks*
VERY EFFECTIVE TREATMENT OF INFECTIONS due to susceptible microorganisms	BONE MARROW DEPRESSION APLASTIC ANEMIA (see Glossary) Peripheral neuritis (see Glossary) Liver damage, jaundice

---

▷ **Principal Uses**

As a Single Drug Product: This drug is quite effective in a broad spectrum of serious infections. However, because of its potential for serious toxicity (fatal aplastic anemia), its use is now reserved for life-threatening infections caused by organisms that are resistant to safer antibiotics, and for infections in individuals who, for one reason or another, cannot take other appropriate anti-infective drugs.

How This Drug Works: This drug prevents the growth and multiplication of susceptible microorganisms by interfering with their formation of essential proteins.

Available Dosage Forms and Strengths

Capsules — 250 mg, 500 mg
Cream — 1%
Eye/Ear Solutions — 0.5%
Eye Ointment — 1%
Injection — 100 mg/ml
Oral Suspension — 150 mg per teaspoonful (5 ml)

▷ **Usual Adult Dosage Range:**   Total daily dose is 250 mg for each 10 pounds of body weight, given in 4 equally divided doses, 6 hours apart. Total daily dose should not exceed 500 mg for each 10 pounds of body weight. **Note: Actual dosage and administration schedule must be determined by the physician for each patient individually.**

▷ **Dosing Instructions:**   Take with a full glass of water on an empty stomach, 1 hour before or 2 hours after eating. Capsule may be opened for administration. Shake oral suspension well before measuring dose.

Usual Duration of Use: Continual use on a regular schedule for 3 to 5 days is usually necessary to determine this drug's effectiveness in controlling the infection. Limit use to the time required to eradicate the infection. Avoid repeated courses of treatment if possible.

▷ **This Drug Should Not Be Taken If**
- you have had an allergic reaction to it previously.
- you have an active blood cell or bone marrow disorder.
- it is prescribed for a mild or trivial infection such as a cold, sore throat or "flulike" illness.
- it is prescribed for a premature or newborn infant (under 2 weeks of age).

▷ **Inform Your Physician Before Taking This Drug If**
- you have a history of a blood cell or bone marrow disorder.
- you have impaired liver or kidney function.
- you are taking anticoagulants.

Possible Side-Effects   (natural, expected and unavoidable drug actions)
Superinfections (see Glossary).

▷ **Possible Adverse Effects**   (unusual, unexpected and infrequent reactions)
If any of the following develop, consult your physician promptly.
Mild Adverse Effects
Allergic Reactions: Skin rashes, hives, swelling of face or extremities, fever.
Headache, confusion, peripheral neuritis (see Glossary)—numbness, pain, weakness in hands and/or feet.
Sore mouth or tongue, "black tongue," nausea, vomiting, diarrhea.
Serious Adverse Effects
Allergic Reactions: Anaphylactic reaction (see Glossary), liver damage with jaundice (rare).
Bone marrow depression (see Glossary)—fatigue, weakness, fever, sore throat, abnormal bleeding or bruising.

▷ **Adverse Effects That May Mimic Natural Diseases or Disorders**
Liver reaction with jaundice may suggest viral hepatitis.

CAUTION
1. This drug can cause serious bone marrow depression and aplastic anemia (see Glossary). It must not be used to treat trivial infections or as a preventive medication under any circumstances. Its use must be restricted to the treatment of serious or life-threatening infections that fail to respond to other anti-infective drugs.
2. Troublesome and persistent diarrhea can develop in sensitive individuals. If diarrhea persists for more than 24 hours, discontinue this drug and consult your physician.

Precautions for Use
By Infants and Children: Follow prescribed dosage exactly. Blood cell counts should be monitored twice a week. Long-term use of this drug can cause optic neuritis. This may be prevented by taking supplemental vitamin B complex during treatment. Idiosyncratic aplastic anemia is rare (1 in 40,000 users), but may occur weeks or months after discontinuation of this drug.
By Those over 60 Years of Age: The natural decline in liver and kidney function after 60 may require reduction in dosage and adjustment of dosage interval. Natural changes in the skin after 60 may predispose to severe and prolonged itching reactions in the genital and anal regions. Report such reactions promptly.

▷ **Advisability of Use During Pregnancy**
Pregnancy Category: C (tentative). See Pregnancy Code inside back cover.
Animal studies: Results are inconclusive.
Human studies: Information from adequate studies in pregnant women is

not available. Limited studies (348 exposures) indicate that this drug does not cause birth defects. Ask physician for guidance.

Advisability of Use if Breast-Feeding
Presence of this drug in breast milk: Yes.
Avoid drug or refrain from nursing.

Habit-Forming Potential: None.

Effects of Overdosage: Possible nausea, vomiting, diarrhea.

Possible Effects of Long-Term Use: Superinfections, impaired vision, bone marrow depression.

Suggested Periodic Examinations While Taking This Drug (at physician's discretion)
Complete blood cell counts—before treatment is started and every 2 to 3 days during administration of drug.
Liver and kidney function tests.

▷ **While Taking This Drug, Observe the Following**
Foods: No restrictions.
Nutritional Support: Supplemental vitamins B-2, B-6 and B-12 are recommended.
Beverages: No restrictions. May be taken with milk.
▷ *Alcohol*: Avoid completely if you have liver disease. Use cautiously until the combined effect has been determined. Some sensitive individuals may develop a "disulfiramlike" reaction (see Glossary).
Tobacco Smoking: No interactions expected.
▷ *Other Drugs*
Chloramphenicol may *increase* the effects of
• oral anticoagulants (Coumadin, dicumarol, etc.), and increase the risk of bleeding.
• barbiturates (phenobarbital, etc.), and cause excessive sedation.
• phenytoin (Dilantin), and cause phenytoin toxicity.
• sulfonylureas (Diabinese, Dymelor, Orinase, Tolinase), and cause hypoglycemia (see Glossary).
Chloramphenicol may *decrease* the effects of
• iron preparations, used to treat anemia.
• penicillins.
• vitamin B-12.
The following drugs may *decrease* the effects of chloramphenicol
• barbiturates (phenobarbital, etc.).
• rifampin (Rifadin, Rimactane, etc.).
▷ *Driving, Hazardous Activities*: Usually no restrictions. Be alert to the rare occurrence of confusion, and restrict activities accordingly.
Aviation Note: The use of this drug *may be a disqualification* for piloting. Consult a designated Aviation Medical Examiner.
Exposure to Sun: No restrictions.

CHLORDIAZEPOXIDE
(klor di az e POX ide)

Introduced: 1960

Class: Mild Tranquilizer, Benzodiazepines

Prescription: USA: Yes
Canada: Yes

Controlled Drug: USA: C-IV*
Canada: No

Available as Generic: Yes

Brand Names: A-poxide, ♣Apo-Chlordiazepoxide, Librax [CD], Libritabs, Librium, Limbitrol [CD], Murcil, ♣Novopoxide, SK-Lygen, ♣Solium

---

BENEFITS versus RISKS

Possible Benefits	*Possible Risks*
RELIEF OF ANXIETY AND NERVOUS TENSION in 70% to 80% of users	Habit-forming potential with prolonged use
Wide margin of safety with therapeutic doses	Minor impairment of mental functions
Very few drug interactions	Very rare jaundice
	Very rare blood cell disorders

▷ **Principal Uses**

As a Single Drug Product: Used primarily to (1) provide short-term relief of mild to moderate anxiety, and (2) relieve the symptoms of acute alcohol withdrawal: agitation, tremors, hallucinations, incipient delirium tremens.

As a Combination Drug Product [CD]: Used in combination with amitriptyline (an antidepressant) to allay the anxiety that is often a troublesome feature in the agitated and depressed individual. Also used in combination with clidinium (a synthetic atropinelike antispasmodic) to treat peptic ulcer disease and irritable bowel syndrome.

How This Drug Works: It is thought that this drug produces a calming effect by enhancing the action of the nerve transmitter gamma-aminobutyric acid (GABA), which in turn blocks the arousal of higher brain centers.

Available Dosage Forms and Strengths
Capsules — 5 mg, 10 mg, 25 mg
Injection — 100 mg/ampul
Tablets — 5 mg, 10 mg, 25 mg

▷ **Usual Adult Dosage Range:** 5 to 25 mg, 3 or 4 times daily. Dose may be increased cautiously as needed and tolerated. After 1 week of continual use, the total daily dose may be taken at bedtime. Total daily dose should not exceed 150 mg for anxiety and tension, or 300 mg for alcohol withdrawal. **Note: Actual dosage and administration schedule must be determined by the physician for each patient individually.**

*See Schedules of Controlled Drugs inside back cover.

▷ **Dosing Instructions:** May be taken on empty stomach or with food or milk. Capsule may be opened and tablet may be crushed for administration. Do not discontinue this drug abruptly if taken for more than 4 weeks.

Usual Duration of Use: Continual use on a regular schedule for 3 to 5 days is usually necessary to determine this drug's effectiveness in relieving moderate anxiety. Limit continual use to 1 to 3 weeks. Avoid uninterrupted and prolonged use.

▷ **This Drug Should Not Be Taken If**
  • you have had an allergic reaction to any dosage form of it previously.
  • you have acute narrow-angle glaucoma.
  • it is prescribed for a child under 6 years of age.

▷ **Inform Your Physician Before Taking This Drug If**
  • you are allergic to any benzodiazepine drug (see Drug Class, Section Four).
  • you have a history of alcoholism or drug abuse.
  • you are pregnant or planning pregnancy.
  • you have impaired liver or kidney function.
  • you have a history of serious depression or mental disorder.
  • you have any of the following: asthma, emphysema, epilepsy, myasthenia gravis, porphyria.

Possible Side-Effects   (natural, expected and unavoidable drug actions)
  Drowsiness (3.9%), lethargy, unsteadiness; "hangover" effects on the day following bedtime use.

▷ **Possible Adverse Effects**   (unusual, unexpected and infrequent reactions)
  If any of the following develop, consult your physician promptly.
  Mild Adverse Effects
  Allergic Reactions: Rashes, fixed skin eruptions, bruising.
  Dizziness, fainting, blurred vision, double vision, slurred speech, sweating, nausea, menstrual irregularity.
  Serious Adverse Effects
  Allergic Reactions: Liver damage with jaundice (see Glossary), abnormally low blood platelets.
  Idiosyncratic Reactions: Inappropriate female breast enlargement and milk production (rare). Acute hepatic porphyria.
  Bone marrow depression—impaired production of red and white blood cells.
  Paradoxical responses of excitement, agitation, anger, rage.

▷ **Adverse Effects That May Mimic Natural Diseases or Disorders**
  Liver reaction with jaundice may suggest viral hepatitis.

Natural Diseases or Disorders That May Be Activated by This Drug
  Acute intermittent hepatic porphyria.
  Systemic lupus erythematosuslike syndrome.

CAUTION
1. This drug should not be discontinued abruptly if it has been taken continually for more than 4 weeks.
2. The concurrent use of some over-the-counter drug products that contain antihistamines (allergy and cold preparations, sleep aids) can cause excessive sedation in sensitive individuals.

Precautions for Use

By Infants and Children: Safety and effectiveness for use by those under 6 years of age have not been established. This drug should not be used in the hyperactive or psychotic child of any age.

By Those over 60 Years of Age: It is advisable to use smaller doses at longer intervals to avoid overdosage. Observe for the possible development of lethargy, indifference, fatigue, weakness, unsteadiness, disturbing dreams, nightmares and paradoxical reactions of excitement, agitation, anger, hostility and rage.

▷ **Advisability of Use During Pregnancy**

Pregnancy Category: D (tentative). See Pregnancy Code inside back cover.

Animal studies: Cleft palate reported in mice.

Human studies: Available information is conflicting and inconclusive. Some studies found a fourfold increase in serious birth defects associated with the use of this drug. Other studies have found no significant increase in birth defects.

Frequent use in late pregnancy can cause the "floppy infant" syndrome in the newborn: weakness, lethargy, unresponsiveness, depressed breathing, low body temperature.

Avoid use during entire pregnancy if possible.

Advisability of Use if Breast-Feeding

Presence of this drug in breast milk: Yes, in small amounts.

Monitor nursing infant closely and discontinue drug or nursing if adverse effects develop.

Habit-Forming Potential: This drug can produce psychological and/or physical dependence (see Glossary) if used in large doses for an extended period of time.

Effects of Overdosage: Marked drowsiness, weakness, feeling of drunkenness, staggering gait, tremor, stupor progressing to deep sleep or coma.

Possible Effects of Long-Term Use: Psychological and/or physical dependence, rare blood cell disorders.

Suggested Periodic Examinations While Taking This Drug   (at physician's discretion)

Complete blood cell counts during long-term use.

▷ **While Taking This Drug, Observe the Following**

Foods: No restrictions.

Beverages: Avoid excessive intake of caffeine-containing beverages: coffee, tea, cola. May be taken with milk.

▷   *Alcohol*: Use with extreme caution until the combined effect is determined. Alcohol may increase the absorption of this drug and add to its depressant effects on the brain. It is advisable to avoid alcohol completely—throughout the day and night—if it is necessary to drive or to engage in any hazardous activity.

Tobacco Smoking: Heavy smoking may reduce the calming action of this drug.

Marijuana Smoking: Increased sedation and significant impairment of intellectual and physical performance.

▷   *Other Drugs*

Chlordiazepoxide may *increase* the effects of
- digoxin (Lanoxin), and cause digoxin toxicity.

Chlordiazepoxide may *decrease* the effects of
- levodopa (Sinemet, etc.), and reduce its effectiveness in treating Parkinson's disease.

The following drugs may *increase* the effects of chlordiazepoxide
- cimetidine (Tagamet).
- disulfiram (Antabuse).
- isoniazid (INH, Rifamate, etc.).
- oral contraceptives.
- valproic acid (Depakene).

The following drugs may *decrease* the effects of chlordiazepoxide
- rifampin (Rimactane, etc.).
- theophylline (aminophylline, Theo-Dur, etc.).

▷   *Driving, Hazardous Activities*: This drug can impair mental alertness, judgment, physical coordination and reaction time. Avoid hazardous activities accordingly.

Aviation Note: The use of this drug *is a disqualification* for piloting. Consult a designated Aviation Medical Examiner.

Exposure to Sun: Use caution until sensitivity is determined. A photoallergic skin reaction may occur rarely.

Discontinuation: Avoid sudden discontinuation if this drug has been taken for over 4 weeks. Dosage should be tapered gradually to prevent a withdrawal syndrome that could include depression, confusion, hallucinations, tremor, seizures, muscle cramping, sweating and vomiting.

CHLOROTHIAZIDE
(klor oh THI a zide)

Introduced: 1957

Class: Antihypertensive, Diuretic, Thiazides

Prescription: USA: Yes
 Canada: Yes

Controlled Drug: USA: No
 Canada: No

Available as Generic: USA: Yes
 Canada: No

Brand Names: Aldoclor [CD], Diupres [CD], Diuril, SK-Chlorothiazide

---

BENEFITS versus RISKS

Possible Benefits	*Possible Risks*
EFFECTIVE, WELL-TOLERATED DIURETIC	Loss of body potassium
POSSIBLY EFFECTIVE IN MILD HYPERTENSION	Increased blood sugar
	Increased blood uric acid
	Increased blood calcium
ENHANCES EFFECTIVENESS OF OTHER ANTIHYPERTENSIVES	Rare blood cell disorders
Beneficial in treatment of diabetes insipidus	

▷ **Principal Uses**

As a Single Drug Product: Thiazide diuretics are used primarily to (1) increase the volume of urine (diuresis) to correct the excessive fluid retention associated with congestive heart failure and certain types of liver and kidney disease; and (2) initiate treatment for high blood pressure (hypertension). They are often the first drugs tried in treating mild to moderate hypertension. Less frequent uses include the treatment of diabetes insipidus and the prevention of kidney stones that contain calcium.

As a Combination Drug Product [CD]: When this drug is used alone to treat hypertension, it is referred to as a "step 1" antihypertensive. Should it fail to reduce the blood pressure adequately, a "step 2" antihypertensive drug is added to be taken concurrently with the "step 1" drug. These drugs may be combined into one drug product. Thiazides are available in combination with beta-blockers, hydralazine, methyldopa, reserpine and other diuretics to increase their effectiveness in treating hypertension.

How This Drug Works: By increasing the elimination of salt and water from the body (through increased urine production), this drug reduces the volume of fluid in the blood and body tissues and lowers the sodium content throughout the body. By relaxing the walls of smaller arteries and allowing them to expand, this drug increases the total capacity of the arterial system. The combined effect of these two actions (reduced blood volume in expanded space) results in lowering of the blood pressure.

Available Dosage Forms and Strengths

Injection — 500 mg/20 ml
Oral Suspension — 250 mg per teaspoonful (5 ml)
Tablets — 250 mg, 500 mg

▷ **Usual Adult Dosage Range:** As antihypertensive: 500 to 1000 mg/day initially; 500 to 2000 mg/day for maintenance. As diuretic: 500 to 2000 mg/day initially; the smallest effective dose should be determined. The total daily dose should not exceed 2000 mg. **Note: Actual dosage and administration schedule must be determined by the physician for each patient individually.**

▷ **Dosing Instructions:** May be taken with or following meals to reduce stomach irritation. Best taken in the morning to avoid nighttime urination. The tablet may be crushed for administration.

Usual Duration of Use: Continual use on a regular schedule for 2 to 3 weeks is usually necessary to determine this drug's effectiveness in lowering high blood pressure. Long-term use (months to years) requires periodic evaluation of response and possible dosage adjustment. Use as a diuretic should be intermittent with "drug holidays" (no drug taken) to reduce the risk of sodium and potassium imbalance.

▷ **This Drug Should Not Be Taken If**
  • you have had an allergic reaction to any dosage form of it previously.

▷ **Inform Your Physician Before Taking This Drug If**
  • you are allergic to any form of "sulfa" drug.
  • you are pregnant or planning pregnancy.
  • you have a history of kidney or liver disease.
  • you have diabetes, gout or lupus erythematosus.
  • you are taking any form of cortisone, digitalis, oral antidiabetic drug or insulin.
  • you plan to have surgery under general anesthesia in the near future.

Possible Side-Effects (natural, expected and unavoidable drug actions)
  Light-headedness on arising from sitting or lying position (see orthostatic hypotension in Glossary).
  Increase in blood sugar level, affecting control of diabetes.
  Increase in blood uric acid level, affecting control of gout.
  Decrease in blood potassium level, causing muscle weakness and cramping.

▷ **Possible Adverse Effects** (unusual, unexpected and infrequent reactions)
  If any of the following develop, consult your physician promptly.
  Mild Adverse Effects
  Allergic Reactions: Skin rashes, hives, drug fever.
  Headache, dizziness, blurred or yellow vision.
  Reduced appetite, indigestion, nausea, vomiting, diarrhea.
  Serious Adverse Effects
  Allergic Reactions: Hepatitis with jaundice (see Glossary), anaphylactic reaction (see Glossary), severe skin reactions.
  Inflammation of the pancreas—severe abdominal pain.
  Bone marrow depression (see Glossary)—fatigue, weakness, fever, sore throat, abnormal bleeding or bruising.

▷ **Adverse Effects That May Mimic Natural Diseases or Disorders**
  Liver reaction may suggest viral hepatitis.

Natural Diseases or Disorders That May Be Activated by This Drug
  Diabetes, gout, systemic lupus erythematosus.

CAUTION
  1. Do not exceed recommended doses. Increased dosage can cause exces-

sive loss of sodium and potassium, with resultant loss of appetite, nausea, fatigue, weakness, confusion and tingling in the extremities.

2. If you are also taking a digitalis preparation (digitoxin, digoxin), ensure an adequate intake of high-potassium foods to prevent potassium deficiency—a potential cause of digitalis toxicity. (See Table of High Potassium Foods in Section Six.)

Precautions for Use

By Infants and Children: Avoid overdosage that could cause serious dehydration. Significant potassium loss can occur within the first 2 weeks of drug use.

By Those over 60 Years of Age: Small doses are advisable until your individual response has been determined. You may be more susceptible to the development of impaired thinking, orthostatic hypotension, potassium loss and blood sugar increase. Overdosage and extended use of this drug can cause excessive loss of body water, thickening (increased viscosity) of the blood and an increased tendency for the blood to clot—predisposing to stroke, heart attack or thrombophlebitis (vein inflammation with blood clot).

▷ Advisability of Use During Pregnancy

Pregnancy Category: D (tentative). See Pregnancy Code inside back cover.
Animal studies: No birth defects found in rat studies.
Human studies: Reports are conflicting and inconclusive. This drug does not seem to carry the risk of birth defects that has been found with other related diuretics. However, other types of fetal injury are possible with this drug. It should not be used during pregnancy unless a very serious complication occurs for which this drug is significantly beneficial. Ask physician for guidance.

Advisability of Use if Breast-Feeding

Presence of this drug in breast milk: Yes, in small amounts.
Avoid drug or refrain from nursing.

Habit-Forming Potential: None.

Effects of Overdosage: Dry mouth, thirst, lethargy, weakness, muscle cramping, nausea, vomiting, drowsiness progressing to stupor or coma.

Possible Effects of Long-Term Use: Impaired balance of water, salt and potassium in blood and body tissues. Development of diabetes in predisposed individuals. Pathological changes in parathyroid glands with increased blood calcium levels and decreased blood phosphate levels.

Suggested Periodic Examinations While Taking This Drug   (at physician's discretion)

Complete blood cell counts, measurements of blood levels of sodium, potassium, chloride, sugar and uric acid.
Kidney and liver function tests.

▷ While Taking This Drug, Observe the Following

Foods: Consult your physician regarding the advisability of eating foods rich in potassium. If so advised, see the Table of High Potassium Foods in Section Six. Follow physician's advice regarding the use of salt.

Beverages: No restrictions. This drug may be taken with milk.

▷ *Alcohol*: Use with caution until the combined effects have been determined. Alcohol may exaggerate the blood-pressure-lowering effects of this drug and cause orthostatic hypotension.

Tobacco Smoking: No interactions expected. Follow physician's advice.

▷ *Other Drugs*

Chlorothiazide may *increase* the effects of

- other antihypertensive drugs; dosage adjustments may be necessary to prevent excessive lowering of blood pressure.
- lithium, and cause lithium toxicity.

Chlorothiazide may *decrease* the effects of

- oral antidiabetic drugs (sulfonylureas); dosage adjustments may be necessary for proper control of blood sugar.

Chlorothiazide *taken concurrently* with

- digitalis preparations (digitoxin, digoxin) requires very careful monitoring and dosage adjustments to prevent fluctuations of blood potassium levels and serious disturbances of heart rhythm.

The following drugs may *decrease* the effects of chlorothiazide

- cholestyramine (Cuemid, Questran) may interfere with its absorption.
- colestipol (Colestid) may interfere with its absorption.

Take cholestyramine and colestipol 1 hour before any oral diuretic.

▷ *Driving, Hazardous Activities*: Use caution until the possible occurrence of orthostatic hypotension, dizziness or impaired vision has been determined.

Aviation Note: The use of this drug *may be a disqualification* for piloting. Consult a designated Aviation Medical Examiner.

Exposure to Sun: Use caution until sensitivity has been determined. This drug can cause photosensitivity (see Glossary).

Exposure to Heat: Avoid excessive perspiring, which could cause additional loss of salt and water from the body.

Heavy Exercise or Exertion: Avoid exertion that produces light-headedness, excessive fatigue or muscle cramping. Isometric exercises—the "overload" technique for strengthening individual muscles—can raise blood pressure significantly. Ask physician for guidance regarding participation in this form of exercise.

Occurrence of Unrelated Illness: Illnesses that cause vomiting or diarrhea can produce a serious imbalance of important body chemistry. Consult your physician for guidance.

Discontinuation: This drug should not be stopped abruptly following long-term use; serious thiazide-withdrawal fluid retention (edema) can develop after sudden withdrawal. The dose should be reduced gradually. It may be advisable to discontinue this drug 5 to 7 days before major surgery. Ask your physician, surgeon and/or anesthesiologist for guidance regarding dosage adjustment or drug withdrawal.

CHLORPHENIRAMINE
(klor fen IR a meen)

Introduced: 1949

Class: Antihistamines

Prescription: USA: No
Canada: No

Controlled Drug: USA: No
Canada: No

Available as Generic: USA: Yes
Canada: No

Brand Names: Allerest [CD], ♣Chlorphen, Chlor-Trimeton, ♣Chlor-Tripolon, Contac [CD], Deconamine [CD], Demazin [CD], Hycomine Compound [CD], Isoclor [CD], Naldecon [CD], Novafed A [CD], ♣Novopheniram, Ornade [CD], ♣Ornade-A.F. [CD], ♣Ornade-DM [CD], ♣Ornade Expectorant [CD], Penntuss [CD], Polaramine*, Rynatan [CD], Sine-Off [CD], Singlet [CD], Teldrin

---

BENEFITS versus RISKS

Possible Benefits	*Possible Risks*
EFFECTIVE RELIEF OF ALLERGIC RHINITIS AND ALLERGIC SKIN DISORDERS	Mild sedation Atropinelike effects Very rare blood cell disorders

---

▷ **Principal Uses**

As a Single Drug Product: Used primarily to provide symptomatic relief in allergic and related disorders: seasonal and perennial allergic rhinitis (hay fever), allergic conjunctivitis and vasomotor rhinitis; also in hives and localized swellings (angioedema) of allergic origin.

As a Combination Drug Product [CD]: This drug is combined with a decongestant drug to enhance its ability to reduce tissue swelling and secretions in allergic and infectious disorders of the upper respiratory tract— hay fever, head colds and sinusitis. It is also combined with decongestants, expectorants and codeine to increase their effectiveness in the symptomatic treatment of allergic and infectious disorders of the lower respiratory tract, often with associated coughing.

How This Drug Works: Antihistamines reduce the intensity of the allergic response by blocking the action of histamine after it has been released from sensitized tissue cells in the eyes, nose, respiratory passages and skin.

Available Dosage Forms and Strengths

Capsules, Prolonged-action — 8 mg, 12 mg
Injection — 10 mg, 20 mg, 100 mg per ml
Syrup — 2 mg per 5 ml teaspoonful (7% alcohol)
Tablets — 2 mg, 4 mg
Tablets, chewable — 2 mg
Tablets, prolonged-action — 4 mg, 6 mg, 8 mg, 12 mg

*A brand of the closely related generic drug dexchlorpheniramine.

▷ **Usual Adult Dosage Range:**   4 mg/4 to 6 hrs, or 8 to 12 mg (prolonged-action form)/12 hrs. Total daily dosage should not exceed 24 mg. **Note: Actual dosage and administration schedule must be determined by the physician for each patient individually.**

▷ **Dosing Instructions:**   Take with food or milk to prevent stomach irritation. The prolonged-action forms should be swallowed whole (not crushed or chewed).

Usual Duration of Use: Continual use on a regular schedule for 2 to 3 days is usually necessary to determine this drug's effectiveness in relieving the symptoms of allergic rhinitis and dermatosis. It may be necessary to take this drug throughout the entire pollen season, depending upon individual sensitivity. However, antihistamines should not be taken continually (without interruption) for long-term use. Limit their use to periods that require symptomatic relief.

▷ **This Drug Should Not Be Taken If**
  • you have had an allergic reaction to any dosage form of it previously.
  • you are currently undergoing allergy skin tests.
  • you are taking, or have taken within the past 14 days, any monoamine oxidase (MAO) inhibitor drug (see Drug Class, Section Four).

▷ **Inform Your Physician Before Taking This Drug If**
  • you have had any allergic reactions or unfavorable responses to the previous use of antihistamines.
  • you have glaucoma (narrow-angle type) or asthma.
  • you have epilepsy or a seizure disorder.
  • you have difficulty emptying the urinary bladder, especially if due to prostate gland enlargement.
  • you plan to have surgery under general anesthesia in the near future.

Possible Side-Effects   (natural, expected and unavoidable drug actions)
Drowsiness; sense of weakness; blurred vision; dryness of the nose, mouth and throat; impaired urination.

▷ **Possible Adverse Effects**   (unusual, unexpected and infrequent reactions)
If any of the following develop, consult your physician promptly.
Mild Adverse Effects
Allergic Reactions: Skin rash, hives.
Headache, nervous agitation, dizziness, confusion, tremor, blurred or double vision, ringing in ears.
Reduced tolerance for contact lenses.
Thickening of bronchial secretions in asthma or bronchitis.
Indigestion, nausea, vomiting, diarrhea.
Serious Adverse Effects
Allergic Reactions: Anaphylactic reaction (see Glossary).
Idiosyncratic Reactions: Euphoria, hysteria, depression, nightmares.
Hemolytic anemia (see Glossary).
Abnormally low white blood cells—fever, sore throat, infections.
Abnormally low blood platelets—abnormal bleeding or bruising.

Natural Diseases or Disorders That May Be Activated by This Drug
Latent epilepsy, glaucoma, prostatism (see Glossary).

CAUTION
1. Discontinue this drug 4 days before diagnostic skin testing procedures in order to prevent false negative test results.
2. Do not use this drug if you have active bronchial asthma, bronchitis or pneumonia. It can thicken bronchial mucus and make it more difficult to remove (by absorption or coughing).

Precautions for Use
By Infants and Children: This drug should not be used in premature or full-term newborn infants. Doses for children should be small. The young child is especially sensitive to the effects of antihistamines on the brain and nervous system.
By Those over 60 Years of Age: You may be more susceptible to the development of drowsiness, dizziness and unsteadiness, and to impairment of thinking, judgment and memory. This drug can increase the degree of impaired urination associated with prostate gland enlargement (prostatism). The sedative effects of antihistamines in the elderly can cause a syndrome of underactivity that may be misinterpreted as senility or emotional depression.

▷ **Advisability of Use During Pregnancy**
Pregnancy Category: B (tentative). See Pregnancy Code inside back cover.
Animal studies: No birth defects reported in mice.
Human studies: Information from studies in pregnant women indicates no significant increase in defects in 3931 exposures to this drug.
Ask physician for guidance.

Advisability of Use if Breast-Feeding
Presence of this drug in breast milk: Yes, in small amounts. Avoid drug or refrain from nursing.

Habit-Forming Potential: None.

Effects of Overdosage: Drowsiness; unsteadiness; faintness; marked dryness of mouth, nose and throat; flushing of face; shortness of breath; hallucinations; convulsions; stupor progressing to coma.

Possible Effects of Long-Term Use: Tardive dyskinesia (see Glossary) has been reported in association with the long-term use of several widely used antihistamines. It is advisable to avoid the prolonged, continual use of antihistamines without interruption.

Suggested Periodic Examinations While Taking This Drug   (at physician's discretion)
Complete blood cell counts.

▷ **While Taking This Drug, Observe the Following**
Foods: No restrictions.

Beverages: No restrictions. May be taken with milk.

▷ *Alcohol*: Use with extreme caution until the combined effects have been determined. The combination of antihistamine and alcohol can produce rapid and marked sedation.

Tobacco Smoking: No interactions expected.

▷ *Other Drugs*

Chlorpheniramine may *increase* the effects of
- all sedatives, sleep-inducing drugs, tranquilizers, analgesics and narcotic drugs, and produce oversedation.

Chlorpheniramine *taken concurrently* with
- phenytoin (Dantoin, Dilantin) may cause phenytoin toxicity, and may alter the pattern of seizures. Dosage adjustments may be necessary.

The following drugs may *increase* the effects of chlorpheniramine
- monoamine oxidase (MAO) inhibitor drugs (see Drug Class, Section Four) may prolong the action of antihistamines.

▷ *Driving, Hazardous Activities*: This drug can impair mental alertness, judgment, coordination and reaction time. Avoid hazardous activities until the full sedative effects have been determined.

Aviation Note: The use of this drug *is a disqualification* for piloting. Consult a designated Aviation Medical Examiner.

Exposure to Sun: Use caution. Some drugs of this class can cause photosensitivity (see Glossary).

CHLORPROMAZINE
(klor PROH ma zeen)

Introduced: 1952

Class: Strong Tranquilizer, Phenothiazines

Prescription: USA: Yes
Canada: Yes

Controlled Drug: USA: No
Canada: No

Available as Generic: Yes

Brand   Names: ✤Apo-Chlorpromazine,   ✤Chlor-Promanyl,   ✤Largactil, ✤Novochlorpromazine, Promapar, Sonazine, Thorazine

BENEFITS versus RISKS	
Possible Benefits	*Possible Risks*
EFFECTIVE CONTROL OF ACUTE MENTAL DISORDERS in the majority of patients	SERIOUS TOXIC EFFECTS ON BRAIN with long-term use
Beneficial effects on thinking, mood and behavior	Liver damage with jaundice (less than 0.5%)
Moderately effective control of nausea and vomiting	Rare blood cell disorders: hemolytic anemia, abnormally low white blood cells

▷ **Principal Uses**

As a Single Drug Product: This antipsychotic drug is used primarily to treat acute and chronic psychotic disorders such as agitated depression, schizophrenia and similar states of mental dysfunction. It may be used as a tranquilizer in the management of agitated and disruptive behavior in the absence of true psychosis. Less frequently it may be used to relieve severe nausea or vomiting.

How This Drug Works: Not completely established. Present theory is that by inhibiting the action of dopamine, this drug acts to correct an imbalance of nerve impulse transmissions that is thought to be responsible for certain mental disorders.

Available Dosage Forms and Strengths

Capsules, prolonged-action — 30 mg, 75 mg, 150 mg, 200 mg, 300 mg
Concentrate — 30 mg per ml, 100 mg per ml
Injection — 25 mg per ml
Suppositories — 25 mg, 100 mg
Syrup — 10 mg per teaspoonful (5 ml)
Tablets — 10 mg, 25 mg, 50 mg, 100 mg, 200omg

▷ **Usual Adult Dosage Range:**   Initially 10 to 25 mg 3 or 4 times daily. Dose may be increased by 20 to 50 mg at 3- to 4-day intervals as needed and tolerated. Usual dosage range is 300 to 800 mg daily. Extreme range is 25 to 2000 mg daily. Total daily dosage should not exceed 2000 mg. **Note: Actual dosage and administration schedule must be determined by the physician for each patient individually.**

▷ **Dosing Instructions:**   May be taken with or following meals to reduce stomach irritation. Tablets may be crushed for administration. Prolonged-action capsules may be opened, but do not crush or chew contents.

Usual Duration of Use: Continual use on a regular schedule for several weeks is usually necessary to determine this drug's effectiveness in controlling psychotic disorders. If not significantly beneficial within 6 weeks, it should be discontinued. Long-term use (months to years) requires periodic evaluation of response, appropriate dosage adjustment and consideration of continued need.

▷ **This Drug Should Not Be Taken If**
• you are allergic to any of the drugs bearing the brand names listed above.
• you have active liver disease.
• you have cancer of the breast.
• you have a current blood cell or bone marrow disorder.

▷ **Inform Your Physician Before Taking This Drug If**
• you are allergic or abnormally sensitive to any phenothiazine drug (see Drug Class, Section Four).
• you have impaired liver or kidney function.
• you have any type of seizure disorder.

- you have diabetes, glaucoma or heart disease.
- you have a history of lupus erythematosus.
- you are taking any drug with sedative effects.
- you plan to have surgery under general or spinal anesthesia in the near future.

Possible Side-Effects   (natural, expected and unavoidable drug actions)

Drowsiness (usually during the first 2 weeks), orthostatic hypotension (see Glossary), blurred vision, dry mouth, nasal congestion, constipation, impaired urination.

Pink or purple coloration of urine, of no significance.

▷ **Possible Adverse Effects**   (unusual, unexpected and infrequent reactions)

If any of the following develop, consult your physician promptly.

Mild Adverse Effects

Allergic Reactions: Skin rash, hives, low-grade fever.

Lowering of body temperature, especially in the elderly.

Increased appetite and weight gain.

Breast fullness, tenderness, milk production, menstrual irregularity.

Weakness, agitation, insomnia, impaired day and night vision.

Chronic constipation, fecal impaction.

Serious Adverse Effects

Allergic Reactions: Hepatitis with jaundice (see Glossary), usually between second and fourth week; high fever; asthma; anaphylactic reaction (see Glossary).

Depression, disorientation, seizures.

Disturbances of heart rhythm, rapid heart rate.

Hemolytic anemia (see Glossary), impaired production of white blood cells—fever, sore throat, infections.

Parkinson-like disorders (see Glossary); muscle spasms of face, jaw, neck, back, extremities.

Prolonged drop in blood pressure with weakness, perspiration and fainting.

▷ **Adverse Effects That May Mimic Natural Diseases or Disorders**

Nervous system reactions may suggest Parkinson's disease.

Liver reactions may suggest viral hepatitis.

Reactions resembling systemic lupus erythematosus can occur.

Natural Diseases or Disorders That May Be Activated by This Drug

Latent epilepsy, glaucoma, diabetes mellitus (25%), prostatism (see Glossary).

CAUTION

1. Many over-the-counter medications (see OTC Drugs in Glossary) for allergies, colds and coughs contain drugs that can interact unfavorably with this drug. Ask your physician or pharmacist for guidance before using any such medications.
2. Antacids that contain aluminum and/or magnesium can prevent the absorption of this drug and reduce its effectiveness.

3. Obtain prompt evaluation of any change or disturbance of vision.
4. This drug can cause false positive pregnancy tests.

Precautions for Use
By Infants and Children: Do not use this drug in infants under 6 months of age, or in children of any age with symptoms suggestive of Reye syndrome (see Glossary). Monitor carefully for blood cell changes.

By Those over 60 Years of Age: Small doses are advisable until individual response has been determined. You may be more susceptible to the development of drowsiness, lethargy, constipation, lowering of body temperature (hypothermia) and orthostatic hypotension (see Glossary). This drug can enhance existing prostatism (see Glossary). You may also be more susceptible to the development of Parkinson-like reactions and/or tardive dyskinesia (see discussion of these terms in Glossary). These reactions must be recognized early since they may become unresponsive to treatment and irreversible.

▷ Advisability of Use During Pregnancy
Pregnancy Category: C (tentative). See Pregnancy Code inside back cover.

Animal studies: No birth defects reported in rodent studies.

Human studies: No increase in birth defects reported in 284 exposures. Information from adequate studies in pregnant women is not available.

Limit use to small and infrequent doses. Avoid drug during the last month because of possible effects of the newborn infant.

Advisability of Use if Breast-Feeding
Presence of this drug in breast milk: Yes, in small amounts.

Monitor nursing infant closely and discontinue drug or nursing if adverse effects develop.

Habit-Forming Potential: None.

Effects of Overdosage: Marked drowsiness, weakness, tremor, agitation, unsteadiness, deep sleep, coma, convulsions.

Possible Effects of Long-Term Use: Tardive dyskinesia in 10% to 20% (see Glossary); eye changes—cataracts and pigmentation of retina; gray to violet pigmentation of skin in exposed areas, more common in women; severe ulcerative colitis.

Suggested Periodic Examinations While Taking This Drug   (at physician's discretion)
Complete blood cell counts, especially between the fourth and tenth weeks of treatment.

Liver function tests, electrocardiograms.

Complete eye examinations—eye structures and vision.

Careful inspection of the tongue for early evidence of fine, involuntary, wavelike movements that could indicate the beginning of tardive dyskinesia.

▷ While Taking This Drug, Observe the Following
Foods: No restrictions.

Nutritional Support: A riboflavin (vitamin B-2) supplement should be taken with long-term use.

Beverages: No restrictions. May be taken with milk.

▷ *Alcohol*: Avoid completely. Alcohol can increase the sedative action of phenothiazines and accentuate their depressant effects on brain function and blood pressure. Phenothiazines can increase the intoxicating effects of alcohol.

Tobacco Smoking: Possible reduction of drowsiness from drug.

Marijuana Smoking: Moderate increase in drowsiness; accentuation of orthostatic hypotension; increased risk of precipitating latent psychoses, confusing the interpretation of mental status and drug responses.

▷ *Other Drugs*

Chlorpromazine may *increase* the effects of
- all sedative drugs, especially meperidine (Demerol), and cause excessive sedation.
- all atropinelike drugs, and cause nervous system toxicity.

Chlorpromazine may *decrease* the effects of
- guanethidine (Ismelin, Esimil), and reduce its effectiveness in lowering blood pressure.

Chlorpromazine *taken concurrently* with
- propranolol (Inderal) may cause increased effects of both drugs; monitor drug effects closely and adjust dosages as necessary.

The following drugs may *decrease* the effects of chlorpromazine
- antacids containing aluminum and/or magnesium.
- benztropine (Cogentin).
- trihexyphenidyl (Artane).

▷ *Driving, Hazardous Activities*: This drug can impair mental alertness, judgment and physical coordination. Avoid hazardous activities.

Aviation Note: The use of this drug *is a disqualification* for piloting. Consult a designated Aviation Medical Examiner.

Exposure to Sun: Use caution until sensitivity has been determined. Some phenothiazines can cause photosensitivity (see Glossary).

Exposure to Heat: Use caution and avoid excessive heat as much as possible. This drug may impair the regulation of body temperature and increase the risk of heat stroke.

Exposure to Cold: Use caution and dress warmly. This drug can increase the risk of hypothermia in the elderly.

Discontinuation: After a period of long-term use, do not discontinue this drug suddenly. Gradual withdrawal over 2 to 3 weeks under physician supervision is recommended. Do not discontinue this drug without your physician's knowledge and approval. The relapse rate of schizophrenia after discontinuation is 50% to 60%.

CHLORPROPAMIDE
(klor PROH pa mide)

Introduced: 1958   **Class:** Antidiabetic, Sulfonylureas

Prescription: USA: Yes   **Controlled Drug:** USA: No
Canada: Yes   Canada: No

Available as Generic: Yes

Brand   Names: ❦Apo-Chlorpropamide,   ❦Chloronase,   Diabinese,
❦Novopropamide

BENEFITS versus RISKS

Possible Benefits	*Possible Risks*
Assistance in regulating blood sugar in noninsulin-dependent diabetes (adjunctive to appropriate diet and weight control)	HYPOGLYCEMIA, severe and prolonged Allergic skin reactions (some severe) Water retention Liver damage Rare blood cell and bone marrow disorders

---

▷ **Principal Uses**

As a Single Drug Product: To assist in the control of mild to moderately severe type II diabetes mellitus (adult, maturity-onset) that does not require insulin, but that cannot be adequately controlled by diet alone.

How This Drug Works: It is thought that this drug (1) stimulates the secretion of insulin (by a pancreas that is capable of responding to stimulation), and (2) enhances the utilization of insulin by appropriate tissues.

Available Dosage Forms and Strengths
Tablets — 100 mg, 250 mg

▷ **Usual Adult Dosage Range:**   Initially 250 mg daily with breakfast. After 5 to 7 days, dose may be increased to 500 mg daily if needed and tolerated. Total daily dosage should not exceed 750 mg. A "loading" or priming dose is not necessary and should not be given. **Note: Actual dosage and administration schedule must be determined by the physician for each patient individually.**

▷ **Dosing Instructions:**   May be taken with food to reduce stomach irritation. Tablet may be crushed for administration.

Usual Duration of Use: Continual use on a regular schedule for 1 to 2 weeks is usually necessary to determine this drug's effectiveness in controlling diabetes. Failure to respond to maximal doses within 1 month constitutes a primary failure. Up to 15% of those who respond initially may develop secondary failure of the drug within the first year of use. The duration of effective use can only be determined by periodic measurement of the blood sugar.

▷ **This Drug Should Not Be Taken If**
- you have had an allergic reaction to it previously.
- you have severe impairment of liver or kidney function.
- you are pregnant.

▷ **Inform Your Physician Before Taking This Drug If**
- you are allergic to other sulfonylurea drugs or to "sulfa" drugs.
- your diabetes has been unstable or "brittle" in the past.
- you do not know how to recognize or treat hypoglycemia (see Glossary).
- you have a history of congestive heart failure, peptic ulcer disease, cirrhosis of the liver, hypothyroidism or porphyria.

Possible Side-Effects   (natural, expected and unavoidable drug actions)
If drug dosage is excessive or food intake is delayed or inadequate, abnormally low blood sugar (hypoglycemia) will occur as a predictable drug effect.

▷ **Possible Adverse Effects**   (unusual, unexpected and infrequent reactions)
If any of the following develop, consult your physician promptly.
Mild Adverse Effects
Allergic Reactions: Skin rash, hives, itching, drug fever.
Headache, ringing in ears, weakness, numbness and tingling.
Indigestion, nausea, vomiting, diarrhea (may be severe).
Serious Adverse Effects
Allergic Reactions: Hepatitis with jaundice (see Glossary), severe skin reactions.
Idiosyncratic Reactions: Hemolytic anemia (see Glossary);
Disulfiramlike reaction with concurrent use of alcohol (see Glossary).
Water retention (edema), weight gain.
Bone marrow depression (see Glossary)—fatigue, weakness, fever, sore throat, abnormal bleeding or bruising.

▷ **Adverse Effects That May Mimic Natural Diseases or Disorders**
Liver reactions may suggest viral hepatitis.

Natural Diseases or Disorders That May Be Activated by This Drug
Acute intermittent porphyria, congestive heart failure (in predisposed individuals), peptic ulcer disease.

CAUTION
1. This drug must be regarded as only one part of the total program for the management of your diabetes. It is not a substitute for a properly prescribed diet and regular exercise.
2. Over a period of time (usually several months), this drug may lose its effectiveness in controlling blood sugar levels. Periodic follow-up examinations are necessary to monitor all aspects of response to drug treatment.
3. This drug has a long duration of action (up to 60 hours) and therefore

can be cumulative in its effects. It can produce severe and prolonged hypoglycemia in some individuals, especially the elderly.

Precautions for Use

By Infants and Children: This drug is not effective in type I (juvenile, growth-onset) insulin-dependent diabetes.

By Those over 60 Years of Age: This drug is best avoided in this age group. Due to its long duration of action it can accumulate and cause marked and prolonged hypoglycemia. Repeated episodes of hypoglycemia in the elderly can cause brain damage.

▷ Advisability of Use During Pregnancy

Pregnancy Category: X (tentative). See Pregnancy Code inside back cover.

Animal studies: Results are inconclusive.

Human studies: Information from adequate studies in pregnant women is not available.

The manufacturer states that this drug is contraindicated during entire pregnancy.

Advisability of Use if Breast-Feeding

Presence of this drug in breast milk: Yes.

Avoid drug or refrain from nursing.

Habit-Forming Potential: None.

Effects of Overdosage: Symptoms of mild to severe hypoglycemia: headache, light-headedness, faintness, nervousness, confusion, tremor, sweating, heart palpitation, weakness, hunger, nausea, vomiting, stupor progressing to coma.

Possible Effects of Long-Term Use: Reduced function of the thyroid gland (hypothyroidism). Reports of increased frequency and severity of heart and blood vessel diseases associated with long-term use of this class of drugs are highly controversial and inconclusive. A direct cause-and-effect relationship (see Glossary) is tenuous. Ask your physician for guidance.

Suggested Periodic Examinations While Taking This Drug   (at physician's discretion)

Complete blood cell counts, liver function tests, thyroid function tests, periodic evaluation of heart and circulatory system.

▷ While Taking This Drug, Observe the Following

Foods: Follow the diabetic diet prescribed by your physician.

Beverages: As directed in the diabetic diet. May be taken with milk.

▷   *Alcohol*: Use with extreme caution until the combined effect has been determined. Alcohol can exaggerate this drug's hypoglycemic effect. This drug can cause a marked intolerance of alcohol resulting in a disulfiramlike reaction (see Glossary): facial flushing, sweating, palpitation.

Tobacco Smoking: No interactions expected.

▷   *Other Drugs*

The following drugs may ***increase*** the effects of chlorpropamide
• ammonium chloride.

- aspirin, and other salicylates.
- chloramphenicol (Chloromycetin).
- clofibrate (Atromid S).
- dicumarol.
- fenfluramine (Pondimin).
- monoamine oxidase (MAO) inhibitor drugs (see Drug Class, Section Four).
- phenylbutazone (Butazolidin).
- some "sulfa" drugs: sulfamethoxazole (Gantanol), sulfisoxazole (Gantrisin).

The following drugs may *decrease* the effects of chlorpropamide

- diazoxide (Proglycem).
- propranolol (Inderal).
- rifampin (Rifidin, Rimactane).
- sodium bicarbonate.
- thiazide diuretics (see Drug Class, Section Four).

▷ *Driving, Hazardous Activities*: Regulate your dosage schedule, eating schedule and physical activities very carefully to prevent hypoglycemia. Be able to recognize the early symptoms of hypoglycemia so you can avoid hazardous activities and take corrective measures.

Aviation Note: Diabetes *is a disqualification* for piloting. Consult a designated Aviation Medical Examiner.

Exposure to Sun: Use caution until sensitivity has been determined. Some drugs of this class can cause photosensitivity (see Glossary).

Occurrence of Unrelated Illness: Acute infections, illnesses causing vomiting or diarrhea, serious injuries and surgical procedures can interfere with diabetic control and may require the use of insulin. If any of these conditions occur, consult your physician promptly.

Discontinuation: It is estimated that no more than 12% of patients remain well controlled by this drug for more than 6 to 7 years. Because of the high incidence of secondary failures, it is advisable to evaluate the continued benefit of this drug every 6 months.

CHLORTHALIDONE
(klor THAL i dohn)

Introduced: 1960

Prescription: USA: Yes
Canada: Yes

Available as Generic: USA: Yes
Canada: Yes

Class: Antihypertensive, Diuretic

Controlled Drug: USA: No
Canada: No

Brand Names: ✽Apo-Chlorthalidone, Combipres [CD], Demi-Regroton [CD], Hygroton, ✽Novothalidone, Regroton [CD], Tenoretic [CD], Thalitone, ✽Uridon

```
┌─────────────────────────────────────────────────────────────────────┐
│                      BENEFITS versus RISKS                          │
│                                                                     │
│         Possible Benefits                    Possible Risks         │
│  EFFECTIVE, WELL-TOLERATED        Loss of body potassium            │
│    DIURETIC                       Increased blood sugar             │
│  POSSIBLY EFFECTIVE IN MILD       Increased blood uric acid         │
│    HYPERTENSION                   Increased blood calcium           │
│  ENHANCES EFFECTIVENESS OF        Rare blood cell disorders         │
│    OTHER ANTIHYPERTENSIVES                                          │
│  Beneficial in treatment of diabetes                               │
│    insipidus                                                        │
└─────────────────────────────────────────────────────────────────────┘
```

▷ **Principal Uses**

As a Single Drug Product: Thiazidelike diuretics are used primarily to (1) increase the volume of urine (diuresis) to correct the excessive fluid retention associated with congestive heart failure and certain types of liver and kidney disease; and (2) initiate treatment for high blood pressure (hypertension). They are often the first drugs tried in treating mild to moderate hypertension. Less frequent uses include the treatment of diabetes insipidus and the prevention of kidney stones that contain calcium.

As a Combination Drug Product [CD]: When this drug is used alone to treat hypertension, it is referred to as a "step 1" antihypertensive. Should it fail to reduce the blood pressure adequately, a "step 2" antihypertensive drug is added to be taken concurrently with the "step 1" drug. These drugs may be combined into one drug product. This drug is available in combination with atenolol, clonidine and reserpine to increase their effectiveness in treating hypertension.

How This Drug Works: By increasing the elimination of salt and water from the body (through increased urine production), this drug reduces the volume of fluid in the blood and body tissues and lowers the sodium content throughout the body. By relaxing the walls of smaller arteries and allowing them to expand, this drug increases the total capacity of the arterial system. The combined effect of these two actions (reduced blood volume in expanded space) results in lowering of blood pressure.

Available Dosage Forms and Strengths
Tablets — 25 mg, 50 mg, 100 mg

▷ **Usual Adult Dosage Range:**   As antihypertensive: 25 to 50 mg/day initially; 50 to 100 mg/day for maintenance. As diuretic: 50 to 100 mg/day initially; the smallest effective dose should be determined. The total daily dose should not exceed 200 mg. **Note: Actual dosage and administration schedule must be determined by the physician for each patient individually.**

▷ **Dosing Instructions:**   May be taken with or following meals to reduce stomach irritation. Best taken in the morning to avoid nighttime urination. The tablet may be crushed for administration.

Usual Duration of Use: Continual use on a regular schedule for 2 to 3 weeks is usually necessary to determine this drug's effectiveness in lowering high blood pressure. Long-term use (months to years) requires periodic evaluation of response and possible dosage adjustment. Use as a diuretic should be intermittent with "drug holidays" (no drug taken) to reduce the risk of sodium and potassium imbalance.

▷ **This Drug Should Not Be Taken If**
- you have had an allergic reaction to it previously.

▷ **Inform Your Physician Before Taking This Drug If**
- you are allergic to any form of "sulfa" drug.
- you are pregnant or planning pregnancy.
- you have a history of kidney or liver disease.
- you have diabetes, gout or lupus erythematosus.
- you are taking any form of cortisone, digitalis, oral antidiabetic drug or insulin.
- you plan to have surgery under general anesthesia in the near future.

Possible Side-Effects (natural, expected and unavoidable drug actions)
Light-headedness on arising from sitting or lying position (see orthostatic hypotension in Glossary).
Increase in blood sugar level, affecting control of diabetes.
Increase in blood uric acid level, affecting control of gout.
Decrease in blood potassium level, causing muscle weakness and cramping.

▷ **Possible Adverse Effects** (unusual, unexpected and infrequent reactions)
If any of the following develop, consult your physician promptly.
Mild Adverse Effects
Allergic Reactions: Skin rashes, hives, drug fever.
Headache, dizziness, blurred or yellow vision.
Reduced appetite, indigestion, nausea, vomiting, diarrhea.
Serious Adverse Effects
Allergic Reactions: Hepatitis with jaundice (see Glossary), anaphylactic reaction (see Glossary), severe skin reactions.
Inflammation of the pancreas—severe abdominal pain.
Bone marrow depression (see Glossary)—fatigue, weakness, fever, sore throat, abnormal bleeding or bruising.

▷ **Adverse Effects That May Mimic Natural Diseases or Disorders**
Liver reaction may suggest viral hepatitis.

Natural Diseases or Disorders That May Be Activated by This Drug
Diabetes, gout, systemic lupus erythematosus (questionable).

CAUTION
1. Do not exceed recommended doses. Increased dosage can cause excessive loss of sodium and potassium, with resultant loss of appetite, nausea, fatigue, weakness, confusion and tingling in the extremities.
2. If you are also taking a digitalis preparation (digitoxin, digoxin), ensure

an adequate intake of high-potassium foods to prevent potassium deficiency, a potential cause of digitalis toxicity. (See Table of High Potassium Foods in Section Six.)

Precautions for Use

By Infants and Children: Avoid overdosage that could cause serious dehydration. Significant potassium loss can occur within the first 2 weeks of drug use.

By Those over 60 Years of Age: Small doses are advisable until your individual response has been determined. You may be more susceptible to the development of fatigue (40%), low blood potassium (10%), elevated blood uric acid (30%), impaired thinking, orthostatic hypotension and blood sugar increase. Overdosage and extended use of this drug can cause excessive loss of body water, thickening (increased viscosity) of the blood, and an increased tendency for the blood to clot—predisposing to stroke, heart attack, or thrombophlebitis (vein inflammation with blood clot). Report promptly any type of skin reaction.

▷ **Advisability of Use During Pregnancy**

Pregnancy Category: D (tentative). See Pregnancy Code inside back cover.
Animal studies: No birth defects reported.
Human studies: Information from adequate studies in pregnant women is not available.
It should not be used during pregnancy unless a very serious complication occurs for which this drug is significantly beneficial. Ask physician for guidance.

Advisability of Use if Breast-Feeding

Presence of this drug in breast milk: Yes.
Avoid drug or refrain from nursing.

Habit-Forming Potential: None.

Effects of Overdosage: Dry mouth, thirst, lethargy, weakness, muscle cramping, nausea, vomiting, drowsiness progressing to stupor or coma.

Possible Effects of Long-Term Use: Impaired balance of water, salt and potassium in blood and body tissues. Development of diabetes in predisposed individuals. Pathological changes in parathyroid glands with increased blood calcium levels and decreased blood phosphate levels.

Suggested Periodic Examinations While Taking This Drug   (at physician's discretion)
Complete blood cell counts; measurements of blood levels of sodium, potassium, chloride, sugar and uric acid.
Kidney and liver function tests.

▷ **While Taking This Drug, Observe the Following**

Foods: Consult your physician regarding the advisability of eating foods rich in potassium. If so advised, see the Table of High Potassium Foods in Section Six. Follow physician's advice regarding the use of salt.
Beverages: No restrictions. This drug may be taken with milk.

▷   *Alcohol*: Use with caution until the combined effects have been determined. Alcohol may exaggerate the blood-pressure-lowering effects of this drug and cause orthostatic hypotension (see Glossary).

Tobacco Smoking: No interactions expected. Follow physician's advice.

▷   *Other Drugs*

Chlorthalidone may *increase* the effects of

- other antihypertensive drugs; dosage adjustments may be necessary to prevent excessive lowering of blood pressure.
- lithium, and cause lithium toxicity.

Chlorthalidone may *decrease* the effects of

- oral antidiabetic drugs (sulfonylureas); dosage adjustments may be necessary for proper control of blood sugar.

Chlorthalidone *taken concurrently* with

- digitalis preparations (digitoxin, digoxin) requires very careful monitoring and dosage adjustments to prevent fluctuations of blood potassium levels and serious disturbances of heart rhythm.

The following drugs may *decrease* the effects of chlorthalidone

- cholestyramine (Cuemid, Questran) may interfere with its absorption.
- colestipol (Colestid) may interfere with its absorption.

Take cholestyramine and colestipol 1 hour before any oral diuretic.

▷   *Driving, Hazardous Activities*: Use caution until the possible occurrence of orthostatic hypotension, dizziness or impaired vision has been determined.

Aviation Note: The use of this drug *may be a disqualification* for piloting. Consult a designated Aviation Medical Examiner.

Exposure to Sun: Use caution until sensitivity has been determined. This drug can cause photosensitivity (see Glossary).

Exposure to Heat: Avoid excessive perspiring which could cause additional loss of salt and water from the body.

Heavy Exercise or Exertion: Avoid exertion that produces light-headedness, excessive fatigue or muscle cramping. Isometric exercises—the "overload" technique for strengthening individual muscles—can raise the blood pressure significantly. Ask physician for guidance regarding participation in this form of exercise.

Occurrence of Unrelated Illness: Illnesses that cause vomiting or diarrhea can produce a serious imbalance of important body chemistry. Consult your physician for guidance.

Discontinuation: It may be advisable to discontinue this drug 5 to 7 days before major surgery. Ask your physician, surgeon and/or anesthesiologist for guidance regarding dosage adjustment or drug withdrawal. Following long-term use, this drug should be withdrawn gradually to prevent the occurrence of rebound edema.

CHLORZOXAZONE
(klor ZOX a zohn)

Introduced: 1958

Prescription: USA: Yes
Canada: No

Available as Generic: USA: Yes
Canada: No

Brand Names: Paraflex, Parafon Forte [CD]

Class: Muscle Relaxant

Controlled Drug: USA: No
Canada: No

BENEFITS versus RISKS	
Possible Benefits	*Possible Risks*
Mild to moderate relief of discomfort due to spasm of voluntary muscles	Red and white blood cell disorders Gastrointestinal bleeding Liver damage, jaundice (questionable) (All rare)

▷ **Principal Uses**

As a Single Drug Product: Used primarily to relieve the pain and stiffness associated with spasm of voluntary muscles, such as that resulting from accidental injury of musculoskeletal structures. It is often necessary to supplement the use of this drug with other treatment measures, such as rest, support and physiotherapy.

As a Combination Drug Product [CD]: It is combined with acetaminophen to enhance its effectiveness in relieving discomfort. Acetaminophen is an effective analgesic and may be necessary to control the pain that is not relieved by chlorzoxazone alone.

How This Drug Works: Not completely established. It is thought that this drug may relieve muscle spasm and pain by blocking the transmission of nerve impulses over reflex pathways and/or by producing a sedative effect that decreases the perception of pain.

Available Dosage Forms and Strengths

Tablets — 250 mg

▷ **Usual Adult Dosage Range:** 250 to 750 mg, 3 or 4 times daily; adjust dosage as needed and tolerated. **Note: Actual dosage and administration schedule must be determined by the physician for each patient individually.**

▷ **Dosing Instructions:** Take either on empty stomach or with food to prevent stomach irritation. Tablet may be crushed for administration.

Usual Duration of Use: Continual use on a regular schedule for 2 to 3 days is usually necessary to determine this drug's effectiveness in relieving the discomfort of muscle spasm. Evaluate need for continued use after periods of 7 to 10 days.

▷ **This Drug Should Not Be Taken If**
- you have had an allergic reaction to it previously.
- you have active liver disease.

▷ **Inform Your Physician Before Taking This Drug If**
- you have experienced any unfavorable reactions to muscle relaxants in the past.
- you have a history of liver or kidney disease.

Possible Side-Effects   (natural, expected and unavoidable drug actions)
Drowsiness, orange or reddish purple discoloration of the urine (of no significance).

▷ **Possible Adverse Effects**   (unusual, unexpected and infrequent reactions)
If any of the following develop, consult your physician promptly.
Mild Adverse Effects
Allergic Reactions: Skin rash, hives, itching, spontaneous bruising.
Light-headedness, dizziness, lethargy.
Indigestion, heartburn, nausea.
Serious Adverse Effects
Idiosyncratic Reactions: Nervousness, excitement, irritability.
Anemia, abnormally low white blood cells—weakness, fever, sore throat.
Gastrointestinal bleeding—black or dark colored stools.
Liver reaction with or without jaundice (see Glossary)—yellow eyes and skin, dark colored urine, light colored stools.

▷ **Adverse Effects That May Mimic Natural Diseases or Disorders**
Liver reaction may suggest viral hepatitis.

Precautions for Use
By Infants and Children: Dosage is based on the child's age and weight. Consult your physician for exact dosage schedule.
By Those over 60 Years of Age: Small doses are advisable initially. You may be more susceptible to the development of drowsiness, dizziness, weakness, unsteadiness and falling.

▷ **Advisability of Use During Pregnancy**
Pregnancy Category: C (tentative). See Pregnancy Code inside back cover.
Animal studies: No data available.
Human studies: Information from adequate studies in pregnant women is not available.
Avoid drug if possible; use only if clearly needed.

Advisability of Use if Breast-Feeding
Presence of this drug in breast milk: Yes.
Avoid drug or refrain from nursing.

Habit-Forming Potential: None.

Effects of Overdosage: Nausea, vomiting, diarrhea, headache, drowsiness, dizziness, marked weakness, sense of paralysis of arms and legs, rapid and irregular breathing.

Possible Effects of Long-Term Use: None reported.

Suggested Periodic Examinations While Taking This Drug (at physician's discretion)
Complete blood cell counts, liver function tests.

▷ **While Taking This Drug, Observe the Following**
Foods: No restrictions.
Beverages: No restrictions. May be taken with milk.
▷ *Alcohol*: Use with caution until the combined effect has been determined. This drug may add to the depressant action of alcohol on the brain.
Tobacco Smoking: No interactions expected.
Marijuana Smoking: Moderate to marked drowsiness, muscle weakness, incoordination, accentuation of orthostatic hypotension (see Glossary).
▷ *Other Drugs*
The following drugs may *decrease* the effects of chlorzoxazone
• testosterone is reported to reduce its ability to relax muscles in spasm.
▷ *Driving, Hazardous Activities*: This drug can cause drowsiness, light-headedness or dizziness in susceptible individuals. Avoid hazardous activities if these drug effects occur.
Aviation Note: The use of this drug *is a disqualification* for piloting. Consult a designated Aviation Medical Examiner.
Exposure to Sun: No restrictions.

CIMETIDINE
(si MET i deen)

Introduced: 1976

Class: Antiulcer, H-2 Receptor Blocker

Prescription: USA: Yes
Canada: Yes

Controlled Drug: USA: No
Canada: No

Available as Generic: No

Brand Names: ✤Apo-Cimetidine, ✤Novocimetine, ✤Peptol, Tagamet

---

BENEFITS versus RISKS

Possible Benefits	*Possible Risks*
EFFECTIVE TREATMENT OF PEPTIC ULCER DISEASE	CONFUSIONAL STATES in the elderly and debilitated
Relief of symptoms	Rare blood cell and bone marrow disorders
Acceleration of healing	Rare pancreatitis
Prevention of recurrence	Rare liver damage
CONTROL OF HYPERSECRETORY STOMACH DISORDERS	Rare kidney damage
Beneficial in treatment of reflux esophagitis	

▷ **Principal Uses**

As a Single Drug Product: Used primarily in the treatment of peptic ulcer disease, specifically to hasten the healing of duodenal ulcer and to prevent its recurrence. Also used to control the excessive production of stomach acid in Zollinger-Ellison syndrome. Though its effectiveness has not been fully established, this drug is also widely used in the management of stomach (gastric) ulcer, esophagitis (as with hiatal hernia) and upper gastrointestinal bleeding.

How This Drug Works: By blocking the action of histamine, this drug effectively inhibits the secretion of stomach acid and thus creates a more favorable environment for the healing of peptic ulcers.

Available Dosage Forms and Strengths

Injection — 300 mg per 2 ml
Liquid — 300 mg per 5 ml teaspoonful (2.8% alcohol)
Tablets — 200 mg, 300 mg, 400 mg

▷ **Usual Adult Dosage Range:**   For active peptic ulcer and hypersecretory states—300 mg, 4 times daily, taken with meals and at bedtime. For prevention of recurrent ulcer—400 mg at bedtime. Total daily dosage should not exceed 1200 mg. **Note: Actual dosage and administration schedule must be determined by the physician for each patient individually.**

▷ **Dosing Instructions:**   To obtain the longest period of stomach acid reduction, this drug should be taken with or immediately following meals. The tablet may be crushed for administration.

Usual Duration of Use: Continual use on a regular schedule for 4 to 6 weeks is usually necessary to determine this drug's effectiveness in healing active peptic ulcer. Continual use for up to 1 year is recommended for prevention of ulcer recurrence.

▷ **This Drug Should Not Be Taken If**
  • you have had an allergic reaction to any dosage form of it previously.

▷ **Inform Your Physician Before Taking This Drug If**
  • you have impaired liver or kidney function.
  • you have a low sperm count.
  • you are taking any oral anticoagulant, propranolol or quinidine.

Possible Side-Effects   (natural, expected and unavoidable drug actions)
None reported.

▷ **Possible Adverse Effects**   (unusual, unexpected and infrequent reactions)
If any of the following develop, consult your physician promptly.
Mild Adverse Effects
Allergic Reactions: Skin rash, hives, drug fever (see Glossary).
Headache, dizziness, double vision, fatigue, muscular pains, diarrhea.
Breast milk secretion in women; breast swelling and tenderness in men.

Serious Adverse Effects

Allergic Reactions: Pancreatitis, kidney damage.

Idiosyncratic Reactions: Nervous agitation, confusion, delirium, hallucinations, coma.

Slowed heart rate, liver damage, reduced sperm count and fertility, reduced libido and sexual potency.

Bone marrow depression (see Glossary)—weakness, fever, sore throat, abnormal bleeding or bruising.

▷ **Adverse Effects That May Mimic Natural Diseases or Disorders**
Liver reactions may suggest viral hepatitis.

Natural Diseases or Disorders That May Be Activated by This Drug
Psoriasis (questionable).

CAUTION
1. Do not discontinue this drug abruptly. Ulcer activation and perforation have occurred following abrupt cessation.
2. Hemodialysis can remove from 8% to 14% of this drug. Schedule the dosage to follow completion of each dialysis treatment.

Precautions for Use
By Infants and Children: Safety and effectiveness for use by those under 16 years of age have not been established. If use of this drug is deemed necessary, observe for sedation, confusion, breast enlargement, milk secretion and possible kidney damage.

By Those over 60 Years of Age: Initiate treatment with one-half the usual dose. Observe for the development of nervous agitation, depression, confusion, slurred speech or excessive drowsiness. This drug can contribute to the formation of stomach phytobezoars (masses of undigested vegetable fibers). Individuals with poor chewing ability (missing teeth) and those who have had partial gastrectomy or vagotomy (stomach surgery) are most susceptible. Observe for loss of appetite, stomach fullness, nausea and vomiting.

▷ **Advisability of Use During Pregnancy**
Pregnancy Category: B (tentative). See Pregnancy Code inside back cover.
Animal studies: No birth defects reported.
Human studies: Information from adequate studies in pregnant women is not available.
Use this drug only if clearly needed. Ask physician for guidance.

Advisability of Use if Breast-Feeding
Presence of this drug in breast milk: Yes, in large amounts.
Avoid drug or refrain from nursing.

Habit-Forming Potential: None.

Effects of Overdosage: Confusion, delirium, slurred speech, flushing, sweating, drowsiness, muscle twitching, seizures, coma.

Possible Effects of Long-Term Use: Liver damage (reversible), swelling and tenderness of breast tissue in men.

Suggested Periodic Examinations While Taking This Drug (at physician's discretion)
Complete blood cell counts, liver and kidney function tests, sperm counts, prothrombin times if an anticoagulant is taken concurrently.

▷ **While Taking This Drug, Observe the Following**
Foods: Protein-rich foods produce maximal stomach acid secretion. Follow the diet prescribed to derive optimal benefit from this drug.
Nutritional Support: This drug may inhibit the absorption of vitamin B-12. Consult physician regarding the need for B-12 supplement.
Beverages: No restrictions. May be taken with milk.
▷ *Alcohol*: No interactions with drug. However, alcoholic beverages increase stomach acidity and can reduce the effectiveness of this drug.
Marijuana Smoking: Possible accentuation of reduced sperm production due to this drug.
▷ *Other Drugs*
Cimetidine may *increase* the effects of
• oral anticoagulants, and increase the risk of bleeding.
• benzodiazepines (Librium, Valium, etc.), see Drug Class, Section Four.
• phenytoin (Dilantin).
• procainamide (Procan, Pronestyl).
• propranolol (Inderal).
• quinidine (Quinaglute, etc.).
• theophylline (Theo-Dur, Bronkodyl, Slo-bid, etc.).
Cimetidine *taken concurrently* with
• carmustine (BCNU) may cause severe bone marrow depression. Do not use these drugs concurrently.
▷ *Driving, Hazardous Activities*: This drug can cause erratic driving behavior. Use caution until it has been determined that dizziness, confusion or double vision does not occur.
Aviation Note: The use of this drug *may be a disqualification* for piloting. Consult a designated Aviation Medical Examiner.
Exposure to Sun: No restrictions.
Discontinuation: Do not discontinue this drug suddenly if taken for peptic ulcer disease. Consult physician for withdrawal instructions. This drug does not provide an extended protective effect. Be alert to the possibility of ulcer recurrence anytime after discontinuation.

CLIDINIUM
(kli DIN ee um)

Introduced: 1961

Prescription: USA: Yes
Canada: Yes

Available as Generic: No

Brand Names: Librax [CD], Quarzan

Class: Antispasmodic, Atropinelike

Controlled Drug: USA: No
Canada: No

BENEFITS versus RISKS

Possible Benefits	*Possible Risks*
RELIEF OF SYMPTOMS DUE TO GASTROINTESTINAL SPASM AND OVERACTIVITY as in peptic ulcer disease and irritable bowel syndrome	Skin rash, hives Dizziness, unsteadiness Confusion, delirium

---

▷ **Principal Uses**

As a Single Drug Product: This atropinelike antispasmodic drug is used primarily in the management of peptic ulcer disease and the irritable bowel syndrome. Because it has been replaced by more effective drugs, it is seldom used alone.

As a Combination Drug Product [CD]: The major use of this drug is in combination with chlordiazepoxide. When combined, the tranquilizing effect of chlordiazepoxide and the atropinelike effects of clidinium are more effective than either drug used alone. Their actions complement each other in the treatment of peptic ulcer and functional disorders of the gastrointestinal tract.

How This Drug Works: By blocking the action of the chemical (acetylcholine) that transmits impulses at parasympathetic nerve endings, this drug prevents stimulation of muscular contraction and glandular secretion within the organs involved. This results in reduced overall activity, including the prevention or relief of muscle spasms.

Available Dosage Forms and Strengths

Capsules — 2.5 mg, 5 mg

Capsules [CD] — 2.5 mg and 5 mg of chlordiazepoxide

Note: In Canada this drug is available only in combination with chlordiazepoxide. To be fully informed on the use of Librax, read the Drug Profiles of both components.

▷ **Usual Adult Dosage Range:** For Librax—1 or 2 capsules from 1 to 4 times daily, as needed and tolerated. Total daily dosage should not exceed 8 capsules. **Note: Actual dosage and administration schedule must be determined by the physician for each patient individually.**

▷ **Dosing Instructions:** Take 30 to 60 minutes before meals and also at bedtime if necessary. The capsule may be opened for administration.

Usual Duration of Use: Continual use on a regular schedule for 3 to 5 days is usually necessary to determine this drug's effectiveness in relieving the symptoms of gastrointestinal spasm and overactivity. Long-term use (weeks to months) requires physician supervision and guidance.

▷ **This Drug Should Not Be Taken If**
- you have had an allergic reaction to it previously.
- your stomach cannot empty properly into the intestine (pyloric obstruction).
- you are unable to empty the urinary bladder completely.
- you have narrow-angle-type glaucoma.
- you have severe ulcerative colitis.

▷ **Inform Your Physician Before Taking This Drug If**
- you have open-angle type glaucoma.
- you have angina or coronary heart disease.
- you have a history of peptic ulcer disease.
- you have chronic bronchitis, a hiatal hernia, myasthenia gravis or prostatism (see Glossary).
- you plan to have surgery under general anesthesia in the near future.

Possible Side-Effects (natural, expected and unavoidable drug actions)
Blurred vision (impaired focus), dry mouth and throat, constipation, impaired urination. (Nature and degree of side-effects depend upon individual sensitivity and drug dosage.)

▷ **Possible Adverse Effects** (unusual, unexpected and infrequent reactions)
If any of the following develop, consult your physician promptly.
Mild Adverse Effects
Allergic Reactions: Skin rash, hives.
Light-headedness, dizziness, unsteadiness.
Dilation of pupils, causing sensitivity to light.
Flushing and dryness of skin, reduced sweating.
Rapid heart action.
Serious Adverse Effects
Idiosyncratic Reactions: Confusion, delirium, abnormal behavior.
Development of acute glaucoma (in susceptible individuals).

CAUTION
1. Many over-the-counter medications (see OTC Drugs in Glossary) for allergies, colds and coughs contain drugs that can interact unfavorably with this drug. Ask your physician or pharmacist for guidance before taking these drugs together.
2. Constipation should be treated promptly with stool softeners and effective laxatives.

Precautions for Use
By Infants and Children: Safety, effectiveness and dosage for use by those

under 12 years of age have not been established. Ask physician for guidance.

By Those over 60 Years of Age: Initial dosage should be 1 capsule twice a day until tolerance has been determined. This drug can accentuate the symptoms of prostatism (see Glossary).

▷ **Advisability of Use During Pregnancy**
Pregnancy Category: B (tentative). See Pregnancy Code inside back cover.
Animal studies: No birth defects reported.
Human studies: Information from adequate studies in pregnant women is not available.
Ask physician for guidance.

Advisability of Use if Breast-Feeding
Presence of this drug in breast milk: Yes.
Avoid drug or refrain from nursing.

Habit-Forming Potential: For clidinium—none. For Librax—see Drug Profile of Chlordiazepoxide.

Effects of Overdosage: Dilated pupils, dry mouth, headache, excitement, confusion, hallucinations, delirium, hot skin, high fever, convulsions, coma.

Possible Effects of Long-Term Use: Chronic constipation, severe enough to cause fecal impaction.

Suggested Periodic Examinations While Taking This Drug   (at physician's discretion)
Measurement of internal eye pressure to detect significant increase that could indicate developing glaucoma.

▷ **While Taking This Drug, Observe the Following**
Foods: No interactions with drug. Follow prescribed diet.
Beverages: As allowed by prescribed diet. Drug may be taken with milk.
▷   *Alcohol*: Use caution and observe for increased sedation or dizziness.
Tobacco Smoking: No interactions with clidinium. For Librax—see Drug Profile of Chlordiazepoxide.
▷   *Other Drugs*
Clidinium may *increase* the effects of
  • atenolol (Tenormin), and require reduction of its dosage.
  • other drugs with atropinelike actions (see Drug Class, Section Four).
▷   *Driving, Hazardous Activities*: This drug may cause drowsiness, dizziness or blurred vision. Avoid hazardous activities if these drug effects occur.
Aviation Note: The use of this drug *may be a disqualification* for piloting. Consult a designated Aviation Medical Examiner.
Exposure to Sun: No restrictions.
Exposure to Heat: Use extreme caution. The use of this drug in hot environments may impair the regulation of body temperature and increase the risk of heat stroke.

CLONIDINE
(KLOH ni deen)

Introduced: 1969

Prescription: USA: Yes
Canada: Yes

Available as Generic: No

Brand Names: Catapres, Catapres-TTS, Combipres [CD], ♣Dixarit

Class: Antihypertensive

Controlled Drug: USA: No
Canada: No

BENEFITS versus RISKS

Possible Benefits	*Possible Risks*
EFFECTIVE ANTIHYPER- TENSIVE in mild to moderate high blood pressure Effective control of menopausal hot flashes (in selected cases)	ACUTE WITHDRAWAL SYNDROME and hypertensive "overshoot" with abrupt discontinuation Raynaud's phenomenon (cold fingers or toes)

▷ **Principal Uses**

As a Single Drug Product: This antihypertensive drug is often used as a "step 2" drug in the treatment of mild to moderate high blood pressure. It is generally not used to initiate treatment, but is added when a "step 1" drug proves to be inadequate. It may also be used as a "step 3 or 4" drug in place of drugs that cause marked orthostatic hypotension (see Glossary). It is sometimes used to prevent migraine headache, to prevent hot flashes of the menopause and to treat menstrual cramps.

As a Combination Drug Product [CD]: This "step 2" antihypertensive is available in combination with the "step 1" antihypertensive drug chlorthalidone, a diuretic. The differing methods of action complement each other to make the combination a more effective antihypertensive.

How This Drug Works: By decreasing the activity of the vasomotor center in the brain, this drug reduces the ability of the sympathetic nervous system to maintain the degree of blood vessel constriction responsible for the elevation of blood pressure. This change results in relaxation of blood vessel walls and lowering of blood pressure.

Available Dosage Forms and Strengths
Patches — 0.1 mg, 0.2 mg, 0.3 mg
Tablets — 0.1 mg, 0.2 mg, 0.3 mg

▷ **Usual Adult Dosage Range:** Tablets—initially 0.1 mg twice daily. Increase by 0.1 to 0.2 mg daily as needed and tolerated. Usual range is 0.2 to 0.8 mg daily, taken in 2 doses. Total daily dosage should not exceed 2.4 mg. Medicated patches are applied once a week. **Note: Actual dosage and administration schedule must be determined by the physician for each patient individually.**

▷ **Dosing Instructions:**   Tablets may be taken without regard to eating. The tablet may be crushed for administration.

Usual Duration of Use: Continual use on a regular schedule for 2 to 3 weeks is usually necessary to determine this drug's effectiveness in controlling high blood pressure. Long-term use (months to years) requires supervision and guidance by the physician.

▷ **This Drug Should Not Be Taken If**
- you have had an allergic reaction to it previously.

▷ **Inform Your Physician Before Taking This Drug If**
- you have a circulatory disorder of the brain.
- you have angina or coronary artery disease.
- you have or have had serious emotional depression.
- you have Buerger's disease or Raynaud's phenomenon.
- you are taking any sedative or hypnotic drugs or an antidepressant.
- you plan to have surgery under general anesthesia in the near future.

Possible Side-Effects   (natural, expected and unavoidable drug actions)
Drowsiness (35%), dry nose and mouth (40%), constipation (common), decreased heart rate, mild orthostatic hypotension (see Glossary).

▷ **Possible Adverse Effects**   (unusual, unexpected and infrequent reactions)
If any of the following develop, consult your physician promptly.
Mild Adverse Effects
Allergic Reactions: Skin rash, hives, localized swellings, itching.
Headache, dizziness, fatigue, anxiety, nervousness, dryness and burning of eyes.
Painful parotid (salivary) gland, nausea, vomiting.
Weight gain, breast enlargement and tenderness, sexual impotence, urinary retention.
Serious Adverse Effects
Idiosyncratic Reactions: Raynaud's phenomenon.
Aggravation of congestive heart failure, heart rhythm disorders, vivid dreaming, nightmares, depression, hallucinations.
Corneal ulcers (rare). Acute pancreatitis (rare).

CAUTION
1. ***Do not discontinue this drug suddenly***. Sudden withdrawal can produce a severe and possibly fatal reaction.
2. Hot weather and the fever associated with infection can reduce blood pressure significantly. Dosage adjustments may be necessary.
3. Report the development of any tendency to emotional depression.

Precautions for Use
By Infants and Children: Safety and effectiveness for use by those under 12 years of age have not been established.
By Those over 60 Years of Age: ***Proceed cautiously*** with the use of any antihypertensive drug. Unacceptably high blood pressure should be reduced without creating the risks associated with excessively low blood

pressure. Start treatment with small doses and monitor the blood pressure response frequently. Observe for the development of light-headedness, dizziness, unsteadiness, fainting and falling. Sedation and dry mouth occur in 50% of elderly users. Report promptly any changes in mood or behavior: depression, delusions, hallucinations.

▷ **Advisability of Use During Pregnancy**
Pregnancy Category: C (tentative). See Pregnancy Code inside back cover.
Animal studies: No birth defects reported.
Human studies: Information from adequate studies in pregnant women is not available.
Avoid use of drug during the first 3 months if possible. Ask physician for guidance.

Advisability of Use if Breast-Feeding
Presence of this drug in breast milk: Yes.
This drug may impair milk production. Monitor nursing infant closely and discontinue drug or nursing if adverse effects develop.

Habit-Forming Potential: None.

Effects of Overdosage: Marked drowsiness, weakness, dry mouth, slow pulse, low blood pressure, vomiting, stupor progressing to coma.

Possible Effects of Long-Term Use: Development of tolerance (see Glossary) with loss of drug effectiveness; weight gain due to salt and water retention; temporary sexual impotence.

Suggested Periodic Examinations While Taking This Drug   (at physician's discretion)
Blood pressure measurements, monitoring of body weight.

▷ **While Taking This Drug, Observe the Following**
Foods: Avoid excessive salt. Ask physician for guidance regarding degree of salt restriction.
Beverages: No restrictions. May be taken with milk.
▷ *Alcohol*: Use with extreme caution. The combined effects can cause marked drowsiness and exaggerated reduction of blood pressure.
Tobacco Smoking: No interactions expected. Follow your physician's advice regarding use of tobacco.
▷ *Other Drugs*
Clonidine may *decrease* the effects of
• levodopa (Larodopa, Sinemet, etc.), causing an increase in parkinsonism symptoms.
Clonidine *taken concurrently* with
• beta-adrenergic-blocking drugs (Inderal, Lopressor, etc.) may increase the risk of serious rebound hypertension if clonidine is discontinued first. It is advisable to discontinue the beta blocker first and then withdraw clonidine gradually.
The following drugs may *decrease* the effects of clonidine
• tricyclic antidepressants (Elavil, Sinequan, etc.) may reduce its effectiveness in lowering blood pressure.

▷   *Driving, Hazardous Activities*: Use caution. This drug can cause drowsiness and can impair mental alertness, judgment and coordination.

Aviation Note: Hypertension (high blood pressure) *is a disqualification* for piloting. Consult a designated Aviation Medical Examiner.

Exposure to Sun: No restrictions.

Exposure to Heat: Use caution. Hot environments may reduce the blood pressure significantly; be alert to the possibility of orthostatic hypotension (see Glossary).

Exposure to Cold: Use caution. This drug may cause painful blanching and numbness of the hands and feet on exposure to cold air or water (Raynaud's phenomenon).

Heavy Exercise or Exertion: Use caution. Isometric exercises—the "overload" technique for strengthening individual muscles—can raise blood pressure significantly. The use of this drug may intensify the hypertensive response to isometric exercise. Ask physician for guidance.

Occurrence of Unrelated Illness: Fever associated with infections may lower the blood pressure significantly. Repeated vomiting may prevent the regular use of this drug and result in an acute withdrawal reaction. Consult your physician.

Discontinuation: *Do not discontinue this drug suddenly.* A severe withdrawal reaction can occur within 12 to 48 hours after the last dose. The dose should be reduced gradually over 3 to 4 days, with periodic monitoring of the blood pressure.

CLORAZEPATE
(klor AZ e payt)

Introduced: 1968

Prescription: USA: Yes
Canada: Yes

Available as Generic: No

Class: Mild Tranquilizer, Benzodiazepines

Controlled Drug: USA: C-IV*
Canada: No

Brand Names: Tranxene, Tranxene-SD, Tranxene-SD Half Strength

---

BENEFITS versus RISKS

Possible Benefits	*Possible Risks*
RELIEF OF ANXIETY AND NERVOUS TENSION in 70% to 80% of users	Habit-forming potential with prolonged use
Wide margin of safety with therapeutic doses	Minor impairment of mental functions
Very few drug interactions	

---

*See Schedules of Controlled Drugs inside back cover.

▷ **Principal Uses**

As a Single Drug Product: Used primarily to (1) provide short-term relief of mild to moderate anxiety, and (2) provide adjunctive treatment in controlling "partial" seizures, a type of epilepsy.

How This Drug Works: It is thought that this drug produces a calming effect by enhancing the action of the nerve transmitter gamma-aminobutyric acid (GABA), which in turn blocks the arousal of higher brain centers.

Available Dosage Forms and Strengths

Capsules — 3.75 mg, 7.5 mg, 15 mg
Tablets — 3.75 mg, 7.5 mg, 15 mg
Tablets, single dose — 11.25 mg, 22.5 mg

▷ **Usual Adult Dosage Range:**   15 to 60 mg/24 hrs, in 2 to 4 divided doses or as a single dose at bedtime. The usual dose is 30 mg/24 hrs. Total daily dose should not exceed 90 mg. **Note: Actual dosage and administration schedule must be determined by the physician for each patient individually.**

▷ **Dosing Instructions:**   May be taken on empty stomach or with food or milk. Capsule may be opened and regular tablet may be crushed for administration; the single-dose tablet should not be crushed. Do not discontinue this drug abruptly if taken for more than 4 weeks.

Usual Duration of Use: Continual use on a regular schedule for 5 to 7 days is usually necessary to determine this drug's effectiveness in relieving moderate anxiety. Limit continual use to 1 to 3 weeks. Avoid uninterrupted and prolonged use.

▷ **This Drug Should Not Be Taken If**

• you have had an allergic reaction to any dosage form of it previously.
• you have acute narrow-angle glaucoma.

▷ **Inform Your Physician Before Taking This Drug If**

• you are allergic to any benzodiazepine drug (see Drug Class, Section Four).
• you have a history of alcoholism or drug abuse.
• you are pregnant or planning pregnancy.
• you have impaired liver or kidney function.
• you have a history of serious depression or mental disorder.
• you have any of the following: asthma, emphysema, epilepsy, myasthenia gravis.

Possible Side-Effects   (natural, expected and unavoidable drug actions)

Drowsiness, lethargy, unsteadiness; "hangover" effects on the day following bedtime use.

▷ **Possible Adverse Effects**   (unusual, unexpected and infrequent reactions)

If any of the following develop, consult your physician promptly.

Mild Adverse Effects

Allergic Reactions: Skin rash, hives.

Dizziness, fainting, blurred vision, double vision, slurred speech, sweating, nausea, menstrual irregularity.

Serious Adverse Effects

Idiosyncratic Reactions: Paradoxical responses of excitement, agitation, anger, rage.

CAUTION

1. This drug should not be discontinued abruptly if it has been taken continually for more than 4 weeks.
2. The concurrent use of some over-the-counter drug products that contain antihistamines (allergy and cold preparations, sleep aids) can cause excessive sedation in sensitive individuals.
3. If this drug is taken at bedtime as a hypnotic (see Glossary), significant impairment of intellectual and physical skills may persist into the following day; avoid alcohol and hazardous activities (driving, etc.).

Precautions for Use

By Infants and Children: Safety and effectiveness for use by those under 9 years of age have not been established. This drug should not be used in the hyperactive or psychotic child of any age.

By Those over 60 Years of Age: It is advisable to use smaller doses at longer intervals to avoid overdosage. Observe for the possible development of lethargy, indifference, fatigue, weakness, unsteadiness, disturbing dreams, nightmares and paradoxical reactions of excitement, agitation, anger, hostility and rage.

▷ **Advisability of Use During Pregnancy**

Pregnancy Category: D (tentative). See Pregnancy Code inside back cover.

Animal studies: No birth defects reported in mouse, rat and rabbit studies.

Human studies: Information from adequate studies in pregnant women is not available.

There has been one report of multiple birth defects in a fetus exposed to this drug during the first 3 months. Frequent use in late pregnancy can cause the "floppy infant" syndrome in the newborn: weakness, lethargy, unresponsiveness, depressed breathing, low body temperature. Avoid use during entire pregnancy if possible.

Advisability of Use if Breast-Feeding

Presence of this drug in breast milk: Yes, in small amounts.

Monitor nursing infant closely and discontinue drug or nursing if adverse effects develop.

Habit-Forming Potential: This drug can produce psychological and/or physical dependence (see Glossary) if used in large doses for an extended period of time.

Effects of Overdosage: Marked drowsiness, weakness, feeling of drunkenness, staggering gait, tremor, stupor progressing to deep sleep or coma.

Possible Effects of Long-Term Use: Psychological and/or physical dependence.

Suggested Periodic Examinations While Taking This Drug (at physician's
discretion)
During long-term use: Complete blood cell counts.

While Taking This Drug, Observe the Following
Foods: No restrictions.
Beverages: Avoid excessive intake of caffeine-containing beverages: coffee,
tea, cola. May be taken with milk.
▷ *Alcohol*: Use with extreme caution until the combined effect is determined.
Alcohol may increase the absorption of this drug and add to its depres-
sant effects on the brain. It is advisable to avoid alcohol completely—
throughout the day and night—if it is necessary to drive or to engage in
any hazardous activity.
Tobacco Smoking: Heavy smoking may reduce the calming action of this
drug.
Marijuana Smoking: Increased sedation and significant impairment of intellectual and physical performance.
▷ *Other Drugs*
Clorazepate may *increase* the effects of
• digoxin (Lanoxin), and cause digoxin toxicity.
Clorazepate may *decrease* the effects of
• levodopa (Sinemet, etc.), and reduce its effectiveness in treating Parkinson's disease.
The following drugs may *increase* the effects of clorazepate
• cimetidine (Tagamet).
• disulfiram (Antabuse).
• isoniazid (INH, Rifamate, etc.).
• oral contraceptives.
• valproic acid (Depakene).
The following drugs may *decrease* the effects of clorazepate
• rifampin (Rimactane, etc.).
• theophylline (aminophylline, Theo-Dur, etc.).
▷ *Driving, Hazardous Activities*: This drug can impair mental alertness, judgment, physical coordination and reaction time. Avoid hazardous activities accordingly.
Aviation Note: The use of this drug *is a disqualification* for piloting. Consult a
designated Aviation Medical Examiner.
Exposure to Sun: No restrictions.
Discontinuation: Avoid sudden discontinuation if this drug has been taken
for more than 4 weeks. Dosage should be tapered gradually to prevent a
withdrawal syndrome that could include depression, confusion, hallucinations, tremor, seizures, muscle cramping, sweating and vomiting.

CLOXACILLIN
(klox a SIL in)

Introduced: 1962

Prescription: USA: Yes
Canada: Yes

Class: Antibiotic, Penicillins

Controlled Drug: USA: No
Canada: No

Available as Generic: USA: Yes
Canada: No

Brand Names: ❦Bactopen, Cloxapen, ❦Novocloxin, ❦Orbenin, Tegopen

---

BENEFITS versus RISKS

Possible Benefits	*Possible Risks*
EFFECTIVE TREATMENT OF INFECTIONS due to susceptible microorganisms	ALLERGIC REACTIONS, mild to severe Superinfections (yeast) Drug-induced colitis Rare blood cell disorders

---

▷ **Principal Uses**

As a Single Drug Product: Used primarily to treat infections that are caused by bacteria (principally staphylococcus) that have developed resistance to the original types of penicillin. It is of value in treating infections of the skin and skin structures, the upper and lower respiratory tract (including "strep" throat) and infections that are widely scattered throughout the body.

How This Drug Works: This drug destroys susceptible infecting bacteria by interfering with their ability to produce new protective cell walls as they multiply and grow.

Available Dosage Forms and Strengths
Capsules — 250 mg, 500 mg
Oral solution — 125 mg per 5 ml teaspoonful

▷ **Usual Adult Dosage Range:** 250 to 500 mg/6 hrs (4 doses/24 hrs). The maximal dose is 6000 mg/24 hrs. **Note: Actual dosage and administration schedule must be determined by the physician for each patient individually.**

▷ **Dosing Instructions:** Take on empty stomach, 1 hour before or 2 hours after eating, at same times each day. Capsule may be opened for administration.

Usual Duration of Use: As long as necessary to eradicate the infection. For all streptococcal infections: not less than 10 consecutive days (without interruption) to reduce the possibility of developing rheumatic fever or glomerulonephritis.

▷ **This Drug Should Not Be Taken If**
- you have had an allergic reaction to any dosage form of it previously.
- you are certain you are allergic to *any* form of penicillin.

▷ **Inform Your Physician Before Taking This Drug If**
- you suspect you may be allergic to penicillin or you have a history of a previous "reaction" to penicillin.
- you are allergic to cephalosporin antibiotics (Ancef, Ceporan, Ceporex, Duricef, Kafocin, Keflex, Keflin, Kefzol, Loridine).
- you are allergic by nature—hay fever, asthma, hives, eczema.
- you have a history of kidney disease, regional enteritis or ulcerative colitis.

Possible Side-Effects   (natural, expected and unavoidable drug actions)
Superinfections (see Glossary), often due to yeast organisms.

▷ **Possible Adverse Effects**   (unusual, unexpected and infrequent reactions)
If any of the following develop, consult your physician promptly.
Mild Adverse Effects
Allergic Reactions: Skin rashes, hives, itching.
Irritations of mouth and tongue, unpleasant taste, nausea, vomiting, mild diarrhea.
Serious Adverse Effects
Allergic Reactions: Anaphylactic reaction (see Glossary), severe skin reactions, drug fever, swollen painful joints, sore throat.
Pseudomembranous colitis—severe diarrhea.

CAUTION
1. Take the exact dose and the full course prescribed.
2. This drug should not be used concurrently with antibiotics like erythromycin or tetracycline.

Precautions for Use
By Infants and Children: Dosage is based on age and weight. Consult your physician for precise dosage schedule.
By Those over 60 Years of Age: It is advisable to evaluate kidney function before and during use of this drug to determine the need for dosage adjustment. Natural changes in the skin may predispose to prolonged itching reactions in the genital and anal regions. Report such reactions promptly.

▷ **Advisability of Use During Pregnancy**
Pregnancy Category: B (tentative). See Pregnancy Code inside back cover.
Animal studies: No birth defects reported in rabbit studies.
Human studies: Information from adequate studies in pregnant women indicates no increased risk of birth defects in 3546 pregnancies exposed to penicillin derivatives.
Ask physician for guidance.

Advisability of Use if Breast-Feeding
Presence of this drug in breast milk: Probably yes.
The nursing infant may be sensitized to penicillin. Avoid drug if possible or refrain from nursing.

Habit-Forming Potential: None.

Effects of Overdosage: Possible nausea, vomiting and/or diarrhea.

Possible Effects of Long-Term Use: Superinfections, often due to yeast organisms.

Suggested Periodic Examinations While Taking This Drug   (at physician's discretion)
Complete blood cell counts. Liver and kidney function tests with long-term use.

▷ **While Taking This Drug, Observe the Following**
Foods: No restrictions.
Beverages: No restrictions.
▷ *Alcohol*: No interactions expected.
Tobacco Smoking: No interactions expected.
▷ *Other Drugs*
Cloxacillin may *decrease* the effects of
• oral contraceptives in some women, and impair their effectiveness in preventing pregnancy.
The following drugs may *decrease* the effects of cloxacillin
• antacids may reduce the absorption of cloxacillin.
• chloramphenicol (Chloromycetin).
• erythromycin (Erythrocin, E-Mycin, etc.).
• tetracyclines (Achromycin, Declomycin, Minocin, etc.). (See Drug Class, Section Four.)
▷ *Driving, Hazardous Activities*: Usually no restrictions.
Aviation Note: The use of this drug *may be a disqualification* for piloting. Consult a designated Aviation Medical Examiner.
Exposure to Sun: No restrictions.
Special Storage Instructions: Keep capsules in a tightly closed container at room temperature. Keep oral solution in the refrigerator.
Observe the Following Expiration Times: Oral solution kept refrigerated is good for 14 days; when kept at room temperature, it is good for only 3 days.

CODEINE
(KOH deen)

Introduced: 1886

Class: Analgesic, Narcotic

Prescription: USA: Yes
  Canada: Yes

Controlled Drug: USA: C-II*
  Canada: <N>

Available as Generic: Yes

Brand Names: Bufferin w/Codeine [CD], Empirin No. 2, 3, 4 [CD], Empracet w/Codeine No. 3, 4 [CD], Fiorinal w/Codeine No. 1, 2, 3 [CD], ♣Paveral, Penntuss [CD], Phenaphen w/Codeine No. 2, 3, 4 [CD], SK-APAP w/Codeine [CD], Tylenol w/Codeine No. 1, 2, 3, 4 [CD]

*See Schedules of Controlled Drugs inside back cover.

+---+
| **BENEFITS versus RISKS** |
| |
| *Possible Benefits*   *Possible Risks* |
| EFFECTIVE RELIEF OF   Low potential for habit formation|
| MODERATE TO SEVERE PAIN   (dependence) |
| EFFECTIVE CONTROL OF   Mild allergic reactions (infrequent)|
| COUGH   Nausea, constipation |
+---+

▷ **Principal Uses**

As a Single Drug Product: Used primarily to (1) relieve moderate to severe pain; (2) control cough; (3) control diarrhea. Its widest use is as an ingredient in analgesic preparations and cough remedies. Its constipating effect is sometimes used to treat diarrhea, though better drugs are now available for this purpose.

As a Combination Drug Product [CD]: Codeine is commonly combined with other milder analgesics to enhance their effectiveness, notably aspirin and acetaminophen. It is frequently added to cough mixtures containing antihistamines, decongestants and expectorants to make these "shotgun" preparations more effective in reducing the frequency and severity of cough.

How This Drug Works: Acting primarily as a depressant of certain brain functions, this drug suppresses the perception of pain, calms the emotional response to pain, reduces the sensitivity of the cough reflex and inhibits the activity of brain centers that regulate the intestinal tract.

Available Dosage Forms and Strengths
     Injection — 30 mg per ml, 60 mg per ml
  Oral solution — 15 mg per 5 ml teaspoonful
     Tablets — 15 mg, 30 mg, 60 mg

▷ **Usual Adult Dosage Range:** As analgesic—15 to 60 mg/3 to 6 hrs as needed. For cough—10 to 20 mg/4 to 6 hrs as needed. For diarrhea—30 mg/6 hrs as needed. Total daily dosage should not exceed 200 mg for pain or 120 mg for cough or diarrhea. **Note: Actual dosage and administration schedule must be determined by the physician for each patient individually.**

▷ **Dosing Instructions:** May be taken with or following food to reduce stomach irritation or nausea. Tablet may be crushed for administration.

Usual Duration of Use: As required to control pain, cough or diarrhea. Continual use should not exceed 5 to 7 days without interruption and reassessment of need.

▷ **This Drug Should Not Be Taken If**
  • you have had an allergic reaction to any dosage form of it previously.
  • you are having an acute attack of asthma.

▷ **Inform Your Physician Before Taking This Drug If**
  • you have a history of drug abuse or alcoholism.
  • you have impaired liver or kidney function.

- you have gall-bladder disease, a seizure disorder or an underactive thyroid gland.
- you are taking any other drugs that have a sedative effect.
- you plan to have surgery under general anesthesia in the near future.

Possible Side-Effects   (natural, expected and unavoidable drug actions)
Drowsiness, light-headedness, dry mouth, urinary retention, constipation.

▷ **Possible Adverse Effects**   (unusual, unexpected and infrequent reactions)
If any of the following develop, consult your physician promptly.
Mild Adverse Effects
Allergic Reactions: Skin rash, hives, itching.
Dizziness, impaired concentration, sensation of drunkenness, confusion, depression, blurred or double vision.
Nausea, vomiting.
Serious Adverse Effects
Allergic Reactions: Anaphylaxis (rare), severe skin reactions.
Idiosyncratic Reactions: Delirium, hallucinations, excitement, increased sensitivity to pain after the analgesic effect has worn off.
Seizures (rare), impaired breathing.

▷ **Adverse Effects That May Mimic Natural Diseases or Disorders**
Paradoxical behavioral disturbances may suggest psychotic disorder.

CAUTION
1. If you have asthma, chronic bronchitis or emphysema, excessive use of this drug may cause significant respiratory difficulty, thickening of bronchial secretions and suppression of coughing.
2. The concurrent use of this drug with atropinelike drugs can increase the risk of urinary retention and reduced intestinal function.
3. Do not take this drug following acute head injury.

Precautions for Use
By Infants and Children: Do not use this drug in children under 2 years of age because of their vulnerability to life-threatening respiratory depression.
By Those over 60 Years of Age: Use small doses initially and increase dosage as needed and tolerated. Limit use to short-term treatment only. There may be increased susceptibility to the development of drowsiness, dizziness, unsteadiness, falling, urinary retention and constipation (often leading to fecal impaction).

▷ **Advisability of Use During Pregnancy**
Pregnancy Category: C (tentative). See Pregnancy Code inside back cover.
Animal studies: Skull defects reported in hamster studies.
Human studies: Information from adequate studies in pregnant women is not available. Some studies suggest a possible increase in significant birth defects when this drug is taken during the first 6 months of pregnancy. Codeine taken during the last few weeks before delivery can cause withdrawal symptoms in the newborn infant.
Use this drug only if clearly needed and in small, infrequent doses.

Advisability of Use if Breast-Feeding
    Presence of this drug in breast milk: Yes, in small amounts.
    Avoid drug or refrain from nursing.

Habit-Forming Potential: Psychological and/or physical dependence can develop with use of large doses for an extended period of time. However, true dependence is infrequent and unlikely with prudent use.

Effects of Overdosage: Drowsiness, restlessness, agitation, nausea, vomiting, dry mouth, vertigo, weakness, lethargy, stupor, coma, seizures.

Possible Effects of Long-Term Use: Psychological and physical dependence, chronic constipation.

Suggested Periodic Examinations While Taking This Drug (at physician's discretion)
    None.

▷ **While Taking This Drug, Observe the Following**
    Foods: No restrictions.
    Beverages: No restrictions. May be taken with milk.
▷ *Alcohol*: Use extreme caution until the combined effects have been determined. Codeine can intensify the intoxicating effects of alcohol, and alcohol can intensify the depressant effects of codeine on brain function, breathing and circulation.
    Tobacco Smoking: No interactions expected.
    Marijuana Smoking: Increase in drowsiness and pain relief; impairment of mental and physical performance.
▷ *Other Drugs*
    Codeine may *increase* the effects of
    • other drugs with sedative effects.
    • atropinelike drugs, and increase the risk of constipation and urinary retention.
▷ *Driving, Hazardous Activities*: This drug can impair mental alertness, judgment, reaction time and physical coordination. Avoid hazardous activities accordingly.
    Aviation Note: The use of this drug *is a disqualification* for piloting. Consult a designated Aviation Medical Examiner.
    Exposure to Sun: No restrictions.
    Discontinuation: It is advisable to limit this drug to short-term use. If it is necessary to use it for extended periods of time, discontinuation should be gradual to minimize possible effects of withdrawal (usually mild with codeine).

COLCHICINE
(KOL chi seen)

Introduced: 1763

Prescription: USA: Yes
    Canada: No

Available as Generic: Yes

Brand Names: ColBENEMID [CD], ♣Novocolchine

Class: Antigout

Controlled Drug: USA: No
    Canada: No

BENEFITS versus RISKS	
Possible Benefits	*Possible Risks*
EFFECTIVE RELIEF OF ACUTE GOUT SYMPTOMS	Loss of hair
	Rare bone marrow depression (see Glossary)
Prevention of recurrent gout attacks	
Prevention of attacks of Mediterranean fever	Rare peripheral neuritis (see Glossary)
	Rare liver damage

▷ **Principal Uses**

As a Single Drug Product: Used primarily to reduce the pain, swelling and inflammation associated with acute attacks of gout. It is also used in smaller doses to prevent recurrent gout attacks. An infrequent use is the prevention and control of attacks of familial Mediterranean fever.

As a Combination Drug Product [CD]: Colchicine is combined with probenecid to enhance its ability to prevent recurrent attacks of gout. While colchicine is most effective in relieving the symptoms of acute gout, it has some effect in preventing recurrent and chronic discomfort. Probenecid increases the elimination of uric acid by the kidneys and thereby reduces the blood level of uric acid to a point at which acute episodes of gout will not occur. This dual action is more effective than either drug used alone in the long-term management of gout.

How This Drug Works: It is thought that by decreasing the acidity of joint tissues, this drug reduces the deposit of uric acid crystals that cause acute inflammation and pain. (Colchicine does not lower the level of uric acid in the blood or increase the level of uric acid in the urine.)

Available Dosage Forms and Strengths
    Injection — 1 mg per 2 ml
    Tablets — 0.432 mg, 0.5 mg, 0.54 mg, 0.6 mg, 0.65 mg

▷ **Usual Adult Dosage Range:**   For acute attack—0.5 to 1.3 mg initially, followed by 0.5 to 0.65 mg/1 to 2 hrs until pain is relieved or nausea, vomiting or diarrhea occurs. The total dose should not exceed 10 mg. For prevention of recurrent attacks—0.5 to 0.65 mg, 1 to 3 times/day. **Note: Actual dosage and administration schedule must be determined by the physician for each patient individually.**

▷ **Dosing Instructions:** May be taken either on an empty stomach or with food to reduce nausea or stomach irritation. Start treatment at the earliest indication of an acute attack. Take the exact dose prescribed. The tablet may be crushed for administration.

Usual Duration of Use: For acute attack—discontinue when pain is relieved or when nausea, vomiting or diarrhea occurs; do not resume this drug for 3 days without consulting your physician. For prevention—use the smallest effective dose for long-term management; consult your physician regarding dosage schedule and duration.

▷ **This Drug Should Not Be Taken If**
- you have had an allergic reaction to it previously.
- you have an active stomach or duodenal ulcer.
- you have active ulcerative colitis.

▷ **Inform Your Physician Before Taking This Drug If**
- you have a history of peptic ulcer disease or ulcerative colitis.
- you have any type of heart disease.
- you have impaired liver or kidney function.
- you plan to have surgery in the near future.

Possible Side-Effects (natural, expected and unavoidable drug actions)
Nausea, vomiting, abdominal cramping, diarrhea.

▷ **Possible Adverse Effects** (unusual, unexpected and infrequent reactions)
If any of the following develop, consult your physician promptly.
Mild Adverse Effects
Allergic Reactions: Skin rash, hives, fever.
Serious Adverse Effects
Allergic Reactions: Anaphylactic reaction (see Glossary).
Loss of hair.
Bone marrow depression (see Glossary)—fatigue, weakness, fever, sore throat, abnormal bleeding or bruising.
Peripheral neuritis (see Glossary)—numbness, tingling, pain, weakness in hands and/or feet.
Inflammation of colon with bloody diarrhea.
Liver damage.

Possible Delayed Adverse Effects
Impaired production of sperm, possibly resulting in birth defects of child that was conceived while father was taking this drug.

Natural Diseases or Disorders That May Be Activated by This Drug
Peptic ulcer disease, ulcerative colitis.

CAUTION
1. If this drug causes vomiting and/or diarrhea before relief of joint pain, discontinue it and inform your physician.
2. Try to limit each course of treatment for acute gout to 4 to 8 mg. Do not exceed 3 mg/24 hrs or a total of 10 mg/course.
3. Omit drug for 3 days between courses to avoid toxicity.

4. Carry this drug with you while traveling if you are subject to attacks of acute gout.
5. It is advisable to take colchicine preventively prior to and following surgery if you have recurrent gout. (Surgery often precipitates acute attacks of gout.) Ask your physician for proper dosage schedule.

Precautions for Use
By Infants and Children: Dosage has not been established. Ask physician for guidance.
By Those over 60 Years of Age: This drug has a very narrow margin of safety. Because the total dosage required to relieve the pain of acute gout often causes vomiting and/or diarrhea, extreme caution is advised when this drug is used by anyone with heart or circulatory disorders, reduced liver or kidney function or general debility.

▷ ### Advisability of Use During Pregnancy
Pregnancy Category: D (tentative). See Pregnancy Code inside back cover.
Animal studies: This drug causes significant birth defects in hamsters and rabbits.
Human studies: Information from adequate studies in pregnant women is not available.
Avoid during entire pregnancy if possible.

Advisability of Use if Breast-Feeding
Presence of this drug in breast milk: Unknown.
Avoid drug or refrain from nursing.

Habit-Forming Potential: None.

Effects of Overdosage: Nausea, vomiting, abdominal cramping, diarrhea (may be bloody), burning sensation in throat and skin, weak and rapid pulse, progressive paralysis, inability to breathe.

Possible Effects of Long-Term Use: Hair loss, aplastic anemia (see Glossary), peripheral neuritis (see Glossary).

Suggested Periodic Examinations While Taking This Drug   (at physician's discretion)
Complete blood cell counts, uric acid blood levels to monitor status of gout, sperm analysis for quantity and condition, liver function tests.

▷ ### While Taking This Drug, Observe the Following
Foods: Follow physician's advice regarding the need for a low-purine diet.
Beverages: It is advisable to drink no less than 3 quarts of liquids/24 hrs. This drug may be taken with milk. Some "herbal teas" (promoted as being beneficial for arthritis) contain phenylbutazone and other potentially toxic ingredients. Avoid herbal teas if you are not certain of their source, content and medicinal effects.
▷ *Alcohol*: No interactions expected. However, alcohol may increase the risk of gastrointestinal irritation or bleeding. It also raises uric acid blood levels and could interfere with gout management.
Tobacco Smoking: No interactions expected.

▷   *Other Drugs*
    Colchicine *taken concurrently* with
    - allopurinol (Zyloprim), probenecid (Benemid) or sulfinpyrazone (Anturane) can prevent attacks of acute gout that often occur when treatment with these drugs is first started.
▷   *Driving, Hazardous Activities*: Usually no restrictions when taken continually in small (preventive) doses. Be alert to the possible occurrence of nausea, vomiting and/or diarrhea when taken in larger (treatment) doses.
    Aviation Note: The use of this drug *may be a disqualification* for piloting. Consult a designated Aviation Medical Examiner.
    Exposure to Sun: No restrictions.
    Exposure to Cold: This drug can lower body temperature. Use caution to prevent excessive lowering (hypothermia), especially if you are over 60 years of age.
    Occurrence of Unrelated Illness: Inform your physician if you are injured or if you develop any new illness or disorder. During periods of such stress you may be subject to acute attacks of gout, and it may be necessary to adjust your medication schedule.

CYCLOBENZAPRINE
(si kloh BENZ a preen)

Introduced: 1977

Prescription: USA: Yes
    Canada: Yes

Available as Generic: USA: No
    Canada: No

Brand Names: Flexeril

Class: Muscle Relaxant

Controlled Drug: USA: No
    Canada: No

BENEFITS versus RISKS	
Possible Benefits	*Possible Risks*
Mild to moderate relief of discomfort due to spasm of voluntary muscles	Confusion, depression Impaired urination Allergic reactions: skin rash, hives, swelling of face or tongue

▷ **Principal Uses**
    As a Single Drug Product: Used primarily to relieve the pain and stiffness associated with spasm of voluntary muscles, such as that resulting from accidental injury of musculoskeletal structures. It is often necessary to supplement the use of this drug with other treatment measures, such as rest, support and physiotherapy.

    How This Drug Works: Not completely established. It is thought that this drug may relieve muscle spasm and pain by blocking the transmission of nerve impulses over reflex pathways and/or by producing a sedative effect that decreases the perception of pain.

Available Dosage Forms and Strengths
Tablets — 10 mg

▷ **Usual Adult Dosage Range:**   10 mg, 2 to 4 times daily; adjust dosage as needed and tolerated. Total daily dosage should not exceed 60 mg. **Note: Actual dosage and administration schedule must be determined by the physician for each patient individually.**

▷ **Dosing Instructions:**   Take either on empty stomach or with food to prevent stomach irritation. Tablet may be crushed for administration.

Usual Duration of Use: Continual use on a regular schedule for 7 to 10 days is usually necessary to determine this drug's effectiveness in relieving the discomfort of muscle spasm. Evaluate need for continued use after periods of 2 to 3 weeks.

▷ **This Drug Should Not Be Taken If**
- you have had an allergic reaction to it previously.
- you have taken any monoamine oxidase (MAO) inhibitor drug within the past 14 days (see Drug Class, Section Four).
- you are recovering from a recent heart attack.
- you have congestive heart failure or a serious heart rhythm disorder.
- you have uncorrected hyperthyroidism (overactive thyroid function).

▷ **Inform Your Physician Before Taking This Drug If**
- you have experienced any unfavorable reactions to other muscle relaxants or to tricyclic antidepressants (see Drug Class, Section Four) in the past.
- you have a history of heart disease or heart rhythm disorder.
- you have glaucoma or prostatism (see Glossary).
- you are currently taking any drugs with atropinelike effects or sedative effects.

Possible Side-Effects   (natural, expected and unavoidable drug actions)
Drowsiness (40%), dizziness (11%), dry mouth (28%), constipation (3%).

▷ **Possible Adverse Effects**   (unusual, unexpected and infrequent reactions)
If any of the following develop, consult your physician promptly.
Mild Adverse Effects
Allergic Reactions: Skin rash, hives, swelling of face and tongue.
Headache, fatigue, weakness, numbness, blurred vision, slurred speech, unsteadiness.
Unpleasant taste, indigestion, nausea.
Serious Adverse Effects
Idiosyncratic Reactions: Euphoria, confusion, disorientation, hallucinations, depression.
Impaired urination (urine retention).

▷ **Adverse Effects That May Mimic Natural Diseases or Disorders**
Mental and behavioral reactions may suggest acute psychosis.

Precautions for Use
By Infants and Children: Safety and effectiveness for use by those under 15 years of age have not been established.
By Those over 60 Years of Age: Small doses are advisable initially. You may be more susceptible to the development of drowsiness, dizziness, weakness, unsteadiness and falling. This drug can aggravate existing prostatism (see Glossary).

▷ **Advisability of Use During Pregnancy**
Pregnancy Category: B (tentative). See Pregnancy Code inside back cover.
Animal studies: No birth defects reported in mice, rats or rabbits.
Human studies: Information from adequate studies in pregnant women is not available.
Avoid drug if possible; use only if clearly needed.

Advisability of Use if Breast-Feeding
Presence of this drug in breast milk: Probably yes.
Avoid drug or refrain from nursing.

Habit-Forming Potential: None.

Effects of Overdosage: Excessive drowsiness, confusion, impaired concentration, visual disturbances, vomiting, stupor progressing to coma, seizures, weak and rapid pulse.

Possible Effects of Long-Term Use: None reported.

Suggested Periodic Examinations While Taking This Drug   (at physician's discretion)
Measurements of internal eye pressure (if any predisposition to glaucoma).

▷ **While Taking This Drug, Observe the Following**
Foods: No restrictions.
Beverages: No restrictions. May be taken with milk.
▷ *Alcohol*: Use with caution until the combined effect has been determined. This drug may add to the depressant action of alcohol on the brain.
Tobacco Smoking: No interactions expected.
Marijuana Smoking: Moderate to marked drowsiness, muscle weakness, incoordination, impairment of intellectual and physical performance. All hazardous activities should be avoided.
▷ *Other Drugs*
Cyclobenzaprine may *increase* the effects of
• atropinelike drugs (see Drug Class, Section Four).
• all drugs with sedative effects, and cause excessive sedation.
Cyclobenzaprine *taken concurrently* with
• monoamine oxidase (MAO) inhibitor drugs may cause high fever, seizures and life-threatening reactions (theoretical).

▷ *Driving, Hazardous Activities*: This drug may cause drowsiness, dizziness and incoordination in susceptible individuals. Avoid hazardous activities if these drug effects occur.

Aviation Note: The use of this drug *is a disqualification* for piloting. Consult a designated Aviation Medical Examiner.

Exposure to Sun: Use caution until sensitivity to sun has been determined. Other drugs closely related to this drug can cause photosensitivity (see Glossary).

Exposure to Heat: Use caution in hot environments. This drug may increase the risk of heat stroke.

CYCLOPHOSPHAMIDE
(si kloh FOSS fa mide)

Introduced: 1959

Prescription: USA: Yes
Canada: Yes

Available as Generic: No

Brand Names: Cytoxan, Neosar, ♣Procytox

Class: Anticancer, Immunosuppressive

Controlled Drug: USA: No
Canada: No

BENEFITS versus RISKS

Possible Benefits	*Possible Risks*
CURE OR CONTROL OF CERTAIN TYPES OF CANCER	REDUCED WHITE BLOOD CELLS
PREVENTION OF REJECTION IN ORGAN TRANSPLANTATION	SECONDARY INFECTION
Possibly beneficial in the treatment of rheumatoid arthritis and lupus erythematosus	URINARY BLADDER BLEEDING
	HEART, LUNG, LIVER OR KIDNEY DAMAGE
	Loss of hair

▷ **Principal Uses**

As a Single Drug Product: Used primarily in the treatment of various forms of cancer, notably malignant lymphomas, multiple myeloma, leukemias and cancers of the breast and ovary. Because this drug exerts a suppressant effect on the immune system, it is also used to prevent rejection in organ transplantation and to treat certain autoimmune disorders.

How This Drug Works: Not completely known. Because of its ability to kill cancer cells during all phases of their development and reproduction, this drug suppresses the primary growth and secondary spread (metastasis) of certain types of cancer.

Available Dosage Forms and Strengths
>   Injection — vials of 100 mg, 200 mg, 500 mg, 1 gram, 2 grams
>   Tablets — 25 mg, 50 mg

▷ **Usual Adult Dosage Range:**   1 to 5 mg per kg of body weight daily. **Note: Actual dosage and administration schedule must be determined by the physician for each patient individually.**

▷ **Dosing Instructions:**   It is preferable to take the tablet on an empty stomach. However, if nausea or indigestion occurs, this drug may be taken with or following food. The total liquid intake should be no less than 3 quarts/24 hrs to reduce the risk of bladder irritation. Tablets may be crushed for administration.

Usual Duration of Use: Continual use on a regular schedule is required to achieve and maintain a significant remission of the cancer under treatment. Actual duration of use depends upon the response of the cancer and the tolerance of the patient to the effects of the drug.

▷ **This Drug Should Not Be Taken If**
*   you have had an allergic reaction to any dosage form of it previously.
*   you have an active infection of any kind.
*   you have bloody urine for any reason.

▷ **Inform Your Physician Before Taking This Drug If**
*   you have impaired liver or kidney function.
*   you have a blood cell or bone marrow disorder.
*   you have had previous chemotherapy or X-ray therapy for any type of cancer.
*   you are now taking, or have taken within the past year, any cortisonelike drug (adrenal corticosteroids).
*   you have diabetes.
*   you plan to have surgery under general anesthesia in the near future.

Possible Side-Effects   (natural, expected and unavoidable drug actions)
>   Bone marrow depression (see Glossary)—impaired production of primarily white blood cells and, to a lesser degree, red blood cells and blood platelets (see Glossary). Possible effects include fever, chills, sore throat, fatigue, weakness, abnormal bleeding or bruising.
>   Impairment of natural resistance (immunity) to infection.

▷ **Possible Adverse Effects**   (unusual, unexpected and infrequent reactions)
>   **If any of the following develop, consult your physician promptly.**
>   *Mild Adverse Effects*
>   Allergic Reactions: Skin rash (rare).
>   Headache, dizziness.
>   Loss of scalp hair (50% of users), darkening of skin and fingernails, transverse ridging of nails.
>   Loss of appetite, nausea (30%), vomiting (25%), ulceration of mouth, diarrhea (may be bloody).

Serious Adverse Effects

Idiosyncratic Reactions: Hemolytic anemia (see Glossary).

Liver damage with jaundice—yellow eyes and skin, dark-colored urine, light-colored stools.

Kidney damage—impaired kidney function, reduced urine volume, bloody urine.

Severe inflammation of bladder (10%)—painful urination, bloody urine.

Drug-induced damage of heart and lung tissue.

Suppression of ovarian function—irregular menstrual pattern or cessation of menstruation.

Suppression of testicular function—reduction or cessation of sperm production.

Possible Delayed Adverse Effects

The development of other types of cancer (secondary malignancies). The development of severe cystitis with bleeding from the bladder wall. (This may occur many months after the last dose.)

CAUTION

1. This drug may interfere with the normal healing of wounds.
2. This drug can cause significant changes (mutations) in the chromosome structure of both sperm and eggs (ova). Any man or woman taking this drug should understand its potential for causing serious defects in children that are conceived during or following the course of medication.
3. This drug can suppress natural resistance (immunity) to infection, resulting in life-threatening illness.
4. Avoid live virus vaccines while taking this drug.

Precautions for Use

By Infants and Children: This drug should not be given if the child is dehydrated. Provide adequate fluid intake to ensure a copious urine volume for 4 hours following each dose. Prevent exposure of child to anyone with active chicken pox or shingles. This drug may cause ovarian or testicular sterility.

By Those over 60 Years of Age: To reduce the risk of developing serious chemical cystitis, it is necessary to maintain a copious volume of urine. This may increase the risk of urinary retention in the man with prostatism (see Glossary).

▷ Advisability of Use During Pregnancy

Pregnancy Category: D (tentative). See Pregnancy Code inside back cover.

Animal studies: Significant birth defects reported in mice, rat and rabbit studies.

Human studies: Information from studies in pregnant women indicates that this drug can cause serious birth defects or fetal death.

Avoid completely during the first 3 months. Use of this drug during the last 6 months must be carefully individualized.

Advisability of Use if Breast-Feeding
Presence of this drug in breast milk: Yes.
Avoid drug or refrain from nursing.

Habit-Forming Potential: None.

Effects of Overdosage: Nausea, vomiting, diarrhea, bloody urine, water retention, weight gain, severe bone marrow depression, severe infections.

Possible Effects of Long-Term Use: Development of fibrous tissue in lungs; secondary malignancies.

Suggested Periodic Examinations While Taking This Drug (at physician's discretion)
Complete blood cell counts, every 2 to 4 days during initial treatment; then every 3 to 4 weeks during maintenance treatment.
Liver and kidney function tests. Thyroid function tests (if symptoms warrant).

▷ **While Taking This Drug, Observe the Following**
Foods: No restrictions.
Beverages: No restrictions. May be taken with milk.
▷ *Alcohol*: No interactions expected.
Tobacco Smoking: No interactions expected.
▷ *Other Drugs*
Cyclophosphamide *taken concurrently* with
• allopurinol (Zyloprim) may increase the degree of bone marrow depression.
▷ *Driving, Hazardous Activities*: Use caution if dizziness occurs.
Aviation Note: The use of this drug *may be a disqualification* for piloting. Consult a designated Aviation Medical Examiner.
Exposure to Sun: No restrictions.
Occurrence of Unrelated Illness: Report promptly the development of any indications of infection—fever, chills, sore throat, cough, flulike symptoms. It may be necessary to discontinue this drug until the infection is controlled. Consult your physician.

DEMECLOCYCLINE
(dem e kloh SI kleen)

Introduced: 1959

Prescription: USA: Yes
Canada: Yes

Available as Generic: No

Brand Names: Declomycin

Class: Antibiotic, Tetracyclines

Controlled Drug: USA: No
Canada: No

```
┌─────────────────────────────────────────────────────────────┐
│                   BENEFITS versus RISKS                      │
│                                                              │
│      Possible Benefits              Possible Risks           │
│  EFFECTIVE TREATMENT OF         Allergic reactions           │
│    INFECTIONS due to susceptible   Drug-induced colitis      │
│    microorganisms               Drug-induced diabetes insipidus │
│                                    (water diabetes)          │
│                                 Fungal superinfections       │
└─────────────────────────────────────────────────────────────┘
```

▷ **Principal Uses**

As a Single Drug Product: This member of the tetracycline drug class is used primarily to (1) treat a broad range of infections caused by susceptible bacteria and protozoa and (2) treat the syndrome of inappropriate secretion of antidiuretic hormone, a condition that reduces the normal production of urine.

How This Drug Works: This drug prevents the growth and multiplication of susceptible bacteria by interfering with their formation of essential proteins.

Available Dosage Forms and Strengths
Capsules — 150 mg
Tablets — 150 mg

▷ **Usual Adult Dosage Range:**   150 mg/6 hrs or 300 mg/12 hrs. Total daily dosage should not exceed 2400 mg. **Note: Actual dosage and administration schedule must be determined by the physician for each patient individually.**

▷ **Dosing Instructions:**   Preferably taken on an empty stomach, 1 hour before or 2 hours after eating. However, if stomach irritation occurs, it may be taken with crackers or light food (not milk or milk products). Take at same time each day, with a full glass of water. Take the full course prescribed. The tablet may be crushed and the capsule may be opened for administration.

Usual Duration of Use: The time required to control the infection and be free of fever and symptoms for 48 hours. This varies with the nature of the infection.

▷ **This Drug Should Not Be Taken If**
- you are allergic to any tetracycline drug (see Drug Class, Section Four).
- you are pregnant or breast-feeding.

▷ **Inform Your Physician Before Taking This Drug If**
- it is prescribed for a child under 8 years of age.
- you have a history of liver or kidney disease.
- you have systemic lupus erythematosus.
- you are taking any penicillin drug.
- you are taking any anticoagulant drug.
- you plan to have surgery under general anesthesia in the near future.

Possible Side-Effects   (natural, expected and unavoidable drug actions)

Superinfections (see Glossary), often due to yeast organisms. These can occur in the mouth, intestinal tract, rectum and/or vagina, resulting in rectal and vaginal itching.

▷ **Possible Adverse Effects**   (unusual, unexpected and infrequent reactions)
If any of the following develop, consult your physician promptly.
Mild Adverse Effects
Allergic Reactions: Skin rash, hives, itching of hands and feet, swelling of face or extremities.
Loss of appetite, nausea, vomiting, diarrhea.
Irritation of mouth or tongue, "black tongue," sore throat, abdominal cramping or pain.
Serious Adverse Effects
Allergic Reactions: Anaphylactic reaction (see Glossary), asthma, fever, swollen joints, abnormal bleeding or bruising, jaundice (see Glossary).
Permanent discoloration and/or malformation of teeth when taken under 8 years of age, including unborn child and infant.
Drug-induced diabetes insipidus (water diabetes).

Natural Diseases or Disorders That May Be Activated by This Drug
Systemic lupus erythematosus.

CAUTION
1. Antacids, dairy products and preparations containing aluminum, bismuth, calcium, iron, magnesium or zinc can prevent adequate absorption of this drug and reduce its effectiveness significantly.
2. Troublesome and persistent diarrhea can develop in sensitive individuals. If diarrhea persists for more than 24 hours, discontinue this drug and consult your physician.
3. If surgery under general anesthesia is required while taking this drug, the choice of anesthetic agent must be considered carefully to prevent serious kidney damage.

Precautions for Use
By Infants and Children: If possible, tetracyclines should not be given to children under 8 years of age because of the risk of permanent discoloration and deformity of the teeth. Rarely, young infants may develop increased intracranial pressure within the first 4 days of receiving this drug. Tetracyclines may inhibit normal bone growth and development.
By Those over 60 Years of Age: Dosage must be carefully individualized and based upon determinations of kidney function. Natural skin changes may predispose to severe and prolonged itching reactions in the genital and anal regions.

▷ **Advisability of Use During Pregnancy**
Pregnancy Category: D (tentative). See Pregnancy Code inside back cover.
Animal studies: Tetracycline causes limb defects in rats, rabbits and chickens.
Human studies: Information from studies in pregnant women indicates

that this drug can cause impaired development and discoloration of teeth and other developmental defects.

It is advisable to avoid this drug completely during entire pregnancy.

Advisability of Use if Breast-Feeding
Presence of this drug in breast milk: Yes.
Avoid drug or refrain from nursing.

Habit-Forming Potential: None.

Effects of Overdosage: Nausea, vomiting, diarrhea, acute liver damage (rare).

Possible Effects of Long-Term Use: Superinfections; rarely, impairment of bone marrow, liver or kidney function.

Suggested Periodic Examinations While Taking This Drug   (at physician's discretion)
Complete blood cell counts, liver and kidney function tests.
During extended use, sputum and stool examinations may detect early superinfection due to yeast organisms.

▷ **While Taking This Drug, Observe the Following**
Foods: Avoid cheeses, yogurt, ice cream, iron-fortified cereals and supplements and meats for 2 hours before and after taking this drug.
Beverages: Avoid all forms of milk for 2 hours before and after taking this drug.
▷ *Alcohol*: No interactions expected. However, it is best avoided if you have active liver disease.
Tobacco Smoking: No interactions expected.
▷ *Other Drugs*
Tetracyclines may *increase* the effects of
• oral anticoagulants, and make it necessary to reduce their dosage.
• digoxin (Lanoxin), and cause digitalis toxicity.
• lithium (Eskalith, Lithane, etc.), and increase the risk of lithium toxicity.
Tetracyclines may *decrease* the effects of
• oral contraceptives, and impair their effectiveness in preventing pregnancy.
• penicillins, and impair their effectiveness in treating infections.
Tetracyclines *taken concurrently* with
• methoxyflurane anesthesia may impair kidney function.
The following drugs may *decrease* the effects of tetracyclines
• antacids (aluminum and magnesium preparations, sodium bicarbonate, etc.) may reduce drug absorption.
• iron and mineral preparations may reduce drug absorption.
▷ *Driving, Hazardous Activities*: Usually no restrictions. Be alert to the possible occurrence of nausea or diarrhea.
Aviation Note: The use of this drug *may be a disqualification* for piloting. Consult a designated Aviation Medical Examiner.
Exposure to Sun: Use caution until sensitivity has been determined. Tetracyclines can cause photosensitivity (see Glossary).

DEXAMETHASONE
(dex a METH a sohn)

Introduced: 1958

Prescription: USA: Yes
Canada: Yes

Available as Generic: USA: Yes
Canada: Yes

Class: Cortisonelike Drugs

Controlled Drug: USA: No
Canada: No

Brand Names: Decaderm, Decadron, Decadron-LA, Decadron Phosphate Ophthalmic, Decadron Phosphate Respihaler, Decadron w/Xylocaine [CD], Decaspray, ❧Deronil, Dexasone, Dexone, Hexadrol, Maxidex, SK-dexamethasone, Turbinaire Decadron Phosphate

---

BENEFITS versus RISKS

Possible Benefits

EFFECTIVE RELIEF OF SYMPTOMS IN A WIDE VARIETY OF INFLAMMATORY AND ALLERGIC DISORDERS
EFFECTIVE IMMUNO-SUPPRESSION in selected benign and malignant disorders

Possible Risks

Short-term use (up to 10 days) is usually well tolerated. Long-term use (exceeding 2 weeks) is associated with many possible adverse effects:
ALTERED MOOD AND PERSONALITY
CATARACTS, GLAUCOMA
HYPERTENSION
OSTEOPOROSIS
ASEPTIC BONE NECROSIS
INCREASED SUSCEPTIBILITY TO INFECTIONS
(See Possible Adverse Effects and Possible Effects of Long-Term Use below)

▷ **Principal Uses**

As a Single Drug Product: This potent drug of the cortisone class is used in the treatment of a wide variety of allergic and inflammatory conditions. It is used most commonly in the management of serious skin disorders, asthma, regional enteritis, ulcerative colitis and all types of major rheumatic disorders including bursitis, tendonitis and most forms of arthritis.

How This Drug Works: Not fully established. It is thought that this drug's anti-inflammatory effect is due to its ability to inhibit the normal defensive functions of certain white blood cells. Its immunosuppressant effect is attributed to a reduced production of lymphocytes and antibodies.

Available Dosage Forms and Strengths
Aerosol — 0.01%, 0.04%
Aerosol inhaler — 84 mcg per spray

Cream — 0.1%
Elixir — 0.5 mg per 5 ml teaspoonful
Gel — 0.1%
Injection — 4 mg per ml, 8 mg per ml, 10 mg per ml, 16 mg per ml,
20 mg per ml, 24 mg per ml
Oral solution — 0.5 mg per 0.5 ml, 0.5 mg per 5 ml
Solution — 0.1%
Suspension — 0.1%
Tablets — 0.25 mg, 0.5 mg, 0.75 mg, 1 mg, 1.5 mg, 2 mg, 4 mg,
6 mg

▷ **Usual Adult Dosage Range:**   0.5 to 9 mg daily as a single dose or in divided doses. **Note: Actual dosage and administration schedule must be determined by the physician for each patient individually.**

▷ **Dosing Instructions:**   Take with or following food to prevent stomach irritation, preferably in the morning. The tablet may be crushed for administration.

Usual Duration of Use: For acute disorders: 4 to 10 days. For chronic disorders: according to individual requirements. The duration of use should not exceed the time necessary to obtain adequate symptomatic relief in acute self-limiting conditions; or the time required to stabilize a chronic condition and permit gradual withdrawal. Because of its long duration of action, this drug is not appropriate for alternate day administration.

▷ **This Drug Should Not Be Taken If**
 • you have had an allergic reaction to any dosage form of it previously.
 • you have active peptic ulcer disease.
 • you have an active infection of the eye caused by the herpes simplex virus.
 • you have active tuberculosis.

▷ **Inform Your Physician Before Taking This Drug If**
 • you have had an unfavorable reaction to any cortisonelike drug in the past.
 • you have a history of peptic ulcer disease, thrombophlebitis or tuberculosis.
 • you have any of the following: diabetes, glaucoma, high blood pressure, deficient thyroid function or myasthenia gravis.
 • you plan to have surgery of any kind in the near future.

Possible Side-Effects   (natural, expected and unavoidable drug actions)
Increased appetite, weight gain, retention of salt and water, excretion of potassium, increased susceptibility to infection.

▷ **Possible Adverse Effects**   (unusual, unexpected and infrequent reactions)
If any of the following develop, consult your physician promptly.
Mild Adverse Effects
Allergic Reactions: Skin rash.
Headache, dizziness, insomnia.

Acid indigestion, abdominal distention.

Muscle cramping and weakness.

Irregular or altered menstruation.

Acne, excessive growth of facial hair.

Serious Adverse Effects

Mental and emotional disturbances of serious magnitude.

Reactivation of latent tuberculosis.

Development of peptic ulcer.

Increased blood pressure.

Development of inflammation of the pancreas.

Thrombophlebitis (inflammation of a vein with the formation of blood clot)—pain or tenderness in thigh or leg, with or without swelling of the foot, ankle or leg.

Pulmonary embolism (movement of a blood clot to the lung)—sudden shortness of breath, pain in the chest, coughing, bloody sputum.

▷ **Adverse Effects That May Mimic Natural Diseases or Disorders**

Pattern of symptoms and signs resembling Cushing's syndrome.

Natural Diseases or Disorders That May Be Activated by This Drug

Latent diabetes, glaucoma, peptic ulcer disease, tuberculosis.

CAUTION

1. It is advisable to carry a card of personal identification with a notation that you are taking this drug, if your course of treatment is to exceed 1 week.
2. Do not discontinue this drug abruptly if you are using it for long-term treatment.
3. If vaccination against measles, rabies, smallpox or yellow fever is required, discontinue this drug 72 hours before vaccination and do not resume it for at least 14 days after vaccination.

Precautions for Use

By Infants and Children: Avoid prolonged use if possible. During long-term use, observe for suppression of normal growth and the possibility of increased intracranial pressure. Following long-term use, the child may be at risk for adrenal gland deficiency during stress for as long as 18 months after cessation of this drug.

By Those over 60 Years of Age: Cortisonelike drugs should be used very sparingly after 60 and only when the disorder under treatment is unresponsive to adequate trials of unrelated drugs. Avoid prolonged use of this drug. Continual use (even in small doses) can increase the severity of diabetes, enhance fluid retention, raise blood pressure, weaken resistance to infection, induce stomach ulcer and accelerate the development of cataract and osteoporosis.

▷ **Advisability of Use During Pregnancy**

Pregnancy Category: C (tentative). See Pregnancy Code inside back cover.

Animal studies: Birth defects reported in mice, rats and rabbits.

Human studies: Information from adequate studies in pregnant women is not available.

Avoid completely during the first 3 months. Limit use during the last 6 months as much as possible. If used, examine infant for possible deficiency of adrenal gland function.

Advisability of Use if Breast-Feeding

Presence of this drug in breast milk: Yes.

Avoid drug or refrain from nursing.

Habit-Forming Potential: Use of this drug to suppress symptoms over an extended period of time may produce a state of functional dependence (see Glossary). In the treatment of conditions like asthma and rheumatoid arthritis, it is advisable to keep the dose as small as possible and to attempt drug withdrawal after periods of reasonable improvement. Such procedures may reduce the degree of "steroid rebound"—the return of symptoms as the drug is withdrawn.

Effects of Overdosage: Fatigue, muscle weakness, stomach irritation, acid indigestion, excessive sweating, facial flushing, fluid retention, swelling of extremities, increased blood pressure.

Possible Effects of Long-Term Use: Increased blood sugar (possible diabetes), increased fat deposits on the trunk of the body ("buffalo hump"), rounding of the face ("moon face"), thinning and fragility of skin, loss of texture and strength of bones (osteoporosis, aseptic necrosis), cataracts, glaucoma, retarded growth and development in children.

Suggested Periodic Examinations While Taking This Drug (at physician's discretion)

Measurements of blood pressure, blood sugar and potassium levels.

Complete eye examinations at regular intervals.

Chest X-ray if history of tuberculosis.

Determination of the rate of development of the growing child to detect retardation of normal growth.

▷ **While Taking This Drug, Observe the Following**

Foods: No interactions expected. Ask physician regarding need to restrict salt intake or to eat potassium-rich foods. During long-term use of this drug, it is advisable to eat a high-protein diet.

Nutritional Support: During long-term use, take a vitamin D supplement. During wound repair, take a zinc supplement.

Beverages: No restrictions. Drink all forms of milk liberally.

▷ *Alcohol*: No interactions expected. Use caution if you are prone to peptic ulcer disease.

Tobacco Smoking: Nicotine increases the blood levels of naturally produced cortisone and related hormones. Heavy smoking may add to the expected actions of this drug and requires close observation for excessive effects.

Marijuana Smoking: May cause additional impairment of immunity.

▷ *Other Drugs*

Dexamethasone may *decrease* the effects of
- isoniazid (INH, Niconyl, etc.)
- salicylates (aspirin, sodium salicylate, etc.)

Dexamethasone *taken concurrently* with
- oral anticoagulants may either increase or decrease their effectiveness; consult physician regarding the need for prothrombin time testing and dosage adjustment.

The following drugs may *decrease* the effects of dexamethasone
- antacids may reduce its absorption.
- barbiturates (Amytal, Butisol, phenobarbital, etc.).
- phenytoin (Dilantin, etc.).
- rifampin (Rifadin, Rimactane, etc.).

▷ *Driving, Hazardous Activities*: Usually no restrictions. Be alert to the rare occurrence of dizziness.

Aviation Note: The use of this drug *may be a disqualification* for piloting. Consult a designated Aviation Medical Examiner.

Exposure to Sun: No restrictions.

Occurrence of Unrelated Illness: This drug may decrease natural resistance to infection. Inform your physician if you develop an infection of any kind. It may also reduce your body's ability to respond to the stress of acute illness, injury or surgery. Keep your physician fully informed of any significant changes in your state of health.

Discontinuation: If you have been taking this drug for an extended period of time, do not discontinue it abruptly. Ask physician for guidance regarding gradual withdrawal. For a period of 2 years after discontinuing this drug, it is essential in the event of illness, injury or surgery that you inform attending medical personnel that you have used this drug in the past. The period of impaired response to stress following the use of cortisonelike drugs may last for 1 to 2 years.

DIAZEPAM
(di AZ e pam)

Introduced: 1963

Class: Mild Tranquilizer, Benzodiazepines

Prescription: USA: Yes
Canada: Yes

Controlled Drug: USA: C-IV*
Canada: No

Available as Generic: Yes

Brand Names: ✦Apo-Diazepam, ✦E-Pam, ✦Meval, ✦Neo-Calme, ✦Novodipam, ✦Rival, ✦Serenack, ✦Stress-Pam, Valium, Valrelease, ✦Vivol

*See Schedules of Controlled Drugs inside back cover.

BENEFITS versus RISKS	
Possible Benefits	*Possible Risks*
RELIEF OF ANXIETY AND NERVOUS TENSION in 70% to 80% of users	Habit-forming potential with prolonged use
Wide margin of safety with therapeutic doses	Minor impairment of mental functions
Very few drug interactions	Very rare jaundice
	Very rare blood cell disorders

▷ **Principal Uses**

As a Single Drug Product: Used primarily to (1) provide short-term relief of mild to moderate anxiety; (2) relieve the symptoms of acute alcohol withdrawal: agitation, tremors, hallucinations, incipient delirium tremens; (3) relieve skeletal muscle spasm; (4) provide short-term control of certain types of seizures (epilepsy).

How This Drug Works: It is thought that this drug produces a calming effect by enhancing the action of the nerve transmitter gamma-aminobutyric acid (GABA), which in turn blocks the arousal of higher brain centers.

Available Dosage Forms and Strengths

Capsules, prolonged action — 15 mg

Injection — 5 mg per ml

Tablets — 2 mg, 5 mg, 10 mg

▷ **Usual Adult Dosage Range:**   2 to 10 mg, 2 to 4 times daily. Dose may be increased cautiously as needed and tolerated. After 1 week of continual use, the total daily dose may be taken at bedtime. Total daily dose should not exceed 60 mg. **Note: Actual dosage and administration schedule must be determined by the physician for each patient individually.**

▷ **Dosing Instructions:**   May be taken on empty stomach or with food or milk. The prolonged-action capsule should not be opened, but the tablet may be crushed for administration. Do not discontinue this drug abruptly if taken for more than 4 weeks.

Usual Duration of Use: Continual use on a regular schedule for 3 to 5 days is usually necessary to determine this drug's effectiveness in relieving moderate anxiety. Limit continual use to 1 to 3 weeks. Avoid uninterrupted and prolonged use.

▷ **This Drug Should Not Be Taken If**

- you have had an allergic reaction to any dosage form of it previously.
- you have acute narrow-angle glaucoma.
- it is prescribed for a child under 6 months of age.

▷ **Inform Your Physician Before Taking This Drug If**

- you are allergic to any benzodiazepine drug (see Drug Class, Section Four).
- you have a history of alcoholism or drug abuse.
- you are pregnant or planning pregnancy.

- you have impaired liver or kidney function.
- you have a history of serious depression or mental disorder.
- you have any of the following: asthma, emphysema, epilepsy, myasthenia gravis.

Possible Side-Effects   (natural, expected and unavoidable drug actions)
Drowsiness (5%), lethargy, unsteadiness (0.2%), "hangover" effects on the day following bedtime use.

▷ **Possible Adverse Effects**   (unusual, unexpected and infrequent reactions)
If any of the following develop, consult your physician promptly.
Mild Adverse Effects
Allergic Reactions: Rashes (0.4%), hives.
Dizziness, fainting, blurred vision, double vision, slurred speech, sweating, nausea, menstrual irregularity.
Serious Adverse Effects
Allergic Reactions: Liver damage with jaundice (see Glossary), abnormally low blood platelets.
Bone marrow depression—impaired production of white blood cells, fever, sore throat.
Paradoxical responses of excitement, agitation, anger, rage.

▷ **Adverse Effects That May Mimic Natural Diseases or Disorders**
Liver reaction with jaundice may suggest viral hepatitis.

CAUTION
1. This drug should not be discontinued abruptly if it has been taken continually for more than 4 weeks.
2. The concurrent use of some over-the-counter drug products that contain antihistamines (allergy and cold preparations, sleep aids) can cause excessive sedation in sensitive individuals.

Precautions for Use
By Infants and Children: Safety and effectiveness for use by those under 6 months of age have not been established. This drug should not be used in the hyperactive or psychotic child of any age. Observe for excessive sedation and incoordination.
By Those over 60 Years of Age: It is advisable to use smaller doses at longer intervals to avoid overdosage. Observe for the possible development of lethargy, indifference, fatigue, weakness, unsteadiness, disturbing dreams, nightmares and paradoxical reactions of excitement, agitation, anger, hostility and rage.

▷ **Advisability of Use During Pregnancy**
Pregnancy Category: D (tentative). See Pregnancy Code inside back cover.
Animal studies: Cleft palate reported in mice; skeletal defects reported in rats.
Human studies: Available information is conflicting and inconclusive. Some studies found an increase in serious birth defects associated with the use of this drug. Other studies have found no significant increase in birth defects.

Frequent use in late pregnancy can cause the "floppy infant" syndrome in the newborn: weakness, lethargy, unresponsiveness, depressed breathing, low body temperature.

Avoid use during entire pregnancy if possible.

Advisability of Use if Breast-Feeding
Presence of this drug in breast milk: Yes.
Avoid drug or refrain from nursing.

Habit-Forming Potential: This drug can produce psychological and/or physical dependence (see Glossary) if used in large doses for an extended period of time.

Effects of Overdosage: Marked drowsiness, weakness, feeling of drunkenness, staggering gait, tremor, stupor progressing to deep sleep or coma.

Possible Effects of Long-Term Use: Psychological and/or physical dependence, rare blood cell disorders.

Suggested Periodic Examinations While Taking This Drug   (at physician's discretion)
Complete blood cell counts during long-term use.

▷ **While Taking This Drug, Observe the Following**
Foods: No restrictions.
Beverages: Avoid excessive intake of caffeine-containing beverages: coffee, tea, cola. May be taken with milk.
▷ *Alcohol*: Use with extreme caution until the combined effect is determined. Alcohol may increase the absorption of this drug and add to its depressant effects on the brain. It is advisable to avoid alcohol completely—throughout the day and night—if it is necessary to drive or to engage in any hazardous activity.
Tobacco Smoking: Heavy smoking may reduce the calming action of this drug.
Marijuana Smoking: Increased sedation and significant impairment of intellectual and physical performance.
▷ *Other Drugs*
Diazepam may *increase* the effects of
• digoxin (Lanoxin), and cause digoxin toxicity.
• phenytoin (Dilantin), and cause phenytoin toxicity.
Diazepam may *decrease* the effects of
• levodopa (Sinemet, etc.), and reduce its effectiveness in treating Parkinson's disease.
The following drugs may *increase* the effects of diazepam
• cimetidine (Tagamet).
• disulfiram (Antabuse).
• isoniazid (INH, Rifamate, etc.).
• oral contraceptives.
• valproic acid (Depakene).

The following drugs may **decrease** the effects of diazepam
- rifampin (Rimactane, etc.).
- theophylline (aminophylline, Theo-Dur, etc.).

▷ *Driving, Hazardous Activities*: This drug can impair mental alertness, judgment, physical coordination and reaction time. Avoid hazardous activities accordingly.

Aviation Note: The use of this drug *is a disqualification* for piloting. Consult a designated Aviation Medical Examiner.

Exposure to Sun: No restrictions.

Exposure to Heat: Use caution until the effect of excessive perspiration is determined. Because of reduced urine volume, this drug may accumulate in the body and produce effects of overdosage.

Discontinuation: Avoid sudden discontinuation if this drug has been taken for over 4 weeks without interruption. Dosage should be tapered gradually to prevent a withdrawal syndrome that could include depression, confusion, hallucinations, tremor, seizures, muscle cramping, sweating and vomiting.

DICYCLOMINE
(di SI kloh meen)

Introduced: 1952

Class: Antispasmodic, Atropinelike Drugs

Prescription: USA: Yes
Canada: No

Controlled Drug: USA: No
Canada: No

Available as Generic: Yes

Brand Names: Bentyl, ✝Bentylol, ✝Formulex, ✝Lomine, Nospaz, ✝Protylol, ✝Spasmoban, ✝Viscerol

---

BENEFITS versus RISKS

Possible Benefits	*Possible Risks*
EFFECTIVE RELIEF OF GASTROINTESTINAL SPASM	Increased internal eye pressure (important in glaucoma) Constipation Urinary retention (in predisposed persons)

▷ **Principal Uses**

As a Single Drug Product: Used primarily for its atropinelike antispasmodic effect in the management of functional disorders of the gastrointestinal tract, notably the irritable bowel syndrome (spastic colon). It is also used to relieve cramping and pain in infant colic.

How This Drug Works: Not completely established. It has been suggested that this drug may relax gastrointestinal muscle by means of a local anesthetic action that blocks reflex activity responsible for contraction and motility.

Available Dosage Forms and Strengths
Capsules — 10 mg, 20 mg
Injection — 10 mg per ml
   Syrup — 10 mg per 5 ml teaspoonful
Tablets — 20 mg

▷ **Usual Adult Dosage Range:**   10 to 20 mg, 3 or 4 times daily. Total daily dosage should not exceed 160 mg. **Note: Actual dosage and administration schedule must be determined by the physician for each patient individually.**

▷ **Dosing Instructions:**   May be taken with or following food to prevent stomach irritation. The syrup may be diluted with an equal amount of water. The capsule may be opened and the tablet may be crushed for administration.

Usual Duration of Use: Continual use on a regular schedule for 2 to 5 days is usually necessary to determine this drug's effectiveness in relieving the symptoms of spastic disorders of the digestive system. Limit use to the relief of symptoms as necessary. Ask physician for guidance regarding long-term use.

▷ **This Drug Should Not Be Taken If**
• you have had an allergic reaction to any dosage form of it previously.
• your stomach cannot empty properly into the intestine (pyloric obstruction).
• you are unable to empty the urinary bladder completely.
• you have ulcerative colitis.

▷ **Inform Your Physician Before Taking This Drug If**
• you have a history of peptic ulcer disease.
• you have impaired liver or kidney function.
• you have glaucoma, myasthenia gravis or prostatism (see Glossary).

Possible Side-Effects   (natural, expected and unavoidable drug actions)
Dryness of the mouth, blurred vision, constipation.

▷ **Possible Adverse Effects**   (unusual, unexpected and infrequent reactions)
If any of the following develop, consult your physician promptly.
Mild Adverse Effects
Allergic Reactions: Skin rash, hives.
Headache, dizziness, drowsiness, weakness.
Reduced appetite, nausea, vomiting.
Difficult urination, impaired sexual function.
Serious Adverse Effects
Allergic Reactions: Anaphylactic reaction (see Glossary).
Idiosyncratic Reactions: Excitement, confusion, disturbed behavior.
Increased internal eye pressure (significant in glaucoma).

Natural Diseases or Disorders That May Be Activated by This Drug
Glaucoma, prostatism (see Glossary).

CAUTION
Many over-the-counter medications (see OTC drugs in Glossary) for allergies, colds and coughs contain drugs that can interact unfavorably with this drug. Ask your physician or pharmacist for guidance before using any such medications.

Precautions for Use
By Infants and Children: Use extreme care in giving syrup to infants so as to prevent aspiration (inhalation) of the drug. Serious reactions have occurred as a result of this accident during administration.
By Those over 60 Years of Age: Begin treatment with small doses until tolerance is determined. You may be more susceptible to the development of confusion, excitement, constipation and prostatism.

▷ **Advisability of Use During Pregnancy**
Pregnancy Category: B (tentative). See Pregnancy Code inside back cover.
Animal studies: No birth defects reported.
Human studies: Information from adequate studies in pregnant women is not available.
Use only if clearly needed. Ask physician for guidance.

Advisability of Use if Breast-Feeding
Presence of this drug in breast milk: Unknown.
Avoid drug or refrain from nursing.

Habit-Forming Potential: None.

Effects of Overdosage: Headache, dizziness, nausea, dry mouth, difficulty in swallowing, excitement, restlessness, dilated pupils, hot and dry skin.

Possible Effects of Long-Term Use: None reported.

Suggested Periodic Examinations While Taking This Drug   (at physician's discretion)
Measurements of internal eye pressure (in presence of glaucoma or suspected glaucoma).

▷ **While Taking This Drug, Observe the Following**
Foods: No interactions. Follow prescribed diet.
Beverages: No interactions. May be taken with milk.
▷ *Alcohol*: Use caution until combined effects have been determined. Observe for increased drowsiness.
Tobacco Smoking: No interactions expected. Follow physician's advice regarding smoking.
Marijuana Smoking: Possible increase in drowsiness and dryness of mouth.
▷ *Other Drugs*
Dicyclomine may *increase* the effects of
• other drugs that have atropinelike actions (see Drug Class, Section Four).
Dicyclomine may *decrease* the effects of
• levodopa (Larodopa, Sinemet, etc.).

▷ *Driving, Hazardous Activities*: This drug may cause drowsiness, dizziness or blurred vision. Restrict activities accordingly.

Aviation Note: The use of this drug *may be a disqualification* for piloting. Consult a designated Aviation Medical Examiner.

Exposure to Sun: No restrictions.

Exposure to Heat: Use caution. The use of this drug in hot environments may impair normal perspiration and interfere with the regulation of body temperature, thus increasing the risk of heat stroke.

DIFLUNISAL
(di FLOO ni sal)

Introduced: 1977

Class: Mild Analgesic, Anti-inflammatory

Prescription: USA: Yes
Canada: Yes

Controlled Drug: USA: No
Canada: No

Available as Generic: No

Brand Names: Dolobid

BENEFITS versus RISKS

Possible Benefits	*Possible Risks*
EFFECTIVE RELIEF OF MILD TO MODERATE PAIN AND INFLAMMATION	Gastrointestinal pain, ulceration, bleeding (rare)
	Rare liver or kidney damage
	Rare fluid retention

▷ **Principal Uses**

As a Single Drug Product: Used primarily to relieve mild to moderately severe pain associated with (1) musculoskeletal injuries; (2) acute and chronic rheumatoid arthritis and osteoarthritis; and (3) dental, obstetrical and orthopedic surgery.

How This Drug Works: Not completely established. It is thought that this drug reduces the tissue concentrations of prostaglandins (and related compounds), chemicals involved in the production of inflammation and pain.

Available Dosage Forms and Strengths
Tablets — 250 mg, 500 mg

▷ **Usual Adult Dosage Range:** Initially 500 to 1000 mg (loading dose), then 250 to 500 mg/8 to 12 hrs. Total daily dosage should not exceed 1500 mg. **Note: Actual dosage and administration schedule must be determined by the physician for each patient individually.**

▷ **Dosing Instructions:** Take either on an empty stomach or with food or milk to prevent stomach irritation. Swallow tablets whole; do not crush or chew. Take with a full glass of water and remain upright (do not lie down) for 30 minutes.

Usual Duration of Use: Continual use on a regular schedule for 1 to 2 weeks is usually necessary to determine this drug's effectiveness in relieving the discomfort of arthritis. Long-term use requires supervision and periodic evaluation by the physician.

▷ **This Drug Should Not Be Taken If**
- you have had an allergic reaction to it previously.
- you are subject to asthma or nasal polyps caused by aspirin.
- you have active peptic ulcer disease or any form of gastrointestinal bleeding.

▷ **Inform Your Physician Before Taking This Drug If**
- you are allergic to aspirin or to other aspirin substitutes.
- you have a history of peptic ulcer disease or any type of bleeding disorder.
- you have impaired liver or kidney function.
- you have high blood pressure or a history of heart failure.
- you are pregnant.
- you are taking any of the following: acetaminophen, aspirin or other aspirin substitutes, anticoagulants, oral antidiabetic drugs.

Possible Side-Effects (natural, expected and unavoidable drug actions)
Drowsiness, ringing in ears, fluid retention.

▷ **Possible Adverse Effects** (unusual, unexpected and infrequent reactions)
If any of the following develop, consult your physician promptly.
Mild Adverse Effects
Allergic Reactions: Skin rash, hives, itching.
Headache, dizziness, altered or blurred vision, depression.
Mouth sores, indigestion, nausea, vomiting, constipation, diarrhea.
Serious Adverse Effects
Allergic Reactions: Severe skin reactions, swollen lymph glands, drug fever (see Glossary), asthma, anaphylaxis (see Glossary).
Active peptic ulcer, with or without bleeding.
Liver damage with jaundice (see Glossary).
Kidney damage with painful urination, bloody urine, reduced urine formation.
Reduced blood platelets (see Glossary) with abnormal bleeding or bruising.

▷ **Adverse Effects That May Mimic Natural Diseases or Disorders**
Liver reaction may suggest viral hepatitis.

Natural Diseases or Disorders That May Be Activated by This Drug
Peptic ulcer disease, ulcerative colitis.

CAUTION
1. Inform your physician promptly if flulike symptoms develop in association with a skin rash; this could represent a serious allergic reaction.
2. This drug may mask early indications of infection. Inform your physician if you think you are developing an infection of any kind.

Precautions for Use
By Infants and Children: Safety and effectiveness for use by those under 12 years of age have not been established.
By Those over 60 Years of Age: Small doses are advisable until tolerance is determined. Observe for any indications of liver or kidney toxicity.

▷ **Advisability of Use During Pregnancy**
Pregnancy Category: C (tentative). See Pregnancy Code inside back cover.
Animal studies: Skeletal birth defects reported in rabbits.
Human studies: Information from adequate studies in pregnant women is not available.
Avoid this drug during the first and last 3 months. Use it during the middle 3 months only if clearly needed. Ask physician for guidance.

Advisability of Use if Breast-Feeding
Presence of this drug in breast milk: Yes.
Avoid drug or refrain from nursing.

Habit-Forming Potential: None.

Effects of Overdosage: Drowsiness, confusion, disorientation, nausea, vomiting, stupor.

Possible Effects of Long-Term Use: None reported.

Suggested Periodic Examinations While Taking This Drug   (at physician's discretion)
Complete blood cell counts, liver and kidney function tests.
Complete eye examinations if vision is altered in any way.

▷ **While Taking This Drug, Observe the Following**
Foods: No restrictions.
Beverages: No restrictions. May be taken with milk.
▷ *Alcohol*: Use with caution. The irritant action of alcohol on the stomach lining, added to the irritant action of this drug in sensitive individuals, can increase the risk of stomach ulceration and/or bleeding.
Tobacco Smoking: No interactions expected.
▷ *Other Drugs*
Diflunisal may *increase* the effects of
- acetaminophen (Tylenol, etc.), and increase the risk of liver damage; avoid this combination.
- anticoagulants (Coumadin, etc.), and increase the risk of bleeding; monitor prothrombin time, adjust dose accordingly.
- hydrochlorothiazide (Esidrix, HydroDiuril, etc.).

Diflunisal *taken concurrently* with the following drugs may increase the risk of bleeding; avoid these combinations:
- aspirin.
- dipyridamole (Persantine).
- indomethacin (Indocin).
- sulfinpyrazone (Anturane).
- valproic acid (Depakene).

The following drugs may *decrease* the effects of diflunisal
- aluminum antacids may decrease its absorption.

▷ *Driving, Hazardous Activities*: This drug may cause drowsiness, dizziness or altered vision. Restrict activities as necessary.

Aviation Note: The use of this drug *may be a disqualification* for piloting. Consult a designated Aviation Medical Examiner.

Exposure to Sun: Use caution until sensitivity is determined. This drug may cause photosensitivity (see Glossary).

DIGOXIN
(di JOX in)

Introduced: 1934

Prescription: USA: Yes
Canada: No

Available as Generic: Yes

Class: Digitalis Preparations

Controlled Drug: USA: No
Canada: No

Brand Names: Lanoxicaps, Lanoxin, ♣Natigoxine, ♣Novodigoxin

BENEFITS versus RISKS

Possible Benefits	*Possible Risks*
EFFECTIVE HEART STIMULANT IN CONGESTIVE HEART FAILURE	NARROW TREATMENT RANGE (Treatment dose is 60% of toxic dose)
EFFECTIVE PREVENTION AND TREATMENT OF CERTAIN HEART RHYTHM DISORDERS	Frequent and sometimes serious disturbances of heart rhythm

---

▷ **Principal Uses**

As a Single Drug Product: This drug has two primary uses: (1) the treatment of congestive heart failure; (2) the restoration and maintenance of normal heart rate and rhythm in such disorders as atrial fibrillation, atrial flutter and atrial/supraventricular tachycardia.

How This Drug Works: By increasing the availability of calcium within the heart muscle, this drug improves the efficiency of the conversion of chemical energy to mechanical energy, thus increasing the force of heart muscle contraction. By slowing the activity of the pacemaker and delaying the transmission of electrical impulses through the conduction system of the heart, this drug assists in restoring normal heart rate and rhythm.

Available Dosage Forms and Strengths
Elixir, pediatric — 0.05 mg per ml
Capsules — 0.05 mg, 0.1 mg, 0.2 mg
Injection — 0.1 mg per ml, 0.25 mg per ml
Tablets — 0.125 mg, 0.25 mg, 0.5 mg

▷ **Usual Adult Dosage Range:**   Rapid digitalization—1 to 1.5 mg divided into 2 or 3 doses given every 6 to 8 hours in 1 day. Slow digitalization—0.125 to 0.5 mg/day for 7 days. Maintenance—0.125 to 0.5 mg/day. Total daily dosage should not exceed 2 mg. **Note: Actual dosage and administration schedule must be determined by the physician for each patient individually.**

▷ **Dosing Instructions:**   Take at the same time each day, preferably on an empty stomach to ensure uniform absorption. May be taken with or following food if desired (not milk or dairy products). The tablet may be crushed for administration; the capsule should be swallowed whole.

Usual Duration of Use: Continual use on a regular schedule for 7 to 10 days is usually necessary to determine this drug's effectiveness in relieving heart failure or controlling heart rhythm disorders. Long-term use requires physician supervision and periodic assessment of continued need. The use of this drug is not necessarily "for life."

▷ **This Drug Should Not Be Taken If**
  • you have had an allergic reaction to any dosage form of it previously.

▷ **Inform Your Physician Before Taking This Drug If**
  • you have experienced any unfavorable reaction to a digitalis preparation in the past.
  • you have taken any digitalis preparation within the past 2 weeks.
  • you are now taking (or have recently taken) any diuretic (urine-producing) drug.
  • you have impaired liver or kidney function.
  • you have a history of thyroid function disorder.

Possible Side-Effects   (natural, expected and unavoidable drug actions)
Slow heart rate, rare enlargement and/or sensitivity of the male breast tissue.

▷ **Possible Adverse Effects**   (unusual, unexpected and infrequent reactions)
If any of the following develop, consult your physician promptly.
Mild Adverse Effects
Allergic Reactions: Skin rash, hives.
Headache, drowsiness, lethargy, confusion, changes in vision: "halo" effect, blurring, spots, double vision, yellow-green vision.
Loss of appetite, nausea, vomiting, diarrhea—early indications of toxicity in adults.

Serious Adverse Effects

Idiosyncratic Reactions: Hallucinations, facial neuralgias, peripheral neuralgias, blindness (very rare).

Disorientation, most common in the elderly.

Heart rhythm disturbances.

▷ **Adverse Effects That May Mimic Natural Diseases or Disorders**

Drug-induced mental disturbances in the elderly may be mistaken for senile dementia or psychosis.

Natural Diseases or Disorders That May Be Activated by This Drug

Digitalis may induce a systemic lupus-erythematosuslike syndrome.

CAUTION

1. This drug has a narrow margin of safe use. Adhere strictly to prescribed dosage schedules. Do not raise or lower the dose without first consulting your physician.
2. If you are taking calcium supplements, ask your physician for guidance. Avoid large doses.
3. It is advisable to carry a card of personal identification with a notation that you are taking this drug.

Precautions for Use

By Infants and Children: Observe carefully for indications of toxicity: slow heart rate (below 60 beats/minute), irregular heart rhythms.

By Those over 60 Years of Age: You may have a reduced tolerance for this drug; smaller doses are advisable. Observe for indications of early toxicity: headache, dizziness, fatigue, weakness, lethargy, depression, confusion, nervousness, agitation, delusions, difficulty with reading. Report the development of any of these effects promptly to your physician.

▷ **Advisability of Use During Pregnancy**

Pregnancy Category: B (tentative). See Pregnancy Code inside back cover.

Animal studies: No birth defects reported.

Human studies: Information from adequate studies in pregnant women is not available. However, no birth defects attributable to the therapeutic use of this drug have been reported.

Use this drug only if clearly needed.

Advisability of Use if Breast-Feeding

Presence of this drug in breast milk: Yes.

Monitor nursing infant closely and discontinue drug or nursing if adverse effects develop.

Habit-Forming Potential: None.

Effects of Overdosage: Loss of appetite, excessive saliva, nausea, vomiting, diarrhea, serious disturbances of heart rate and rhythm, intestinal bleeding, drowsiness, headache, confusion, delirium, hallucinations, convulsions.

Possible Effects of Long-Term Use: None reported.

Suggested Periodic Examinations While Taking This Drug   (at physician's discretion)
> Measurements of blood levels of digoxin, calcium, magnesium and potassium; electrocardiograms.

▷ **While Taking This Drug, Observe the Following**
> *Foods*: Avoid all cheeses, yogurt and ice cream for 2 hours before and after taking this drug. Consult physician regarding the advisability of eating high-potassium foods.
> *Beverages*: Avoid all forms of milk for 2 hours before and after taking this drug. Avoid excessive amounts of caffeine-containing beverages: coffee, tea, cola.

▷ *Alcohol*: No interactions expected.
> *Tobacco Smoking*: Nicotine can cause irritability of the heart muscle and can predispose to serious rhythm disturbances. It is advisable to abstain from all forms of tobacco.
> *Marijuana Smoking*: Possible accentuation of heart failure; reduced digoxin effect; possible changes in electrocardiogram, confusing interpretation.

▷ *Other Drugs*
> Digoxin *taken concurrently* with
> - diuretics (other than spironolactone and triamterene) may result in serious heart rhythm disturbances due to excessive loss of potassium.
> - quinidine may result in decreased digoxin effectiveness and increased digoxin toxicity; careful dosage adjustments are necessary.
>
> The following drugs may *increase* the effects of digoxin
> - amiodarone (Cordarone).
> - benzodiazepines (Librium, Valium, etc.; see Drug Class, Section Four).
> - diltiazem (Cardizem).
> - erythromycin (EES, Erythrocin, etc.).
> - methimazole (Tapazole).
> - propylthiouracil (Propacil).
> - quinine.
> - tetracyclines (see Drug Class, Section Four).
> - verapamil (Isoptin).
>
> The following drugs may *decrease* the effects of digoxin
> - aluminum-containing antacids (Amphojel, Maalox, etc.).
> - bleomycin (Blenoxane).
> - carmustine (Bicnu).
> - cholestyramine (Questran).
> - colestipol (Colestid).
> - cyclophosphamide (Cytoxan).
> - cytarabine (Cytosar).
> - doxorubicin (Adriamycin).
> - methotrexate (Mexate).
> - penicillamine (Cuprimine, Depen).
> - procarbazine (Matulane).

- thyroid hormones.
- vincristine (Oncovin).

▷ *Driving, Hazardous Activities*: Usually no restrictions. However, this drug may cause drowsiness, vision changes and nausea. Restrict activities as necessary.

Aviation Note: Heart function disorders *are a disqualification* for piloting. Consult a designated Aviation Medical Examiner.

Exposure to Sun: No restrictions.

Occurrence of Unrelated Illness: Any illness that causes vomiting or diarrhea can seriously alter this drug's effectiveness. Notify your physician promptly.

Discontinuation: This drug must be continued indefinitely (possibly for life). Do not discontinue it without consulting your physician.

DILTIAZEM ✗
(dil TI a zem)

Introduced: 1977

Class: Antianginal, Calcium Channel Blocker

Prescription: USA: Yes
Canada: Yes

Controlled Drug: USA: No
Canada: No

Available as Generic: No

Brand Names: Cardizem

BENEFITS versus RISKS	
Possible Benefits	*Possible Risks*
EFFECTIVE PREVENTION OF BOTH MAJOR TYPES OF ANGINA	Depression, confusion
	Low blood pressure
	Heart rhythm disturbance (2%)
	Fluid retention (2.4%)
	Liver damage (very rare)

▷ **Principal Uses**

As a Single Drug Product: Used primarily to treat (1) angina pectoris due to coronary artery spasm (Prinzmetal's variant angina) that occurs spontaneously and is not associated with exertion; and (2) classical angina-of-effort (due to atherosclerotic disease of the coronary arteries) in individuals who have not responded to or cannot tolerate the nitrates and "beta blocker" drugs customarily used to treat this disorder.

How This Drug Works: Not completely established. It is thought that by blocking the normal passage of calcium through certain cell walls (which is necessary for the function of nerve and muscle tissue), this drug slows the spread of electrical activity through the conduction system of the heart and inhibits the contraction of coronary arteries and peripheral arterioles. As a result of these combined effects, this drug

- prevents spontaneous spasm of the coronary arteries (Prinzmetal's type of angina).
- reduces the rate and contraction force of the heart during exertion, thus lowering the oxygen requirement of the heart muscle; this reduces the occurrence of effort-induced angina (classical angina pectoris).
- reduces the degree of contraction of peripheral arterial walls, resulting in their relaxation and consequent lowering of blood pressure. This further reduces the work load of the heart during exertion and contributes to the prevention of angina.

Available Dosage Forms and Strengths
Tablets — 30 mg, 60 mg

▷ **Usual Adult Dosage Range:** Initially 30 mg, 3 or 4 times daily. Dose may be increased gradually at 1- to 2-day intervals as needed and tolerated. Total daily dosage should not exceed 240 mg. **Note: Actual dosage and administration schedule must be determined by the physician for each patient individually.**

▷ **Dosing Instructions:** Preferably taken before meals and at bedtime. Tablet may be crushed for administration.

Usual Duration of Use: Continual use on a regular schedule for 2 to 4 weeks is usually necessary to determine this drug's effectiveness in reducing the frequency and severity of angina. For long-term use (months to years), determine the smallest effective dose.

▷ **This Drug Should Not Be Taken If**
- you have had an allergic reaction to it previously.
- you have a "sick sinus" syndrome (and are not wearing an artificial pacemaker).
- you have been told that you have a second-degree or third-degree heart block.
- you have low blood pressure—systolic pressure below 90.

▷ **Inform Your Physician Before Taking This Drug If**
- you have had an unfavorable response to any "calcium blocker" drug in the past.
- you are currently taking any form of digitalis or a "beta blocker" drug (see Drug Class, Section Four).
- you have a history of congestive heart failure.
- you have impaired liver or kidney function.
- you have a history of drug-induced liver damage.

Possible Side-Effects (natural, expected and unavoidable drug actions)
Fatigue (1.2%), light-headedness, heart rate and rhythm changes in predisposed individuals (1.1%).

▷ **Possible Adverse Effects** (unusual, unexpected and infrequent reactions)
If any of the following develop, consult your physician promptly.
Mild Adverse Effects
Allergic Reactions: Skin rash (1.3%), hives, itching.
Headache (2.1%), drowsiness, dizziness (1.5%), nervousness, insomnia, depression, confusion, hallucinations.
Flushing, palpitations, fainting, slow heart rate, low blood pressure.
Nausea (1.9%), indigestion, heartburn, vomiting, diarrhea, constipation.
Serious Adverse Effects
Serious disturbances of heart rate and/or rhythm, fluid retention (edema) (2.4%), congestive heart failure.
Drug-induced liver damage (very rare).

CAUTION
1. Be sure to inform all physicians and dentists you consult that you are taking this drug. Note the use of this drug on your card of personal identification.
2. You may use nitroglycerin and other nitrate drugs as needed to relieve acute episodes of angina pain. However, if you detect that your angina attacks are becoming more frequent or intense, notify your physician promptly.

Precautions for Use
By Infants and Children: Safety and effectiveness for use by those under 12 years of age have not been established.
By Those over 60 Years of Age: You may be more susceptible to the development of weakness, dizziness, fainting and falling. Take necessary precautions to prevent injury. Report promptly any changes in your pattern of thirst and urination.

▷ **Advisability of Use During Pregnancy**
Pregnancy Category: C (tentative). See Pregnancy Code inside back cover.
Animal studies: Embryo and fetal deaths and skeletal birth defects reported in mice, rats and rabbits.
Human studies: Information from adequate studies in pregnant women is not available.
Avoid this drug during the first 3 months.
Use during the last 6 months only if clearly needed. Ask physician for guidance.

Advisability of Use if Breast-Feeding
Presence of this drug in breast milk: Possibly yes.
Avoid drug or refrain from nursing.

Habit-Forming Potential: None.

Effects of Overdosage: Weakness, light-headedness, fainting, slow pulse, low blood pressure, shortness of breath, congestive heart failure.

Possible Effects of Long-Term Use: None reported.

Suggested Periodic Examinations While Taking This Drug (at physician's discretion)

Evaluations of heart function, including electrocardiograms; liver and kidney function tests, with long-term use.

▷ **While Taking This Drug, Observe the Following**

Foods: No restrictions. Avoid excessive salt intake.

Beverages: No restrictions. May be taken with milk.

▷　*Alcohol*: Use with caution until combined effects have been determined. Alcohol may exaggerate the drop in blood pressure experienced by some individuals.

Tobacco Smoking: Nicotine may reduce the effectiveness of this drug. Follow your physician's advice regarding smoking.

Marijuana Smoking: Possible reduced effectiveness of this drug; mild to moderate increase in angina; possible changes in electrocardiogram, confusing interpretation.

▷　*Other Drugs*

Diltiazem *taken concurrently* with

- "beta blocker" drugs or digitalis preparations (see Drug Classes, Section Four) may affect heart rate and rhythm adversely. Careful monitoring by your physician is necessary if these drugs are taken concurrently.

The following drugs may *increase* the effects of diltiazem

- cimetidine (Tagamet).

▷　*Driving, Hazardous Activities*: Usually no restrictions. This drug may cause drowsiness or dizziness. Restrict activities as necessary.

Aviation Note: Coronary artery disease *is a disqualification* for piloting. Consult a designated Aviation Medical Examiner.

Exposure to Sun: Use caution until sensitivity has been determined. This drug may cause photosensitivity (see Glossary).

Exposure to Heat: Caution advised. Hot environments can exaggerate the blood-pressure-lowering effects of this drug. Observe for light-headedness or weakness.

Heavy Exercise or Exertion: This drug may improve your ability to be more active without resulting angina pain. Use caution and avoid excessive exercise that could impair heart function in the absence of warning pain.

Discontinuation: Do not discontinue this drug abruptly. Consult your physician regarding gradual withdrawal.

DIPHENHYDRAMINE
(di fen HI dra meen)

Introduced: 1946

Prescription: USA: Varies
Canada: No

Available as Generic: Yes

Class: Hypnotic, Antihistamines

Controlled Drug: USA: No*
Canada: No

Brand Names: ♣Allerdryl, ♣Ambenyl Expectorant [CD], Ambenyl Syrup [CD], Benadryl, Benylin, ♣Benylin Decongestant Cough Syrup [CD], Compoz, ♣Insomnal, Nytol w/DPH, Sominex 2, Twilite

---

BENEFITS versus RISKS

Possible Benefits	*Possible Risks*
EFFECTIVE RELIEF OF ALLERGIC RHINITIS AND ALLERGIC SKIN DISORDERS	Marked sedation (50%)
	Atropinelike effects
EFFECTIVE, NONADDICTIVE SEDATIVE AND HYPNOTIC	Accentuation of prostatism (see Glossary)
Prevention and relief of motion sickness	Rare blood cell disorders: abnormally low white blood cells and platelets
Partial relief of symptoms of Parkinson's disease	

▷ **Principal Uses**

As a Single Drug Product: This versatile antihistamine is used primarily for (1) the safe and effective induction of sleep (mild to moderate sedation); (2) the prevention and treatment of motion sickness (control of dizziness, nausea and vomiting); (3) the relief of symptoms associated with Parkinson's disease; (4) the treatment of drug-induced parkinsonian reactions, especially in children and the elderly.

As a Combination Drug Product [CD]: This drug may have a mild suppressant effect on coughing, but its actual effectiveness is questionable. It is combined with expectorants and either codeine or dextromethorphan in some cough preparations.

How This Drug Works: This drug reduces the intensity of allergic response by blocking the action of histamine after it has been released from sensitized tissue cells. Its natural side-effects are used to advantage: its sedative action is used to induce drowsiness and sleep; its atropinelike action is used in the management of motion sickness and Parkinson-related disorders.

Available Dosage Forms and Strengths
Capsules — 25 mg, 50 mg
Elixir — 12.5 mg per 5 ml teaspoonful

*Ambenyl Syrup is C-V. See Schedules of Controlled Drugs inside back cover.

Syrup — 12.5 mg per 5 ml teaspoonful
Tablets — 25 mg, 50 mg

▷ **Usual Adult Dosage Range:**   25 to 50 mg/4 to 6 hrs. Total daily dosage should not exceed 300 mg. **Note: Actual dosage and administration schedule must be determined by the physician for each patient individually.**

▷ **Dosing Instructions:**   Preferably taken with or following food to reduce stomach irritation. Tablet may be crushed and capsule may be opened for administration.

Usual Duration of Use: Continual use on a regular schedule for 2 to 3 days is usually necessary to determine this drug's effectiveness in relieving the symptoms of allergic rhinitis and dermatosis. If not effective after 5 days, this drug should be discontinued. As a bedtime sedative (hypnotic), use only as needed. Avoid long-term use without interruption.

▷ **This Drug Should Not Be Taken If**
- you have had an allergic reaction to any dosage form of it previously.
- you are taking, or have taken during the past 2 weeks, any monoamine oxidase (MAO) inhibitor drug (see Drug Class, Section Four).

▷ **Inform Your Physician Before Taking This Drug If**
- you have had an unfavorable response to any antihistamine drug in the past.
- you have narrow-angle glaucoma.
- you have peptic ulcer disease, with any degree of pyloric obstruction.
- you have prostatism (see Glossary).
- you are subject to bronchial asthma or seizures (epilepsy).

Possible Side-Effects   (natural, expected and unavoidable drug actions)
Drowsiness; sense of weakness; dryness of nose, mouth and throat; constipation.

▷ **Possible Adverse Effects**   (unusual, unexpected and infrequent reactions)
If any of the following develop, consult your physician promptly.
Mild Adverse Effects
Allergic Reactions: Skin rash, hives.
Headache, dizziness, inability to concentrate, nervousness, blurred or double vision, difficult urination.
Reduced tolerance for contact lenses.
Nausea, vomiting, diarrhea.
Serious Adverse Effects
Allergic Reactions: Anaphylactic reaction (see Glossary).
Idiosyncratic Reactions: Insomnia, excitement, confusion.
Hemolytic anemia (see Glossary).
Reduced white blood cells—fever, sore throat, infections.
Blood platelet destruction (see Glossary)—abnormal bleeding or bruising.

Natural Diseases or Disorders That May Be Activated by This Drug
Latent epilepsy, glaucoma, prostatism.

CAUTION
1. Discontinue this drug 5 days before diagnostic skin testing procedures in order to prevent false negative test results.
2. Do not use this drug if you have active bronchial asthma, bronchitis or pneumonia. It can thicken bronchial mucous and make it more difficult to remove (by absorption or coughing).

Precautions for Use

By Infants and Children: This drug should not be used in premature or full-term newborn infants. Doses for children should be small. The young child is especially sensitive to the effects of antihistamines on the brain and nervous system. Avoid the use of this drug in the child with chicken pox or a flulike infection; although unproven, this drug may adversely affect the course of Reye syndrome should the child develop it during the course of illness.

By Those over 60 Years of Age: You may be more susceptible to the development of drowsiness, dizziness and unsteadiness, and to impairment of thinking, judgment and memory. This drug can increase the degree of impaired urination associated with prostate gland enlargement (prostatism). The sedative effects of antihistamines in the elderly can cause a syndrome of underactivity that may be misinterpreted as senility or emotional depression.

▷ **Advisability of Use During Pregnancy**

Pregnancy Category: B (tentative). See Pregnancy Code inside back cover.

Animal studies: No birth defects reported in rats or rabbits.

Human studies: Information from studies in pregnant women indicates no significant increase in birth defects in 2948 exposures to this drug.

A withdrawal syndrome of tremor and diarrhea has been reported in a 5-day-old infant whose mother used this drug (150 mg daily) during pregnancy.

Avoid drug during the last 3 months. Use sparingly during the first 6 months only if clearly needed.

Advisability of Use if Breast-Feeding

Presence of this drug in breast milk: Yes.

Habit-Forming Potential: None.

Effects of Overdosage: Marked drowsiness, confusion, incoordination, unsteadiness, muscle tremors, stupor, coma, seizures, fever, flushed face, dilated pupils, weak pulse, shallow breathing.

Possible Effects of Long-Term Use: The development of tolerance (see Glossary) and reduced effectiveness of drug.

Suggested Periodic Examinations While Taking This Drug   (at physician's discretion)

Complete blood cell counts.

▷ **While Taking This Drug, Observe the Following**

Foods: No restrictions.

Beverages: No restrictions. May be taken with milk.

▷   *Alcohol*: Use with extreme caution until the combined effect has been determined. The combination of alcohol and antihistamines can cause rapid and marked sedation.

Tobacco Smoking: No interactions expected.

Marijuana Smoking: Increased drowsiness and mouth dryness; possible accentuation of impaired thinking.

▷   *Other Drugs*

Diphenhydramine may *increase* the effects of
- all drugs with a sedative effect, and cause oversedation.
- atropine and atropinelike drugs (see Drug Class, Section Four).

The following drugs may *increase* the effects of diphenhydramine
- monoamine oxidase (MAO) inhibitor drugs (see Drug Class, Section Four) may delay its elimination, thus exaggerating and prolonging its action.

▷   *Driving, Hazardous Activities*: This drug may impair mental alertness, judgment, physical coordination and reaction time. Restrict activities as necessary.

Aviation Note: The use of this drug *is a disqualification* for piloting. Consult a designated Aviation Medical Examiner.

Exposure to Sun: Use caution until sensitivity has been determined. This drug may cause photosensitivity (see Glossary).

Exposure to Environmental Chemicals: The insecticides Aldrin, Dieldrin and Chlordane may decrease the effectiveness of this drug. The insecticide Sevin may increase the sedative effects of this drug.

DIPHENOXYLATE
(di fen OX i layt)

Introduced: 1960   **Class:** Antidiarrheal

Prescription: USA: Yes   **Controlled Drug:** USA: C-V*
Canada: Yes   Canada: <N>

Available as Generic: USA: Yes
Canada: No

Brand Names: Enoxa [CD], Lomotil [CD], SK-Diphenoxylate [CD]

BENEFITS versus RISKS	
Possible Benefits	*Possible Risks*
EFFECTIVE RELIEF OF	Drowsiness
INTESTINAL CRAMPING AND	Constipation
DIARRHEA	Low habit-forming potential

*See Schedules of Controlled Drugs inside back cover.

▷ **Principal Uses**

As a Single Drug Product: Used primarily for the control of overactivity of the intestinal tract, cramping and diarrhea. Because of its potential for abuse, this drug is not marketed as a single-entity product in the USA.

As a Combination Drug Product [CD]: This drug, in therapeutically effective dosage, is combined with a small amount of atropine to discourage abusive overdosage. The accumulative effects of atropine overdosage would make the combination intolerable.

How This Drug Works: Not completely established. It is thought that this drug acts directly on the nerve supply of the gastrointestinal tract to reduce its motility and propulsive contractions, thus relieving cramping and diarrhea.

Available Dosage Forms and Strengths

Liquid — 2.5 mg (+ 0.025 mg atropine) per 5-ml teaspoonful
Tablets — 2.5 mg (+ 0.025 mg atropine)

▷ **Usual Adult Dosage Range:** Initially 2.5 to 5 mg/4 hrs as needed for acute diarrhea; then 2.5 mg/6 to 8 hrs as needed for chronic diarrhea. **Note: Actual dosage and administration schedule must be determined by the physician for each patient individually.**

▷ **Dosing Instructions:** May be taken on an empty stomach or with food if stomach irritation occurs. Tablet may be crushed for administration.

Usual Duration of Use: Continual use on a regular schedule for 24 to 36 hours is usually necessary to determine this drug's effectiveness in controlling acute diarrhea. If diarrhea persists, consult your physician. Avoid prolonged and uninterrupted use.

▷ **This Drug Should Not Be Taken If**
• you are allergic to either component of this combination drug. (Single component in Canada.)
• you have active liver disease.
• it is prescribed for a child under 2 years of age.

▷ **Inform Your Physician Before Taking This Drug If**
• you have a history of liver disease or impaired liver function.
• you have regional enteritis or ulcerative colitis.
• you have chronic lung disease of any kind.

Possible Side-Effects   (natural, expected and unavoidable drug actions)
Drowsiness, constipation.

▷ **Possible Adverse Effects**   (unusual, unexpected and infrequent reactions)
If any of the following develop, consult your physician promptly.
Mild Adverse Effects
Allergic Reactions: Skin rash, hives, localized swellings, itching.
Headache, dizziness, weakness, euphoria.
Reduced appetite, nausea, vomiting, bloating.

Serious Adverse Effects
"Toxic megacolon" (distended, immobile colon with fluid retention) may develop in acute ulcerative colitis.

CAUTION
1. Do not exceed recommended doses.
2. Use with caution in the presence of chronic lung disease (asthma, bronchitis, emphysema). This drug may impair respiration.
3. If used to treat chronic diarrhea, report promptly any development of bloating, abdominal distension, nausea, vomiting, constipation or abdominal pain.

Precautions for Use
By Infants and Children: Do not use in those under 2 years of age. Use with caution (especially in children with Down's syndrome); observe closely for any indications of atropine overdosage: excitement, overactivity, hallucinations, fever, flushed face, dilated pupils.

By Those over 60 Years of Age: Start treatment with small doses. You may be more sensitive to the sedative and constipating effects of this drug.

▷ Advisability of Use During Pregnancy
Pregnancy Category: C (tentative). See Pregnancy Code inside back cover.
Animal studies: No information available.
Human studies: Information from adequate studies in pregnant women is not available.
Use sparingly and only if clearly needed. Ask physician for guidance.

Advisability of Use if Breast-Feeding
Presence of this drug in breast milk: Yes.
Avoid drug or refrain from nursing.

Habit-Forming Potential: Because of its similarity to meperidine, this drug may cause physical dependence (see Glossary) if used in large doses over an extended period of time.

Effects of Overdosage: Marked drowsiness, lethargy, depression, numbness in arms and legs, dry skin and mouth, flushing, fever, rapid pulse, slow and shallow breathing, stupor progressing to coma.

Possible Effects of Long-Term Use: The development of tolerance with loss of drug effectiveness. Physical dependence is a remote possibility.

Suggested Periodic Examinations While Taking This Drug (at physician's discretion)
None required.

▷ While Taking This Drug, Observe the Following
Foods: No restrictions. Follow prescribed diet.
Beverages: No restrictions. May be taken with milk.
▷   *Alcohol*: Use with extreme caution until combined effects have been determined. This drug may increase the depressant action of alcohol on the brain.
Tobacco Smoking: No interactions expected.

▷   *Other Drugs*

Diphenoxylate may *increase* the effects of

• all drugs with a sedative effect, and cause oversedation.

Diphenoxylate *taken concurrently* with

• monoamine oxidase (MAO) inhibitor drugs (see Drug Class, Section Four) will require close observation for excessive rise in blood pressure.

▷   *Driving, Hazardous Activities*: This drug may cause drowsiness or dizziness. Restrict activities as necessary.

Aviation Note: The use of this drug *is a disqualification* for piloting. Consult a designated Aviation Medical Examiner.

Exposure to Sun: No restrictions.

DIPYRIDAMOLE
(di peer ID a mohl)

Introduced: 1959

Class: Antianginal, Platelet Inhibitor

Prescription: USA: Yes
Canada: No

Controlled Drug: USA: No
Canada: No

Available as Generic: USA: Yes
Canada: No

Brand Names: ✚Apo-Dipyridamole, Persantine, SK-Dipyridamole

BENEFITS versus RISKS	
Possible Benefits	*Possible Risks*
EFFECTIVE PREVENTION OF THROMBOEMBOLISM (BLOOD CLOTS) FOLLOWING HEART SURGERY Possibly effective in the long-term treatment of chronic, stable angina	Mild low blood pressure with dizziness and fainting (infrequent) Mild indigestion

▷ **Principal Uses**

As a Single Drug Product: This drug is used primarily for (1) the prevention of thromboembolism (blood clot formation and migration) following heart surgery; (2) the prevention of thromboembolism thought to be responsible for transient ischemic attacks in brain circulation (ministrokes); (3) the long-term treatment of chronic angina pectoris. (This drug does not relieve the pain of acute anginal episodes. It is used to reduce the frequency and severity of angina attacks.)

How This Drug Works: Not completely established. It is thought that by inhibiting the actions of certain enzymes, this drug (1) prevents the aggregation of blood platelets (see Glossary) and thereby reduces the tendency to blood clot formation; and (2) selectively dilates small coronary arteries and thereby increases the flow of blood and the supply of oxygen to working heart muscle.

Available Dosage Forms and Strengths
Tablets — 25 mg, 50 mg, 75 mg

▷ **Usual Adult Dosage Range:** 50 to 100 mg, 3 or 4 times daily. Total daily dosage should not exceed 400 mg. **Note: Actual dosage and administration schedule must be determined by the physician for each patient individually.**

▷ **Dosing Instructions:** Preferably taken with a full glass of water on an empty stomach, 1 hour before or 2 hours after eating. However, it may be taken with or following food to reduce stomach irritation. Tablet may be crushed for administration.

Usual Duration of Use: Continual use on a regular schedule for 2 to 3 months is usually necessary to determine this drug's effectiveness in reducing the frequency and severity of angina attacks. Significant reduction in platelet aggregation is thought to occur in 1 week. Long-term use (months to years) requires supervision and periodic evaluation by your physician.

▷ **This Drug Should Not Be Taken If**
- you have had an allergic reaction to it previously.
- you have just experienced an acute heart attack (myocardial infarction).
- you have uncontrolled high blood pressure.

▷ **Inform Your Physician Before Taking This Drug If**
- you have low blood pressure.
- you have impaired liver function.
- you have any type of bleeding disorder.

Possible Side-Effects (natural, expected and unavoidable drug actions)
Flushing, light-headedness, weakness.

▷ **Possible Adverse Effects** (unusual, unexpected and infrequent reactions)
If any of the following develop, consult your physician promptly.
Mild Adverse Effects
Allergic Reactions: Skin rash.
Headache, dizziness, fainting.
Stomach irritation, nausea, diarrhea.
Serious Adverse Effects
Significant low blood pressure with large doses.
Paradoxical increase in angina on starting treatment (infrequent).
Aggravation of migraine headaches.

CAUTION
1. Occasionally this drug may cause an *increase* in the frequency and/or severity of angina attacks during the initial trial of treatment. If this

response occurs, discontinue this drug promptly and inform your physician.

2. Anyone with low blood pressure should avoid large doses of this drug.

Precautions for Use

By Infants and Children: Observe closely for indications of excessively low blood pressure.

By Those over 60 Years of Age: Begin treatment with small doses (25 mg twice daily) to evaluate effect on blood pressure. Avoid doses that cause excessively low blood pressure. Observe for any tendency to develop hypothermia (see Glossary) in cold environments.

▷ **Advisability of Use During Pregnancy**

Pregnancy Category: C (tentative). See Pregnancy Code inside back cover.

Animal studies: No information available.

Human studies: Information from adequate studies in pregnant women is not available.

Use this drug only if clearly needed. If possible, avoid use during the last month of pregnancy and during labor and delivery because of possible prolongation of bleeding following delivery.

Advisability of Use if Breast-Feeding

Presence of this drug in breast milk: Yes, in small amounts.

Monitor nursing infant closely and discontinue drug or nursing if adverse effects develop.

Habit-Forming Potential: None.

Effects of Overdosage: Flushing, stomach irritation, nausea, vomiting, stomach cramps, diarrhea, rapid heart rate, low blood pressure, weakness, fainting.

Possible Effects of Long-Term Use: None reported.

Suggested Periodic Examinations While Taking This Drug (at physician's discretion)

Measurements of blood pressure in lying, sitting and standing positions.

▷ **While Taking This Drug, Observe the Following**

Foods: No restrictions.

Beverages: No restrictions. May be taken with milk.

▷ *Alcohol*: Use with caution until the combined effect has been determined. Alcohol may enhance the ability of this drug to lower blood pressure.

Tobacco Smoking: Nicotine can reduce the effectiveness of this drug. Follow physician's advice regarding smoking.

Marijuana Smoking: Possible reduced effectiveness of this drug; mild to moderate increase in angina; possible changes in electrocardiogram, confusing interpretation.

▷ *Other Drugs*

Dipyridamole may *increase* the effects of

• oral anticoagulants (warfarin, etc.), when doses of dipyridamole

approach or exceed 400 mg/day; observe for abnormal bleeding or bruising.
- other drugs that inhibit platelet activity; observe for abnormal bleeding or bruising.

Dipyridamole *taken concurrently* with
- aspirin makes it possible to reduce the dose of dipyridamole and thus lessen any side-effects that may occur.

▷ *Driving, Hazardous Activities*: This drug may cause light-headedness or dizziness. Restrict activities as necessary.

Aviation Note: Cerebral circulatory disorders and coronary artery disease *are disqualifications* for piloting. Consult a designated Aviation Medical Examiner.

Exposure to Sun: No restrictions.

Exposure to Heat: Use caution. Hot environments can cause a significant drop in blood pressure.

Exposure to Cold: Use caution. Cold environments can provoke angina. Also, this drug may increase the risk of hypothermia in the elderly.

Discontinuation: Following long-term use, this drug should not be discontinued abruptly. It should be withdrawn gradually over a period of 2 to 3 weeks. Ask your physician for guidance.

DISOPYRAMIDE
(di so PEER a mide)

Introduced: 1969

Class: Antiarrhythmic

Prescription: USA: Yes
Canada: Yes

Controlled Drug: USA: No
Canada: No

Available as Generic: USA: Yes
Canada: No

Brand Names: Norpace, Norpace CR, ✤Rythmodan, ✤Rythmodan-LA

BENEFITS versus RISKS	
Possible Benefits	*Possible Risks*
EFFECTIVE TREATMENT OF SELECTED HEART RHYTHM DISORDERS	NARROW TREATMENT RANGE FREQUENT ADVERSE EFFECTS (10%–40%) LOW BLOOD PRESSURE CONGESTIVE HEART FAILURE Heart conduction and rhythm abnormalities Frequent atropinelike side-effects

▷ **Principal Uses**

As a Single Drug Product: This drug is classified as a Type 1 antiarrhythmic agent, similar to procainamide and quinidine in its actions. It is used primarily to abolish and prevent the recurrence of premature beats arising in the atria (upper chambers) and the ventricles (lower chambers) of the heart. It is also useful in the treatment and prevention of abnormally rapid heart rates (tachycardia) that originate in the atria or the ventricles.

How This Drug Works: By slowing the activity of the pacemaker and delaying the transmission of electrical impulses through the conduction system and muscle of the heart, this drug assists in restoring normal heart rate and rhythm.

Available Dosage Forms and Strengths
Capsules — 100 mg, 150 mg
Capsules, prolonged-action — 100 mg, 150 mg

▷ **Usual Adult Dosage Range:** 100 to 200 mg/6 hrs. Dosage should not exceed 200 mg/6 hrs or 800 mg/24 hrs (1600 mg/24 hrs have been used occasionally). **Note: Actual dosage and administration schedule must be determined by the physician for each patient individually.**

▷ **Dosing Instructions:** Preferably taken on an empty stomach, 1 hour before or 2 hours after eating. However, it may be taken with or following food to reduce stomach irritation. The regular capsules may be opened for administration; however, the prolonged-action capsules should not be opened, chewed or crushed.

Usual Duration of Use: Continual use on a regular schedule for 2 to 4 days is usually necessary to determine this drug's effectiveness in correcting or preventing responsive rhythm disorders. Long-term use requires supervision and periodic evaluation by your physician.

▷ **This Drug Should Not Be Taken If**
  • you have had an allergic reaction to it previously.
  • you have second-degree or third-degree heart block (determined by electrocardiogram).

▷ **Inform Your Physician Before Taking This Drug If**
  • you have had any unfavorable reactions to other antiarrhythmic drugs in the past.
  • you have a history of heart disease of any kind, especially "heart block."
  • you have a history of low blood pressure.
  • you have impaired liver or kidney function.
  • you have glaucoma, or a family history of glaucoma.
  • you have an enlarged prostate gland.
  • you have myasthenia gravis.
  • you are taking any form of digitalis or any diuretic drug that can cause excessive loss of body potassium (ask physician).

Possible Side-Effects (natural, expected and unavoidable drug actions)
Drop in blood pressure in susceptible individuals.

Dry mouth (32%), constipation (11%), blurred vision (3%–9%), impaired urination (14%).

▷ **Possible Adverse Effects**   (unusual, unexpected and infrequent reactions)
If any of the following develop, consult your physician promptly.
Mild Adverse Effects
Allergic Reactions: Skin rash (1%–3%), itching.
Headache, nervousness, fatigue, muscular weakness, mild aches.
Loss of appetite, indigestion, nausea, vomiting, diarrhea.
Lowered blood sugar level (hypoglycemia).
Serious Adverse Effects
Idiosyncratic Reactions: Acute psychotic behavior (rare).
Severe drop in blood pressure, fainting.
Progressive heart weakness, predisposing to congestive heart failure.
Inability to empty urinary bladder, prostatism (see Glossary).
Sexual impotence.
Jaundice (see Glossary).
Abnormally low white blood cells (rare).

▷ **Adverse Effects That May Mimic Natural Diseases or Disorders**
Reversible jaundice may suggest viral hepatitis.

Natural Diseases or Disorders That May Be Activated by This Drug
Glaucoma, myasthenia gravis.

CAUTION
1. Thorough evaluation of your heart function (including electrocardiograms) is necessary prior to using this drug.
2. Periodic evaluation of your heart function is necessary to determine your response to this drug. Some individuals may experience worsening of their heart rhythm disorder and/or deterioration of heart function. Close monitoring of heart rate, rhythm and overall performance is essential.
3. Dosage must be adjusted carefully for each individual. Do not change your dosage without the knowledge and supervision of your physician.
4. Do not take any other antiarrhythmic drug while taking this drug unless directed to do so by your physician.

Precautions for Use
By Infants and Children: Safety and effectiveness for use by those under 12 years of age have not been established. Initial use of this drug requires hospitalization and supervision by a qualified pediatrician.
By Those over 60 Years of Age: Reduced kidney function may require reduction in dosage. This drug can aggravate existing prostatism (see Glossary) and promote constipation. Observe carefully for lightheadedness, dizziness, unsteadiness and tendency to fall.

▷ **Advisability of Use During Pregnancy**
Pregnancy Category: B (tentative). See Pregnancy Code inside back cover.
Animal studies: No birth defects reported in rats and rabbits.

Human studies: Information from adequate studies in pregnant women is not available.

Use this drug only if clearly needed.

Advisability of Use if Breast-Feeding
Presence of this drug in breast milk: Yes.
Avoid drug or refrain from nursing.

Habit-Forming Potential: None.

Effects of Overdosage: Dryness of eyes, nose, mouth and throat; impaired urination; constipation; marked drop in blood pressure; abnormal heart rhythms; congestive heart failure.

Possible Effects of Long-Term Use: None reported.

Suggested Periodic Examinations While Taking This Drug (at physician's discretion)
Electrocardiograms, complete blood cell counts, measurements of potassium blood levels.

▷ **While Taking This Drug, Observe the Following**
Foods: No restrictions. Ask physician regarding need for salt restriction and advisability of eating potassium-rich foods.
Beverages: No restrictions. May be taken with milk.
▷ *Alcohol*: Use caution until the combined effects have been determined. Alcohol can increase the blood-pressure-lowering effects and the blood-sugar-lowering effects of this drug.
Tobacco Smoking: Nicotine can cause irritability of the heart and reduce the effectiveness of this drug. Follow physician's advice regarding smoking.
▷ *Other Drugs*
Disopyramide may *increase* the effects of
• antihypertensive drugs, and cause excessive lowering of blood pressure.
• atropinelike drugs (see Drug Class, Section Four).
• warfarin (Coumadin, etc.); monitor prothrombin times, adjust dosage accordingly.
Disopyramide may *decrease* the effects of
• ambenonium (Mytelase).
• neostigmine (Prostigmin).
• pyridostigmine (Mestinon).
The beneficial effects of these three drugs in the treatment of myasthenia gravis may be reduced.
The following drugs may *decrease* the effects of disopyramide
• all diuretics that promote potassium loss.
• rifampin (Rimactane, Rifadin).
▷ *Driving, Hazardous Activities*: This drug may cause dizziness or blurred vision. Restrict activities as necessary.
Aviation Note: The use of this drug *may be a disqualification* for piloting. Consult a designated Aviation Medical Examiner.
Exposure to Sun: Use caution. This drug is reported to cause photosensitization (see Glossary) in susceptible individuals.

Exposure to Heat: Use caution. The use of this drug in hot environments may increase the risk of heat stroke.

Occurrence of Unrelated Illness: Disorders that cause vomiting, diarrhea or dehydration can affect this drug's action adversely. Report such developments promptly.

Discontinuation: This drug should not be discontinued abruptly following long-term use. Ask your physician for guidance regarding gradual dose reduction.

DISULFIRAM
(di SULF i ram)

Introduced: 1948

Prescription: USA: Yes
    Canada: Yes

Available as Generic: Yes

Brand Names: Antabuse

Class: Antialcoholism

Controlled Drug: USA: No
    Canada: No

BENEFITS versus RISKS

Possible Benefits	*Possible Risks*
EFFECTIVE ADJUNCT IN THE TREATMENT OF CHRONIC ALCOHOLISM	DANGEROUS REACTIONS WITH ALCOHOL INGESTION Acute psychotic reactions (uncommon) Drug-induced liver damage (rare) Drug-induced optic and/or peripheral neuritis (rare)

▷ **Principal Uses**

As a Single Drug Product: This drug is used for one purpose only—to deter the abusive drinking of alcoholic beverages. It does not abolish the craving or impulse to drink. It is of value in the treatment of alcoholism because of the psychological reinforcement it provides by reminding the patient of the dire consequences of ingesting alcohol.

How This Drug Works: Following the ingestion of alcohol, this drug interrupts normal liver enzyme activity after the conversion of alcohol to acetaldehyde. This causes excessive accumulation of acetaldehyde, a highly toxic substance that produces the disulfiram (Antabuse) reaction (see Glossary).

Available Dosage Forms and Strengths
    Tablets — 250 mg, 500 mg

▷ **Usual Adult Dosage Range:** In the absence of all signs of alcoholic intoxication and no less than 12 hours after the last ingestion of alcohol, treatment is started with a single dose of 500 mg/day for 1 to 2 weeks. This is followed by a maintenance dose of 250 mg/day. The range of the maintenance dose is 125 mg to 500 mg/day and is determined by experience with each patient individually. The total daily dosage should not exceed 1000 mg. **Note: Actual dosage and administration schedule must be determined by the physician for each patient individually.**

▷ **Dosing Instructions:**   May be taken with or following food to reduce stomach irritation. Tablet may be crushed for administration.

Usual Duration of Use: Continual use on a regular schedule for several months is usually necessary to determine this drug's effectiveness in deterring the drinking of alcohol. If tolerated well, use should continue until a basis for permanent self-control and sobriety is established.

▷ **This Drug Should Not Be Taken If**
- you have experienced a severe allergic reaction to disulfiram in the past. (Note: The interaction of disulfiram and alcohol is *not an allergic* reaction.)
- you have ingested any form of alcohol in any amount within the past 12 hours.
- you are pregnant.
- you are taking (or have taken recently) metronidazole (Flagyl).
- you have coronary heart disease or a serious heart rhythm disorder.

▷ **Inform Your Physician Before Taking This Drug If**
- you have used disulfiram in the past.
- you do not intend to avoid alcohol completely while taking this drug.
- you have not been given a full explanation of the reaction you will experience if you drink alcohol while taking this drug.
- you are planning pregnancy in the near future.
- you have a history of diabetes, epilepsy, kidney or liver disease.
- you are currently taking oral anticoagulants, digitalis, isoniazid, paraldehyde or phenytoin (Dilantin).
- you plan to have surgery under general anesthesia while taking this drug.

Possible Side-Effects   (natural, expected and unavoidable drug actions)
Drowsiness, lethargy during early use.
Offensive breath and body odor.

▷ **Possible Adverse Effects**   (unusual, unexpected and infrequent reactions)
If any of the following develop, consult your physician promptly.
Mild Adverse Effects
Allergic Reactions: Skin rash, hives.
Headache, dizziness, restlessness, tremor.
Metallic or garliclike taste, indigestion. (These usually subside after 2 weeks of use.)
Serious Adverse Effects
Allergic Reactions: Severe skin rashes, drug-induced hepatitis (rare).
Idiosyncratic Reactions: Acute toxic effect on brain; psychotic behavior.
Optic or peripheral neuritis (see Glossary), reduced sexual potency.

▷ **Adverse Effects That May Mimic Natural Diseases or Disorders**
Liver reaction may suggest viral hepatitis.
Brain toxicity may suggest spontaneous psychosis.

CAUTION
1. This drug should never be taken by anyone who is in a state of alcoholic intoxication.
2. The patient should be fully informed regarding the purpose and actions of this drug *before* treatment is started.
3. During long-term use of this drug, examine for any indication of reduced thyroid function.
4. Carry a card of personal identification with the notation that you are taking this drug.

Precautions for Use
By Infants and Children: Safety and effectiveness for use by those under 12 years of age have not been established.
By Those over 60 Years of Age: Observe for excessive sedation during the early use of this drug. *Do not* perform an "alcohol trial" to determine the effects of this drug.

▷ **Advisability of Use During Pregnancy**
Pregnancy Category: X (tentative). See Pregnancy Code inside back cover.
Animal studies: No defects reported in rats and hamsters.
Human studies: Two reports indicate that 4 of 8 fetuses exposed to this drug had serious birth defects. Information from adequate studies in pregnant women is not available.
Avoid this drug completely if possible.

Advisability of Use if Breast-Feeding
Presence of this drug in breast milk: Unknown.
Avoid drug or refrain from nursing.

Habit-Forming Potential: None.

Effects of Overdosage: Marked lethargy, impaired memory, altered behavior, confusion, unsteadiness, weakness, stomach pain, nausea, vomiting, diarrhea.

Possible Effects of Long-Term Use: Decreased function of thyroid gland.

Suggested Periodic Examinations While Taking This Drug   (at physician's discretion)
Visual acuity, liver function tests.

▷ **While Taking This Drug, Observe the Following**
Foods: Avoid all foods prepared with alcohol, including sauces, marinades, vinegars, desserts, etc. Inquire when dining out regarding the use of alcohol in food preparation.
Beverages: Avoid all punches, fruit drinks, etc., that may contain alcohol. This drug may be taken with milk.
▷   *Alcohol*: *Avoid completely in all forms* while taking this drug and for 14 days

following the last dose. The combination of disulfiram and alcohol—even in small amounts—produces the "disulfiram (Antabuse) reaction." This begins within 5 to 10 minutes after ingesting alcohol and consists of intense flushing and warming of the face, a severe throbbing headache, shortness of breath, chest pains, nausea, repeated vomiting, sweating and weakness. If the amount of alcohol ingested is large enough, the reaction may progress to blurred vision, vertigo, confusion, marked drop in blood pressure and loss of consciousness. Severe reactions may lead to convulsions and death. The reaction may last from 30 minutes to several hours, depending upon the amount of alcohol and disulfiram in the body. As the symptoms subside, the individual is exhausted and usually sleeps for several hours.

Tobacco Smoking: No interactions expected.

Marijuana Smoking: Possible increase in drowsiness and lethargy.

▷ *Other Drugs*

Disulfiram may *increase* the effects of

- oral anticoagulants (warfarin, etc.), and increase the risk of bleeding; dosage adjustments may be necessary.
- barbiturates, and cause oversedation (see Drug Class, Section Four).
- chlordiazepoxide (Librium) and diazepam (Valium), and cause oversedation.
- paraldehyde, and cause excessive depression of brain function.
- phenytoin (Dilantin), and cause toxic effects on the brain; dosage adjustments may be necessary.

Disulfiram may *decrease* the effects of

- perphenazine (Tilafon, etc.).

Disulfiram *taken concurrently* with

- isoniazid (INH, etc.) may cause acute mental disturbance and incoordination, making it necessary to discontinue treatment.
- metronidazole (Flagyl) may cause acute mental and behavioral disturbances, making it necessary to discontinue treatment.
- OTC cough syrups, tonics, etc., containing alcohol may cause a disulfiram (Antabuse) reaction; avoid concurrent use. (See OTC Drugs in Glossary.)

The following drugs may *increase* the effects of disulfiram

- amitriptyline (Elavil) may enhance the disulfiram + alcohol interaction; avoid concurrent use of these drugs.

▷ *Driving, Hazardous Activities*: This drug may cause drowsiness or dizziness. Restrict activities as necessary.

Aviation Note: Alcoholism *is a disqualification* for piloting. Consult a designated Aviation Medical Examiner.

Exposure to Sun: No restrictions.

Exposure to Environmental Chemicals: Thiram, a pesticide, and carbon disulfide, a pesticide and industrial solvent, can have additive toxic effects during use of this drug. Observe for toxic effects on the brain and nervous system.

Discontinuation: Treatment with this drug is only part of your total treatment program. Do not discontinue it without the knowledge and guidance of your physician. Abrupt withdrawal does not cause any symptoms. However, no alcohol should be ingested for 14 days following discontinuation.

DOXEPIN ✗
(DOX e pin)

Introduced: 1969

Prescription: USA: Yes
Canada: Yes

Available as Generic: Yes

Brand Names: Adapin, Sinequan

Class: Antidepressant

Controlled Drug: USA: No
Canada: No

BENEFITS versus RISKS	
Possible Benefits	*Possible Risks*
EFFECTIVE RELIEF OF ENDOGENOUS DEPRESSION	ADVERSE BEHAVIORAL EFFECTS: Confusion, disorientation, hallucinations, delusions
EFFECTIVE RELIEF OF ANXIETY AND NERVOUS TENSION	
Possibly beneficial in other depressive disorders	CONVERSION OF DEPRESSION TO MANIA in manic-depressive disorder
	Aggravation of schizophrenia and paranoia
	Rare blood cell disorders

▷ **Principal Uses**

As a Single Drug Product: To relieve the symptoms associated with spontaneous (endogenous) depression, and to initiate the restoration of normal mood. This drug should be used only when a diagnosis of a true, primary depression of significant degree has been established. It should not be used to treat the symptoms of mild and transient (reactive) depression that may be associated with many life situations in the absence of a bona fide affective illness.

How This Drug Works: Not completely established. It is thought that this drug relieves depression by slowly restoring to normal levels certain constituents of brain tissue (norepinephrine and serotonin) that transmit nerve impulses.

Available Dosage Forms and Strengths

Capsules — 10 mg, 25 mg, 50 mg, 75 mg, 100 mg, 150 mg
Oral concentrate — 10 mg per ml

▷ **Usual Adult Dosage Range:** Initially 25 mg 2 to 4 times daily. Dose may be increased cautiously as needed and tolerated by 10 to 25 mg daily at intervals of 1 week. Usual maintenance dose is 75 to 150 mg/24 hrs. Total dose should not exceed 300 mg/24 hrs. When the optimal requirement is determined, it may be taken at bedtime as one dose. **Note: Actual dosage and administration schedule must be determined by the physician for each patient individually.**

▷ **Dosing Instructions:** May be taken without regard to meals. Capsule may be opened for administration.

Usual Duration of Use: Some benefit may be apparent within 1 to 2 weeks, but adequate response may require continual use for 10 to 12 weeks or longer. Long-term use should not exceed 6 months without evaluation regarding the need for continuation of the drug.

▷ **This Drug Should Not Be Taken If**
- you have had an allergic reaction to it previously.
- you are taking or have taken within the past 14 days any monoamine oxidase (MAO) inhibitor drug (see Drug Class, Section Four).
- you are recovering from a recent heart attack.
- you have narrow-angle glaucoma.

▷ **Inform Your Physician Before Taking This Drug If**
- you are allergic or sensitive to any other tricyclic antidepressant (see Drug Class, Section Four).
- you have a history of any of the following: diabetes, epilepsy, glaucoma, heart diseae, prostate gland enlargement or overactive thyroid function.
- you plan to have surgery under general anesthesia in the near future.

Possible Side-Effects (natural, expected and unavoidable drug actions)
Drowsiness, blurred vision, dry mouth, constipation, impaired urination.

▷ **Possible Adverse Effects** (unusual, unexpected and infrequent reactions)
If any of the following develop, consult your physician promptly.
Mild Adverse Effects
Allergic Reactions: Skin rash, hives, swelling of face or tongue, drug fever (see Glossary).
Headache, dizziness, weakness, fainting, unsteady gait, tremors.
Peculiar taste, irritation of tongue or mouth, nausea, indigestion.
Breast enlargement, milk formation, swelling of testicles.
Fluctuation of blood sugar levels.
Serious Adverse Effects
Allergic Reactions: Hepatitis, with or without jaundice (see Glossary).
Confusion, hallucinations, agitation, restlessness, delusions.
Bone marrow depression (see Glossary)—fatigue, weakness, fever, sore throat, abnormal bleeding or bruising (reported for other drugs of this class).
Peripheral neuritis (see Glossary)—numbness, tingling, pain, loss of strength in arms and legs.

Parkinson-like disorders (see Glossary)—usually mild and infrequent; more likely to occur in the elderly.

▷ **Adverse Effects That May Mimic Natural Diseases or Disorders**
Liver toxicity may suggest viral hepatitis.

Natural Diseases or Disorders That May Be Activated by This Drug
Latent diabetes, epilepsy, glaucoma, impaired urination due to prostate gland enlargement (prostatism, see Glossary).

CAUTION
1. Dosage must be adjusted for each person individually. Report for follow-up evaluation and laboratory tests as directed by your physician.
2. It is advisable to withhold this drug if electroconvulsive therapy (ECT, "shock" treatment) is to be used to treat your depression.

Precautions for Use
By Infants and Children: Safety and effectiveness for use by those under 12 years of age have not been established.
By Those over 60 Years of Age: During the first 2 weeks of treatment, observe for the development of confusion, agitation, forgetfulness, disorientation, delusions and hallucinations. Reduction of dosage or discontinuation may be necessary. Unsteadiness may predispose to falling and injury. This drug can increase the degree of impaired urination associated with prostate gland enlargement (prostatism).

▷ **Advisability of Use During Pregnancy**
Pregnancy Category: B (tentative). See Pregnancy Code inside back cover.
Animal studies: No birth defects reported in rats, rabbits, dogs or monkeys.
Human studies: Information from adequate studies in pregnant women is not available.
Use this drug only if clearly needed. If possible, avoid use during the first 3 months and the last month. Ask physician for guidance.

Advisability of Use if Breast-Feeding
Presence of this drug in breast milk: Yes, in small amounts.
Monitor nursing infant closely and discontinue drug or nursing if adverse effects develop.

Habit-Forming Potential: None.

Effects of Overdosage: Confusion, hallucinations, marked drowsiness, heart palpitations, dilated pupils, tremors, stupor, deep sleep, coma, convulsions.

Suggested Periodic Examinations While Taking This Drug   (at physician's discretion)
Complete blood cell counts, liver function tests, serial blood pressure readings and electrocardiograms.

▷ **While Taking This Drug, Observe the Following**
Foods: No restrictions. This drug may increase the appetite and cause excessive weight gain.

Beverages: No restrictions. May be taken with milk.

▷ *Alcohol*: Avoid completely. This drug can markedly increase the intoxicating effects of alcohol and accentuate its depressant action on brain function.

Tobacco Smoking: May hasten the elimination of this drug. Higher doses may be necessary.

▷ *Other Drugs*

Doxepin may *increase* the effects of
- atropinelike drugs (see Drug Class, Section Four).
- dicumarol, and increase the risk of bleeding; dosage adjustments may be necessary.
- thyroid hormones.

Doxepin may *decrease* the effects of
- clonidine (Catapres).
- guanethidine (Ismelin).

Doxepin *taken concurrently* with
- monoamine oxidase (MAO) inhibitor drugs may cause high fever, delirium and convulsions (see Drug Class, Section Four).

▷ *Driving, Hazardous Activities*: This drug may impair mental alertness, judgment, physical coordination and reaction time. Avoid hazardous activities.

Aviation Note: The use of this drug *is a disqualification* for piloting. Consult a designated Aviation Medical Examiner.

Exposure to Sun: Use caution until sensitivity to sun has been determined. This drug may cause photosensitivity (see Glossary).

Exposure to Heat: This drug can inhibit sweating and impair the body's adaptation to hot environments, increasing the risk of heat stroke. Avoid saunas.

Exposure to Cold: The elderly should use caution and avoid conditions conducive to hypothermia (see Glossary).

Discontinuation: It is advisable to discontinue this drug gradually. Abrupt withdrawal after long-term use can cause headache, malaise and nausea.

DOXYCYCLINE ႘
(dox ee SI kleen)

Introduced: 1967   **Class:** Antibiotic, Tetracyclines

Prescription: USA: Yes   **Controlled Drug:** USA: No
Canada: Yes   Canada: No

Available as Generic: USA: Yes
Canada: No

Brand Names: Doryx, Doxychel, SK-Doxycycline, Vibramycin, Vibra-Tabs

---

BENEFITS versus RISKS

Possible Benefits	*Possible Risks*
EFFECTIVE TREATMENT OF INFECTIONS due to susceptible microorganisms	ALLERGIC REACTIONS, mild to severe
	Liver reaction with jaundice (rare)
	Fungal superinfections
	Drug-induced colitis
	Blood cell disorders

▷ **Principal Uses**

As a Single Drug Product: This member of the tetracycline drug class is used primarily to (1) treat a broad range of infections caused by susceptible bacteria and protozoa; (2) treat and prevent "traveler's diarrhea." It is often used to treat acute and chronic sinusitis and bronchitis.

How This Drug Works: This drug prevents the growth and multiplication of susceptible bacteria by interfering with their formation of essential proteins.

Available Dosage Forms and Strengths

Capsules — 50 mg, 100 mg
Injection — 100 mg per vial, 200 mg per vial
Oral suspension — 25 mg per 5 ml teaspoonful
Syrup — 50 mg per 5 ml teaspoonful
Tablets — 50 mg, 100 mg

▷ **Usual Adult Dosage Range:**   100 mg/12 hrs the first day; then 100 to 200 mg once daily or 50 to 100 mg/12 hrs. Total daily dosage should not exceed 300 mg. **Note: Actual dosage and administration schedule must be determined by the physician for each patient individually.**

▷ **Dosing Instructions:**   Preferably taken on an empty stomach, 1 hour before or 2 hours after eating. However, if stomach irritation occurs, it may be taken with food or milk. Take at same time each day, with a full glass of water. Take the full course prescribed. The tablet may be crushed and the capsule may be opened for administration.

Usual Duration of Use: The time required to control the infection and be free of fever and symptoms for 48 hours. This varies with the nature of the infection.

▷ **This Drug Should Not Be Taken If**
- you are allergic to any tetracycline drug (see Drug Class, Section Four).
- you are pregnant or breast-feeding.

▷ **Inform Your Physician Before Taking This Drug If**
- it is prescribed for a child under 8 years of age.
- you have a history of liver or kidney disease.
- you have systemic lupus erythematosus.
- you are taking any penicillin drug.

- you are taking any anticoagulant drug.
- you plan to have surgery under general anesthesia in the near future.

Possible Side-Effects   (natural, expected and unavoidable drug actions)
   Superinfections (see Glossary), often due to yeast organisms. These can occur in the mouth, intestinal tract, rectum and/or vagina, resulting in rectal and vaginal itching.

▷ **Possible Adverse Effects**   (unusual, unexpected and infrequent reactions)
   If any of the following develop, consult your physician promptly.
   Mild Adverse Effects
   Allergic Reactions: Skin rash, hives, itching of hands and feet, swelling of face or extremities.
   Loss of appetite, nausea, vomiting, diarrhea.
   Irritation of mouth or tongue, "black tongue," sore throat, abdominal cramping or pain.
   Serious Adverse Effects
   Allergic Reactions: Anaphylactic reaction (see Glossary), asthma, fever, swollen joints, abnormal bleeding or bruising, jaundice (see Glossary).
   Permanent discoloration and/or malformation of teeth when taken by children under 8 years of age, including unborn child and infant.

Natural Diseases or Disorders That May Be Activated by This Drug
   Systemic lupus erythematosus.

CAUTION
   1. Antacids and preparations containing aluminum, bismuth, iron, magnesium or zinc can prevent adequate absorption of this drug and reduce its effectiveness significantly.
   2. Troublesome and persistent diarrhea can develop in sensitive individuals. If diarrhea persists for more than 24 hours, discontinue this drug and consult your physician.

Precautions for Use
   By Infants and Children: If possible, tetracyclines should not be given to children under 8 years of age because of the risk of permanent discoloration and deformity of the teeth. Rarely, young infants may develop increased intracranial pressure within the first 4 days of receiving this drug. Tetracyclines may inhibit normal bone growth and development.
   By Those over 60 Years of Age: Natural skin changes may predispose to severe and prolonged itching reactions in the genital and anal regions.

▷ **Advisability of Use During Pregnancy**
   Pregnancy Category: D (tentative). See Pregnancy Code inside back cover.
   Animal studies: Tetracycline causes limb defects in rats, rabbits and chickens.
   Human studies: Information from studies in pregnant women indicates that drugs of this class can cause impaired development and discoloration of teeth and other developmental defects.
   It is advisable to avoid this drug completely during entire pregnancy.

Advisability of Use if Breast-Feeding
Presence of this drug in breast milk: Yes.
Avoid drug or refrain from nursing.

Habit-Forming Potential: None.

Effects of Overdosage: Nausea, vomiting, diarrhea, acute liver damage (rare).

Possible Effects of Long-Term Use: Superinfections (see Glossary), prolongation of prothrombin time.

Suggested Periodic Examinations While Taking This Drug (at physician's discretion)
Complete blood cell counts, liver and kidney function tests.
During extended use, sputum and stool examinations may detect early superinfection due to yeast organisms.

▷ **While Taking This Drug, Observe the Following**
Foods: Avoid meats and iron-fortified cereals and supplements for 2 hours before and after taking this drug.
Beverages: No restrictions. May be taken with milk.
▷ *Alcohol*: No interactions expected. However, it is best avoided if you have active liver disease.
Tobacco Smoking: No interactions expected.
▷ *Other Drugs*
Doxycycline may *increase* the effects of
- oral anticoagulants, and make it necessary to reduce their dosage.
- digoxin (Lanoxin), and cause digitalis toxicity.
- lithium (Eskalith, Lithane, etc.), and increase the risk of lithium toxicity.

Doxycycline may *decrease* the effects of
- oral contraceptives, and impair their effectiveness in preventing pregnancy.
- penicillins, and impair their effectiveness in treating infections.

The following drugs may *decrease* the effects of doxycycline
- antacids (aluminum and magnesium preparations, sodium bicarbonate, etc.) may reduce drug absorption.
- barbiturates (see Drug Class, Section Four).
- bismuth preparations (Pepto-Bismol, etc.).
- carbamazepine (Tegretol).
- cimetidine (Tagamet).
- phenytoin (Dilantin).
- iron and mineral preparations may reduce drug absorption.

▷ *Driving, Hazardous Activities*: Usually no restrictions. Be alert to the possible occurrence of nausea or diarrhea.
Aviation Note: The use of this drug *may be a disqualification* for piloting. Consult a designated Aviation Medical Examiner.
Exposure to Sun: Use caution until sensitivity has been determined. Tetracyclines can cause photosensitivity (see Glossary).

ENALAPRIL
(e NAL a pril)

Introduced: 1981

Class: Antihypertensive, ACE Inhibitor

Prescription: USA: Yes

Controlled Drug: USA: No

Available as Generic: No

Brand Names: Vasotec

BENEFITS versus RISKS

Possible Benefits	*Possible Risks*
EFFECTIVE CONTROL OF MILD TO SEVERE HIGH BLOOD PRESSURE	Headache (4.8%), dizziness (4.6%), fatigue (2.8%) Low blood pressure (2.3%) Bone marrow depression (rare) Allergic swelling of face, tongue or vocal cords (0.2%)

▷ **Principal Uses**

As a Single Drug Product: Used primarily to treat all degrees of high blood pressure. Mild to moderate high blood pressure usually responds to low doses; severe high blood pressure may require higher doses, with greater risk of serious adverse effects.

How This Drug Works: Not completely known. It is thought that by blocking certain enzyme systems that influence arterial function, this drug contributes to the relaxation of arterial walls throughout the body and thus lowers the resistance to blood flow that causes high blood pressure. This, in turn, reduces the workload of the heart and improves its performance.

Available Dosage Forms and Strengths

Tablets — 5 mg, 10 mg, 20 mg

▷ **Usual Adult Dosage Range:**   Initially 5 mg once daily for 2 weeks. Usual maintenance dose is 10 to 40 mg/day in a single dose or in 2 divided doses. Total daily dose should not exceed 40 mg if kidney function is impaired. **Note: Actual dosage and administration schedule must be determined by the physician for each patient individually.**

▷ **Dosing Instructions:**   Take on an empty stomach or with food, at same time each day. Tablet may be crushed for administration.

Usual Duration of Use: Continual use on a regular schedule for several weeks is usually necessary to determine this drug's effectiveness in controlling high blood pressure. The proper treatment of high blood pressure usually requires the long-term use of effective medications. Consult your physician before stopping this drug.

▷ **This Drug Should Not Be Taken If**
  • you have had an allergic reaction to it previously.
  • you currently have a blood cell or bone marrow disorder.
  • you have active liver disease.
  • you have an abnormally high level of blood potassium.

▷ **Inform Your Physician Before Taking This Drug If**
  • you have a history of kidney disease or impaired kidney function.
  • you have scleroderma or systemic lupus erythematosus.
  • you have any form of heart disease.
  • you have diabetes.
  • you are taking any of the following drugs: other antihypertensives, diuretics, nitrates or potassium supplements.
  • you plan to have surgery under general anesthesia in the near future.

Possible Side-Effects   (natural, expected and unavoidable drug actions)
  Dizziness, light-headedness, fainting (excessive drop in blood pressure).

▷ **Possible Adverse Effects**   (unusual, unexpected and infrequent reactions)
  If any of the following develop, consult your physician promptly.
  Mild Adverse Effects
  Allergic Reactions: Skin rash, itching.
  Headache, fatigue, drowsiness, nervousness, numbness and tingling, insomnia.
  Rapid heart rate, palpitation.
  Indigestion, stomach pain, nausea, vomiting, diarrhea.
  Excessive sweating, muscle cramps.
  Serious Adverse Effects
  Allergic Reactions: Swelling (angioedema) of face, tongue and/or vocal cords: can be life threatening.
  Bone marrow depression—fatigue, weakness, fever, sore throat, abnormal bleeding or bruising.

CAUTION
  1. Consult your physician regarding the advisability of discontinuing other antihypertensive drugs (especially diuretics) for 1 week before starting this drug.
  2. **Report promptly** any indications of infection (fever, sore throat), and any indications of water retention (weight gain, puffiness, swollen feet or ankles).
  3. Do not use a salt substitute without your physician's knowledge and approval. (Many salt substitutes contain potassium.)
  4. It is advisable to obtain blood cell counts and urine analyses **before** starting this drug.

Precautions for Use
  By Infants and Children: Safety and effectiveness for use by those in this age group have not been established.
  By Those over 60 Years of Age: Small doses are advisable until tolerance has been determined. Sudden and excessive lowering of blood pressure can

predispose to stroke or heart attack in those with impaired brain circulation or coronary artery heart disease.

▷ **Advisability of Use During Pregnancy**
   Pregnancy Category: C (tentative). See Pregnancy Code inside back cover.
   Animal studies: No birth defects found in rat or rabbit studies.
   Human studies: Information from adequate studies in pregnant women is not available.
   Avoid during first 3 months if possible.

Advisability of Use if Breast-Feeding
   Presence of this drug in breast milk: Not known.
   Monitor nursing infant closely and discontinue drug or nursing if adverse effects develop.

Habit-Forming Potential: None.

Effects of Overdosage: Excessive drop in blood pressure—light-headedness, dizziness, fainting.

Possible Effects of Long-Term Use: Gradual increase in blood potassium level.

Suggested Periodic Examinations While Taking This Drug   (at physician's discretion)
   Before starting drug: Complete blood cell counts; urine analysis with measurement of protein content; blood potassium level.
   During use of drug: Blood cell counts; measurements of blood potassium.

▷ **While Taking This Drug, Observe the Following**
   Foods: Consult physician regarding salt intake.
   Nutritional Support: **Do not take** potassium supplements unless directed by your physician.
   Beverages: No restrictions. May be taken with milk.
▷   *Alcohol*: Use caution until combined effect has been determined. Alcohol may enhance the blood-pressure-lowering effect of this drug.
   Tobacco Smoking: No interactions expected.
▷   *Other Drugs*
      Enalapril *taken concurrently* with
      • potassium preparations (K-Lyte, Slow-K, etc.) may cause increased blood levels of potassium with risk of serious heart rhythm disturbances.
      • potassium-sparing diuretics: amiloride (Moduretic), spironolactone (Aldactazide), triamterene (Dyazide) may cause increased blood levels of potassium with risk of serious heart rhythm disturbances.
▷   *Driving, Hazardous Activities*: Usually no restrictions. Be aware of possible drops in blood pressure with resultant dizziness or faintness.
   Aviation Note: The use of this drug **may be a disqualification** for piloting. Consult a designated Aviation Medical Examiner.
   Exposure to Sun: Caution advised. A similar drug of this class can cause photosensitivity.

Exposure to Heat: Caution advised. Avoid excessive perspiring with resultant loss of body water and drop in blood pressure.

Occurrence of Unrelated Illness: Report promptly any disorder that causes nausea, vomiting or diarrhea. Fluid and chemical imbalances must be corrected as soon as possible.

EPINEPHRINE
(ep i NEF rin)

Other Names: Adrenaline

Introduced: 1900

Class: Antiasthmatic, Antiglaucoma, Decongestant

Prescription: USA: Varies
Canada: No

Controlled Drug: USA: No
Canada: No

Available as Generic: USA: Yes
Canada: No

Brand Names: Adrenalin, ♣Bronkaid Mistometer, ♣Dysne-Inhal, Epifrin, Glaucon, Medihaler-Epi, Primatene Mist, Sus-Phrine, Vaponefrin

---

BENEFITS versus RISKS

Possible Benefits	*Possible Risks*
EFFECTIVE RELIEF OF SEVERE ALLERGIC (ANAPHYLACTIC) REACTIONS TEMPORARY RELIEF OF ACUTE BRONCHIAL ASTHMA Reduction of internal eye pressure (treatment of glaucoma) Relief of allergic congestion of the nose and sinuses	Significant increase in blood pressure (in sensitive individuals) Idiosyncratic Reaction: pulmonary edema (fluid formation in lungs) Heart rhythm disorders (in sensitive individuals)

▷ **Principal Uses**

As a Single Drug Product: This drug is used most commonly by inhalation to relieve acute attacks of bronchial asthma. It is used less frequently as a decongestant for symptomatic relief of allergic nasal congestion and as eye drops in the management of glaucoma.

How This Drug Works: By stimulating certain sympathetic nerve terminals, this drug acts to

- contract blood vessel walls and raise the blood pressure.
- inhibit the release of harmful amounts of histamine into the skin and internal organs.
- dilate those bronchial tubes that are in sustained constriction, thereby increasing the size of the airways and improving the ability to breathe.

- decrease the formation of fluid within the eye, increase its outflow from the eye and thereby reduce internal eye pressure.
- decrease the volume of blood in nasal tissue, thereby shrinking the tissue mass (decongestion) and expanding the nasal airway.

Available Dosage Forms and Strengths

Aerosol — 0.3 mg per spray
Eye drops — 0.1%, 0.25%, 0.5%, 1%, 2%
Nose drops — 0.1%
Solution for nebulizer — 1%, 1.25%, 2.25%
Solution for injection — 0.01 mg per ml, 0.1 mg per ml, 1 mg per ml

▷ **Usual Adult Dosage Range:** Aerosols: 1 inhalation, repeated in 1 to 2 minutes if needed; wait 4 hours before next inhalation. Eye drops: 1 drop/12 hrs. Dosage may vary with product; follow printed instructions and label directions. **Note: Actual dosage and administration schedule must be determined by the physician for each patient individually.**

▷ **Dosing Instructions:** Aerosols and inhalation solutions: After first inhalation, wait 1 to 2 minutes to determine if a second inhalation is necessary. If relief does not occur within 20 minutes of use, and difficult breathing persists, discontinue this drug and seek medical attention promptly. Avoid prolonged and excessive use. Eye drops: During instillation of drops and for 2 minutes following, press finger against the tear sac (inner corner of eye) to prevent rapid absorption of drug into body circulation.

Usual Duration of Use: According to individual needs. Long-term use requires supervision and periodic evaluation by your physician.

▷ **This Drug Should Not Be Taken If**
- you have had an allergic reaction to any dosage form of it previously.
- you have narrow-angle glaucoma.
- you have experienced a recent stroke or heart attack.

▷ **Inform Your Physician Before Taking This Drug If**
- you have any degree of high blood pressure.
- you have any form of heart disease, especially coronary heart disease (with or without angina), or a heart rhythm disorder.
- you have diabetes or overactive thyroid function (hyperthyroidism).
- you have a history of stroke.
- you are taking any of the following drugs: monoamine oxidase (MAO) inhibitors, phenothiazines (see Drug Classes, Section Four), digitalis preparations or quinidine.

Possible Side-Effects (natural, expected and unavoidable drug actions)
In sensitive individuals—restlessness, anxiety, headache, tremor, palpitation, coldness of hands and feet, dryness of mouth and throat (with use of aerosol).

▷ **Possible Adverse Effects** (unusual, unexpected and infrequent reactions)
If any of the following develop, consult your physician promptly.

Mild Adverse Effects

Allergic Reactions: Skin rash; eye drops may cause redness, swelling and itching of the eyelids.

Weakness, dizziness, pallor.

Serious Adverse Effects

Idiosyncratic Reactions: Sudden development of excessive fluid in the lungs (pulmonary edema).

In predisposed individuals—excessive rise in blood pressure with risk of stroke (cerebral hemorrhage).

CAUTION

1. The frequently repeated use of this drug at short intervals can produce a condition of unresponsiveness and result in medication failure. If this develops, avoid use completely for 12 hours, at which time a normal response should return.

2. Excessive use of aerosol preparations in the treatment of asthma has been associated with sudden death.

3. This drug can cause significant irritability of the nerve pathways (conduction system) and muscles of the heart, predisposing to serious heart rhythm disorders. If you have any form of heart disorder, consult your physician.

4. This drug can increase the blood sugar level. If you have diabetes, test for urine sugar frequently to detect significant changes.

5. If you become unresponsive to this drug and you intend to substitute isoproterenol (Isuprel), allow an interval of 4 hours between using these two drugs.

6. Promptly discard all preparations of this drug at the first appearance of discoloration (pink to red to brown) or cloudiness (precipitation). Such changes indicate drug deterioration.

Precautions for Use

By Infants and Children: Use cautiously in small doses until tolerance is determined. Observe for any indications of weakness, light-headedness or inclination to faint.

By Those over 60 Years of Age: Use cautiously in small doses until tolerance is determined. Observe for excessive stimulation: nervousness, headache, tremor, rapid heart rate. If you have hardening of the arteries (arteriosclerosis), heart disease, high blood pressure, Parkinson's disease or prostatism (see Glossary), this drug may aggravate your disorder. Ask your physician for guidance.

▷ **Advisability of Use During Pregnancy**

Pregnancy Category: C (tentative). See Pregnancy Code inside back cover.

Animal studies: Birth defects reported in rats.

Human studies: Information from adequate studies in pregnant women is not available.

This drug can cause significant reduction of oxygen supply to the fetus. Use it only if clearly needed and in small, infrequent doses. Avoid during the first 3 months and during labor and delivery.

Advisability of Use if Breast-Feeding
> Presence of this drug in breast milk: Yes.
> Avoid drug or refrain from nursing.

Habit-Forming Potential: Tolerance to this drug can develop with frequent use (see Glossary), but dependence does not occur.

Effects of Overdosage: Nervousness, throbbing headache, dizziness, tremor, palpitation, disturbance of heart rhythm, difficult breathing, abdominal pain, vomiting of blood.

Possible Effects of Long-Term Use: "Epinephrine-fastness": loss of ability to respond to this drug's bronchodilator effect. With long-term treatment of glaucoma: pigment deposits on eyeball and eyelids, possible damage to retina, impaired vision, blockage of tear ducts.

Suggested Periodic Examinations While Taking This Drug (at physician's discretion)
> Blood pressure measurements; blood or urine sugar measurements in presence of diabetes; vision testing and measurement of internal eye pressure in presence of glaucoma.

▷ **While Taking This Drug, Observe the Following**
> *Foods*: No restrictions, except those that have been shown to cause you to have asthma.
> *Beverages*: No restrictions.
▷ *Alcohol*: Alcoholic beverages can increase the urinary excretion of this drug.
> *Tobacco Smoking*: No interactions expected. Follow physician's advice regarding smoking as it affects the condition under treatment.
▷ *Other Drugs*
> Epinephrine *taken concurrently* with
> - certain beta-blocker drugs (nadolol, propranolol) may cause increased blood pressure and decreased heart rate.
> - chlorpromazine (Thorazine) may cause decreased blood pressure and increased heart rate.
> - furazolidone (Furoxone) may cause increased blood pressure and high fever.
> - guanethidine (Esimil, Ismelin) may cause increased blood pressure.
> - tricyclic antidepressants (amitriptyline, etc.) may cause increased blood pressure and heart rhythm disturbances.
▷ *Driving, Hazardous Activities*: This drug may cause dizziness or excessive nervousness. Restrict activities as necessary.
> *Aviation Note*: The use of this drug *may be a disqualification* for piloting. Consult a designated Aviation Medical Examiner.
> *Exposure to Sun*: No restrictions.
> *Heavy Exercise or Exertion*: No interactions expected. However, exercise can induce asthma in sensitive individuals.
> *Occurrence of Unrelated Illness:* Use caution in presence of severe burns. This drug can increase drainage from burned tissue and cause significant loss of tissue fluids and blood proteins.

Discontinuation: If this drug fails to provide relief after an adequate trial, discontinue it and consult your physician. It is dangerous to increase the dosage or frequency of use.

Special Storage Instructions: Protect drug from exposure to air, light and heat. Keep in a cool place, preferably in the refrigerator.

ERGOLOID MESYLATES
(ER goh loyd MESS i lates)

Other Names: Dihydrogenated Ergot Alkaloids

Introduced: 1949   **Class:** Ergot Preparations

Prescription: USA: Yes   **Controlled Drug:** USA: No
Canada: Yes   Canada: No

Available as Generic: USA: Yes
Canada: No

Brand Names: Circanol, Deapril-ST, Hydergine, Hydergine LC

BENEFITS versus RISKS

Possible Benefits	*Possible Risks*
Limited relief of symptoms associated with deteriorating brain function (in some individuals)	Low blood pressure, fainting Slow heart rate Worsening of symptoms (instead of relief)

▷ **Principal Uses**

As a Single Drug Product: The use of this drug is limited to the treatment of the aging individual with symptoms indicative of deteriorating brain function. Its benefit is unpredictable, and its use must be monitored carefully and adjusted appropriately for each individual.

How This Drug Works: Not completely established. Present theory is that by stimulating brain cell metabolism, this drug increases the brain's ability to utilize oxygen and nutrients. The resulting improvement in brain function is thought to contribute to the benefit seen in responsive individuals.

Available Dosage Forms and Strengths

       Capsules, liquid — 1 mg
             Liquid — 1 mg per ml
          Tablets — 0.5 mg, 1 mg
    Tablets, sublingual — 0.5 mg, 1 mg

▷ **Usual Adult Dosage Range:** 1 to 2 mg, 3 times/day. **Note: Actual dosage and administration schedule must be determined by the physician for each patient individually.**

▷ **Dosing Instructions:**   May be taken on an empty stomach or with food to reduce stomach irritation. The regular tablet may be crushed for administration. The sublingual tablet should be dissolved under the tongue and not swallowed. The liquid capsule should be taken whole (unopened).

Usual Duration of Use: Continual use on a regular schedule for 3 to 4 weeks is usually necessary to determine this drug's effectiveness in relieving the symptoms of mental deterioration. Long-term use requires supervision and periodic evaluation by your physician.

▷ **This Drug Should Not Be Taken If**
  • you have had an allergic reaction to any dosage form of it previously.
  • your pulse rate is below 60 beats/minute or your systolic blood pressure is consistently below 100.
  • you have an active psychosis.

▷ **Inform Your Physician Before Taking This Drug If**
  • you have a history of low blood pressure.
  • you are taking any of the following: antihypertensive drugs, a beta-blocker drug or any form of digitalis.

Possible Side-Effects   (natural, expected and unavoidable drug actions)
  Orthostatic hypotension (see Glossary).

▷ **Possible Adverse Effects**   (unusual, unexpected and infrequent reactions)
  If any of the following develop, consult your physician promptly.
  Mild Adverse Effects
  Allergic Reactions: Skin rash, drug fever (see Glossary).
  Headache, dizziness, flushing, blurred vision.
  Nasal stuffiness, reduced appetite, nausea, vomiting, stomach cramping.
  Serious Adverse Effects
  Marked drop in blood pressure, falling, fainting.
  Marked slowing of the heart rate (40 to 50 beats/minute).
  Reduced activity, sluggishness, drowsiness, emotional withdrawal, apathy.

Natural Diseases or Disorders That May Be Activated by This Drug
  Ergot alkaloids can precipitate attacks of acute intermittent porphyria in susceptible individuals.

CAUTION
  While numerous studies have demonstrated that this drug can be beneficial in relieving many complaints of the elderly related to memory, intellectual performance and social adjustment, others have not confirmed this. It is important to remember that the causes of such symptoms are poorly understood, that they can occur whether or not drugs are being taken and that behavioral changes in the elderly are often frequent and unpredictable. It is therefore advisable to monitor the response to this drug very closely and to notify the physician if any significant adverse personality changes occur. In some instances, the development of ner-

vousness, hostility, confusion and depression may be related to the use of this drug.

Precautions for Use

By Those over 60 Years of Age: It is not possible to predict in advance the nature of your response to this drug. It may relieve your symptoms, have no significant effect or make your symptoms worse. Dosage must be carefully individualized.

Habit-Forming Potential: None.

Effects of Overdosage: Headache, flushing, nasal stuffiness, weakness, nausea, vomiting, collapse, coma.

Possible Effects of Long-Term Use: None reported.

Suggested Periodic Examinations While Taking This Drug (at physician's discretion)
Pulse counts and blood pressure measurements on a regular basis.

▷ **While Taking This Drug, Observe the Following**
Foods: No restrictions.
Beverages: No restrictions.
▷   *Alcohol*: Use with caution until the combined effects have been determined. Sensitive individuals may experience an excessive drop in blood pressure.
Tobacco Smoking: No interactions expected.
▷   *Other Drugs*
Ergoloid mesylates may *increase* the effects of
• antihypertensive drugs, and cause excessive lowering of blood pressure.
Ergoloid mesylates *taken concurrently* with
• beta-blocker drugs (see Drug Class, Section Four) may cause excessive slowing of heart rate and/or excessive lowering of blood pressure.
• digitalis preparations (Lanoxin, etc.) may cause excessive slowing of heart rate.
▷   *Driving, Hazardous Activities*: This drug may cause dizziness or blurred vision. Restrict activities as necessary.
Aviation Note: Brain function disorder *is a disqualification* for piloting. Consult a designated Aviation Medical Examiner.
Exposure to Sun: No restrictions.
Exposure to Cold: Use caution. Avoid exposure that could lower body temperature, impair metabolism and induce hypothermia (see Glossary).

ERGOTAMINE
(er GOT a meen)

Introduced: 1926

Class: Antimigraine, Ergot Preparations

Prescription: USA: Yes
Canada: Yes

Controlled Drug: USA: No
Canada: No

Available as Generic: No

Brand Names: Bellergal [CD], Bellergal-S [CD], Cafergot [CD], Cafergot P-B [CD], ♣Ergodryl [CD], Ergomar, Ergostat, ♣Gynergen, Medihaler Ergotamine, Wigraine [CD],

BENEFITS versus RISKS	
Possible Benefits	*Possible Risks*
PREVENTION AND RELIEF OF VASCULAR HEADACHES: MIGRAINE, MIGRAINELIKE AND HISTAMINE HEADACHES	GANGRENE OF THE FINGERS, TOES OR INTESTINE AGGRAVATION OF CORONARY ARTERY DISEASE (ANGINA) ABORTION

▷ **Principal Uses**

As a Single Drug Product: This drug is used primarily in the treatment of vascular headaches, especially migraine and "cluster" headaches. It should not be used on a continual basis to prevent migraine attacks, but it is often effective in terminating the headache if taken within the first hour following the onset of pain. It may be used on a short-term basis in an attempt to prevent or abort "cluster" headaches during the period of their occurrence. The inhalation form provides rapid onset of action.

As a Combination Drug Product [CD]: This drug is combined with caffeine to take advantage of caffeine's ability to enhance its absorption. This permits a smaller dose of ergotamine to be effective and reduces the risk of adverse effects with repeated use. This drug is also combined with belladonna (atropine) and one of the barbiturates to provide preparations that are useful in relieving the symptoms of premenstrual tension and the menopausal syndrome: nervousness, nausea, hot flushes and sweating.

How This Drug Works: Not completely established. It is thought that by constricting the walls of blood vessels in the head, this drug prevents or relieves the excessive expansion (dilation) that is responsible for the pain of migrainelike headaches.

Available Dosage Forms and Strengths

Aerosol inhaler — 9 mg per ml (0.36 mg/inhalation)
Suppositories — 2 mg (in combination with caffeine)
Tablets — 1 mg
Tablets, sublingual — 2 mg

▷ **Usual Adult Dosage Range:**   Inhalation: 1 spray (0.36 mg) at the onset of headache; repeat 1 spray every 5 to 10 minutes as needed for relief, up to a
maximum of 6 sprays/24 hrs. Do not exceed 15 sprays/week. Sublingual
tablets: Dissolve 1 mg under tongue at the onset of headache; repeat 1
mg every 30 to 60 minutes as needed, up to a maximum of 5 mg/attack.
Do not exceed 5 mg/24 hrs or 10 mg/week. Try to determine the optimal
dose required (up to 5 mg) that will abort the headache when taken as a
single dose at the onset of pain. **Note: Actual dosage and administration
schedule must be determined by the physician for each patient individually.**

▷ **Dosing Instructions:**   Follow written instructions carefully. Do not exceed prescribed doses. The regular tablets (combination drug) may be crushed
for administration; the sustained-release tablets should be taken whole
(not crushed). Sublingual tablets should be dissolved under the tongue,
not swallowed.

Usual Duration of Use: Continual use on a regular schedule for several episodes of headache is usually necessary to determine this drug's effectiveness in aborting or relieving the pain of vascular headache. Do not
exceed recommended dosage schedules. If headaches are not controlled
after several trials of maximal doses, consult your physician for alternative treatment.

▷ **This Drug Should Not Be Taken If**
  • you have had an allergic reaction to any dosage form of it previously.
  • you are pregnant.
  • you have a severe infection.
  • you have any of the following conditions:
  angina pectoris (coronary artery disease)
  Buerger's disease
  hardening of the arteries (arteriosclerosis)
  high blood pressure (severe hypertension)
  kidney disease or impaired kidney function
  liver disease or impaired liver function
  Raynaud's phenomenon
  thrombophlebitis
  severe itching

▷ **Inform Your Physician Before Taking This Drug If**
  • you are allergic or overly sensitive to *any* ergot preparation.

Possible Side-Effects   (natural, expected and unavoidable drug actions)
  Usually infrequent and mild with recommended doses.
  Susceptible individuals may notice a sensation of cold hands and feet, with
  mild numbness and tingling.

▷ **Possible Adverse Effects**   (unusual, unexpected and infrequent reactions)
  If any of the following develop, consult your physician promptly.
  Mild Adverse Effects
  Allergic Reactions: Localized swellings (angioedema), itching.

Headache, drowsiness, dizziness, confusion.

Chest pain, numbness and tingling of fingers and toes, muscle pains in arms or legs.

Nausea, vomiting, diarrhea.

Serious Adverse Effects

Gangrene of the extremities—coldness; numbness; pain; dark discoloration; eventual loss of fingers, toes or feet.

Gangrene of the intestine—severe abdominal pain and swelling; emergency surgery required.

Natural Diseases or Disorders That May Be Activated by This Drug

Angina pectoris (coronary artery insufficiency), Buerger's disease, Raynaud's syndrome.

CAUTION

1. The excessive use of this drug can actually provoke migraine headache and increase the frequency of its occurrence.
2. Do not exceed a total dose of 5 mg/24 hrs or 10 mg/week.
3. Individual sensitivity to the effects of this drug vary greatly. Some may experience early toxic effects even while taking recommended doses. Report promptly any indications of impaired circulation: numbness in fingers or toes, muscle cramping, chest pain.

Precautions for Use

By Infants and Children: Safety and effectiveness for use by those under 12 years of age have not been established.

By Those over 60 Years of Age: Natural changes in blood vessels and circulation may make you more susceptible to the serious adverse effects of this drug. See the preceding list of disorders that are contraindications for the use of this drug.

▷ **Advisability of Use During Pregnancy**

Pregnancy Category: X. See Pregnancy Code inside back cover.

Animal studies: No information available.

Human studies: Information from studies in pregnant women indicates that this drug can cause abortion.

This drug should be avoided during the entire pregnancy.

Advisability of Use if Breast-Feeding

Presence of this drug in breast milk: Yes.

Avoid drug or refrain from nursing.

Habit-Forming Potential: None.

Effects of Overdosage: Manifestations of "ergotism": coldness of skin, severe muscle pains, tingling and burning pain in hands and feet, loss of blood supply to extremities resulting in tissue death (gangrene) in fingers and toes. Acute ergot poisoning: nausea, vomiting, diarrhea, cold skin, numbness of extremities, confusion, seizures, coma.

Possible Effects of Long-Term Use: A form of functional dependence (see Glossary) may develop, resulting in withdrawal headaches when the drug is discontinued.

Suggested Periodic Examinations While Taking This Drug (at physician's discretion)
Evaluation of circulation (blood flow) to the extremities.

▷ **While Taking This Drug, Observe the Following**
Foods: No interactions expected. Avoid all foods to which you are allergic; some migraine headaches are due to food allergies.
Beverages: No restrictions.
▷ *Alcohol*: Best avoided; alcohol can intensify vascular headache.
Tobacco Smoking: Best avoided; nicotine can further reduce the restricted blood flow produced by this drug.
Marijuana Smoking: Best avoided; additive effects can increase the coldness of hands and feet.
▷ *Other Drugs*
Ergotamine may *decrease* the effects of
• nitroglycerin, and reduce its effectiveness in preventing or relieving angina pain.
The following drugs may *increase* the effects of ergotamine
• erythromycin (E-Mycin, Eryc, etc.).
• troleandomycin (TAO).
▷ *Driving, Hazardous Activities*: This drug may cause drowsiness or dizziness. Restrict activities as necessary.
Aviation Note: Vascular headache *is a disqualification* for piloting. Consult a designated Aviation Medical Examiner.
Exposure to Sun: No restrictions.
Exposure to Cold: Avoid as much as possible. Cold environments and handling cold objects will further reduce the restricted blood flow to the extremities.
Discontinuation: Following long-term use, it may be necessary to withdraw this drug gradually to prevent withdrawal headache. Ask physician for guidance.

ERYTHROMYCIN
(er ith roh MY sin)

Introduced: 1952	**Class:** Antibiotic, Erythromycins
Prescription: USA: Yes	**Controlled Drug:** USA: No
Canada: Yes	Canada: No

Available as Generic: Yes

Brand Names: ❦Apo-Erythro-S, Bristamycin, E.E.S., E-Mycin, E-Mycin E, Eryc, Erypar, Eryped, Ery-Tab, Erythrocin, ❦Erythromid, Erythril,

Ilosone, Ilotycin, ✤Novorythro, Pediamycin, Pfizer-E, Robimycin, RP-Mycin, SK-Erythromycin, Wyamycin E, Wyamycin S

BENEFITS versus RISKS	
Possible Benefits	*Possible Risks*
EFFECTIVE TREATMENT OF INFECTIONS DUE TO SUSCEPTIBLE MICROORGANISMS	Allergic reactions, mild and infrequent
	Liver reaction (most common with erythromycin estolate)
	Drug-induced colitis (rare)
	Superinfections (rare)

▷ **Principal Uses**

As a Single Drug Product: This well-tolerated and versatile antibiotic is used to treat a broad variety of common infections. The more important among these are (1) skin and skin structure infections; (2) upper and lower respiratory tract infections, including "strep" throat, diphtheria and several types of pneumonia; (3) gonorrhea and syphilis; and (4) amebic dysentery. It is also used for the long-term prevention of recurrences of rheumatic fever. Effective use requires the precise identification of the causative organism and determination of its sensitivity to erythromycin.

How This Drug Works: This drug prevents the growth and multiplication of susceptible organisms by interfering with their formation of essential proteins.

Available Dosage Forms and Strengths

Capsules —	125 mg, 250 mg
Capsules, enteric coated —	250 mg
Capsules, prolonged action —	250 mg
Drops —	100 mg per ml
Ointment, eye —	5 mg per gram
Ointment, skin —	2%
Solution, skin —	1.5%, 2%
Suspension, oral —	100 mg per 2.5 ml, 100 mg per ml, 125 mg per 5 ml, 200 mg per 5 ml, 250 mg per 5 ml, 400 mg per 5 ml
Tablets —	250 mg, 500 mg
Tablets, chewable —	125 mg, 200 mg, 250 mg
Tablets, enteric coated —	250 mg, 333 mg, 500 mg
Tablets, film coated —	250 mg, 400 mg, 500 mg

▷ **Usual Adult Dosage Range:** 250 to 1000 mg/6 hrs, according to nature and severity of infection. Total daily dosage should not exceed 8 grams. **Note: Actual dosage and administration schedule must be determined by the physician for each patient individually.**

▷ **Dosing Instructions:** Nonenteric-coated preparations should be taken 1 hour before or 2 hours after eating. Enteric-coated preparations may be taken without regard to food. Regular uncoated capsules may be opened and tablets may be crushed for administration; coated and prolonged-action preparations should be swallowed whole. Ask pharmacist for guidance.

Usual Duration of Use: Continual use on a regular schedule for 3 to 5 days is usually necessary to determine this drug's effectiveness in controlling responsive infections. For streptococcal infections: not less than 10 consecutive days (without interruption) to reduce the possibility of developing rheumatic fever or glomerulonephritis. The duration of use should not exceed the time required to eliminate the infection.

▷ **This Drug Should Not Be Taken If**
- you have had an allergic reaction to any form of erythromycin previously.
- you have active liver disease.

▷ **Inform Your Physician Before Taking This Drug If**
- you have a history of a previous "reaction" to erythromycin.
- you are allergic by nature: hay fever, asthma, hives, eczema.
- you have taken the estolate form of erythromycin previously.

Possible Side-Effects   (natural, expected and unavoidable drug actions)
Superinfections (see Glossary).

▷ **Possible Adverse Effects**   (unusual, unexpected and infrequent reactions)
If any of the following develop, consult your physician promptly.
Mild Adverse Effects
Allergic Reactions: Skin rash, hives, itching.
Nausea, vomiting, diarrhea, abdominal cramping.
Serious Adverse Effects
Allergic Reactions: Rare anaphylactic reaction (see Glossary).
Idiosyncratic Reactions: Liver reaction—nausea, vomiting, fever, jaundice (usually but not exclusively associated with erythromycin estolate).
Drug-induced colitis, transient loss of hearing.

▷ **Adverse Effects That May Mimic Natural Diseases or Disorders**
Liver toxicity may resemble acute gallbladder disease or viral hepatitis.

CAUTION
1. Take the full dosage prescribed to prevent the possible emergence of resistant bacterial strains.
2. If you have a history of liver disease or impaired liver function, avoid any form of erythromycin estolate.
3. If diarrhea develops and continues for more than 24 hours, consult your physician promptly.

Precautions for Use
By Infants and Children: Observe allergic children closely for indications of developing allergy to this drug. Observe also for evidence of gastrointestinal irritation.
By Those over 60 Years of Age: Observe for indications of itching reactions in

the genital and anal regions, often due to yeast superinfections. Observe also for evidence of hearing loss. Report such developments promptly.

▷ **Advisability of Use During Pregnancy**
Pregnancy Category: B (tentative). See Pregnancy Code inside back cover.
Animal studies: Studies in rats are inconclusive.
Human studies: No increase in birth defects reported in 230 exposures. Information from adequate studies in pregnant women is not available.
Generally thought to be safe during entire pregnancy, *except for erythromycin estolate*; this form of erythromycin can cause toxic liver reactions during pregnancy and should be avoided.

Advisability of Use if Breast-Feeding
Presence of this drug in breast milk: Yes.
Monitor nursing infant closely and discontinue drug or nursing if adverse effects develop.

Habit-Forming Potential: None.

Effects of Overdosage: Possible nausea, vomiting, diarrhea and abdominal discomfort.

Possible Effects of Long-Term Use: Superinfections (see Glossary).

Suggested Periodic Examinations While Taking This Drug (at physician's discretion)
Liver function tests if the estolate form is used.

▷ **While Taking This Drug, Observe the Following**
Foods: No restrictions.
Beverages: Avoid fruit juices and carbonated beverages for 1 hour after taking any nonenteric-coated preparation. May be taken with milk.
▷ *Alcohol*: Avoid if you have impaired liver function or are taking the estolate form of this drug.
Tobacco Smoking: No interactions expected.
▷ *Other Drugs*
Erythromycin may *increase* the effects of
- carbamazepine (Tegretol), and cause toxicity.
- digoxin (Lanoxin), and cause toxicity.
- ergotamine (Cafergot, Ergostat, etc.), and cause impaired circulation to extremities.
- methylprednisolone (Medrol), and cause excess steroid effects.
- theophylline (aminophylline, Theo-Dur, etc.), and cause toxicity.
- warfarin (Coumadin), and increase the risk of bleeding.
Erythromycin may *decrease* the effects of
- clindamycin.
- lincomycin.
- penicillins.
▷ *Driving, Hazardous Activities*: This drug may cause nausea and/or diarrhea. Restrict activities as necessary.
Aviation Note: The use of this drug *may be a disqualification* for piloting. Consult a designated Aviation Medical Examiner.

Exposure to Sun: No restrictions.

Special Storage Instructions: Keep liquid forms refrigerated.

Observe the Following Expiration Times: Freshly mixed oral suspension—14 days. Premixed oral suspension—18 months. Ask pharmacist for guidance.

ESTROGENS
(ES troh jenz)

Other Names: chlorotrianisene, conjugated estrogens, esterified estrogens, estradiol, estriol, estrone, estropipate, quinestrol

Introduced: 1933

Class: Female Sex Hormones

Prescription: USA: Yes
Canada: Yes

Controlled Drug: USA: No
Canada: No

Available as Generic: USA: Yes
Canada: No

Brand Names: ♣C.E.S., ♣Climestrone, ♣Delestrogen, ♣Estinyl, Estrace, Estraderm-50, Estraderm-100, Estratab, ♣Estromed, Estrovis, ♣Femogen, ♣Femogex, Menest, Menrium [CD], Milprem [CD], ♣Oestrilin, Ogen, PMB [CD], Premarin, TACE, Theogen

---

BENEFITS versus RISKS

Possible Benefits	*Possible Risks*
EFFECTIVE RELIEF OF MENOPAUSAL HOT FLUSHES AND NIGHT SWEATS	INCREASED RISK OF CANCER OF THE UTERUS with 3+ years of continual use
PREVENTION OR RELIEF OF ATROPHIC VAGINITIS, ATROPHY OF THE VULVA AND URETHRA	Increased frequency of gallstones
	Accelerated growth of preexisting fibroid tumors of the uterus
PREVENTION OF OSTEOPOROSIS	Fluid retention
Prevention of thinning of the skin	Postmenopausal bleeding
Mental tonic effect	Deep vein thrombophlebitis and thromboembolism (less likely with conjugated estrogens, more likely with synthetic unconjugated hormones)
	Increased blood pressure (rare)
	Decreased sugar tolerance (rare)

▷ **Principal Uses**

As a Single Drug Product: This widely used hormone is very effective when administered in proper dosage and carefully supervised. Its primary use is supplemental ("replacement" therapy) when used to treat the following conditions: (1) ovarian failure or removal in the young woman; (2) the menopausal syndrome; (3) postmenopausal atrophy of genital tissues; and (4) postmenopausal osteoporosis. It is also used in selected cases of breast cancer and prostate cancer.

As a Combination Drug Product [CD]: Estrogen is available in combination with chlordiazepoxide (Librium) and with meprobamate (Equanil, Miltown). These mild tranquilizers are added to provide a calming effect that makes the combination more effective in treating selected cases of the menopausal syndrome. See the Drug Profile of the Oral Contraceptives for a discussion of the combination of estrogens and progestins.

How This Drug Works: When used to correct hormonal deficiency states, estrogens restore normal cellular activity by increasing the synthesis of chromatin, RNA and cellular proteins. The frequency and intensity of menopausal symptoms are significantly reduced when normal tissue levels of estrogen are restored.

Available Dosage Forms and Strengths
> Capsules — 12 mg, 25 mg, 72 mg (TACE)
> Cream, vaginal — 0.1 mg per gram, 0.625 mg per gram, 1.5 mg per gram
> Tablets — 0.1 mg, 0.3 mg, 0.625 mg, 0.75 mg, 0.9 mg, 1 mg, 1.25 mg, 1.5 mg, 2 mg, 2.5 mg, 3 mg, 6 mg
> Transdermal patch — 0.05 mg, 0.1 mg

▷ **Usual Adult Dosage Range:** For conjugated and esterified estrogens: 0.3 to 1.25 mg daily for 21 days. Omit for 7 days. Repeat cyclically as needed. For other forms of estrogen: consult your physician. **Note: Actual dosage and administration schedule must be determined by the physician for each patient individually.**

▷ **Dosing Instructions:** May be taken without regard to food. The tablets may be crushed for administration. The capsules should be taken whole.

Usual Duration of Use: Continual use on a regular schedule for 10 to 20 days is usually necessary to determine this drug's effectiveness in relieving menopausal symptoms. Long-term use requires supervision and periodic evaluation by your physician every 6 months.

▷ **This Drug Should Not Be Taken If**
- you have had a significant allergic reaction to any dosage form of it previously.
- you have a history of thrombophlebitis, embolism, heart attack or stroke.
- you have seriously impaired liver function.
- you have abnormal and unexplained vaginal bleeding.
- you have sickle cell disease.
- you are pregnant.

▷ **Inform Your Physician Before Taking This Drug If**
- you have had an unfavorable reaction to estrogen therapy previously.
- you have a history of cancer of the breast or reproductive organs.
- you have any of the following conditions: fibrocystic breast changes, fibroid tumors of the uterus, endometriosis, migrainelike headaches, epilepsy, asthma, heart disease, high blood pressure, gallbladder disease, diabetes or porphyria.
- you smoke tobacco on a regular basis.
- you plan to have surgery in the near future.

Possible Side-Effects   (natural, expected and unavoidable drug actions)
> Fluid retention, weight gain, "breakthrough" bleeding (spotting in middle of menstrual cycle), altered menstrual pattern, resumption of menstrual flow (bleeding from the uterus) after a period of natural cessation (postmenopausal bleeding), increased susceptibility to yeast infection of the genital tissues.

▷ **Possible Adverse Effects**   (unusual, unexpected and infrequent reactions)
If any of the following develop, consult your physician promptly.
Mild Adverse Effects
> Allergic Reactions: Skin rash, hives, itching.
> Headache, nervous tension, irritability, accentuation of migraine headaches.
> Nausea, vomiting, bloating, diarrhea.
> Breast enlargement, tenderness, milk production.
> Tannish pigmentation of the face.

Serious Adverse Effects
> Idiosyncratic Reactions: Cutaneous porphyria—fragility and scarring of the skin.
> Emotional depression, rise in blood pressure (in susceptible individuals).
> Gallbladder disease, benign liver tumors, jaundice, rise in blood sugar.
> Erosion of uterine cervix, enlargement of uterine fibroid tumors.
> Thrombophlebitis (inflammation of a vein with formation of blood clot)—pain or tenderness in thigh or leg, with or without swelling of foot or leg.
> Pulmonary embolism (movement of blood clot to lung)—sudden shortness of breath, pain in chest, coughing, bloody sputum.
> Stroke (blood clot in brain)—headaches, blackout, sudden weakness or paralysis of any part of the body, severe dizziness, altered vision, slurred speech, inability to speak.
> Retinal thrombosis (blood clot in eye vessels)—sudden impairment or loss of vision.
> Heart attack (blood clot in coronary artery)—sudden pain in chest, neck, jaw or arm; weakness; sweating; nausea.

Possible Delayed Adverse Effects
> Estrogens taken during pregnancy can predispose the female child to the later development of cancer of the vagina or cervix following puberty.

▷ **Adverse Effects That May Mimic Natural Diseases or Disorders**
> Liver reactions may suggest viral hepatitis.

Natural Diseases or Disorders That May Be Activated by This Drug
Latent hypertension, diabetes mellitus, acute intermittent porphyria.

CAUTION
1. To avoid prolonged (uninterrupted) stimulation of breast and uterine tissues, estrogen should be taken in cycles of 3 weeks on and 1 week off of medication.
2. The estrogen in estrogen vaginal creams is absorbed systemically by the woman. It may also be absorbed through the penis during sexual intercourse and can cause enlargement and tenderness of male breast tissue.

Precautions for Use
By Those over 60 Years of Age: This drug has very limited usefulness after 60. Its use should be restricted to those women who are at increased risk for developing osteoporosis. In this age group, it is advisable to attempt relief of hot flushes with nonestrogenic medications. During use, report promptly any indications of impaired circulation: speech disturbances, altered vision, sudden hearing loss, vertigo, sudden weakness or paralysis, angina, leg pains.

▷ **Advisability of Use During Pregnancy**
Pregnancy Category: X. See Pregnancy Code inside back cover.
Animal studies: Genital defects reported in mice and guinea pigs; cleft palate reported in rodents.
Human studies: Information from studies in pregnant women indicates that estrogens can masculinize the female fetus. In addition, limb defects and heart malformations have been reported.
It is now known that estrogens taken during pregnancy can predispose the female child to the development of cancer of the vagina or cervix following puberty.
Avoid estrogens completely during entire pregnancy.

Advisability of Use if Breast-Feeding
Presence of this drug in breast milk: Yes, in minute amounts.
Estrogens in large doses can suppress milk formation.
Breast-feeding is considered to be safe during the use of estrogens.

Habit-Forming Potential: None.

Effects of Overdosage: Headache, drowsiness, nausea, vomiting, fluid retention, abnormal vaginal bleeding, breast enlargement and discomfort.

Possible Effects of Long-Term Use: High blood pressure, gallbladder disease with gallstone formation, increased growth of benign fibroid tumors of the uterus. Several reports suggest a possible association between the long-term use (3+ years) of estrogens and the development of cancer of the lining of the uterus. Further studies are needed to establish a definite cause-and-effect relationship (see Glossary). Prudence dictates that women with uterus intact should use estrogens only when symptoms justify it and with proper supervision.

Suggested Periodic Examinations While Taking This Drug (at physician's discretion)

Regular (every 6 months) evaluation of the breasts and pelvic organs, including Pap smears. Liver function tests as indicated.

▷ **While Taking This Drug, Observe the Following**

Foods: Avoid excessive use of salt if fluid retention occurs.

Beverages: No restrictions. May be taken with milk.

▷ *Alcohol*: No interactions expected.

Tobacco Smoking: Recent studies indicate that heavy smoking (15 or more cigarettes daily) in association with the use of estrogen-containing oral contraceptives significantly increases the risk of heart attack (coronary thrombosis). Avoid heavy smoking during long-term estrogen therapy.

▷ *Other Drugs*

Estrogens *taken concurrently* with

- antidiabetic drugs may cause unpredictable fluctuations of blood sugar.
- tricyclic antidepressants (Elavil, Sinequan, etc.) may enhance their adverse effects and reduce their antidepressant effectiveness.
- warfarin (Coumadin) may cause unpredictable alterations of prothrombin activity.

The following drugs may *decrease* the effects of estrogens

- carbamazepine (Tegretol).
- phenobarbital.
- phenytoin (Dilantin).
- primidone (Mysoline).
- rifampin (Rifadin, Rimactane).

▷ *Driving, Hazardous Activities*: Usually no restrictions. Consult your physician for assessment of individual risk and for guidance regarding specific restrictions.

Aviation Note: Usually no restrictions. However, it is advisable to observe for the rare occurrence of disturbed vision and to restrict activities accordingly. Consult a designated Aviation Medical Examiner.

Exposure to Sun: Use caution until full effect is known. These drugs can cause photosensitivity (see Glossary).

Discontinuation: It is advisable to discontinue estrogens periodically to determine if a need for them still exists. Reduce the dose gradually to prevent acute withdrawal hot flushes. Avoid continual, uninterrupted use of large doses. Discontinue altogether when a definite indication for replacement therapy no longer exists. Ask your physician for guidance.

ETHOSUXIMIDE
(eth oh SUX i mide)

Introduced: 1960

Prescription: USA: Yes
Canada: Yes

Available as Generic: No

Brand Names: Zarontin

Class: Anticonvulsant, Succinimides

Controlled Drug: USA: No
Canada: No

BENEFITS versus RISKS

Possible Benefits	*Possible Risks*
EFFECTIVE CONTROL OF ABSENCE SEIZURES (PETIT MAL EPILEPSY) in 70% of cases	RARE APLASTIC ANEMIA (See Aplastic Anemia and Bone Marrow Depression in Glossary)
EFFECTIVE CONTROL OF MYOCLONIC AND AKINETIC EPILEPSY in some individuals	Rare decrease in white blood cells and blood platelets

---

▷ **Principal Uses**

As a Single Drug Product: This is the drug of first choice by many physicians for the management of absence seizures. It causes serious adverse effects less frequently than other drugs used for this disorder, and it is quite effective in the presence of structural abnormalities of the brain.

How This Drug Works: Not completely established. It is thought that by altering the transmission of certain nerve impulses, this drug suppresses the abnormal showers of electrical activity responsible for the absence seizures of petit mal epilepsy.

Available Dosage Forms and Strengths
Capsules — 250 mg
Syrup — 250 mg per 5 ml teaspoonful

▷ **Usual Adult Dosage Range:** 20 to 40 mg per kilogram of body weight/24 hrs. Initially 500 mg/24 hrs. Dosage may be increased cautiously by 250 mg every 4 to 7 days until satisfactory control is achieved. The total daily dosage should not exceed 1500 mg. **Note: Actual dosage and administration schedule must be determined by the physician for each patient individually.**

▷ **Dosing Instructions:** May be taken with food to reduce stomach irritation. Capsule may be opened for administration.

Usual Duration of Use: Continual use on a regular schedule for 1 to 2 weeks is usually necessary to determine this drug's effectiveness in reducing the frequency of absence seizures. Long-term use requires supervision and periodic evaluation by your physician.

▷ **This Drug Should Not Be Taken If**
  • you are allergic to this or any other succinimide drug (See Drug Class, Section Four).
  • you have active liver disease.
  • you currently have a blood cell or bone marrow disorder.

▷ **Inform Your Physician Before Taking This Drug If**
  • you have a history of liver or kidney disease.
  • you have a history of any type of blood cell disorder, especially one induced by drugs.
  • you have a history of serious depression or other mental illness.

  Possible Side-Effects   (natural, expected and unavoidable drug actions)
  Drowsiness, lethargy, fatigue.

▷ **Possible Adverse Effects**   (unusual, unexpected and infrequent reactions)
  If any of the following develop, consult your physician promptly.
  Mild Adverse Effects
  Allergic Reactions: Skin rash, hives.
  Headache, dizziness, unsteadiness, euphoria, impaired vision, numbness and tingling in extremities.
  Loss of appetite, nausea, vomiting, hiccups, stomach pain, diarrhea.
  Excessive growth of hair.
  Serious Adverse Effects
  Allergic Reactions: Swelling of tongue.
  Thickening and overgrowth of gums.
  Nervousness, hyperactivity, disturbed sleep, night terrors.
  Aggravation of emotional depression and paranoid mental disorders.
  Severe bone marrow depression—fatigue, weakness, fever, sore throat, abnormal bleeding or bruising.

  Natural Diseases or Disorders That May Be Activated by This Drug
  Latent psychosis, systemic lupus erythematosus.

  CAUTION
  1. This drug may increase the frequency of grand mal seizures in individuals with mixed seizure disorders.
  2. It is mandatory that you comply with your physician's request for periodic blood counts and other tests that are deemed necessary.

  Precautions for Use
  By Infants and Children: If a single daily dose causes nausea or vomiting, give in 2 or 3 divided doses 8 to 12 hours apart. Marked individual variation in response occurs; the use of blood levels for monitoring is advised. Observe for a possible lupuslike reaction: fever, rash, arthritis.
  By Those over 60 Years of Age: Rarely used in this age group.

▷ **Advisability of Use During Pregnancy**
  Pregnancy Category: C (tentative). See Pregnancy Code inside back cover.
  Animal studies: Bone defects reported in rodents.

Human studies: Three instances of birth defects have been reported. Information from adequate studies in pregnant women is not available.

Avoid during first 3 months. Use only if clearly needed during the last 6 months.

Advisability of Use if Breast-Feeding

Presence of this drug in breast milk: Yes.

Monitor nursing infant closely and discontinue drug or nursing if adverse effects develop. If mother requires high doses, refrain from nursing. Ask physician for guidance.

Habit-Forming Potential: None.

Effects of Overdosage: Increased drowsiness, lethargy, weakness, dizziness, unsteadiness, nausea, vomiting, stupor progressing to coma.

Possible Effects of Long-Term Use: Systemic lupus erythematosus.

Suggested Periodic Examinations While Taking This Drug (at physician's discretion)

Complete blood cell counts every 2 weeks during the first 3 months of use, then monthly thereafter; liver and kidney function tests.

▷ **While Taking This Drug, Observe the Following**

Foods: No restrictions.

Beverages: No restrictions. May be taken with milk.

▷　*Alcohol*: Use caution until the combined effects have been determined. This drug may increase the sedative effects of alcohol. Excessive alcohol may precipitate seizures.

Tobacco Smoking: No interactions expected.

▷　*Other Drugs*

Ethosuximide may *increase* the effects of
- phenytoin (Dilantin), by slowing its elimination.

Ethosuximide *taken concurrently* with
- valproic acid (Depakene) may alter the effects of ethosuximide unpredictably.

The following drugs may *increase* the effects of ethosuximide
- isoniazid (INH, Niconyl, etc.).

▷　*Driving, Hazardous Activities*: This drug may cause drowsiness, dizziness, unsteadiness and impaired vision. Restrict activities as necessary.

Aviation Note: Seizure disorders and the use of this drug *are disqualifications* for piloting. Consult a designated Aviation Medical Examiner.

Exposure to Sun: No restrictions.

Discontinuation: Do not stop taking this drug abruptly. Ask your physician for guidance regarding gradual reduction of dosage.

FENOPROFEN
(fen oh PROH fen)

Introduced: 1976

Prescription: USA: Yes
  Canada: Yes

Available as Generic: No

Brand Names: Nalfon

Class: Mild Analgesic, Anti-
  inflammatory

Controlled Drug: USA: No
  Canada: No

BENEFITS versus RISKS

Possible Benefits	*Possible Risks*
EFFECTIVE RELIEF OF MILD TO MODERATE PAIN AND INFLAMMATION	Gastrointestinal pain, ulceration, bleeding (rare)
	Rare liver or kidney damage
	Rare fluid retention
	Rare bone marrow depression

▷ **Principal Uses**

  As a Single Drug Product: Used primarily to relieve mild to moderately severe pain associated with (1) musculoskeletal injuries; (2) acute and chronic gout, rheumatoid arthritis and osteoarthritis; (3) dental, obstetrical and orthopedic surgery; (4) menstrual cramps; and (5) vascular (migraine-like) headaches.

How This Drug Works: Not completely established. It is thought that this drug reduces the tissue concentrations of prostaglandins (and related compounds), chemicals involved in the production of inflammation and pain.

Available Dosage Forms and Strengths
  Capsules — 200 mg, 300 mg
  Tablets — 600 mg

▷ **Usual Adult Dosage Range:** 300 to 600 mg 3 or 4 times/day. Total daily dosage should not exceed 3200 mg. **Note: Actual dosage and administration schedule must be determined by the physician for each patient individually.**

▷ **Dosing Instructions:** Take either on an empty stomach or with food or milk to prevent stomach irritation. Take with a full glass of water and remain upright (do not lie down) for 30 minutes. The tablet may be crushed and the capsule may be opened for administration.

Usual Duration of Use: Continual use on a regular schedule for 2 to 3 weeks is usually necessary to determine this drug's effectiveness in relieving the discomfort of arthritis. Long-term use requires supervision and periodic evaluation by the physician.

▷ **This Drug Should Not Be Taken If**
- you have had an allergic reaction to it previously.
- you are subject to asthma or nasal polyps caused by aspirin.
- you have active peptic ulcer disease or any form of gastrointestinal bleeding.
- you have a bleeding disorder or a blood cell disorder.
- you have severe impairment of kidney function.

▷ **Inform Your Physician Before Taking This Drug If**
- you are allergic to aspirin or to other aspirin substitutes.
- you have a history of peptic ulcer disease or any type of bleeding disorder.
- you have impaired liver or kidney function.
- you have high blood pressure or a history of heart failure.
- you are taking any of the following: acetaminophen, aspirin or other aspirin substitutes, anticoagulants, oral antidiabetic drugs.

Possible Side-Effects   (natural, expected and unavoidable drug actions)
Drowsiness (15%), ringing in ears, fluid retention.

▷ **Possible Adverse Effects**   (unusual, unexpected and infrequent reactions)
If any of the following develop, consult your physician promptly.
Mild Adverse Effects
Allergic Reactions: Skin rash, hives, itching (9%).
Headache (15%), dizziness, altered or blurred vision, depression.
Mouth sores, indigestion, nausea, vomiting, constipation, diarrhea.
Serious Adverse Effects
Allergic Reactions: Anaphylaxis (see Glossary).
Blurred vision, impaired hearing.
Active peptic ulcer, with or without bleeding.
Liver damage with jaundice (see Glossary).
Kidney damage with painful urination, bloody urine, reduced urine formation.
Rare bone marrow depression (see Glossary)—fatigue, weakness, fever, sore throat, abnormal bleeding or bruising.

Possible Delayed Adverse Effects
Mild anemia due to "silent" blood loss from the stomach (less than that caused by aspirin).

▷ **Adverse Effects That May Mimic Natural Diseases or Disorders**
Liver reaction may suggest viral hepatitis.

Natural Diseases or Disorders That May Be Activated by This Drug
Peptic ulcer disease, ulcerative colitis.

CAUTION
1. Dosage should always be limited to the smallest amount that produces reasonable improvement.
2. This drug may mask early indications of infection. Inform your physician if you think you are developing an infection of any kind.

Precautions for Use

By Infants and Children: Safety and effectiveness for use by those under 12 years of age have not been established.

By Those over 60 Years of Age: Small doses are advisable until tolerance is determined. Observe for any indications of liver or kidney toxicity, fluid retention, dizziness, confusion, impaired memory, stomach bleeding or constipation.

▷ **Advisability of Use During Pregnancy**

Pregnancy Category: B (tentative). See Pregnancy Code inside back cover.

Animal studies: No birth defects reported.

Human studies: Information from adequate studies in pregnant women is not available.

Avoid this drug during the last 3 months. Use it during the first 6 months only if clearly needed. Ask physician for guidance.

The manufacturer does not recommend the use of this drug during pregnancy.

Advisability of Use if Breast-Feeding

Presence of this drug in breast milk: Yes, in minute amounts. Avoid drug or refrain from nursing.

Habit-Forming Potential: None.

Effects of Overdosage: Drowsiness, nausea, vomiting, diarrhea.

Possible Effects of Long-Term Use: Cataracts have been reported, but a definite cause-and-effect relationship (see Glossary) has not been established.

Suggested Periodic Examinations While Taking This Drug   (at physician's discretion)

Complete blood cell counts, liver and kidney function tests, complete eye examinations if vision is altered in any way.

▷ **While Taking This Drug, Observe the Following**

Foods: No restrictions.

Beverages: No restrictions. May be taken with milk.

▷   *Alcohol*: Use with caution. The irritant action of alcohol on the stomach lining, added to the irritant action of this drug in sensitive individuals, can increase the risk of stomach ulceration and/or bleeding.

Tobacco Smoking: No interactions expected.

▷   *Other Drugs*

Fenoprofen may *increase* the effects of

- acetaminophen (Tylenol, etc.), and increase the risk of kidney damage; avoid prolonged use of this combination.
- anticoagulants (Coumadin, etc.), and increase the risk of bleeding; monitor prothrombin time, adjust dose accordingly.

Fenoprofen *taken concurrently* with the following drugs may increase the risk of bleeding; avoid these combinations:

- aspirin.
- dipyridamole (Persantine).

- indomethacin (Indocin).
- sulfinpyrazone (Anturane).
- valproic acid (Depakene).

▷ *Driving, Hazardous Activities*: This drug may cause drowsiness or dizziness. Restrict activities as necessary.

Aviation Note: The use of this drug *may be a disqualification* for piloting. Consult a designated Aviation Medical Examiner.

Exposure to Sun: No restrictions.

FLECAINIDE
(FLEK a nide)

Introduced: 1982

Prescription: USA: Yes

Available as Generic: USA: No

Brand Names: Tambocor

Class: Antiarrhythmic

Controlled Drug: USA: No

BENEFITS versus RISKS	
Possible Benefits	*Possible Risks*
EFFECTIVE TREATMENT (72%) OF SELECTED HEART RHYTHM DISORDERS	DRUG-INDUCED HEART RHYTHM DISORDERS (7%) CONGESTIVE HEART FAILURE (5%) Rare blood cell disorders Rare liver damage with jaundice

▷ **Principal Uses**

As a Single Drug Product: This drug is classified as a Type 1 antiarrhythmic agent, similar to procainamide and quinidine in its actions. It is used primarily to correct and prevent the recurrence of (1) abnormally rapid heart rates (tachycardia) that arise in the ventricles (lower heart chambers); and (2) premature beats arising in the ventricles.

How This Drug Works: By slowing the transmission of electrical impulses throughout the conduction system of the heart, this drug assists in restoring normal heart rate and rhythm.

Available Dosage Forms and Strengths
Tablets — 100 mg

▷ **Usual Adult Dosage Range:** Do not take a loading dose. Initiate treatment with 100 mg/12 hrs. At intervals of 4 days, increase dose by 50-mg increments to 150 mg/12 hrs, then to 200 mg/12 hrs if necessary. Total daily dosage should not exceed 400 mg. Measurement of drug blood levels is advised to determine the optimal dose and schedule. **Note: Actual dos-**

age and administration schedule must be determined by the physician for each patient individually.

▷ **Dosing Instructions:**   May be taken without regard to meals. Take at same time each day to obtain uniform results. Tablet may be crushed for administration.

Usual Duration of Use: Continual use on a regular schedule for 1 to 2 weeks is usually necessary to determine this drug's effectiveness in correcting or preventing responsive rhythm disorders. Long-term use requires supervision and periodic evaluation by your physician.

▷ **This Drug Should Not Be Taken If**
- you have had an allergic reaction to it previously.
- you have second-degree or third-degree heart block (determined by electrocardiogram).

▷ **Inform Your Physician Before Taking This Drug If**
- you have had any unfavorable reactions to other antiarrhythmic drugs in the past.
- you have a history of heart disease of any kind, especially "heart block."
- you have impaired liver or kidney function.
- you are taking any form of digitalis, a potassium supplement or any diuretic drug that can cause excessive loss of body potassium (ask physician).

Possible Side-Effects   (natural, expected and unavoidable drug actions)
Flushing, increased sweating, light-headedness.

▷ **Possible Adverse Effects**   (unusual, unexpected and infrequent reactions)
If any of the following develop, consult your physician promptly.
Mild Adverse Effects
Allergic Reactions: Skin rash (1% to 3%), hives, itching.
Headache (9%), dizziness (18%), visual disturbance (15%), fatigue (7%), weakness (4%), tremor (4%).
Loss of appetite, indigestion, nausea (8%), vomiting, constipation (4%), abdominal pain (3%).
Serious Adverse Effects
Idiosyncratic Reactions: Depression, confusion, amnesia, euphoria (less than 1%).
Drug-induced heart rhythm disorders (7%), congestive heart failure (5%), shortness of breath (10%), palpitations (6%), chest pain (5%), swelling of feet (3%).
Sexual impotence, urinary retention.
Jaundice (see Glossary).
Abnormally low white blood cells and blood platelets (rare): fever, sore throat, abnormal bleeding or bruising.

▷ **Adverse Effects That May Mimic Natural Diseases or Disorders**
Reversible jaundice may suggest viral hepatitis.

CAUTION
1. Thorough evaluation of your heart function (including electrocardiograms) is necessary prior to using this drug.
2. Periodic evaluation of your heart function is necessary to determine your response to this drug. Some individuals may experience worsening of their heart rhythm disorder and/or deterioration of heart function. Close monitoring of heart rate, rhythm and overall performance is essential.
3. Dosage must be adjusted carefully for each individual. Do not change your dosage without the knowledge and supervision of your physician.
4. Do not take any other antiarrhythmic drug while taking this drug unless directed to do so by your physician.

Precautions for Use
By Infants and Children: Safety and effectiveness for use by those under 18 years of age have not been established. Initial use of this drug requires hospitalization and supervision by a qualified cardiologist.
By Those over 60 Years of Age: Reduced kidney function may require reduction in dosage. Observe carefully for light-headedness, dizziness, unsteadiness and tendency to fall.

▷ **Advisability of Use During Pregnancy**
Pregnancy Category: C (tentative). See Pregnancy Code inside back cover.
Animal studies: Birth defects reported in one species of rabbit.
Human studies: Information from adequate studies in pregnant women is not available.
Avoid during first 3 months. Use this drug only if clearly needed. Ask physician for guidance.

Advisability of Use if Breast-Feeding
Presence of this drug in breast milk: Unknown.
Avoid drug or refrain from nursing.

Habit-Forming Potential: None.

Effects of Overdosage: Impaired urination, constipation, marked drop in blood pressure, abnormal heart rhythms, slow heart rate, congestive heart failure.

Possible Effects of Long-Term Use: None reported.

Suggested Periodic Examinations While Taking This Drug   (at physician's discretion)
Electrocardiograms, complete blood cell counts, measurements of potassium blood levels.

▷ **While Taking This Drug, Observe the Following**
Foods: No restrictions. Ask physician regarding need for salt restriction and advisability of eating potassium-rich foods.
Beverages: No restrictions. May be taken with milk.

▷   *Alcohol*: Use caution until the combined effects have been determined. Alcohol can increase the blood-pressure-lowering effects of this drug.

Tobacco Smoking: Nicotine can cause irritability of the heart and reduce the effectiveness of this drug. Follow physician's advice regarding smoking.

▷   *Other Drugs*

Flecainide may *increase* the effects of

- antihypertensive drugs, and cause excessive lowering of blood pressure.
- beta-blocker drugs (see Drug Class, Section Four).

The following drugs may *decrease* the effects of flecainide

- diuretics that promote potassium loss.

▷   *Driving, Hazardous Activities*: This drug may cause drowsiness, dizziness or blurred vision. Restrict activities as necessary.

Aviation Note: The use of this drug *may be a disqualification* for piloting. Consult a designated Aviation Medical Examiner.

Exposure to Sun: No restrictions.

Occurrence of Unrelated Illness: Disorders that cause vomiting, diarrhea or dehydration can affect this drug's action adversely. Report such developments promptly.

Discontinuation: This drug should not be discontinued abruptly following long-term use. Ask your physician for guidance regarding gradual dose reduction.

FLUPHENAZINE
(flu FEN a zeen)

Introduced: 1959

Class: Strong Tranquilizer, Phenothiazines

Prescription: USA: Yes
Canada: Yes

Controlled Drug: USA: No
Canada: No

Available as Generic: USA: No
Canada: Yes

Brand Names: ❦Apo-Fluphenazine, ❦Modecate, ❦Moditen, Permitil, Prolixin

---

BENEFITS versus RISKS	
Possible Benefits	*Possible Risks*
EFFECTIVE CONTROL OF ACUTE MENTAL DISORDERS in the majority of patients	SERIOUS TOXIC EFFECTS ON BRAIN with long-term use
Beneficial effects on thinking, mood and behavior	Liver damage with jaundice (less than 0.5%)
	Rare blood cell disorders: abnormally low white blood cells

▷ **Principal Uses**

As a Single Drug Product: This antipsychotic drug is used primarily to treat acute and chronic psychotic disorders such as schizophrenia, mania and similar states of mental dysfunction.

How This Drug Works: Not completely established. Present theory is that by inhibiting the action of dopamine, this drug acts to correct an imbalance of nerve impulse transmissions that is thought to be responsible for certain mental disorders.

Available Dosage Forms and Strengths

Concentrate — 5 mg per ml (1% alcohol)
Elixir — 2.5 mg per 5 ml teaspoonful (14% alcohol)
Injection — 2.5 mg per ml, 25 mg per ml
Tablets — 0.25 mg, 1 mg, 2.5 mg, 5 mg, 10 mg
Tablets, prolonged action — 1 mg

▷ **Usual Adult Dosage Range:**   0.5 to 2.5 mg 1 to 4 times/day; adjust dosage as needed and tolerated. Total daily dosage should not exceed 20 mg. **Note: Actual dosage and administration schedule must be determined by the physician for each patient individually.**

▷ **Dosing Instructions:**   May be taken with or following meals to reduce stomach irritation. Regular tablets may be crushed for administration. Prolonged-action tablets should be swallowed whole (not crushed). The concentrate must be diluted in 4 to 6 ounces of water, milk, fruit juice or carbonated beverage.

Usual Duration of Use: Continual use on a regular schedule for several weeks is usually necessary to determine this drug's effectiveness in controlling psychotic disorders. If not significantly beneficial within 6 weeks, it should be discontinued. Long-term use (months to years) requires periodic evaluation of response, appropriate dosage adjustment and consideration of continued need.

▷ **This Drug Should Not Be Taken If**

- you are allergic to any of the drugs bearing the brand names listed above.
- you have a history of brain damage.
- you have active liver disease.
- you have cancer of the breast.
- you have a current blood cell or bone marrow disorder.

▷ **Inform Your Physician Before Taking This Drug If**

- you are allergic or abnormally sensitive to any phenothiazine drug (see Drug Class, Section Four).
- you have impaired liver or kidney function.
- you have any type of seizure disorder.
- you have diabetes, glaucoma, heart disease or chronic lung disease.
- you have a history of lupus erythematosus.

- you are taking any drug with sedative effects.
- you plan to have surgery under general or spinal anesthesia in the near future.

Possible Side-Effects   (natural, expected and unavoidable drug actions)

Drowsiness (usually during the first 2 weeks), orthostatic hypotension (see Glossary), blurred vision, dry mouth, nasal congestion, constipation, impaired urination (all mild).

▷ **Possible Adverse Effects**   (unusual, unexpected and infrequent reactions)

If any of the following develop, consult your physician promptly.

Mild Adverse Effects

Allergic Reactions: Skin rash, hives, itching.

Lowering of body temperature, especially in the elderly.

Headache, dizziness, weakness, excitement, restlessness, unusual dreaming.

Increased appetite and weight gain.

Breast fullness, tenderness, milk production, menstrual irregularity.

Serious Adverse Effects

Allergic Reactions: Hepatitis with jaundice (see Glossary), usually between second and fourth week; anaphylactic reaction (see Glossary).

Idiosyncratic Reactions: High fever.

Impaired production of white blood cells—fever, sore throat, infections.

Parkinson-like disorders (see Glossary); muscle spasms of face, jaw, neck, back, extremities.

Prolonged drop in blood pressure with weakness, perspiration and fainting.

▷ **Adverse Effects That May Mimic Natural Diseases or Disorders**

Nervous system reactions may suggest Parkinson's disease.

Liver reactions may suggest viral hepatitis.

Reactions resembling systemic lupus erythematosus may occur.

Natural Diseases or Disorders That May Be Activated by This Drug

Latent epilepsy, glaucoma, prostatism (see Glossary).

CAUTION

1. Many over-the-counter medications (see OTC Drugs in Glossary) for allergies, colds and coughs contain drugs that can interact unfavorably with this drug. Ask your physician or pharmacist for guidance before using any such medications.
2. Antacids that contain aluminum and/or magnesium can prevent the absorption of this drug and reduce its effectiveness.
3. Obtain prompt evaluation of any change or disturbance of vision.

Precautions for Use

By Infants and Children: Do not use this drug in infants under 6 months of age, or in children of any age with symptoms suggestive of Reye syndrome (see Glossary). Monitor carefully for blood cell changes.

By Those over 60 Years of Age: Small doses are advisable until individual response has been determined. You may be more susceptible to the development of drowsiness, lethargy, constipation, lowering of body temperature (hypothermia) and orthostatic hypotension (see Glossary). This drug can enhance existing prostatism (see Glossary). You may also be more susceptible to the development of parkinson-like reactions and/or tardive dyskinesia (see discussion of these terms in Glossary). These reactions must be recognized early since they may become unresponsive to treatment and irreversible.

▷ **Advisability of Use During Pregnancy**

Pregnancy Category: C (tentative). See Pregnancy Code inside back cover.

Animal studies: Significant birth defects reported in mice.

Human studies: Information from adequate studies in pregnant women is not available.

Avoid drug during the first 3 months and during the last month because of possible effects on the newborn infant.

Advisability of Use if Breast-Feeding

Presence of this drug in breast milk: Unknown.

Avoid drug or refrain from nursing.

Habit-Forming Potential: None.

Effects of Overdosage: Marked drowsiness, weakness, tremor, agitation, unsteadiness, deep sleep, coma, convulsions.

Possible Effects of Long-Term Use: Tardive dyskinesia (see Glossary); eye changes—cataracts and pigmentation of retina; gray to violet pigmentation of skin in exposed areas, more common in women.

Suggested Periodic Examinations While Taking This Drug (at physician's discretion)

Complete blood cell counts, especially between the fourth and tenth weeks of treatment.

Liver function tests, electrocardiograms.

Complete eye examinations—eye structures and vision.

Careful inspection of the tongue for early evidence of fine, involuntary, wavelike movements that could indicate the beginning of tardive dyskinesia.

▷ **While Taking This Drug, Observe the Following**

Foods: No restrictions.

Beverages: No restrictions. May be taken with milk.

▷ *Alcohol*: Avoid completely. Alcohol can increase the sedative action of phenothiazines and accentuate their depressant effects on brain function and blood pressure. Phenothiazines can increase the intoxicating effects of alcohol.

Tobacco Smoking: Possible reduction of drowsiness from drug.

Marijuana Smoking: Moderate increase in drowsiness; accentuation of orthostatic hypotension; increased risk of precipitating latent psychoses, confusing the interpretation of mental status and drug responses.

▷ *Other Drugs*

Fluphenazine may *increase* the effects of

- all sedative drugs, and cause excessive sedation.
- all atropinelike drugs, and cause nervous system toxicity.

Fluphenazine may *decrease* the effects of

- guanethidine (Ismelin, Esimil), and reduce its effectiveness in lowering blood pressure.

Fluphenazine *taken concurrently* with

- beta-blocker drugs (see Drug Class, Section Four) may cause increased effects of both drugs; monitor drug effects closely and adjust dosages as necessary.

The following drugs may *decrease* the effects of fluphenazine

- antacids containing aluminum and/or magnesium.
- benztropine (Cogentin).
- trihexyphenidyl (Artane).

▷ *Driving, Hazardous Activities*: This drug can impair mental alertness, judgment and physical coordination. Avoid hazardous activities.

Aviation Note: The use of this drug *is a disqualification* for piloting. Consult a designated Aviation Medical Examiner.

Exposure to Sun: Use caution until sensitivity has been determined. Some phenothiazines can cause photosensitivity (see Glossary).

Exposure to Heat: Use caution and avoid excessive heat as much as possible. This drug may impair the regulation of body temperature and increase the risk of heat stroke.

Exposure to Cold: Use caution and dress warmly. This drug can increase the risk of hypothermia in the elderly.

Discontinuation: After a period of long-term use, do not discontinue this drug suddenly. Gradual withdrawal over 2 to 3 weeks under physician supervision is recommended. Do not discontinue this drug without your physician's knowledge and approval. The relapse rate of schizophrenia after discontinuation is 50% to 60%.

FLURAZEPAM
(floor AZ e pam)

Introduced: 1970

Prescription: USA: Yes
Canada: Yes

Available as Generic: USA: Yes
Canada: No

Class: Hypnotic, Benzodiazepines

Controlled Drug: USA: C-IV*
Canada: No

Brand Names: ✚Apo-Flurazepam, <u>Dalmane,</u> ✚Novoflupam, ✚Somnol, ✚Som-Pam

*See Schedules of Controlled Drugs inside back cover.

```
┌─────────────────────────────────────────────────────────────────┐
│                   BENEFITS versus RISKS                           │
│                                                                   │
│      Possible Benefits                 Possible Risks             │
│  EFFECTIVE HYPNOTIC after 2       Habit-forming potential with long- │
│    weeks of continual use           term use                      │
│  NO SUPPRESSION OF REM            Minor impairment of mental       │
│    (RAPID EYE MOVEMENT)             functions ("hangover" effect)  │
│    SLEEP                           Very rare jaundice              │
│  NO REM SLEEP REBOUND after       Very rare blood cell disorder    │
│    discontinuation                 Suppression of stage-4 sleep with │
│  Wide margin of safety with         reduced "quality" of sleep     │
│    therapeutic doses                                              │
└─────────────────────────────────────────────────────────────────┘
```

▷ **Principal Uses**

As a Single Drug Product: This member of the benzodiazepine class of "minor tranquilizers" is used exclusively as a bedtime sedative to induce sleep.

How This Drug Works: It is thought that this drug produces a calming effect by enhancing the action of the nerve transmitter gamma-aminobutyric acid (GABA), which in turn blocks the arousal of higher brain centers and helps to induce sleep.

Available Dosage Forms and Strengths
Capsules — 15 mg, 30 mg

▷ **Usual Adult Dosage Range:** 15 to 30 mg at bedtime. Total daily dosage should not exceed 90 mg. **Note: Actual dosage and administration schedule must be determined by the physician for each patient individually.**

▷ **Dosing Instructions:** May be taken on an empty stomach or with food or milk. The capsule may be opened for administration. Do not discontinue this drug abruptly if taken for more than 4 weeks.

Usual Duration of Use: Periods of 3 to 5 nights intermittently, repeated as needed with appropriate dosage adjustment. Avoid uninterrupted and prolonged use. The duration of use should not exceed 2 weeks without reappraisal of continued need.

▷ **This Drug Should Not Be Taken If**
- you have had an allergic reaction to it previously.
- you have acute narrow-angle glaucoma.

▷ **Inform Your Physician Before Taking This Drug If**
- you are allergic to any benzodiazepine drug (see Drug Class, Section Four).
- you have a history of alcoholism or drug abuse.
- you are pregnant or planning pregnancy.
- you have impaired liver or kidney function.
- you have a history of serious depression or mental disorder.
- you are taking other drugs with sedative effects.
- you have any of the following: asthma, emphysema, epilepsy, myasthenia gravis.

Possible Side-Effects   (natural, expected and unavoidable drug actions)
"Hangover" effects on arising: drowsiness, lethargy and unsteadiness.

Possible Adverse Effects   (unusual, unexpected and infrequent reactions)
If any of the following develop, consult your physician promptly.
Mild Adverse Effects
Allergic Reactions: Skin rash, hives, burning eyes, swelling of tongue.
Dizziness, fainting, blurred vision, double vision, slurred speech, nausea,
indigestion.
Serious Adverse Effects
Allergic Reactions: Liver damage with jaundice (see Glossary).
Idiosyncratic Reactions: Nervousness, talkativeness, irritability, apprehension, euphoria, excitement, hallucinations.
Bone marrow depression—impaired production of white blood cells, fever,
sore throat.

▷ **Adverse Effects That May Mimic Natural Diseases or Disorders**
Liver reaction with jaundice may suggest viral hepatitis.

CAUTION
1. This drug should not be discontinued abruptly if it has been taken continually for more than 4 weeks.
2. The concurrent use of some over-the-counter drug products that contain antihistamines (allergy and cold preparations, sleep aids) can cause excessive sedation in sensitive individuals.
3. Regular nightly use of any hypnotic drug should be avoided.
4. This drug is transformed by the liver into long-acting forms that can persist in the body for 24 hours or more. With continual use of this drug daily, these active drug forms accumulate and produce increasing sedation. If you experience a "hangover" effect, avoid hazardous activities (driving, etc.) and the use of alcohol.

Precautions for Use
By Infants and Children: Safety and effectiveness for use by those under 15
years of age have not been established.
By Those over 60 Years of Age: It is advisable to use smaller doses at longer
intervals to avoid overdosage. Observe for the possible development of
lethargy, indifference, fatigue, weakness, unsteadiness, disturbing
dreams, nightmares and paradoxical reactions of excitement, agitation,
anger, hostility and rage.

▷ **Advisability of Use During Pregnancy**
Pregnancy Category: C (tentative). See Pregnancy Code inside back cover.
Animal studies: No birth defects reported in rat and rabbit studies.
Human studies: Information from adequate studies in pregnant women is
not available.
Frequent use in late pregnancy can cause the "floppy infant" syndrome in
the newborn: weakness, lethargy, unresponsiveness, depressed breathing, low body temperature.
Avoid use during entire pregnancy if possible. Ask physician for guidance.

Advisability of Use if Breast-Feeding
Presence of this drug in breast milk: Probably yes.
Avoid drug or refrain from nursing.

Habit-Forming Potential: This drug can produce psychological and/or physical dependence (see Glossary) if used in large doses for an extended period of time. Avoid continual use.

Effects of Overdosage: Marked drowsiness, weakness, feeling of drunkenness, staggering gait, tremor, stupor progressing to deep sleep or coma.

Possible Effects of Long-Term Use: Psychological and/or physical dependence, impaired liver function.

Suggested Periodic Examinations While Taking This Drug   (at physician's discretion)
Complete blood cell counts and liver function tests during long-term use.

▷ **While Taking This Drug, Observe the Following**
Foods: No restrictions.
Beverages: Avoid excessive intake of caffeine-containing beverages (coffee, tea, cola) within 4 hours of taking this drug. May be taken with milk.
▷ *Alcohol*: Use with extreme caution until the combined effect is determined. Alcohol may increase the absorption of this drug and add to its depressant effects on the brain. It is advisable to avoid alcohol completely—throughout the day and night—if it is necessary to drive or to engage in any hazardous activity.
Tobacco Smoking: Heavy smoking may reduce the hypnotic action of this drug.
Marijuana Smoking: Increased sedation and significant impairment of intellectual and physical performance.
▷ *Other Drugs*
Flurazepam may *increase* the effects of
- digoxin (Lanoxin), and cause digoxin toxicity.
- phenytoin (Dilantin), and cause phenytoin toxicity.
Flurazepam may *decrease* the effects of
- levodopa (Sinemet, etc.), and reduce its effectiveness in treating Parkinson's disease.
The following drugs may *increase* the effects of flurazepam
- cimetidine (Tagamet).
- disulfiram (Antabuse).
- isoniazid (INH, Rifamate, etc.).
- oral contraceptives.
- valproic acid (Depakene).
The following drugs may *decrease* the effects of flurazepam
- rifampin (Rimactane, etc.).
- theophylline (aminophylline, Theo-Dur, etc.).
▷ *Driving, Hazardous Activities*: This drug can impair mental alertness, judgment, physical coordination and reaction time. Avoid hazardous activities accordingly.

Aviation Note: The use of this drug *is a disqualification* for piloting. Consult a designated Aviation Medical Examiner.

Exposure to Sun: No restrictions.

Exposure to Heat: Use caution until the effect of excessive perspiration is determined. Because of reduced urine volume, this drug may accumulate in the body and produce effects of overdosage.

Discontinuation: Avoid sudden discontinuation if this drug has been taken for over 4 weeks without interruption. Dosage should be tapered gradually to prevent a withdrawal syndrome that could include depression, confusion, hallucinations, tremor, seizures, muscle cramping, sweating and vomiting.

FUROSEMIDE
(fur OH se mide)

Introduced: 1964

Class: Antihypertensive, Diuretic

Prescription: USA: Yes
Canada: Yes

Controlled Drug: USA: No
Canada: No

Available as Generic: USA: Yes
Canada: Yes

Brand Names: ♣Apo-Furosemide, ♣Furoside, Lasix, ♣Neo-Renal, ♣Novosemide, SK-Furosemide, ♣Uritol

---

BENEFITS versus RISKS

Possible Benefits	*Possible Risks*
PROMPT, EFFECTIVE, RELIABLE DIURETIC	WATER AND ELECTROLYTE DEPLETION with excessive use
MODEST ANTIHYPERTENSIVE IN MILD TO MODERATE HYPERTENSION	Excessive potassium loss
	Increased blood sugar level
	Increased blood uric acid level
ENHANCES EFFECTIVENESS OF OTHER ANTIHYPERTENSIVES	Decreased blood calcium level
	Rare liver damage
	Rare blood cell disorder

▷ **Principal Uses**

As a Single Drug Product: This powerful diuretic is used primarily to increase the volume of urine and thereby relieve the body of excessive water retention (edema) that is commonly associated with congestive heart failure and some forms of liver disease and kidney disease. It is also used in the treatment of high blood pressure, but usually in conjunction with other antihypertensive drugs. A less frequent use is to increase the amount of calcium excreted in the urine when the blood level of calcium is abnormally high.

How This Drug Works: By increasing the elimination of salt and water from the body (through increased urine production), this drug reduces the volume of fluid in the blood and body tissues and lowers the sodium content throughout the body. These changes contribute to lowering blood pressure.

Available Dosage Forms and Strengths
Injection — 10 mg per ml
Oral Solution — 10 mg per ml
Tablets — 20 mg, 40 mg, 80 mg

▷ **Usual Adult Dosage Range:**   As antihypertensive: 40 mg/12 hrs initially; increase dose as needed and tolerated. As diuretic: 20 to 80 mg in a single dose initially; if necessary, increase the dose by 20 to 40 mg/6 to 8 hrs. The smallest effective dose should be determined. The total daily dose should not exceed 600 mg. **Note: Actual dosage and administration schedule must be determined by the physician for each patient individually.**

▷ **Dosing Instructions:**   May be taken with or following meals to reduce stomach irritation. Best taken in the morning to avoid nighttime urination. The tablet may be crushed for administration.

Usual Duration of Use: Continual use on a regular schedule for 2 to 3 weeks is usually necessary to determine this drug's effectiveness in lowering high blood pressure. Long-term use (months to years) requires periodic evaluation of response and possible dosage adjustment. Use as a diuretic should be intermittent with "drug holidays" (no drug taken) to reduce the risk of sodium and potassium imbalance.

▷ **This Drug Should Not Be Taken If**
• you have had an allergic reaction to any dosage form of it previously.

▷ **Inform Your Physician Before Taking This Drug If**
• you are allergic to any form of "sulfa" drug.
• you are pregnant or planning pregnancy.
• you have a history of kidney or liver disease.
• you have diabetes, gout or lupus erythematosus.
• you are taking any form of cortisone, digitalis, oral antidiabetic drug or insulin.
• you plan to have surgery under general anesthesia in the near future.

Possible Side-Effects   (natural, expected and unavoidable drug actions)
Light-headedness on arising from sitting or lying position (see orthostatic hypotension in Glossary).
Increase in blood sugar level, affecting control of diabetes.
Increase in blood uric acid level, affecting control of gout.
Decrease in blood potassium level, causing muscle weakness and cramping.

▷ **Possible Adverse Effects**   (unusual, unexpected and infrequent reactions)
If any of the following develop, consult your physician promptly.
Mild Adverse Effects
Allergic Reactions: Skin rashes, hives, drug fever.
Headache, dizziness, blurred or yellow vision, ringing in ears, numbness and tingling.
Reduced appetite, indigestion, nausea, vomiting, diarrhea.
Serious Adverse Effects
Allergic Reactions: Hepatitis with jaundice (see Glossary), anaphylactic reaction (see Glossary), severe skin reactions.
Idiosyncratic Reactions: Fluid accumulation in lungs.
Temporary hearing loss.
Inflammation of the pancreas—severe abdominal pain.
Bone marrow depression (see Glossary)—fatigue, weakness, fever, sore throat, abnormal bleeding or bruising.

▷ **Adverse Effects That May Mimic Natural Diseases or Disorders**
Liver reaction may suggest viral hepatitis.

Natural Diseases or Disorders That May Be Activated by This Drug
Diabetes, gout, systemic lupus erythematosus.

CAUTION
1. Do not exceed recommended doses. Increased dosage can cause excessive loss of sodium and potassium, with resultant loss of appetite, nausea, fatigue, weakness, confusion and tingling in the extremities.
2. If you are also taking a digitalis preparation (digitoxin, digoxin), ensure an adequate intake of high-potassium foods to prevent potassium deficiency—a potential cause of digitalis toxicity. (See Table of High Potassium Foods in Section Six.)

Precautions for Use
By Infants and Children: Avoid overdosage that could cause serious dehydration. Significant potassium loss can occur within the first 2 weeks of drug use.
By Those over 60 Years of Age: Small doses are advisable until your individual response has been determined. You may be more susceptible to the development of impaired thinking, orthostatic hypotension, potassium loss and blood sugar increase. Overdosage and extended use of this drug can cause excessive loss of body water, thickening (increased viscosity) of the blood and an increased tendency for the blood to clot—predisposing to stroke, heart attack or thrombophlebitis (vein inflammation with blood clot).

▷ **Advisability of Use During Pregnancy**
Pregnancy Category: C (tentative). See Pregnancy Code inside back cover.
Animal studies: Significant birth defects have been reported.
Human studies: Information from adequate studies in pregnant women is not available.
It should not be used during pregnancy unless a very serious complication

occurs for which this drug is significantly beneficial. Avoid completely during the first 3 months. Ask physician for guidance.

Advisability of Use if Breast-Feeding
Presence of this drug in breast milk: Yes.
Avoid drug or refrain from nursing.

Habit-Forming Potential: None.

Effects of Overdosage: Dry mouth, thirst, lethargy, weakness, muscle cramping, nausea, vomiting, drowsiness progressing to stupor or coma.

Possible Effects of Long-Term Use: Impaired balance of water, salt and potassium in blood and body tissues; dehydration and increased blood coagulability, with predisposition to thromboembolic disorders. Development of diabetes in predisposed individuals.

Suggested Periodic Examinations While Taking This Drug (at physician's discretion)
Complete blood cell counts, measurements of blood levels of sodium, potassium, chloride, sugar and uric acid.
Kidney and liver function tests.

▷ **While Taking This Drug, Observe the Following**
Foods: Consult your physician regarding the advisability of eating foods rich in potassium. If so advised, see the Table of High Potassium Foods in Section Six. Follow physician's advice regarding the use of salt.
Beverages: No restrictions. This drug may be taken with milk.
▷ *Alcohol*: Use with caution until the combined effects have been determined. Alcohol may exaggerate the blood-pressure-lowering effects of this drug and cause orthostatic hypotension.
Tobacco Smoking: No interactions expected. Follow physician's advice.
▷ *Other Drugs*
Furosemide may *increase* the effects of
- other antihypertensive drugs; dosage adjustments may be necessary to prevent excessive lowering of blood pressure.
- lithium, and cause lithium toxicity.
Furosemide may *decrease* the effects of
- oral antidiabetic drugs (sulfonylureas); dosage adjustments may be necessary for proper control of blood sugar.
Furosemide *taken concurrently* with
- digitalis preparations (digitoxin, digoxin) requires very careful monitoring and dosage adjustments to prevent fluctuations of blood potassium levels and serious disturbances of heart rhythm.
The following drugs may *decrease* the effects of furosemide
- indomethacin (Indocin).
▷ *Driving, Hazardous Activities*: Use caution until the possible occurrence of orthostatic hypotension, dizziness or impaired vision has been determined.
Aviation Note: The use of this drug *may be a disqualification* for piloting. Consult a designated Aviation Medical Examiner.

Exposure to Sun: Use caution until sensitivity has been determined. This drug may cause photosensitivity (see Glossary).

Exposure to Heat: Avoid excessive perspiring, which could cause additional loss of salt and water from the body.

Heavy Exercise or Exertion: Avoid exertion that produces light-headedness, excessive fatigue or muscle cramping. Isometric exercises—the "overload" technique for strengthening individual muscles—can raise blood pressure significantly. Ask physician for guidance regarding participation in this form of exercise.

Occurrence of Unrelated Illness: Illnesses that cause vomiting or diarrhea can produce a serious imbalance of important body chemistry. Consult your physician for guidance.

Discontinuation: It may be advisable to discontinue this drug 5 to 7 days before major surgery. Ask your physician, surgeon and/or anesthesiologist for guidance regarding dosage adjustment or drug withdrawal.

GLIPIZIDE
(GLIP i zide)

Introduced: 1972

Prescription: USA: Yes

Available as Generic: No

Brand Names: Glucotrol

Class: Antidiabetic, Sulfonylureas

Controlled Drug: USA: No

BENEFITS versus RISKS

Possible Benefits	*Possible Risks*
Assistance in regulating blood sugar in noninsulin-dependent diabetes (adjunctive to appropriate diet and weight control)	HYPOGLYCEMIA, severe and prolonged
	Allergic skin reactions (some severe)
	Water retention
	Rare liver damage
	Rare blood cell and bone marrow disorders

▷ **Principal Uses**

As a Single Drug Product: To assist in the control of mild to moderately severe type II diabetes mellitus (adult, maturity-onset) that does not require insulin, but that cannot be adequately controlled by diet alone.

How This Drug Works: It is thought that this drug (1) stimulates the secretion of insulin (by a pancreas that is capable of responding to stimulation), and (2) enhances the utilization of insulin by appropriate tissues.

Available Dosage Forms and Strengths

Tablets — 5 mg, 10 mg

▷ **Usual Adult Dosage Range:**   Initially 5 mg daily with breakfast. At 7 day intervals, the dose may be increased by increments of 2.5 to 5 mg daily as
needed and tolerated. Total daily dosage should not exceed 40 mg. A
"loading" or priming dose is not necessary and should not be given.
**Note: Actual dosage and administration schedule must be determined
by the physician for each patient individually.**

Dosing Instructions: If the daily maintenance dose is found to be 15 mg or
more, the total dose should be divided into 2 equal doses: the first taken
with the morning meal, the second with the evening meal. The tablet
may be crushed for administration.

Usual Duration of Use: Continual use on a regular schedule for 1 to 2 weeks is
usually necessary to determine this drug's effectiveness in controlling
diabetes. Failure to respond to maximal doses within 1 month constitutes
a primary failure. Up to 10% of those who respond initially may develop
secondary failure of the drug later. The duration of effective use can only
be determined by periodic measurement of the blood sugar.

▷ **This Drug Should Not Be Taken If**
  • you have had an allergic reaction to it previously.
  • you have severe impairment of liver or kidney function.
  • you are pregnant.

▷ **Inform Your Physician Before Taking This Drug If**
  • you are allergic to other sulfonylurea drugs or to "sulfa" drugs.
  • your diabetes has been unstable or "brittle" in the past.
  • you do not know how to recognize or treat hypoglycemia (see Glossary).
  • you have a history of congestive heart failure, peptic ulcer disease, cir-
    rhosis of the liver, hypothyroidism or porphyria.

Possible Side-Effects   (natural, expected and unavoidable drug actions)
    If drug dosage is excessive or food intake is delayed or inadequate, abnor-
    mally low blood sugar (hypoglycemia) will occur as a predictable drug
    effect.

▷ **Possible Adverse Effects**   (unusual, unexpected and infrequent reactions)
    If any of the following develop, consult your physician promptly.
    Mild Adverse Effects
    Allergic Reactions: Skin rash, hives, itching.
    Headache (1.25%), drowsiness (1.75%), dizziness (2.25%), fatigue (2.13%),
      sweating (1.25%).
    Indigestion, nausea (1.38%), vomiting, diarrhea (1.25%).
    Serious Adverse Effects
    Allergic Reactions: Hepatitis with jaundice (see Glossary), severe skin reac-
      tions.
    Idiosyncratic Reactions: Hemolytic anemia (see Glossary).
    Disulfiramlike reaction with concurrent use of alcohol (see Glossary), infre-
      quent with this drug.
    Water retention (edema), weight gain.

Bone marrow depression (see Glossary)—fatigue, weakness, fever, sore throat, abnormal bleeding or bruising.

▷ **Adverse Effects That May Mimic Natural Diseases or Disorders**
Liver reactions may suggest viral hepatitis.

CAUTION
1. This drug must be regarded as only one part of the total program for the management of your diabetes. It is not a substitute for a properly prescribed diet and regular exercise.
2. Over a period of time (usually several months), this drug may lose its effectiveness in controlling blood sugar levels. Periodic follow-up examinations are necessary to monitor all aspects of response to drug treatment.

Precautions for Use
By Infants and Children: This drug is not effective in type I (juvenile, growth-onset) insulin-dependent diabetes.
By Those over 60 Years of Age: This drug should be used with caution in this age group. Start treatment with 2.5 mg/day; increase dosage cautiously and monitor closely to prevent hypoglycemic reactions. Repeated episodes of hypoglycemia in the elderly can cause brain damage.

▷ **Advisability of Use During Pregnancy**
Pregnancy Category: C (tentative). See Pregnancy Code inside back cover.
Animal studies: No birth defects reported in rats and rabbits.
Human studies: Information from adequate studies in pregnant women is not available.
Because uncontrolled blood sugar levels during pregnancy are associated with a higher incidence of birth defects, many experts recommend that insulin (instead of an oral agent) be used as necessary to control diabetes during the entire pregnancy.

Advisability of Use if Breast-Feeding
Presence of this drug in breast milk: Unknown.
Avoid drug or refrain from nursing.

Habit-Forming Potential: None.

Effects of Overdosage: Symptoms of mild to severe hypoglycemia: headache, light-headedness, faintness, nervousness, confusion, tremor, sweating, heart palpitation, weakness, hunger, nausea, vomiting, stupor progressing to coma.

Possible Effects of Long-Term Use: Reduced function of the thyroid gland (hypothyroidism). Reports of increased frequency and severity of heart and blood vessel diseases associated with long-term use of this class of drugs are highly controversial and inconclusive. A direct cause-and-effect relationship (see Glossary) is tenuous. Ask your physician for guidance.

Suggested Periodic Examinations While Taking This Drug (at physician's discretion)

Complete blood cell counts, liver function tests, thyroid function tests, periodic evaluation of heart and circulatory system.

▷ **While Taking This Drug, Observe the Following**

Foods: Follow the diabetic diet prescribed by your physician.

Beverages: As directed in the diabetic diet. May be taken with milk.

▷ *Alcohol*: Use with extreme caution until the combined effect has been determined. Alcohol can exaggerate this drug's hypoglycemic effect. This drug infrequently causes a marked intolerance of alcohol, resulting in a disulfiramlike reaction (see Glossary): facial flushing, sweating, palpitation.

Tobacco Smoking: No interactions expected.

▷ *Other Drugs*

The following drugs may *increase* the effects of glipizide

- aspirin, and other salicylates.
- cimetidine (Tagamet).
- clofibrate (Atromid S).
- fenfluramine (Pondimin).
- monoamine oxidase (MAO) inhibitor drugs (see Drug Class, Section Four).
- phenylbutazone (Butazolidin).
- ranitidine (Zantac).

The following drugs may *decrease* the effects of glipizide

- beta-blocker drugs (see Drug Class, Section Four).
- bumetanide (Bumex).
- diazoxide (Proglycem).
- ethacrynic acid (Edecrin).
- furosemide (Lasix).
- phenytoin (Dilantin).
- thiazide diuretics (see Drug Class, Section Four).

▷ *Driving, Hazardous Activities*: Regulate your dosage schedule, eating schedule and physical activities very carefully to prevent hypoglycemia. Be able to recognize the early symptoms of hypoglycemia so you can avoid hazardous activities and take corrective measures.

Aviation Note: Diabetes *is a disqualification* for piloting. Consult a designated Aviation Medical Examiner.

Exposure to Sun: Use caution until sensitivity has been determined. Some drugs of this class can cause photosensitivity (see Glossary).

Occurrence of Unrelated Illness: Acute infections, illnesses causing vomiting or diarrhea, serious injuries and surgical procedures can interfere with diabetic control and may require the use of insulin. If any of these conditions occur, consult your physician promptly.

Discontinuation: Because of the possibility of secondary failure, it is advisable to evaluate the continued benefit of this drug every 6 months.

GLYBURIDE
(GLI byoor ide)

Other Names: Glibenclamide

Introduced: 1970

Prescription: USA: Yes
    Canada: Yes

Available as Generic: No

Brand Names: DiaBeta, ✦Euglucon, Micronase

Class: Antidiabetic, Sulfonylureas

Controlled Drug: USA: No
    Canada: No

BENEFITS versus RISKS	
Possible Benefits	*Possible Risks*
Assistance in regulating blood sugar in noninsulin-dependent diabetes (adjunctive to appropriate diet and weight control)	HYPOGLYCEMIA, severe and prolonged Allergic skin reactions (some severe) Rare liver damage Rare blood cell and bone marrow disorders

---

▷ **Principal Uses**

As a Single Drug Product: To assist in the control of mild to moderately severe type II diabetes mellitus (adult, maturity-onset) that does not require insulin, but that cannot be adequately controlled by diet alone.

How This Drug Works: It is thought that this drug (1) stimulates the secretion of insulin (by a pancreas that is capable of responding to stimulation), and (2) enhances the utilization of insulin by appropriate tissues.

Available Dosage Forms and Strengths

Tablets — 1.25 mg, 2.5 mg, 5 mg

▷ **Usual Adult Dosage Range:** Initially 2.5 to 5 mg daily with breakfast. At 7-day intervals the dose may be increased by increments of 2.5 mg daily as needed and tolerated. Total daily dosage should not exceed 20 mg. A "loading" or priming dose is not necessary and should not be given. **Note: Actual dosage and administration schedule must be determined by the physician for each patient individually.**

Dosing Instructions: If the daily maintenance dose is found to be 10 mg or more, the total dose should be divided into 2 equal doses: the first taken with the morning meal, the second with the evening meal. The tablet may be crushed for administration.

Usual Duration of Use: Continual use on a regular schedule for 1 to 2 weeks is usually necessary to determine this drug's effectiveness in controlling diabetes. Failure to respond to maximal doses within 1 month constitutes a primary failure. Up to 10% of those who respond initially may develop secondary failure of the drug later. The duration of effective use can only be determined by periodic measurement of the blood sugar.

▷ **This Drug Should Not Be Taken If**
- you have had an allergic reaction to it previously.
- you have severe impairment of liver and kidney function.
- you are pregnant.

▷ **Inform Your Physician Before Taking This Drug If**
- you are allergic to other sulfonylurea drugs or to "sulfa" drugs.
- your diabetes has been unstable or "brittle" in the past.
- you do not know how to recognize or treat hypoglycemia (see Glossary).
- you have a history of congestive heart failure, peptic ulcer disease, cirrhosis of the liver, hypothyroidism or porphyria.

Possible Side-Effects   (natural, expected and unavoidable drug actions)

If drug dosage is excessive or food intake is delayed or inadequate, abnormally low blood sugar (hypoglycemia) will occur as a predictable drug effect.

▷ **Possible Adverse Effects**   (unusual, unexpected and infrequent reactions)
If any of the following develop, consult your physician promptly.

Mild Adverse Effects

Allergic Reactions: Skin rash, hives, itching.

Headache, drowsiness, dizziness, fatigue.

Indigestion, heartburn, nausea.

Serious Adverse Effects

Allergic Reactions: Hepatitis with jaundice (see Glossary), severe skin reactions.

Idiosyncratic Reactions: Hemolytic anemia (see Glossary).

Disulfiramlike reaction with concurrent use of alcohol (see Glossary), infrequent with this drug.

Bone marrow depression (see Glossary)—fatigue, weakness, fever, sore throat, abnormal bleeding or bruising.

▷ **Adverse Effects That May Mimic Natural Diseases or Disorders**

Liver reactions may suggest viral hepatitis.

CAUTION
1. This drug must be regarded as only one part of the total program for the management of your diabetes. It is not a substitute for a properly prescribed diet and regular exercise.
2. Over a period of time (usually several months), this drug may lose its effectiveness in controlling blood sugar levels. Periodic follow-up examinations are necessary to monitor all aspects of response to drug treatment.

Precautions for Use

By Infants and Children: This drug is not effective in type I (juvenile, growth-onset) insulin-dependent diabetes.

By Those over 60 Years of Age: This drug should be used with caution in this age group. Start treatment with 1.25 mg/day; increase dosage cautiously and monitor closely to prevent hypoglycemic reactions. Repeated episodes of hypoglycemia in the elderly can cause brain damage.

▷ **Advisability of Use During Pregnancy**

    Pregnancy Category: B (tentative). See Pregnancy Code inside back cover.

    Animal studies: No birth defects reported in rats and rabbits.

    Human studies: Information from adequate studies in pregnant women is not available.

    Because uncontrolled blood sugar levels during pregnancy are associated with a higher incidence of birth defects, many experts recommend that insulin (instead of an oral agent) be used as necessary to control diabetes during the entire pregnancy.

Advisability of Use if Breast-Feeding

    Presence of this drug in breast milk: Unknown.

    Avoid drug or refrain from nursing.

Habit-Forming Potential: None.

Effects of Overdosage: Symptoms of mild to severe hypoglycemia: headache, light-headedness, faintness, nervousness, confusion, tremor, sweating, heart palpitation, weakness, hunger, nausea, vomiting, stupor progressing to coma.

Possible Effects of Long-Term Use: Reduced function of the thyroid gland (hypothyroidism). Reports of increased frequency and severity of heart and blood vessel diseases associated with long-term use of this class of drugs are highly controversial and inconclusive. A direct cause-and-effect relationship (see Glossary) is tenuous. Ask your physician for guidance.

Suggested Periodic Examinations While Taking This Drug   (at physician's discretion)

    Complete blood cell counts, liver function tests, thyroid function tests, periodic evaluation of heart and circulatory system.

▷ **While Taking This Drug, Observe the Following**

    Foods: Follow the diabetic diet prescribed by your physician.

    Beverages: As directed in the diabetic diet. May be taken with milk.

▷   *Alcohol*: Use with extreme caution until the combined effect has been determined. Alcohol can exaggerate this drug's hypoglycemic effect. This drug infrequently causes a marked intolerance of alcohol, resulting in a disulfiramlike reaction (see Glossary): facial flushing, sweating, palpitation.

    Tobacco Smoking: No interactions expected.

▷   *Other Drugs*

      The following drugs may *increase* the effects of glyburide

- aspirin, and other salicylates.
- cimetidine (Tagamet).
- clofibrate (Atromid S).
- fenfluramine (Pondimin).
- monoamine oxidase (MAO) inhibitor drugs (see Drug Class, Section Four).
- phenylbutazone (Butazolidin).
- ranitidine (Zantac).

      The following drugs may *decrease* the effects of glyburide

- beta-blocker drugs (see Drug Class, Section Four).

- bumetanide (Bumex).
- diazoxide (Proglycem).
- ethacrynic acid (Edecrin).
- furosemide (Lasix).
- phenytoin (Dilantin).
- thiazide diuretics (see Drug Class, Section Four).

▷ *Driving, Hazardous Activities*: Regulate your dosage schedule, eating schedule and physical activities very carefully to prevent hypoglycemia. Be able to recognize the early symptoms of hypoglycemia so you can avoid hazardous activities and take corrective measures.

Aviation Note: Diabetes *is a disqualification* for piloting. Consult a designated Aviation Medical Examiner.

Exposure to Sun: Use caution until sensitivity has been determined. Some drugs of this class can cause photosensitivity (see Glossary).

Occurrence of Unrelated Illness: Acute infections, illnesses causing vomiting or diarrhea, serious injuries and surgical procedures can interfere with diabetic control and may require the use of insulin. If any of these conditions occur, consult your physician promptly.

Discontinuation: Because of the possibility of secondary failure, it is advisable to evaluate the continued benefit of this drug every 6 months.

HALOPERIDOL
(hal oh PER i dohl)

Introduced: 1958

Class: Strong Tranquilizer, Butyrophenones

Prescription: USA: Yes
Canada: Yes

Controlled Drug: USA: No
Canada: No

Available as Generic: No

Brand Names: ♣Apo-Haloperidol, Haldol, ♣Novoperidol, ♣Peridol

---

BENEFITS versus RISKS

Possible Benefits	*Possible Risks*
EFFECTIVE CONTROL OF ACUTE FREQUENT PSYCHOSES in majority of patients: beneficial effects on thinking, mood and behavior	FREQUENT PARKINSON-LIKE SIDE-EFFECTS
	SERIOUS TOXIC EFFECTS ON BRAIN with long-term use
EFFECTIVE CONTROL OF SOME CASES OF TOURETTE'S DISORDER	Rare blood cell disorders
	Abnormally low white blood cells
Beneficial in the management of the hyperactive child	

▷ **Principal Uses**

As a Single Drug Product: Used primarily to control the psychotic thinking and abnormal behavior associated with acute psychosis of unknown nature, acute schizophrenia, paranoid states and the manic phase of manic-depressive disorders. It is also used to treat the hyperactivity syndrome in children. A less frequent use is to control the tics and offensive language characteristic of Gilles de la Tourette's syndrome.

How This Drug Works: Not completely established. It is thought that by interfering with the action of dopamine as a nerve impulse transmitter in certain areas of the brain, this drug reduces anxiety and agitation, improves coherence and organization of thinking and abolishes delusions and hallucinations.

Available Dosage Forms and Strengths

> Concentrate — 2 mg per ml
> Injection — 5 mg per ml
> Tablets — 0.5 mg, 1 mg, 2 mg, 5 mg, 10 mg, 20 mg

▷ **Usual Adult Dosage Range:** Initially 0.5 to 2 mg 2 or 3 times daily. Dose may be increased by 0.5 mg/day at 3- to 4-day intervals as needed and tolerated. The usual dosage range is 0.5 to 30 mg/24 hrs. The total daily dosage should not exceed 100 mg. **Note: Actual dosage and administration schedule must be determined by the physician for each patient individually.**

▷ **Dosing Instructions:** May be taken with or following food to reduce stomach irritation. The concentrate may be diluted in 2 ounces of water or fruit juice; do not add it to coffee or tea. The tablet may be crushed for administration.

Usual Duration of Use: Continual use on a regular schedule for several weeks is usually necessary to determine this drug's effectiveness in controlling the symptoms of psychotic or psychoneurotic behavior. If not significantly beneficial within 6 weeks, it should be discontinued. Long-term use requires supervision and periodic evaluation by your physician.

▷ **This Drug Should Not Be Taken If**
- you have had an allergic reaction to any dosage form of it previously.
- you are experiencing mental depression.
- you have any form of Parkinson's disease.
- you have cancer of the breast.
- you have active liver disease.
- you currently have a bone marrow or blood cell disorder.

▷ **Inform Your Physician Before Taking This Drug If**
- you are allergic or abnormally sensitive to phenothiazine drugs.
- you have a history of mental depression.
- you have any type of heart disease.
- you have impaired liver or kidney function.
- you have low blood pressure, epilepsy or glaucoma.
- you are taking any drugs with a sedative effect.

- you plan to have surgery under general or spinal anesthesia in the near future.

Possible Side-Effects   (natural, expected and unavoidable drug actions)

Mild drowsiness, low blood pressure, blurred vision, dry mouth, constipation, marked and frequent Parkinson-like reactions (see Glossary).

▷ **Possible Adverse Effects**   (unusual, unexpected and infrequent reactions)

If any of the following develop, consult your physician promptly.

Mild Adverse Effects

Allergic Reactions: Skin rash, hives.

Dizziness, weakness, agitation, insomnia.

Loss of appetite, indigestion, nausea, vomiting, diarrhea.

Altered menstrual pattern, urinary retention.

Serious Adverse Effects

Allergic Reactions: Rare liver reaction with jaundice, asthma, spasm of vocal cords.

Idiosyncratic Reactions: High fever, weakness, fast heart rate, muscle stiffness, seizures (rare neuroleptic malignant syndrome).

Depression, disorientation, eye damage (deposits in cornea, lens and retina).

Breast enlargement, milk production, sexual impotence.

Blood cell disorders: anemia, fluctuation in number of white blood cells.

Nervous system reactions: rigidity of extremities, tremors, restlessness, constant movement, facial grimacing, eye-rolling, spasm of neck muscles, tardive dyskinesia (see Glossary).

▷ **Adverse Effects That May Mimic Natural Diseases or Disorders**

Liver reaction may suggest viral hepatitis.

Nervous system reactions may suggest Parkinson's disease or Reye syndrome.

Natural Diseases or Disorders That May Be Activated by This Drug

Latent epilepsy, glaucoma, diabetes.

CAUTION

1. It is advisable to use the smallest dose that is effective for long-term treatment.
2. Use with extreme caution in epilepsy; this drug can alter the pattern of seizures.
3. Individuals with lupus erythematosus and those taking prednisone are more susceptible to nervous system reactions.
4. Do not use levodopa to treat Parkinson-like reactions; it can cause agitation and worsening of the psychotic disorder.
5. Obtain prompt evaluation of any change or disturbance in vision.

Precautions for Use

By Infants and Children: This drug should not be used in children under 3 years of age or 15 kilograms in weight. Avoid this drug in the presence of symptoms suggestive of Reye syndrome. Children are quite susceptible to nervous system reactions induced by this drug.

By Those over 60 Years of Age: Initiate treatment with small doses. This drug can cause significant changes in mood and behavior; observe for confusion, disorientation, agitation, restlessness, aggression and paranoia. You may be more susceptible to the development of drowsiness, lethargy, orthostatic hypotension (see Glossary), hypothermia (see Glossary), Parkinson-like reactions and prostatism (see Glossary).

▷ **Advisability of Use During Pregnancy**
Pregnancy Category: C (tentative). See Pregnancy Code inside back cover.
Animal studies: Cleft palate reported in mouse studies.
Human studies: No increase in birth defects reported in 100 exposures. Information from adequate studies in pregnant women is not available.
Avoid during the first trimester. Use only if clearly needed. Ask physician for guidance.

Advisability of Use if Breast-Feeding
Presence of this drug in breast milk: Yes.
Monitor nursing infant closely and discontinue drug or nursing if adverse effects develop.

Habit-Forming Potential: None.

Effects of Overdosage: Marked drowsiness, weakness, tremor, unsteadiness, agitation, stupor, coma, convulsions.

Possible Effects of Long-Term Use: Eye damage: deposits in cornea, lens or retina; tardive dyskinesia (see Glossary).

Suggested Periodic Examinations While Taking This Drug (at physician's discretion)
Complete blood cell counts, liver function tests, eye examinations, electrocardiograms.
Careful inspection of the tongue for early evidence of fine, involuntary, wavelike movements that could indicate the beginning of tardive dyskinesia.

▷ **While Taking This Drug, Observe the Following**
Foods: No restrictions.
Beverages: No restrictions. May be taken with milk.
▷ *Alcohol*: Avoid completely. Alcohol can increase the sedative action of haloperidol and accentuate its depressant effects on brain function. Haloperidol can increase the intoxicating effects of alcohol.
Tobacco Smoking: No interactions expected.
Marijuana Smoking: Moderate increase in drowsiness; accentuation of orthostatic hypotension; increased risk of precipitating latent psychosis, confusing interpretation of mental status and of drug response.
▷ *Other Drugs*
Haloperidol may *increase* the effects of
• all drugs with sedative actions, and cause excessive sedation.
• some antihypertensive drugs, and cause excessive lowering of blood pressure; monitor the combined effects carefully.
Haloperidol may *decrease* the effects of
• guanethidine (Esimil, Ismelin), and reduce its antihypertensive effect.
Haloperidol *taken concurrently* with
• beta-blocker drugs may cause excessive lowering of blood pressure.

- lithium may cause toxic effects on the brain and nervous system.
- methyldopa (Aldomet) may cause serious dementia.

The following drugs may *decrease* the effects of haloperidol

- antacids containing aluminum and/or magnesium may reduce its absorption.
- barbiturates.
- benztropine (Cogentin).
- phenytoin (Dilantin).
- trihexyphenidyl (Artane).

▷ *Driving, Hazardous Activities*: This drug may impair mental alertness, judgment and physical coordination. Restrict activities as necessary.

Aviation Note: The use of this drug *is a disqualification* for piloting. Consult a designated Aviation Medical Examiner.

Exposure to Sun: Use caution until sensitivity has been determined. This drug can cause photosensitivity.

Exposure to Heat: Use caution in hot environments. This drug may impair the regulation of body temperature and increase the risk of heat stroke.

Exposure to Cold: The elderly are advised to use caution; this drug can increase the risk of hypothermia (see Glossary).

Discontinuation: This drug should not be discontinued abruptly following long-term use. Gradual withdrawal over a period of 2 to 3 weeks is advised. Ask physician for guidance.

HYDRALAZINE
(hi DRAL a zeen)

Introduced: 1950

Prescription: USA: Yes
Canada: Yes

Available as Generic: USA: Yes
Canada: No

Class: Antihypertensive

Controlled Drug: USA: No
Canada: No

Brand Names: Apresazide [CD], Apresoline, Apresoline-Esidrix [CD], Hydral [CD], Ser-Ap-Es [CD], Serpasil-Apresoline [CD], Unipres [CD]

BENEFITS versus RISKS

Possible Benefits	*Possible Risks*
EFFECTIVE STEP 2 OR 3 ANTIHYPERTENSIVE FOR MODERATE TO SEVERE HYPERTENSION when used adjunctively with other antihypertensive drugs	DRUG-INDUCED LUPUS ERYTHEMATOSUSLIKE SYNDROME (up to 13%)
Possibly beneficial in the management of severe congestive heart failure	Intensification of angina pectoris Rare blood cell disorders Rare liver damage

---

▷ **Principal Uses**

    As a Single Drug Product: Used primarily as a step 2 or 3 antihypertensive drug in conjunction with other antihypertensives in the treatment of moderate to severe high blood pressure.

    As a Combination Drug Product [CD]: This drug is available in combination with hydrochlorothiazide (a diuretic) and with reserpine (another type of antihypertensive). When used in combination, several different types of drug action occur concurrently to reduce blood pressure: hydralazine relaxes and expands blood vessel walls; the diuretic reduces the amount of water and sodium in the body; reserpine reduces the rate and contraction force of the heart and enhances the expansion of blood vessels.

How This Drug Works: By causing direct relaxation of arterial walls (mechanism unknown), this drug dilates peripheral blood vessels, with resultant lowering of blood pressure. The dilation of blood vessels can also be beneficial in some cases of heart failure by reducing the workload of the heart and increasing its output.

Available Dosage Forms and Strengths
    Tablets — 10 mg, 25 mg, 50 mg, 100 mg

▷ **Usual Adult Dosage Range:**   Initially 10 mg 4 times daily for 2 to 4 days; then increase to 25 mg 4 times daily for the balance of the first week. During the second week the dose may be increased to 50 mg 4 times daily if needed and tolerated. The total daily dosage should not exceed 300 mg for fast acetylators or 200 mg for slow acetylators. Ask your physician for guidance. **Note: Actual dosage and administration schedule must be determined by the physician for each patient individually.**

▷ **Dosing Instructions:**   Preferably taken with or following meals to enhance absorption and reduce stomach irritation. The tablet may be crushed and the capsule [CD] may be opened for administration.

Usual Duration of Use: Continual use on a regular schedule for several weeks is usually necessary to determine this drug's effectiveness in lowering blood pressure. Long-term use requires supervision and periodic evaluation by your physician.

▷ **This Drug Should Not Be Taken If**
- you have had an allergic reaction to it previously.
- you have active angina pectoris.
- you have mitral valvular heart disease.

▷ **Inform Your Physician Before Taking This Drug If**
- you have a history of any type of heart disease.
- you have lupus erythematosus.
- you have impaired brain circulation.
- you are subject to migraine headaches.
- you have impaired kidney function.
- you have a history of liver sensitivity to other drugs.
- you plan to have surgery under general anesthesia in the near future.

Possible Side-Effects (natural, expected and unavoidable drug actions)
Orthostatic hypotension (see Glossary), nasal congestion, constipation, delayed or impaired urination, increased heart rate of 10 to 25 beats/minute.

▷ **Possible Adverse Effects** (unusual, unexpected and infrequent reactions)
If any of the following develop, consult your physician promptly.
Mild Adverse Effects
Allergic Reactions: Skin rash, hives, itching, drug fever.
Headache, dizziness, flushing of face, palpitation.
Loss of appetite, nausea, vomiting, diarrhea.
Tremors, muscle cramps.
Serious Adverse Effects
Allergic Reactions: Liver reaction, with or without jaundice.
Idiosyncratic Reactions: Behavioral changes: nervousness, confusion, emotional depression. Bleeding into lung tissue: densities found on X-ray examination. A syndrome resembling rheumatoid arthritis or lupus erythematosus (see Glossary).
Intensification of coronary artery disease.
Peripheral neuropathy (see Glossary): weakness, numbness and/or pain in extremities.
Rare bone marrow depression (see Glossary): fatigue, weakness, fever, sore throat, abnormal bleeding or bruising.

▷ **Adverse Effects That May Mimic Natural Diseases or Disorders**
Drug fever may suggest systemic infection. Liver reaction may suggest viral hepatitis. Skin and joint symptoms may suggest lupus erythematosus.

Natural Diseases or Disorders That May Be Activated by This Drug
Latent coronary artery disease.

CAUTION
1. Toxic reactions are more likely to occur with large doses. Adhere strictly to prescribed dosage schedules. Keep appointments for periodic follow-up examinations.
2. Report the development of any tendency to emotional depression.
3. This drug can cause salt and water retention if a diuretic is not taken concurrently.
4. This drug can provoke migraine headache.

Precautions for Use
By Infants and Children: Dosage is based upon age, weight and kidney function status. Observe for the possible development of a lupus erythematosuslike reaction.
By Those over 60 Years of Age: Initiate treatment with low doses and proceed cautiously. Unacceptably high blood pressure should be reduced without creating the risks associated with excessively low blood pressure. Sudden, rapid and excessive reduction of blood pressure can predispose to stroke or heart attack. Observe for possible dizziness, unsteadiness, faint-

ing or falling. Headache, palpitation and rapid heart rates are more common in the elderly and can mimic acute anxiety states.

▷ **Advisability of Use During Pregnancy**

Pregnancy Category: C (tentative). See Pregnancy Code inside back cover.
Animal studies: Birth defects of head and facial bones reported in mice.
Human studies: Information from adequate studies in pregnant women is not available.
Avoid use during the first and last 3 months; if taken late in pregnancy, this drug can cause a deficiency of blood platelets (see Glossary) in the newborn infant.

Advisability of Use if Breast-Feeding

Presence of this drug in breast milk: Yes.
Avoid drug or refrain from nursing.

Habit-Forming Potential: None.

Effects of Overdosage: Marked light-headedness, dizziness, headache, flushing of skin, nausea, vomiting, collapse of circulation: loss of consciousness, cold and sweaty skin, weak and rapid pulse, irregular heart rhythm.

Possible Effects of Long-Term Use: An acute or subacute syndrome resembling rheumatoid arthritis or lupus erythematosus, usually seen in slow acetylators taking daily doses of over 200 mg.

Suggested Periodic Examinations While Taking This Drug (at physician's discretion)
Complete blood cell counts, liver function tests, blood tests for evidence of lupus erythematosus.

▷ **While Taking This Drug, Observe the Following**

Foods: No restrictions.
Nutritional Support: Monitor for peripheral neuropathy and take a supplement of pyridoxine (vitamin B-6) as needed. Ask physician for guidance.
Beverages: No restrictions. May be taken with milk.
▷   *Alcohol*: Use with extreme caution until the combined effect has been determined. Alcohol can exaggerate the blood-pressure-lowering effect of this drug and cause excessive reduction.
Tobacco Smoking: Avoid completely. Nicotine can contribute significantly to this drug's ability to intensify angina in susceptible individuals.
▷   *Other Drugs*
Hydralazine may *increase* the effects of
- metoprolol (Lopressor).
- oxprenolol (Trasicor).
- propranolol (Inderal).
▷   *Driving, Hazardous Activities*: This drug may cause light-headedness or dizziness. Restrict activities as necessary.
Aviation Note: Hypertension and the use of this drug *are disqualifications* for piloting. Consult a designated Aviation Medical Examiner.
Exposure to Sun: No restrictions.

Exposure to Heat: Caution advised. Hot environments may reduce blood pressure significantly.

Exposure to Cold: Caution advised. Cold environments may increase this drug's ability to cause angina in susceptible individuals.

Heavy Exercise or Exertion: Caution advised. Excessive exertion can increase this drug's ability to cause angina in susceptible individuals. Also, isometric exercises can raise blood pressure significantly.

HYDROCHLOROTHIAZIDE
(hi droh klor oh THI a zide)

Introduced: 1959

Class: Antihypertensive, Diuretic, Thiazides

Prescription: USA: Yes
Canada: Yes

Controlled Drug: USA: No
Canada: No

Available as Generic: USA: Yes
Canada: Yes

Brand Names: Aldactazide [CD], Aldoril [CD], ♣Apo-Hydro, Apresazide [CD], Apresoline-Esidrix [CD], Capozide [CD], ♣Diuchlor H, Dyazide [CD], Esidrix, Hydral [CD], HydroDIURIL, Hydro Plus [CD], Hydropres [CD], Hydro-Z-50, Inderide [CD], Moduretic [CD], ♣Natrimax, ♣Nefrol, ♣Neo-Codema, ♣Novohydrazide, Oretic, Ser-Ap-Es [CD], Serpasil-Esidrix [CD], SK-Hydrochlorothiazide, Thiuretic, Timolide [CD], Unipres [CD], ♣Urozide, Zide

---

BENEFITS versus RISKS

Possible Benefits	*Possible Risks*
EFFECTIVE, WELL-TOLERATED DIURETIC	Loss of body potassium
	Increased blood sugar
POSSIBLY EFFECTIVE IN MILD HYPERTENSION	Increased blood uric acid
	Increased blood calcium
ENHANCES EFFECTIVENESS OF OTHER ANTIHYPERTENSIVES	Rare blood cell disorders
Beneficial in treatment of diabetes insipidus	

▷ **Principal Uses**

As a Single Drug Product: Thiazide diuretics are used primarily to (1) increase the volume of urine (diuresis) to correct the excessive fluid retention associated with congestive heart failure and certain types of liver and kidney disease; and (2) initiate treatment for high blood pressure (hypertension). They are often the first drugs tried in treating mild to moderate hypertension. Less frequent uses include the treatment of diabetes insipidus and the prevention of kidney stones that contain calcium.

As a Combination Drug Product [CD]: When this drug is used alone to treat hypertension, it is referred to as a "step 1" antihypertensive. Should it fail to reduce the blood pressure adequately, a "step 2" antihypertensive drug is added to be taken concurrently with the "step 1" drug. These drugs may be combined into one drug product. Thiazides are available in combination with beta-blockers, hydralazine, methyldopa, reserpine and other diuretics to increase their effectiveness in treating hypertension.

How This Drug Works: By increasing the elimination of salt and water from the body (through increased urine production), this drug reduces the volume of fluid in the blood and body tissues and lowers the sodium content throughout the body. By relaxing the walls of smaller arteries and allowing them to expand, this drug increases the total capacity of the arterial system. The combined effect of these two actions (reduced blood volume in expanded space) results in lowering of the blood pressure.

Available Dosage Forms and Strengths
>   Solution — 50 mg per 5 ml teaspoonful
>   Solution, intensol — 100 mg per ml
>   Tablets — 25 mg, 50 mg, 100 mg

▷ **Usual Adult Dosage Range:**   As antihypertensive: 50 to 100 mg/day initially; 50 to 200 mg/day for maintenance. As diuretic: 50 to 200 mg/day initially; the smallest effective dose should be determined. The total daily dose should not exceed 200 mg. **Note: Actual dosage and administration schedule must be determined by the physician for each patient individually.**

▷ **Dosing Instructions:**   May be taken with or following meals to reduce stomach irritation. Best taken in the morning to avoid nighttime urination. The tablet may be crushed for administration.

Usual Duration of Use: Continual use on a regular schedule for 2 to 3 weeks is usually necessary to determine this drug's effectiveness in lowering high blood pressure. Long-term use (months to years) requires periodic evaluation of response and possible dosage adjustment. Use as a diuretic should be intermittent with "drug holidays" (no drug taken) to reduce the risk of sodium and potassium imbalance.

▷ **This Drug Should Not Be Taken If**
  • you have had an allergic reaction to any dosage form of it previously.

▷ **Inform Your Physician Before Taking This Drug If**
  • you are allergic to any form of "sulfa" drug.
  • you are pregnant or planning pregnancy.
  • you have a history of kidney or liver disease.
  • you have a history of pancreatitis.
  • you have diabetes, gout or lupus erythematosus.
  • you are taking any form of cortisone, digitalis, oral antidiabetic drug or insulin.
  • you plan to have surgery under general anesthesia in the near future.

Possible Side-Effects   (natural, expected and unavoidable drug actions)

Light-headedness on arising from sitting or lying position (see orthostatic hypotension in Glossary).

Increase in blood sugar level, affecting control of diabetes.

Increase in blood uric acid level, affecting control of gout.

Decrease in blood potassium level, causing muscle weakness and cramping.

▷ **Possible Adverse Effects**   (unusual, unexpected and infrequent reactions)

If any of the following develop, consult your physician promptly.

Mild Adverse Effects

Allergic Reactions: Skin rashes, hives, drug fever.

Headache, dizziness, blurred or yellow vision.

Reduced appetite, indigestion, nausea, vomiting, diarrhea.

Serious Adverse Effects

Allergic Reactions: Hepatitis with jaundice (see Glossary), anaphylactic reaction (see Glossary), severe skin reactions.

Inflammation of the pancreas—severe abdominal pain.

Bone marrow depression (see Glossary)—fatigue, weakness, fever, sore throat, abnormal bleeding or bruising.

▷ **Adverse Effects That May Mimic Natural Diseases or Disorders**

Liver reaction may suggest viral hepatitis.

Natural Diseases or Disorders That May Be Activated by This Drug

Diabetes, gout, systemic lupus erythematosus.

CAUTION

1. Do not exceed recommended doses. Increased dosage can cause excessive loss of sodium and potassium, with resultant loss of appetite, nausea, fatigue, weakness, confusion and tingling in the extremities.

2. If you are also taking a digitalis preparation (digitoxin, digoxin), ensure an adequate intake of high-potassium foods to prevent potassium deficiency—a potential cause of digitalis toxicity. (See Table of High Potassium Foods in Section Six.)

Precautions for Use

By Infants and Children: Avoid overdosage that could cause serious dehydration. Significant potassium loss can occur within the first 2 weeks of drug use.

By Those over 60 Years of Age: Small doses are advisable until your individual response has been determined. You may be more susceptible to the development of impaired thinking, orthostatic hypotension, potassium loss and blood sugar increase. Overdosage and extended use of this drug can cause excessive loss of body water, thickening (increased viscosity) of the blood and an increased tendency for the blood to clot—predisposing to stroke, heart attack or thrombophlebitis (vein inflammation with blood clot).

▷ **Advisability of Use During Pregnancy**

Pregnancy Category: D (tentative). See Pregnancy Code inside back cover.

Animal studies: No birth defects found in rat studies.

Human studies: Reports are conflicting and inconclusive. This drug does not seem to carry the risk of birth defects that has been found with other related diuretics. However, other types of fetal injury are possible with this drug. It should not be used during pregnancy unless a very serious complication occurs for which this drug is significantly beneficial. Ask physician for guidance.

Advisability of Use if Breast-Feeding

Presence of this drug in breast milk: Yes.

Avoid drug or refrain from nursing.

Habit-Forming Potential: None.

Effects of Overdosage: Dry mouth, thirst, lethargy, weakness, muscle cramping, nausea, vomiting, drowsiness progressing to stupor or coma.

Possible Effects of Long-Term Use: Impaired balance of water, salt and potassium in blood and body tissues. Development of diabetes in predisposed individuals. Pathological changes in parathyroid glands with increased blood calcium levels and decreased blood phosphate levels.

Suggested Periodic Examinations While Taking This Drug   (at physician's discretion)

Complete blood cell counts, measurements of blood levels of sodium, potassium, chloride, sugar and uric acid.

Kidney and liver function tests.

▷ **While Taking This Drug, Observe the Following**

Foods: Consult your physician regarding the advisability of eating foods rich in potassium. If so advised, see the Table of High Potassium Foods in Section Six. Follow physician's advice regarding the use of salt.

Beverages: No restrictions. This drug may be taken with milk.

▷   *Alcohol*: Use with caution until the combined effects have been determined. Alcohol may exaggerate the blood-pressure-lowering effects of this drug and cause orthostatic hypotension.

Tobacco Smoking: No interactions expected. Follow physician's advice.

▷   *Other Drugs*

Hydrochlorothiazide may *increase* the effects of

- other antihypertensive drugs; dosage adjustments may be necessary to prevent excessive lowering of blood pressure.
- lithium, and cause lithium toxicity.

Hydrochlorothiazide may *decrease* the effects of

- oral antidiabetic drugs (sulfonylureas); dosage adjustments may be necessary for proper control of blood sugar.

Hydrochlorothiazide *taken concurrently* with

- digitalis preparations (digitoxin, digoxin) requires very careful monitoring and dosage adjustments to prevent fluctuations of blood potassium levels and serious disturbances of heart rhythm.

The following drugs may *decrease* the effects of hydrochlorothiazide
- cholestyramine (Cuemid, Questran) may interfere with its absorption.
- colestipol (Colestid) may interfere with its absorption.

Take cholestyramine and colestipol 1 hour before any oral diuretic.

▷ *Driving, Hazardous Activities*: Use caution until the possible occurrence of orthostatic hypotension, dizziness or impaired vision has been determined.

Aviation Note: The use of this drug *may be a disqualification* for piloting. Consult a designated Aviation Medical Examiner.

Exposure to Sun: Use caution until sensitivity has been determined. This drug can cause photosensitivity (see Glossary).

Exposure to Heat: Avoid excessive perspiring, which could cause additional loss of salt and water from the body.

Heavy Exercise or Exertion: Avoid exertion that produces light-headedness, excessive fatigue or muscle cramping. Isometric exercises—the "overload" technique for strengthening individual muscles—can raise blood pressure significantly. Ask physician for guidance regarding participation in this form of exercise.

Occurrence of Unrelated Illness: Illnesses that cause vomiting or diarrhea can produce a serious imbalance of important body chemistry. Consult your physician for guidance.

Discontinuation: This drug should not be stopped abruptly following long-term use; sudden discontinuation can cause serious thiazide-withdrawal fluid retention (edema). The dose should be reduced gradually. It may be advisable to discontinue this drug 5 to 7 days before major surgery. Ask your physician, surgeon and/or anesthesiologist for guidance regarding dosage adjustment or drug withdrawal.

HYDROCODONE
(hi droh KOH dohn)

Other Names: Dihydrocodeinone

Introduced: 1951

Class: Analgesic, Narcotic; Cough Suppressant

Prescription: USA: Yes
Canada: Yes

Controlled Drug: USA: C-III*
Canada: <N>

Available as Generic: No

Brand Names: ✤Hycodan, Hycodan [CD], ✤Hycomine [CD], Hycomine Compound [CD], Hycomine Pediatric Syrup [CD], ✤Hycomine-S [CD], Hycomine Syrup [CD], Hycotuss Expectorant [CD], ✤Robidone, Triaminic Expectorant DH [CD], Tussend [CD], Tussend Expectorant [CD], Tussionex [CD], Vicodin [CD]

*See Schedules of Controlled Drugs inside back cover.

BENEFITS versus RISKS

Possible Benefits	*Possible Risks*
EFFECTIVE RELIEF OF MILD TO MODERATE PAIN	Low potential for habit formation (dependence)
EFFECTIVE CONTROL OF COUGH	Mild allergic reactions (infrequent)
	Nausea, constipation

▷ **Principal Uses**

As a Single Drug Product: Used primarily to (1) control cough; (2) relieve mild to moderate pain. Its widest use is as an ingredient in cough remedies.

As a Combination Drug Product [CD]: Hydrocodone is frequently added to cough mixtures containing antihistamines, decongestants and expectorants to make these "shotgun" preparations more effective in reducing the frequency and severity of cough. It is also combined with milder analgesics, such as acetaminophen and aspirin, to enhance pain relief.

How This Drug Works: Acting primarily as a depressant of certain brain functions, this drug suppresses the perception of pain, calms the emotional response to pain and reduces the sensitivity of the cough reflex.

Available Dosage Forms and Strengths

Syrup — 5 mg per 5 ml teaspoonful

Tablets — 5 mg

▷ **Usual Adult Dosage Range:** As analgesic—5 to 10 mg/4 to 6 hrs as needed. For cough—5 mg/4 to 6 hrs as needed. Total daily dosage should not exceed 60 mg. **Note: Actual dosage and administration schedule must be determined by the physician for each patient individually.**

▷ **Dosing Instructions:** May be taken with or following food to reduce stomach irritation or nausea. Tablet may be crushed for administration.

Usual Duration of Use: As required, to control pain or cough. Continual use should not exceed 5 to 7 days without interruption and reassessment of need.

▷ **This Drug Should Not Be Taken If**
- you have had an allergic reaction to any dosage form of it previously.
- you are having an acute attack of asthma.

▷ **Inform Your Physician Before Taking This Drug If**
- you have had an unfavorable reaction to any narcotic drug in the past.
- you have a history of drug abuse or alcoholism.
- you have chronic lung disease with impaired breathing.
- you have impaired liver or kidney function.
- you have gallbladder disease, a seizure disorder or an underactive thyroid gland.
- you have difficulty emptying the urinary bladder.
- you are taking any other drugs that have a sedative effect.
- you plan to have surgery under general anesthesia in the near future.

Possible Side-Effects   (natural, expected and unavoidable drug actions)
Drowsiness, light-headedness, dry mouth, urinary retention, constipation.

▷ **Possible Adverse Effects**   (unusual, unexpected and infrequent reactions)
If any of the following develop, consult your physician promptly.
Mild Adverse Effects
Allergic Reactions: Skin rash, hives, itching.
Dizziness, impaired concentration, sensation of drunkenness, confusion, depression, blurred or double vision, facial flushing, sweating.
Nausea, vomiting.
Serious Adverse Effects
Allergic Reactions: Anaphylaxis (rare), severe skin reactions.
Idiosyncratic Reactions: Delirium, hallucinations, excitement, increased sensitivity to pain after the analgesic effect has worn off.
Seizures (rare), impaired breathing.

▷ **Adverse Effects That May Mimic Natural Diseases or Disorders**
Paradoxical behavioral disturbances may suggest psychotic disorder.

CAUTION
1. If you have asthma, chronic bronchitis or emphysema, the excessive use of this drug may cause significant respiratory difficulty, thickening of bronchial secretions and suppression of coughing.
2. The concurrent use of this drug with atropinelike drugs can increase the risk of urinary retention and reduced intestinal function.
3. Do not take this drug following acute head injury.

Precautions for Use
By Infants and Children: Do not use this drug in children under 2 years of age because of their vulnerability to life-threatening respiratory depression.
By Those over 60 Years of Age: Use small doses initially and increase dosage as needed and tolerated. Limit use to short-term treatment only. There may be increased susceptibility to the development of drowsiness, dizziness, unsteadiness, falling, urinary retention and constipation (often leading to fecal impaction).

▷ **Advisability of Use During Pregnancy**
Pregnancy Category: C (tentative). See Pregnancy Code inside back cover.
Animal studies: Birth defects reported in hamster studies.
Human studies: Information from adequate studies in pregnant women is not available. Hydrocodone taken repeatedly during the last few weeks before delivery may cause withdrawal symptoms in the newborn infant.
Use this drug only if clearly needed and in small, infrequent doses.

Advisability of Use if Breast-Feeding
Presence of this drug in breast milk: Unknown.
Monitor nursing infant closely and discontinue drug or nursing if adverse effects develop. Ask physician for guidance.

Habit-Forming Potential: Psychological and/or physical dependence can develop with use of large doses for an extended period of time. However, true dependence is infrequent and unlikely with prudent use.

Effects of Overdosage: Drowsiness, restlessness, agitation, nausea, vomiting, dry mouth, vertigo, weakness, lethargy, stupor, coma, seizures.

Possible Effects of Long-Term Use: Psychological and physical dependence, chronic constipation.

Suggested Periodic Examinations While Taking This Drug   (at physician's discretion)
None.

▷ **While Taking This Drug, Observe the Following**
Foods: No restrictions.
Beverages: No restrictions. May be taken with milk.
▷   *Alcohol*: Use extreme caution until the combined effects have been determined. Hydrocodone can intensify the intoxicating effects of alcohol, and alcohol can intensify the depressant effects of hydrocodone on brain function, breathing and circulation.
Tobacco Smoking: No interactions expected.
Marijuana Smoking: Increase in drowsiness and pain relief; impairment of mental and physical performance.
▷   *Other Drugs*
Hydrocodone may *increase* the effects of
- other drugs with sedative effects.
- atropinelike drugs, and increase the risk of constipation and urinary retention.
▷   *Driving, Hazardous Activities*: This drug can impair mental alertness, judgment, reaction time and physical coordination. Avoid hazardous activities accordingly.
Aviation Note: The use of this drug *is a disqualification* for piloting. Consult a designated Aviation Medical Examiner.
Exposure to Sun: No restrictions.
Discontinuation: It is advisable to limit this drug to short-term use. If it is necessary to use it for extended periods of time, discontinuation should be gradual to minimize possible effects of withdrawal (usually mild with this drug).

HYDROXYZINE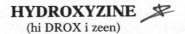
(hi DROX i zeen)

Introduced: 1953

Class: Mild Tranquilizer, Antihistamines

Prescription: USA: Yes
Canada: Yes

Controlled Drug: USA: No
Canada: No

Available as Generic: USA: Yes
Canada: No

Brand Names: Atarax, Enarax [CD], Marax [CD], Marax DF [CD], ✦Multipax, Vistaril, Vistrax [CD]

BENEFITS versus RISKS

Possible Benefits	*Possible Risks*
EFFECTIVE RELIEF OF ITCHING DUE TO HIVES	Mild atropinelike effects
	Potentiation of other sedative drugs
Moderately effective relief of itching due to allergic skin disorders	Impaired control of seizure disorders (epilepsy)
Moderately effective relief of mild to moderate anxiety and nervous tension	

▷ **Principal Uses**

As a Single Drug Product: Used primarily as a mild tranquilizer to relieve anxiety and nervous tension, whether occurring independently or in association with a physical disorder. Also used frequently to relieve itching due to allergic skin conditions.

As a Combination Drug Product [CD]: Combined with antispasmodic drugs, this drug helps to allay the anxiety that is conducive to functional disorders of the gastrointestinal tract. Combined with ephedrine and theophylline (bronchodilator drugs), this drug controls the anxiety that is often associated with bronchial spasm in asthma, bronchitis and emphysema.

How This Drug Works: Not completely established. It is thought that this drug may reduce excessive activity in those brain systems that determine the emotional state.

Available Dosage Forms and Strengths
```
        Capsules — 25 mg, 50 mg, 100 mg
      Injections — 25 mg per ml, 50 mg per ml
  Suspension, oral — 25 mg per 5ml teaspoonful
           Syrup — 10 mg per 5 ml teaspoonful
         Tablets — 10 mg, 25 mg, 50 mg, 100 mg
```

▷ **Usual Adult Dosage Range:**   25 to 100 mg 3 or 4 times daily. The total daily dosage should not exceed 600 mg. **Note: Actual dosage and administration schedule must be determined by the physician for each patient individually.**

▷ **Dosing Instructions:**   May be taken without regard to eating. The tablet may be crushed and the capsule may be opened for administration.

Usual Duration of Use: Continual use on a regular schedule for 1 to 3 weeks is usually necessary to determine this drug's effectiveness in relieving anxiety and tension. Relief of itching is usually apparent in 2 to 3 days. Duration of use as a tranquilizer should not exceed 4 months without reappraisal of continued need.

▷ **This Drug Should Not Be Taken If**
- you have had an allergic reaction to any dosage form of it previously.

▷ **Inform Your Physician Before Taking This Drug If**
- you have a seizure disorder (epilepsy).
- you have prostatism (see Glossary).
- you are taking any drugs with sedative effects.
- you plan to have surgery under general anesthesia in the near future.

Possible Side-Effects (natural, expected and unavoidable drug actions)
Drowsiness (may subside with continued use); "hangover" effect if taken at bedtime for sleep; dry mouth.

▷ **Possible Adverse Effects** (unusual, unexpected and infrequent reactions)
If any of the following develop, consult your physician promptly.
Mild Adverse Effects
Allergic Reactions: Itching.
Headache.
Serious Adverse Effects
Idiosyncratic Reactions: Involuntary movements, tremors, seizures (with excessive dosage).

Natural Diseases or Disorders That May Be Activated by This Drug
Latent epilepsy.

CAUTION
1. This drug can cause excessive sedation if taken concurrently with other sedative drugs.
2. Use very cautiously if you have a seizure disorder. This drug may increase the frequency of seizures.
3. If pregnancy occurs, discontinue this drug immediately and inform your physician.

Precautions for Use
By Infants and Children: Observe for evidence of excessive sedation.
By Those over 60 Years of Age: There may be increased susceptibility to the development of drowsiness, dizziness and lethargy, and to impairment of thinking, judgment and memory. A pattern of underactivity may be misinterpreted as senility or emotional depression. Observe also for orthostatic hypotension and prostatism (see Glossary).

▷ **Advisability of Use During Pregnancy**
Pregnancy Category: C (tentative). See Pregnancy Code inside back cover.
Animal studies: Facial bone defects reported in mice, rats and dogs.
Human studies: Information from adequate studies in pregnant women is not available.
Avoid completely during the first 3 months. During the last 6 months, use only if clearly needed. Ask physician for guidance.

Advisability of Use if Breast-Feeding
Presence of this drug in breast milk: Yes.
Monitor nursing infant closely and discontinue drug or nursing if adverse effects (sedation, poor feeding) develop.

Habit-Forming Potential: None.

Effects of Overdosage: Drowsiness, unsteadiness, dry mouth, delirium, stupor, tremors, seizures.

Possible Effects of Long-Term Use: Loss of drug effectiveness due to development of tolerance (see Glossary).

Suggested Periodic Examinations While Taking This Drug   (at physician's discretion)
   None required.

▷ **While Taking This Drug, Observe the Following**
   Foods: No restrictions.
   Beverages: Avoid large amounts of caffeine-containing beverages: coffee, tea, cola, chocolate. May be taken with milk.
▷   *Alcohol*: Use with extreme caution until the combined effects have been determined. Alcohol can increase the sedative action of hydroxyzine. Hydroxyzine can increase the intoxicating effect of alcohol.
   Tobacco Smoking: No interactions expected.
   Marijuana Smoking: Increased sedative effects.
▷   *Other Drugs*
   Hydroxyzine may *increase* the effects of
   • ketamine (intravenous anesthetic), and prolong the recovery time.
   • other drugs with sedative effects, and cause excessive sedation.
   Hydroxyzine may *decrease* the effects of
   • phenothiazines (see Drug Class, Section Four), and reduce their antipsychotic effectiveness.
▷   *Driving, Hazardous Activities*: This drug may impair mental alertness, judgment, coordination and reaction time. Restrict activities as necessary.
   Aviation Note: The use of this drug *is a disqualification* for piloting. Consult a designated Aviation Medical Examiner.
   Exposure to Sun: No restrictions.

IBUPROFEN ⌧
(i BYU proh fen)

Introduced: 1969	**Class:** Mild Analgesic, Anti-inflammatory
Prescription: USA: Varies Canada: Yes	**Controlled Drug:** USA: No Canada: No

Available as Generic: Yes

Brand Names: Advil, ✤Amersol, ✤Apo-Ibuprofen, Motrin, ✤Novoprofen, Nuprin, Rufen

---

BENEFITS versus RISKS

Possible Benefits	*Possible Risks*
EFFECTIVE RELIEF OF MILD TO MODERATE PAIN AND INFLAMMATION	Gastrointestinal pain, ulceration, bleeding (rare) Rare kidney damage Rare fluid retention Rare bone marrow depression (less than 1%)

▷ **Principal Uses**

As a Single Drug Product: Used primarily to relieve mild to moderately severe pain associated with (1) musculoskeletal injuries; (2) acute and chronic gout, rheumatoid arthritis and osteoarthritis; (3) dental, obstetrical and orthopedic surgery; (4) menstrual cramps; (5) vascular (migrainelike) headaches; and (6) to reduce fever.

How This Drug Works: Not completely established. It is thought that this drug reduces the tissue concentrations of prostaglandins (and related compounds), chemicals involved in the production of inflammation and pain.

Available Dosage Forms and Strengths

Tablets — 200 mg, 300 mg, 400 mg, 600 mg, 800 mg

▷ **Usual Adult Dosage Range:**   200 to 800 mg 3 or 4 times/day. Total daily dosage should not exceed 3200 mg (3600 mg in selected individuals). **Note: Actual dosage and administration schedule must be determined by the physician for each patient individually.**

▷ **Dosing Instructions:**   Take either on an empty stomach or with food or milk to prevent stomach irritation. Take with a full glass of water and remain upright (do not lie down) for 30 minutes. The tablet may be crushed for administration.

Usual Duration of Use: Continual use on a regular schedule for 1 to 2 weeks is usually necessary to determine this drug's effectiveness in relieving the discomfort of arthritis. Long-term use requires supervision and periodic evaluation by the physician.

▷ **This Drug Should Not Be Taken If**
- you have had an allergic reaction to it previously.
- you are subject to asthma or nasal polyps caused by aspirin.
- you have active peptic ulcer disease or any form of gastrointestinal bleeding.
- you have a bleeding disorder or a blood cell disorder.
- you have severe impairment of kidney function.

▷ **Inform Your Physician Before Taking This Drug If**
- you are allergic to aspirin or to other aspirin substitutes.
- you have a history of peptic ulcer disease or any type of bleeding disorder.
- you have impaired liver or kidney function.

- you have high blood pressure or a history of heart failure.
- you are taking any of the following: acetaminophen, aspirin or other aspirin substitutes, anticoagulants, oral antidiabetic drugs.

Possible Side-Effects   (natural, expected and unavoidable drug actions)
Fluid retention (weight gain); pink, red, purple or rust coloration of urine (of no significance).

▷ **Possible Adverse Effects**   (unusual, unexpected and infrequent reactions)
If any of the following develop, consult your physician promptly.
Mild Adverse Effects
Allergic Reactions: Skin rash, hives, itching.
Headache, dizziness, altered or blurred vision, ringing in the ears, depression.
Mouth sores, indigestion, nausea, vomiting, constipation, diarrhea.
Serious Adverse Effects
Allergic Reactions: Anaphylaxis (see Glossary), severe skin reactions.
Idiosyncratic Reactions: Drug-induced meningitis with fever and coma.
Active peptic ulcer, with or without bleeding.
Liver damage with jaundice (see Glossary).
Kidney damage with painful urination, bloody urine, reduced urine formation.
Rare bone marrow depression (see Glossary)—fatigue, weakness, fever, sore throat, abnormal bleeding or bruising.

Possible Delayed Adverse Effects
Mild anemia due to "silent" blood loss from the stomach (less than that caused by aspirin).

▷ **Adverse Effects That May Mimic Natural Diseases or Disorders**
Liver reaction may suggest viral hepatitis.

Natural Diseases or Disorders That May Be Activated by This Drug
Peptic ulcer disease, ulcerative colitis.

CAUTION
1. Dosage should always be limited to the smallest amount that produces reasonable improvement.
2. This drug may mask early indications of infection. Inform your physician if you think you are developing an infection of any kind.

Precautions for Use
By Infants and Children: Safety and effectiveness for use by those under 12 years of age have not been established.
By Those over 60 Years of Age: Small doses are advisable until tolerance is determined. Observe for any indications of liver or kidney toxicity, fluid retention, dizziness, confusion, impaired memory, stomach bleeding or constipation.

▷ **Advisability of Use During Pregnancy**
Pregnancy Category: B (tentative). See Pregnancy Code inside back cover.
Animal studies: No birth defects reported in rats or rabbits.

Human studies: Information from adequate studies in pregnant women is not available.

Avoid this drug during the last 3 months. Use it during the first 6 months only if clearly needed. Ask physician for guidance.

The manufacturer does not recommend the use of this drug during pregnancy.

Advisability of Use if Breast-Feeding

Presence of this drug in breast milk: Yes, in minute amounts.

Avoid drug or refrain from nursing.

Habit-Forming Potential: None.

Effects of Overdosage: Drowsiness, dizziness, ringing in the ears, nausea, vomiting, diarrhea, confusion, unsteadiness, stupor progressing to coma.

Possible Effects of Long-Term Use: Fluid retention.

Suggested Periodic Examinations While Taking This Drug (at physician's discretion)

Complete blood cell counts, liver and kidney function tests, complete eye examinations if vision is altered in any way.

▷ **While Taking This Drug, Observe the Following**

Foods: No restrictions.

Beverages: No restrictions. May be taken with milk.

▷ *Alcohol*: Use with caution. The irritant action of alcohol on the stomach lining, added to the irritant action of this drug in sensitive individuals, can increase the risk of stomach ulceration and/or bleeding.

Tobacco Smoking: No interactions expected.

▷ *Other Drugs*

Ibuprofen may *increase* the effects of

- acetaminophen (Tylenol, etc.), and increase the risk of kidney damage; avoid prolonged use of this combination.
- anticoagulants (Coumadin, etc.), and increase the risk of bleeding; monitor prothrombin time, adjust dose accordingly.

Ibuprofen *taken concurrently* with the following drugs may increase the risk of bleeding; avoid these combinations:

- aspirin.
- dipyridamole (Persantine).
- indomethacin (Indocin).
- sulfinpyrazone (Anturane).
- valproic acid (Depakene).

▷ *Driving, Hazardous Activities*: This drug may cause drowsiness or dizziness. Restrict activities as necessary.

Aviation Note: The use of this drug *may be a disqualification* for piloting. Consult a designated Aviation Medical Examiner.

Exposure to Sun: Use caution until sensitivity is determined. Questionable photosensitivity (see Glossary) has been reported.

INDAPAMIDE
(in DAP a mide)

Introduced: 1974

Prescription: USA: Yes
     Canada: Yes

Available as Generic: No

Brand Names: ♣Lozide, Lozol

Class: Antihypertensive, Diuretic

Controlled Drug: USA: No
     Canada: No

BENEFITS versus RISKS

Possible Benefits	*Possible Risks*
EFFECTIVE ONCE-A-DAY TREATMENT OF MILD TO MODERATE HYPERTENSION EFFECTIVE, MILD DIURETIC	Excessive loss of blood potassium (14%) Increased blood sugar level Increased blood uric acid level

---

▷ **Principal Uses**

As a Single Drug Product: Used primarily to (1) increase the volume of urine (diuresis) to correct the excessive fluid retention associated with congestive heart failure; and (2) initiate treatment for high blood pressure (hypertension). It may be the first drug tried in treating mild to moderate hypertension.

How This Drug Works: By increasing the elimination of salt and water from the body (through increased urine production), this drug reduces the volume of fluid in the blood and body tissues and lowers the sodium content throughout the body. By relaxing the walls of smaller arteries and allowing them to expand, this drug increases the total capacity of the arterial system. The combined effect of these two actions (reduced blood volume in expanded space) results in lowering of blood pressure.

Available Dosage Forms and Strengths

Tablets — 2.5 mg

▷ **Usual Adult Dosage Range:** Initially 2.5 mg/day, taken as a single dose in the morning. If necessary, the dose may be increased to 5 mg/day after 1 week (for diuresis) or after 4 weeks (for hypertension). The total daily dosage should not exceed 5 mg. (In Canada, the total daily dosage limit is given as 2.5 mg.) **Note: Actual dosage and administration schedule must be determined by the physician for each patient individually.**

▷ **Dosing Instructions:** May be taken with or following food to reduce stomach irritation. Best taken in the morning to avoid nighttime urination. The tablet may be crushed for administration.

Usual Duration of Use: Continual use on a regular schedule for 2 to 4 weeks is usually necessary to determine this drug's effectiveness in lowering high blood pressure. Long-term use (months to years) requires periodic evaluation of response and possible dosage adjustment. Use as a diuretic should be intermittent with "drug holidays" (no drug taken) to reduce the risk of sodium and potassium imbalance.

▷ **This Drug Should Not Be Taken If**
- you have had an allergic reaction to it previously.

▷ **Inform Your Physician Before Taking This Drug If**
- you are allergic to any form of "sulfa" drug.
- you are pregnant or planning pregnancy.
- you have a history of kidney or liver disease.
- you have diabetes, gout or lupus erythematosus.
- you are taking any form of cortisone, digitalis, oral antidiabetic drug or insulin.
- you plan to have surgery under general anesthesia in the near future.

Possible Side-Effects   (natural, expected and unavoidable drug actions)
Light-headedness on arising from sitting or lying position (see orthostatic hypotension in Glossary).
Increase in blood sugar level, affecting control of diabetes.
Increase in blood uric acid level, affecting control of gout.
Decrease in blood potassium level, causing muscle weakness and cramping.

▷ **Possible Adverse Effects**   (unusual, unexpected and infrequent reactions)
If any of the following develop, consult your physician promptly.
Mild Adverse Effects
Allergic Reactions: Skin rashes, hives, itching.
Headache, dizziness, drowsiness, weakness, lethargy, visual disturbance.
Reduced appetite, indigestion, nausea, vomiting, diarrhea.
Reduced sexual interest and potency (less than 1%).
Serious Adverse Effects
None reported.

Natural Diseases or Disorders That May Be Activated by This Drug
Diabetes, gout, systemic lupus erythematosus.

CAUTION
1. Do not exceed recommended doses. Increased dosage can cause excessive loss of sodium and potassium, with resultant loss of appetite, nausea, fatigue, weakness, confusion and tingling in the extremities.
2. If you are also taking a digitalis preparation (digitoxin, digoxin), ensure an adequate intake of high-potassium foods to prevent potassium deficiency—a potential cause of digitalis toxicity. (See Table of High Potassium Foods in Section Six.)

Precautions for Use
By Infants and Children: Safety and effectiveness for use by those under 12 years of age have not been established.
By Those over 60 Years of Age: Small doses are advisable until your individual

response has been determined. You may be more susceptible to the development of impaired thinking, orthostatic hypotension, potassium loss and blood sugar increase. Overdosage and extended use of this drug can cause excessive loss of body water, thickening (increased viscosity) of the blood and an increased tendency for the blood to clot—predisposing to stroke, heart attack or thrombophlebitis (vein inflammation with blood clot).

▷ **Advisability of Use During Pregnancy**
Pregnancy Category: B (tentative). See Pregnancy Code inside back cover.
Animal studies: No birth defects reported.
Human studies: Information from adequate studies in pregnant women is not available.
This drug should not be used during pregnancy unless a very serious complication occurs for which this drug is significantly beneficial. Ask physician for guidance.

Advisability of Use if Breast-Feeding
Presence of this drug in breast milk: Unknown.
Avoid drug or refrain from nursing.

Habit-Forming Potential: None.

Effects of Overdosage: Dry mouth, thirst, lethargy, weakness, muscle cramping, nausea, vomiting, drowsiness progressing to stupor or coma.

Possible Effects of Long-Term Use: Impaired balance of water, salt and potassium in blood and body tissues. Development of diabetes in predisposed individuals.

Suggested Periodic Examinations While Taking This Drug   (at physician's discretion)
Measurements of blood levels of sodium, potassium, chloride, sugar and uric acid.

▷ **While Taking This Drug, Observe the Following**
Foods: Consult your physician regarding the advisability of eating foods rich in potassium. If so advised, see the Table of High Potassium Foods in Section Six. Follow physician's advice regarding the use of salt.
Beverages: No restrictions. This drug may be taken with milk.
▷   *Alcohol*: Use with caution until the combined effects have been determined. Alcohol may exaggerate the blood-pressure-lowering effects of this drug and cause orthostatic hypotension.
Tobacco Smoking: No interactions expected. Follow physician's advice.
▷   *Other Drugs*
Indapamide may *increase* the effects of
• other antihypertensive drugs; dosage adjustments may be necessary to prevent excessive lowering of blood pressure.
• lithium, and cause lithium toxicity.

Indapamide may *decrease* the effects of
- oral antidiabetic drugs (sulfonylureas); dosage adjustments may be necessary for proper control of blood sugar.

Indapamide *taken concurrently* with
- digitalis preparations (digitoxin, digoxin) requires very careful monitoring and dosage adjustments to prevent fluctuations of blood potassium levels and serious disturbances of heart rhythm.

The following drugs may *decrease* the effects of indapamide
- cholestyramine (Cuemid, Questran) may interfere with its absorption.
- colestipol (Colestid) may interfere with its absorption.

Take cholestyramine and colestipol 1 hour before any oral diuretic.

▷ *Driving, Hazardous Activities*: Use caution until the possible occurrence of orthostatic hypotension, drowsiness, dizziness or impaired vision has been determined.

Aviation Note: The use of this drug *may be a disqualification* for piloting. Consult a designated Aviation Medical Examiner.

Exposure to Sun: No restrictions.

Exposure to Heat: Avoid excessive perspiring, which could cause additional loss of salt and water from the body.

Heavy Exercise or Exertion: Avoid exertion that produces light-headedness, excessive fatigue or muscle cramping. Isometric exercises—the "overload" technique for strengthening individual muscles—can raise blood pressure significantly. Ask physician for guidance regarding participation in this form of exercise.

Occurrence of Unrelated Illness: Illnesses that cause vomiting or diarrhea can produce a serious imbalance of important body chemistry. Consult your physician for guidance.

Discontinuation: It may be advisable to discontinue this drug 5 to 7 days before major surgery. Ask your physician, surgeon and/or anesthesiologist for guidance regarding dosage adjustment or drug withdrawal.

INDOMETHACIN ⚕
(in doh METH a sin)

Introduced: 1963	**Class:** Mild Analgesic, Anti-inflammatory
Prescription: USA: Yes Canada: Yes	**Controlled Drug:** USA: No Canada: No
Available as Generic: USA: Yes Canada: No	

Brand Names: ✲Apo-Indomethacin, ✲Indocid, ✲Indocid PDA, ✲Indocid SR, Indocin, Indocin-SR, ✲Novomethacin

BENEFITS versus RISKS	
Possible Benefits	*Possible Risks*
EFFECTIVE RELIEF OF MILD TO MODERATE PAIN AND INFLAMMATION	Gastrointestinal pain, ulceration, bleeding (rare)
	Rare liver or kidney damage
	Rare fluid retention
	Rare bone marrow depression
	Mental depression, confusion

▷ **Principal Uses**

As a Single Drug Product: Used primarily to relieve mild to moderately severe pain associated with (1) musculoskeletal injuries; (2) acute and chronic gout, rheumatoid arthritis and osteoarthritis; (3) dental, obstetrical and orthopedic surgery; (4) menstrual cramps; and (5) vascular (migraine-like) headaches.

How This Drug Works: Not completely established. It is thought that this drug reduces the tissue concentrations of prostaglandins (and related compounds), chemicals involved in the production of inflammation and pain.

Available Dosage Forms and Strengths

Capsules — 25 mg, 50 mg
Capsules, prolonged action — 75 mg
Suppositories — 50 mg
Suspension, oral — 25 mg per 5 ml teaspoonful

▷ **Usual Adult Dosage Range:** For arthritis and related conditions: 25 to 50 mg 2 to 4 times daily. If needed and tolerated, dose may be increased by 25 or 50 mg/day at intervals of 1 week. For acute gout: 100 mg initially; then 50 mg 3 times/day until pain is relieved. Total daily dosage should not exceed 200 mg. **Note: Actual dosage and administration schedule must be determined by the physician for each patient individually.**

▷ **Dosing Instructions:** Take with or following food to prevent stomach irritation. Take with a full glass of water and remain upright (do not lie down) for 30 minutes. The regular capsule may be opened for administration, but not the prolonged-action capsule.

Usual Duration of Use: Continual use on a regular schedule for 1 to 2 weeks is usually necessary to determine this drug's effectiveness in relieving the discomfort of arthritis. The usual length of treatment for bursitis or tendinitis is 7 to 14 days. Long-term use requires supervision and periodic evaluation by the physician.

▷ **This Drug Should Not Be Taken If**
- you have had an allergic reaction to it previously.
- you are subject to asthma or nasal polyps caused by aspirin.
- you are pregnant or breast-feeding.

- you have active peptic ulcer disease or any form of gastrointestinal ulceration or bleeding.
- you have a bleeding disorder or a blood cell disorder.
- you have severe impairment of kidney function.

▷ **Inform Your Physician Before Taking This Drug If**
- you are allergic to aspirin or to other aspirin substitutes.
- you have a history of peptic ulcer disease, Crohn's disease, ulcerative colitis or any type of bleeding disorder.
- you have a history of epilepsy, Parkinson's disease or mental illness (psychosis).
- you have impaired liver or kidney function.
- you have high blood pressure or a history of heart failure.
- you are taking any of the following: acetaminophen, aspirin or other aspirin substitutes, anticoagulants, oral antidiabetic drugs.

Possible Side-Effects   (natural, expected and unavoidable drug actions)
Drowsiness, ringing in ears, fluid retention.

▷ **Possible Adverse Effects**   (unusual, unexpected and infrequent reactions)
If any of the following develop, consult your physician promptly.
Mild Adverse Effects
Allergic Reactions: Skin rash, hives, itching, localized swellings of face and/or extremities.
Headache, dizziness, feelings of detachment.
Mouth sores, indigestion, nausea, vomiting, diarrhea.
Temporary loss of hair.
Serious Adverse Effects
Allergic Reactions: Asthma, difficult breathing, mouth irritation.
Blurred vision, confusion, depression.
Active peptic ulcer, with or without bleeding.
Liver damage with jaundice (see Glossary).
Kidney damage with painful urination, bloody urine, reduced urine formation.
Rare bone marrow depression (see Glossary)—fatigue, weakness, fever, sore throat, abnormal bleeding or bruising.
Peripheral neuritis (see Glossary)—numbness, pain or weakness in extremities.

Possible Delayed Adverse Effects
Mild anemia due to "silent" blood loss from the stomach (less than that caused by aspirin).

▷ **Adverse Effects That May Mimic Natural Diseases or Disorders**
Liver reaction may suggest viral hepatitis.

Natural Diseases or Disorders That May Be Activated by This Drug
Peptic ulcer disease, ulcerative colitis.

CAUTION
1. Dosage should always be limited to the smallest amount that produces reasonable improvement.
2. This drug may mask early indications of infection. Inform your physician if you think you are developing an infection of any kind.

Precautions for Use
By Infants and Children: This drug frequently causes impairment of kidney function in infants. Fatal liver reactions have occurred in children between 6 and 12 years of age; avoid the use of this drug in this age group.

By Those over 60 Years of Age: Adverse effects are very common in this age group. Small doses are advisable until tolerance is determined. Observe for any indications of liver or kidney toxicity, fluid retention, dizziness, confusion, impaired memory, depression, peptic ulcer or diarrhea, often with rectal bleeding.

▷ **Advisability of Use During Pregnancy**
Pregnancy Category: D (tentative). See Pregnancy Code inside back cover.
Animal studies: Significant toxicity and birth defects reported in mice and rats.
Human studies: Information from adequate studies in pregnant women is not available. However, birth defects have been attributed to the use of this drug during pregnancy.
The manufacturer recommends that this drug not be taken during pregnancy.

Advisability of Use if Breast-Feeding
Presence of this drug in breast milk: Yes.
Avoid drug or refrain from nursing.
The manufacturer recommends that this drug not be taken while breast-feeding.

Habit-Forming Potential: None.

Effects of Overdosage: Drowsiness, agitation, confusion, nausea, vomiting, diarrhea, disorientation, seizures, coma.

Possible Effects of Long-Term Use: Eye changes: deposits in the cornea, alterations in the retina.

Suggested Periodic Examinations While Taking This Drug   (at physician's discretion)
Complete blood cell counts, liver and kidney function tests, complete eye examinations if vision is altered in any way.

▷ **While Taking This Drug, Observe the Following**
Foods: No restrictions.
Nutritional Support: Take 50 mg of vitamin C (ascorbic acid) daily.
Beverages: No restrictions. May be taken with milk.

▷   *Alcohol*: Use with caution. The irritant action of alcohol on the stomach lining, added to the irritant action of this drug in sensitive individuals, can increase the risk of stomach ulceration and/or bleeding.

Tobacco Smoking: No interactions expected.

▷   *Other Drugs*

Indomethacin may *increase* the effects of

- acetaminophen (Tylenol, etc.), and increase the risk of kidney damage; avoid prolonged use of this combination.
- anticoagulants (Coumadin, etc.), and increase the risk of bleeding; monitor prothrombin time, adjust dose accordingly.
- lithium, and cause lithium toxicity.

Indomethacin may *decrease* the effects of

- beta-blocker drugs (see Drug Class, Section Four), and reduce their antihypertensive effectiveness.
- bumetanide (Bumex).
- captopril (Capoten).
- ethacrynic acid (Edecrin). furosemide (Lasix).

Indomethacin *taken concurrently* with the following drugs may increase the risk of bleeding; avoid these combinations:

- aspirin.
- diflunisal (Dolobid).
- dipyridamole (Persantine).
- sulfinpyrazone (Anturane).
- valproic acid (Depakene).

▷   *Driving, Hazardous Activities*: This drug may cause drowsiness, dizziness or impaired vision. Restrict activities as necessary.

Aviation Note: The use of this drug *may be a disqualification* for piloting. Consult a designated Aviation Medical Examiner.

Exposure to Sun: No restrictions.

INSULIN ✈
(IN suh lin)

Introduced: 1922

Class: Antidiabetic

Prescription: USA: No
Canada: No

Controlled Drug: USA: No
Canada: No

Available as Generic: Yes

Brand Names: ✤Actrapid MC, Humulin L, Humulin N, Humulin R, ✤Initard, Insulatard NPH, ✤Insulin-Toronto, Lente Iletin I, Lente Iletin II Beef, Lente Iletin II Pork, Lente Insulin, Mixtard, ✤Monotard MC, Novolin L, Novolin N, Novolin R, ✤Novolin-Lente, ✤Novolin-NPH, ✤Novolin-30/70, ✤Novolin-Toronto, ✤Novolin-Ultralente, NPH Iletin I, NPH Iletin II Beef, NPH Iletin II Pork, NPH Insulin, NPH Purified Pork, Protamine, Zinc & Iletin I, Protamine, Zinc & Iletin II Beef, Protamine, Zinc & Iletin II Pork, Protamine Zinc Insulin, ✤Protaphane MC, Regular Iletin I, Regular Iletin II Beef, Regular Iletin II Pork, Regular Insulin, Regular Purified Pork Insulin, Semilente Iletin I, Semilente Insulin, Semilente Purified Pork, Ultralente Iletin I, Ultralente Insulin, Ultralente Purified Beef, Velosulin

---

BENEFITS versus RISKS

Possible Benefits	Possible Risks
EFFECTIVE CONTROL OF TYPE I (INSULIN-DEPENDENT) DIABETES MELLITUS	HYPOGLYCEMIA WITH EXCESSIVE DOSAGE Infrequent allergic reactions

---

▷ **Principal Uses**

As a Single Drug Product: Insulin is used to control diabetes mellitus in those individuals whose diabetes has been shown to be insulin-dependent. Proper use involves selection of the most appropriate type of insulin for the individual and determination of the optimal dosage schedule for the continuous regulation of blood sugar levels.

How This Drug Works: Not completely established. By direct action on certain cell membranes, insulin facilitates the transport of sugar through the cell wall to the interior of the cell where it is utilized. This occurs primarily in the brain, the voluntary muscles, the heart muscle and the liver.

Available Dosage Forms and Strengths

Injections — 40 units per ml, 100 units per ml, 500 units per ml

▷ **Usual Adult Dosage Range:** According to individual requirements for the optimal regulation of blood sugar on a 24-hour basis. **Note: Actual dosage and administration schedule must be determined by the physician for each patient individually.**

▷ **Dosing Instructions:** Inject insulin subcutaneously according to the schedule prescribed by your physician. The timing and frequency of injections will vary with the type of insulin precribed. The following table of insulin actions (according to type) will help you understand the treatment schedule prescribed for you.

Insulin Type	Action Onset	Peak	Duration
Regular	0.5-1 hr	2-4 hrs	5-7 hrs
Isophane (NPH)	3-4 hrs	6-12 hrs	18-28 hrs
Regular 30%/NPH 70%	0.5 hr	4-8 hrs	24 hrs
Semilente	1-3 hrs	2-8 hrs	12-16 hrs
Lente	1-3 hrs	8-12 hrs	18-28 hrs
Ultralente	4-6 hrs	18-24 hrs	36 hrs
Protamine Zinc	4-6 hrs	14-24 hrs	36 hrs

Usual Duration of Use: Type I insulin-dependent (juvenile-onset) diabetes mellitus usually requires insulin treatment for life. Type II noninsulin-dependent (maturity-onset) diabetes is usually controlled by oral antidiabetic drugs and/or diet but may, on occasion, require insulin for adequate control. Such occasions include serious infections, injuries, burns, surgical procedures and other forms of physical stress. Insulin is used as needed on a temporary basis to regulate and normalize the body's use of sugar until recovery is complete and basic health is restored.

▷ **This Drug Should Not Be Taken If**
- the need for it and its correct dosage schedule have not been established by a properly qualified physician.

▷ **Inform Your Physician Before Taking This Drug If**
- you have a history of allergic reaction to any form of insulin on previous use.
- you do not know how to recognize and treat abnormally low blood sugar (see hypoglycemia in Glossary).
- you are taking any of the following drugs: aspirin, beta-blockers, fenfluramine (Pondimin), monoamine oxidase (MAO) inhibitors (see respective Drug Classes, Section Four).

Possible Side-Effects   (natural, expected and unavoidable drug actions)
In the management of stable diabetes, no side-effects occur when insulin dose, diet and physical activity are correctly balanced and maintained. In the management of unstable ("brittle") diabetes, unexpected drops in blood sugar levels can occur, resulting in periods of hypoglycemia (see Glossary).

▷ **Possible Adverse Effects**   (unusual, unexpected and infrequent reactions)
If any of the following develop, consult your physician promptly.
Mild Adverse Effects
Allergic Reactions: Local redness, swelling and itching at site of injection. Occasional hives.
Thinning of subcutaneous tissue at sites of injection.
Serious Adverse Effects
Allergic Reactions: Anaphylactic reactions (see Glossary).
Severe, prolonged hypoglycemia.

▷ **Adverse Effects That May Mimic Natural Diseases or Disorders**
The early manifestations of hypoglycemia may be mistaken for alcoholic intoxication.

CAUTION
1. It is most important that you carry with you a card of personal identification with a notation that you have diabetes and are taking insulin.
2. Be sure that you know how to recognize the onset of hypoglycemia and how to treat it. Always carry with you a readily available form of sugar, such as hard candy or sugar cubes. Report all episodes of hypoglycemia to your physician; it may be necessary to adjust your insulin dosage or schedule.
3. Improvement in vision may occur during the first several weeks of insulin treatment. It is advisable to defer examination for glasses for 6 weeks after starting insulin.

4. The rates of insulin absorption vary significantly from one anatomic site to another. Absorption is 80% greater from the abdominal wall than from the leg, and 30% greater than from the arm. Individuals with unstable diabetes may achieve better control of blood sugar levels by rotating the injection site within the same anatomic region rather than by rotating from one anatomic region to another.

Precautions for Use
By Infants and Children: Insulin dosages and schedules are modified according to patient size. Adhere strictly to the physician's prescribed routine.

By Those over 60 Years of Age: Insulin requirements may change with aging. Periodic evaluation of individual status is necessary to determine correct insulin dosage and scheduling. The aging brain adapts well to higher blood sugar levels. Attempts to maintain strictly "normal" blood sugar levels may result in episodes of unrecognized hypoglycemia that is manifested by confusion and abnormal behavior. Repeated episodes of hypoglycemia (especially if severe) in the elderly may cause brain damage.

▷ **Advisability of Use During Pregnancy**
Pregnancy Category: B (tentative). See Pregnancy Code inside back cover.
Animal studies: Inconclusive.

Human studies: Information from adequate studies in pregnant women is not available. It is known that birth defects occur 2 to 4 times more frequently in infants of diabetic mothers than in infants of mothers who do not have diabetes. The exact causes of this are not known.

Insulin is the drug of choice for managing diabetes during pregnancy. To preserve the health of the mother and the welfare of the fetus, every effort must be made to establish the optimal dosage of insulin necessary for "good control" and to prevent episodes of hypoglycemia.

Advisability of Use if Breast-Feeding
Presence of this drug in breast milk: No.

Insulin treatment of the mother has no adverse effect on the nursing infant.

Breast-feeding may decrease insulin requirements; dosage adjustment may be necessary.

Habit-Forming Potential: None.

Effects of Overdosage: Hypoglycemia: fatigue, weakness, headache, nervousness, irritability, sweating, tremors, hunger, confusion, delirium, abnormal behavior (resembling alcoholic intoxication), loss of consciousness, seizures.

Possible Effects of Long-Term Use: Thinning of subcutaneous fat tissue at sites of insulin injection.

Suggested Periodic Examinations While Taking This Drug   (at physician's discretion)
Monitoring of urine sugar content as a guide to adjustment of diet and insulin dosage. Measurement of blood sugar levels at intervals recommended by physician.

▷ **While Taking This Drug, Observe the Following**

Foods: Follow your prescribed diabetic diet conscientiously. Do not omit snack foods in midafternoon or at bedtime if they are prescribed to prevent hypoglycemia.

Beverages: According to prescribed diabetic diet.

▷ *Alcohol*: Use with caution until the combined effect has been determined. Used excessively, alcohol can induce severe hypoglycemia, resulting in brain damage.

Tobacco Smoking: Regular smoking can decrease insulin absorption and increase insulin requirements by 30%. It is advisable to refrain from smoking altogether.

Marijuana Smoking: Possible increase in blood sugar levels.

▷ *Other Drugs*

The following drugs may *increase* the effects of insulin
- aspirin, and other salicylates.
- some beta-blocker drugs (especially the nonselective ones) may prolong insulin-induced hypoglycemia. (See Drug Class, Section Four.)
- fenfluramine (Pondimin).
- monoamine oxidase (MAO) inhibitor drugs (see Drug Class, Section Four).

The following drugs may *decrease* the effects of insulin (by raising blood sugar levels)
- chlorthalidone (Hygroton).
- cortisonelike drugs (see Drug Class, Section Four).
- furosemide (Lasix).
- oral contraceptives.
- phenytoin (Dilantin, etc.).
- thiazide diuretics (see Drug Class, Section Four).
- thyroid preparations.

▷ *Driving, Hazardous Activities*: Usually no restrictions. However, be prepared to stop and take corrective action if indications of impending hypoglycemia develop.

Aviation Note: Diabetes and the use of this drug *are disqualifications* for piloting. Consult a designated Aviation Medical Examiner.

Exposure to Sun: No restrictions.

Exposure to Heat: Use caution. Sauna baths can signficantly increase the rate of insulin absorption and cause hypoglycemia.

Heavy Exercise or Exertion: Use caution. Periods of unusual or unplanned heavy physical activity will hasten the utilization of blood sugar and predispose to hypoglycemia.

Occurrence of Unrelated Illness: Report all illnesses that prevent regular eating. The omission of meals as a result of nausea, vomiting or injury may lead to hypoglycemia. Untreated infections can increase insulin requirements. Consult physician for guidance.

Discontinuation: Do not discontinue this drug without consulting your physician. Diabetes that is insulin-dependent requires continual treatment on a regular basis. Omission of insulin may result in life-threatening coma.

Special Storage Instructions: Keep in a cool place, preferably in the refrigerator. Protect from freezing. Protect from strong light and high temperatures when not refrigerated.

Observe the Following Expiration Times: Do not use this drug if it is older than the expiration date on the vial. Always use fresh, "within date" insulin.

ISONIAZID ✗
(i soh NI a zid)

Other Names: Isonicotinic acid hydrazide, INH

Introduced: 1956

Class: Antitubercular

Prescription: USA: Yes
Canada: Yes

Controlled Drug: USA: No
Canada: No

Available as Generic: USA: Yes
Canada: No

Brand Names: ✤Isotamine, Laniazid, Nydrazid, P-I-N Forte [CD], ✤PMS Isoniazid, Rifamate [CD], Rimactane/INH Dual Pack [CD], ✤Rimifon, Teebaconin, Teebaconin and Vitamin B-6 [CD], Triniad, Uniad

---

BENEFITS versus RISKS

Possible Benefits	*Possible Risks*
EFFECTIVE PREVENTION AND TREATMENT OF ACTIVE TUBERCULOSIS	ALLERGIC LIVER REACTION (1% to 2%)
	Peripheral neuropathy (see Glossary)
	Bone marrow depression (see Glossary)
	Mental and behavioral disturbances

▷ **Principal Uses**

As a Single Drug Product: Used alone to prevent the development of active tuberculous infection in individuals who are considered to be at high risk because of known exposure to infection or recent conversion of a negative tuberculin skin test to positive.

As a Combination Drug Product [CD]: This drug is available in combination with rifampin, another antitubercular drug that has a different mechanism of action. This combination is more effective than either drug used alone. Isoniazid can cause a deficiency of pyridoxine (vitamin B-6); for this reason, a combination of the two drugs is available in tablet form.

How This Drug Works: Not completely established. It is thought that this drug destroys susceptible tuberculosis organisms by interfering with several of their essential metabolic activities and by disrupting their cell wall.

Available Dosage Forms and Strengths
  Injection — 100 mg per ml
    Syrup — 50 mg per 5 ml teaspoonful
    Tablets — 50 mg, 100 mg, 300 mg

▷ **Usual Adult Dosage Range:**   For prevention: 300 mg once daily. For treatment: 5 mg per kilogram of body weight daily. The total daily dosage should not exceed 600 mg. **Note: Actual dosage and administration schedule must be determined by the physician for each patient individually.**

▷ **Dosing Instructions:**   May be taken with food to prevent stomach irritation. The tablet may be crushed for administration.

Usual Duration of Use: Continual use on a regular schedule for 1 or more years is often necessary, depending upon the nature of the infection. Shorter courses of intermittent high dosage may be adequate in some cases.

▷ **This Drug Should Not Be Taken If**
  • you have had an allergic reaction (especially a liver reaction) to any dosage form of it previously.
  • you have active liver disease.

▷ **Inform Your Physician Before Taking This Drug If**
  • you have serious impairment of liver or kidney function.
  • you drink an alcoholic beverage daily.
  • you have a seizure disorder.
  • you are taking any other drugs on a long-term basis, especially phenytoin (Dilantin).
  • you plan to have surgery under general anesthesia in the near future.

Possible Side-Effects   (natural, expected and unavoidable drug actions)
  None.

▷ **Possible Adverse Effects**   (unusual, unexpected and infrequent reactions)
  If any of the following develop, consult your physician promptly.
  Mild Adverse Effects
  Allergic Reactions: Skin rash, fever, swollen glands, painful muscles and joints.
  Dizziness, indigestion, nausea, vomiting.
  Serious Adverse Effects
  Allergic Reactions: Drug-induced hepatitis (see Glossary): loss of appetite, nausea, fatigue, fever, itching, dark-colored urine, yellow discoloration of eyes and skin.
  Peripheral neuritis (see Glossary): numbness, tingling, pain, weakness in hands and/or feet.
  Acute mental and behavioral disturbances, impaired vision, increase in epileptic seizures.
  Male breast enlargement or discomfort.
  Bone marrow depression (see Glossary): fatigue, weakness, fever, sore throat, abnormal bleeding or bruising.

Possible Delayed Adverse Effects
An increase in the frequency of cirrhosis of the liver has been reported.

▷ **Adverse Effects That May Mimic Natural Diseases or Disorders**
Drug-induced hepatitis may suggest viral hepatitis.

Natural Diseases or Disorders That May Be Activated by This Drug
Latent epilepsy, systemic lupus erythematosus (questionable).

CAUTION
1. Consult your physician regarding the advisability of determining if you are a "slow" or "rapid" inactivator (acetylator) of isoniazid. This has a bearing on your predisposition to developing adverse effects from this drug.
2. Copper sulfate tests for urine sugar may give a false positive test result. (Diabetics please note.)

Precautions for Use
By Infants and Children: Use with caution in children with seizure disorders. "Slow acetylators" are more prone to adverse drug effects. It is advisable to give supplemental pyridoxine (vitamin B-6).
By Those over 60 Years of Age: There is a greater incidence of liver damage in this age group; the liver status should be monitored carefully. Observe for any indications of an "acute brain syndrome" consisting of confusion, delirium and seizures.

▷ **Advisability of Use During Pregnancy**
Pregnancy Category: C (tentative). See Pregnancy Code inside back cover.
Animal studies: No birth defects reported in mice, rats or rabbits.
Human studies: Information from adequate studies in pregnant women is not available.
Earlier reports of human birth defects due to this drug have not been substantiated by later studies. If clearly needed, this drug is now used at any time during pregnancy. Ask your physician for guidance.

Advisability of Use if Breast-Feeding
Presence of this drug in breast milk: Yes.
Avoid drug or refrain from nursing.

Habit-Forming Potential: None.

Effects of Overdosage: Nausea, vomiting, dizziness, blurred vision, hallucinations, slurred speech, stupor, coma, seizures.

Possible Effects of Long-Term Use: Peripheral neuritis due to a deficiency of pyridoxine (vitamin B-6).

Suggested Periodic Examinations While Taking This Drug (at physician's discretion)
Complete blood cell counts, liver function tests, complete eye examinations.

▷ **While Taking This Drug, Observe the Following**
Foods: Eat the following foods cautiously until your tolerance is determined: Swiss and Cheshire cheeses, tuna fish, skipjack fish and Sardinella spe-

cies. These may interact with the drug to produce skin rash, itching, sweating, chills, headache, light-headedness or rapid heart rate.

Nutritional Support: It is advisable to take a supplement of pyridoxine (vitamin B-6) to prevent peripheral neuritis. Ask your physician for dosage.

Beverages: No restrictions. May be taken with milk.

▷   *Alcohol*: Avoid completely or use very sparingly. Alcohol may reduce the effectiveness of this drug and increase the risk of liver toxicity.

Tobacco Smoking: No interactions expected.

▷   *Other Drugs*

Isoniazid may *increase* the effects of
- carbamazepine (Tegretol), and cause toxicity.
- phenytoin (Dilantin), and cause toxicity.

The following drugs may *decrease* the effects of isoniazid
- cortisonelike drugs (see Drug Class, Section Four).

▷   *Driving, Hazardous Activities*: Usually no restrictions. This drug may cause dizziness. Restrict activities as necessary.

Aviation Note: The use of this drug *may be a disqualification* for piloting. Consult a designated Aviation Medical Examiner.

Exposure to Sun: No restrictions.

Discontinuation: Long-term treatment is required. Do not discontinue this drug without consulting your physician.

ISOSORBIDE DINITRATE
(i soh SOHR bide di NI trayt)

Other Names: Sorbide Nitrate

Introduced: 1959   **Class:** Antianginal, Nitrates

Prescription: USA: Yes   **Controlled Drug:** USA: No
Canada: No   Canada: No

Available as Generic: USA: Yes
Canada: No

Brand Names: ✤Apo-ISDN, ✤Coronex, Dilatrate-SR, Isordil, Isordil Tembids, Isordil Titradose, ✤Novosorbide, Sorbitrate

---

BENEFITS versus RISKS

Possible Benefits	*Possible Risks*
EFFECTIVE RELIEF AND PREVENTION OF ANGINA	Orthostatic hypotension (see Glossary)
EFFECTIVE ADJUNCTIVE TREATMENT IN SELECTED CASES OF CONGESTIVE HEART FAILURE	Rare skin reactions (severe peeling)

▷ **Principal Uses**

As a Single Drug Product: The sublingual (under-the-tongue) tablets and the chewable tablets are used to prevent and to relieve acute attacks of anginal pain. The longer-acting tablets and capsules are used to prevent the development of angina, but are not effective in relieving acute episodes of anginal pain. This drug is also used to improve heart function in selected cases of congestive heart failure.

How This Drug Works: By direct action on the muscle in blood vessel walls, this drug relaxes and dilates both arteries and veins. It is thought that its beneficial effects in treating angina and heart failure are due to (1) dilation of coronary arteries, and (2) dilation of systemic veins with consequent reduction of volume and pressure of blood in the heart. The net effects are improved blood flow to the heart muscle and reduced workload of the heart.

Available Dosage Forms and Strengths

Capsules — 40 mg
Capsules, prolonged-action — 40 mg
Tablets — 5 mg, 10 mg, 20 mg, 30 mg, 40 mg
Tablets, chewable — 5 mg, 10 mg
Tablets, prolonged-action — 40 mg
Tablets, sublingual — 2.5 mg, 5 mg, 10 mg

▷ **Usual Adult Dosage Range**

Sublingual tablets: 5 to 10 mg dissolved under tongue every 2 to 3 hours; use for relief of acute attack and for prevention of anticipated attack.

Chewable tablets: Initially, 5 mg chewed to evaluate tolerance; increase dose to 5 or 10 mg every 2 to 3 hours as needed and tolerated; use for relief of acute attack and for prevention of anticipated attack.

Tablets: 5 to 30 mg 4 times daily to prevent acute attack; usual dose is 10 to 20 mg 4 times/day.

Prolonged-action capsules and tablets: 40 mg/6 to 12 hours as needed to prevent acute attacks.

The total daily dosage should not exceed 120 mg.

Note: Actual dosage and administration schedule must be determined by the physician for each patient individually.

▷ **Dosing Instructions:** Capsules and tablets to be swallowed are best taken on an empty stomach to achieve maximal blood levels. Regular tablets may be crushed for administration; prolonged-action capsules and tablets should be taken whole and not altered.

Usual Duration of Use: Continual use on a regular schedule for 3 to 7 days is usually necessary to (1) determine this drug's effectiveness in preventing or relieving acute anginal pain, and (2) establish the optimal dosage shedule. Long-term use (months to years) requires supervision and periodic evaluation by your physician.

▷ **This Drug Should Not Be Taken If**
  - you have had an allergic reaction to any dosage form of it previously.
  - you have had a very recent heart attack (myocardial infarction).

▷ **Inform Your Physician Before Taking This Drug If**
  - you have had an unfavorable response to other nitrate drugs or vasodilators in the past.
  - you have a history of low blood pressure.
  - you have any form of glaucoma.

Possible Side-Effects   (natural, expected and unavoidable drug actions)
  Flushing of face, throbbing in head, palpitation, rapid heart rate, orthostatic hypotension (see Glossary).

▷ **Possible Adverse Effects**   (unusual, unexpected and infrequent reactions)
  If any of the following develop, consult your physician promptly.
  Mild Adverse Effects
  Allergic Reactions: Skin rash.
  Headache (may be severe and persistent), dizziness, fainting.
  Nausea, vomiting.
  Serious Adverse Effects
  Allergic Reactions: Severe dermatitis with peeling of skin.
  Transient ischemic attacks (TIAs) in presence of impaired circulation within the brain: dizziness, fainting, impaired vision or speech, localized numbness or weakness.

▷ **Adverse Effects That May Mimic Natural Diseases or Disorders**
  Spells of low blood pressure (due to this drug) may be mistaken for late-onset epilepsy.

CAUTION
  1. The development of tolerance (see Glossary) to long-acting forms of nitrates may render the sublingual tablets of nitroglycerin less effective for the relief of acute anginal attacks. Antianginal effectiveness is restored after 1 week of abstinence from long-acting nitrates.
  2. Many over-the-counter (OTC) medications for allergies, colds and coughs contain drugs that may counteract the desired effects of this drug. Ask your physician or pharmacist for guidance before using such medications.

Precautions for Use
  By Those over 60 Years of Age: Small doses are advisable until your tolerance has been determined. You may be more susceptible to the development of low blood pressure and associated "blackout" spells, fainting and falling. Throbbing headaches and flushing may be more apparent.

▷ **Advisability of Use During Pregnancy**
  Pregnancy Category: C (tentative). See Pregnancy Code inside back cover.
  Animal studies: No information available.

Human studies: Information from adequate studies of pregnant women is not available.

Use this drug only if clearly needed.

Advisability of Use if Breast-Feeding
Presence of this drug in breast milk: Unknown.
If drug is thought to be necessary, monitor the nursing infant for low blood pressure and poor feeding.

Habit-Forming Potential: None.

Effects of Overdosage: Headache, dizziness, marked flushing of face and skin, vomiting, weakness, fainting, difficult breathing, coma.

Possible Effects of Long-Term Use: Development of tolerance with temporary loss of effectiveness at recommended doses. Development of abnormal hemoglobin (red blood cell pigment).

Suggested Periodic Examinations While Taking This Drug   (at physician's discretion)
Measurement of internal eye pressure. Red blood cell counts and hemoglobin evaluation.

▷ **While Taking This Drug, Observe the Following**
Foods: No restrictions.
Beverages: No restrictions. May be taken with milk.
▷ *Alcohol*: Use extreme caution until the combined effects have been determined. Avoid alcohol completely in the presence of any side-effects or adverse effects of this drug. Alcohol may exaggerate the blood-pressure-lowering effect of this drug.
Tobacco Smoking: Nicotine can reduce the effectiveness of this drug. Avoid all forms of tobacco.
Marijuana Smoking: Possible reduced effectiveness of this drug; mild to moderate increase in angina; possible changes in electrocardiogram, confusing interpretation.
▷ *Other Drugs*
Isosorbide dinitrate *taken concurrently* with
• antihypertensive drugs may cause excessive lowering of blood pressure; dosage adjustments may be necessary.
▷ *Driving, Hazardous Activities*: Usually no restrictions. This drug may cause dizziness or spells of low blood pressure. Restrict activities as necessary.
Aviation Note: Coronary artery disease *is a disqualification* for piloting. Consult a designated Aviation Medical Examiner.
Exposure to Sun: No restrictions.
Exposure to Heat: Use caution. Hot environments can cause a significant drop in blood pressure.
Exposure to Cold: Cold environments can increase the need for this drug and limit its effectiveness.

Heavy Exercise or Exertion: This drug may improve your ability to be more active without anginal pain. Use caution and avoid excessive exertion.

Discontinuation: It is advisable to withdraw this drug gradually after long-term use. The dosage and frequency of prolonged-action dosage forms should be reduced gradually over a period of 4 to 6 weeks.

ISOTRETINOIN
(i soh TRET i noin)

Introduced: 1979

Prescription: USA: Yes
   Canada: Yes

Available as Generic: No

Brand Names: Accutane

Class: Antiacne

Controlled Drug: USA: No
   Canada: No

BENEFITS versus RISKS

Possible Benefits	*Possible Risks*
EFFECTIVE TREATMENT OF SEVERE CYSTIC ACNE	MAJOR BIRTH DEFECTS Initial worsening of acne (transient) Inflammation of lips (90%) Dry skin, nose and mouth Musculoskeletal discomfort Corneal opacities (rare)

▷ **Principal Uses**

As a Single Drug Product: This drug is reserved to treat severe nodular and cystic acne that has failed to respond to all other forms of standard therapy. *It should not be used to treat mild forms of acne.* It is also used to treat some less common conditions of the skin that are due to disorders of keratin production.

How This Drug Works: Not completely established. By an unknown action, this drug reduces the size of sebaceous glands and inhibits their production of sebum (skin oil). This helps to correct the major feature of acne and its complications.

Available Dosage Forms and Strengths
   Capsules — 10 mg, 20 mg, 40 mg

▷ **Usual Adult Dosage Range:**   Initial dosage is individualized according to the patient's weight and the severity of the acne; the ususal dose is 1 to 2 mg per kilogram of body weight daily, taken in 2 divided doses for 15 to 20 weeks. After 2 weeks of treatment, the dose should be adjusted according to the response of the acne and the development of adverse effects. **Note: Actual dosage and administration schedule must be determined by the physician for each patient individually.**

▷ **Dosing Instructions:**   Take with meals (morning and evening) to achieve optimal blood levels. The capsule should not be opened for administration.

Usual Duration of Use: Continual use on a regular schedule for 15 to 20 weeks is usually necessary to determine this drug's effectiveness in clearing or improving severe cystic acne. The drug may be discontinued earlier if the total cyst count is reduced by more than 70%. If a repeat course of treatment is necessary, it should not be started until after a period of 2 months without this drug. Long-term use (months to years) requires supervision and periodic evaluation by your physician.

▷ **This Drug Should Not Be Taken If**
- you are allergic to parabens, additives that are used to preserve the drug product.
- you are pregnant, or planning pregnancy.

▷ **Inform Your Physician Before Taking This Drug If**
- you have had an allergic reaction to any form of vitamin A in the past.
- you have diabetes mellitus.
- you have a cholesterol or triglyceride disorder.
- you have a history of liver or kidney disease.

Possible Side-Effects   (natural, expected and unavoidable drug actions)
Dryness of the nose and mouth (80%), inflammation of the lips (90%), dryness of the skin with itching (80%), peeling of the palms and soles (5%).

▷ **Possible Adverse Effects**   (unusual, unexpected and infrequent reactions)
If any of the following develop, consult your physician promptly.
Mild Adverse Effects
Allergic Reactions: Skin rash (less that 10%).
Thinning of hair, conjunctivitis, intolerance of contact lenses, muscular and joint aches, headache, fatigue, indigestion.
Serious Adverse Effects
Skin infections, worsening of arthritis, inflammatory bowel disorders.
Abnormal acceleration of bone development in children.
Development of opacities in the cornea of the eye.
Reduced red blood cell and white blood cell counts; increased blood platelet counts.
Increased pressure within the head, with associated headache, visual disturbances, nausea and vomiting.

CAUTION
1. This drug should not be used to treat mild forms of acne.
2. A transient worsening of your acne may occur during the first few weeks of treatment; this will subside with continued use of the drug.
3. Do not take any other form of vitamin A while taking this drug. (Observe contents of multiple vitamin preparations.)
4. Women with potential for pregnancy should have a pregnancy test before taking this drug and should use an effective form of contraception during its use. It is recommended that contraception be continued until normal menstruation resumes after discontinuing this drug.

5. This drug may cause increased blood levels of cholesterol and triglycerides.
6. If repeated courses of this drug are prescribed, wait a minimum of 2 months between courses before resuming medication.

Precautions for Use

By Infants and Children: Long-term use (6 to 12 months) may cause abnormal acceleration of bone growth and development. Your physician can monitor this possibility by periodic X-ray examination of long bones.

▷ **Advisability of Use During Pregnancy**

Pregnancy Category: X. See Pregnancy Code inside back cover.

Animal studies: Birth defects of skull, brain and vertebral column found in rats; skeletal birth defects found in rabbits.

Human studies: Information from adequate studies of pregnant women is not available. However, serious birth defects of fetal brain development (thought to be due to this drug) have been reported.

Avoid this drug completely during entire pregnancy.

Advisability of Use if Breast-Feeding

Presence of this drug in breast milk: Unknown.

Avoid drug or refrain from nursing.

Habit-Forming Potential: None.

Effects of Overdosage: No experience with overdosage in humans to date.

Suggested Periodic Examinations While Taking This Drug   (at physician's discretion)

Complete blood cell counts, including platelet counts.

Measurements of blood cholesterol and triglyceride levels.

Complete eye examinations.

Liver and kidney function tests.

▷ **While Taking This Drug, Observe the Following**

Foods: No restrictions.

Beverages: No restrictions.

▷ *Alcohol*: No interactions expected.

Tobacco Smoking: No interactions expected.

▷ *Other Drugs*: No interactions reported to date.

▷ *Driving, Hazardous Activities*: No restrictions.

Exposure to Sun: This drug can cause photosensitivity (see Glossary). Avoid excessive exposure to sun until your sensitivity is determined.

KETOPROFEN
(kee toh PROH fen)

Introduced: 1973

Class: Mild Analgesic, Anti-inflammatory

Prescription: USA: Yes
Canada: Yes

Controlled Drug: USA: No
Canada: No

Available as Generic: No

Brand Names: Orudis, ✦Orudis E-50

BENEFITS versus RISKS

Possible Benefits	*Possible Risks*
EFFECTIVE RELIEF OF MILD TO MODERATE PAIN AND INFLAMMATION	Gastrointestinal pain, ulceration, bleeding (rare) Rare liver or kidney damage Rare fluid retention Rare bone marrow depression

---

▷ **Principal Uses**

As a Single Drug Product: Used primarily to relieve mild to moderately severe pain associated with (1) rheumatoid arthritis and osteoarthritis; (2) acute gouty arthritis; (3) acute bursitis, tendinitis and related conditions; and (4) menstrual cramps.

How This Drug Works: Not completely established. It is thought that this drug reduces the tissue concentrations of prostaglandins (and related compounds), chemicals involved in the production of inflammation and pain.

Available Dosage Forms and Strengths
Capsules — 50 mg, 75 mg
Suppositories — 100 mg (in Canada)
Tablets, enteric-coated — 50 mg (in Canada)

▷ **Usual Adult Dosage Range:** Initially, 75 mg 3 times/day or 50 mg 4 times/day. Usual daily dose is 150 to 300 mg divided into 3 or 4 doses. Total daily dosage should not exceed 300 mg. **Note: Actual dosage and administration schedule must be determined by the physician for each patient individually.**

▷ **Dosing Instructions:** Take either on an empty stomach or with food or milk to prevent stomach irritation. Take with a full glass of water and remain upright (do not lie down) for 30 minutes. The capsule may be opened for administration; the tablet should not be crushed or altered.

Usual Duration of Use: Continual use on a regular schedule for 1 to 3 weeks is usually necessary to determine this drug's effectiveness in relieving the discomfort of arthritis. Long-term use (months to years) requires supervision and periodic evaluation by the physician.

▷ **This Drug Should Not Be Taken If**
- you have had an allergic reaction to it previously.
- you are subject to asthma or nasal polyps caused by aspirin.
- you have active peptic ulcer disease or any form of gastrointestinal ulceration or bleeding.
- you have a bleeding disorder or a blood cell disorder.
- you have severe impairment of kidney function.
- you have active liver disease.

▷ **Inform Your Physician Before Taking This Drug If**
- you are allergic to aspirin or to other aspirin substitutes.
- you have a history of peptic ulcer disease or any type of bleeding disorder.
- you have impaired liver or kidney function.
- you have high blood pressure or a history of heart failure.
- you are taking any of the following: acetaminophen, aspirin or other aspirin substitutes, anticoagulants, oral antidiabetic drugs, or probenecid.

Possible Side-Effects   (natural, expected and unavoidable drug actions)
Drowsiness (1% to 3%), ringing in ears (1% to 3%), fluid retention (3%).

▷ **Possible Adverse Effects**   (unusual, unexpected and infrequent reactions)
If any of the following develop, consult your physician promptly.
Mild Adverse Effects
Allergic Reactions: Skin rash (1% to 3%), hives, itching.
Headache (less than 1%), dizziness, altered or blurred vision, depression, confusion, impaired memory.
Mouth sores, indigestion (11%), nausea, vomiting, constipation, diarrhea.
Serious Adverse Effects
Allergic Reactions: Anaphylaxis (see Glossary).
Impaired hearing.
Active peptic ulcer, with or without bleeding (2%).
Rare liver damage with jaundice (see Glossary).
Kidney damage with painful urination, bloody urine, reduced urine formation.
Rare bone marrow depression (see Glossary)—fatigue, weakness, fever, sore throat, abnormal bleeding or bruising.

Possible Delayed Adverse Effects
Mild anemia due to "silent" blood loss from the stomach (less than that caused by aspirin).

▷ **Adverse Effects That May Mimic Natural Diseases or Disorders**
Liver reaction may suggest viral hepatitis.

Natural Diseases or Disorders That May Be Activated by This Drug
Peptic ulcer disease, ulcerative colitis.

CAUTION
1. Dosage should always be limited to the smallest amount that produces reasonable improvement.
2. This drug may mask early indications of infection. Inform your physician if you think you are developing an infection of any kind.

Precautions for Use
By Infants and Children: Safety and effectiveness for use by those under 12 years of age have not been established.
By Those over 60 Years of Age: Small doses are advisable until tolerance is determined. Observe for any indications of liver or kidney toxicity, fluid retention, dizziness, confusion, impaired memory, stomach bleeding or constipation.

▷ **Advisability of Use During Pregnancy**
Pregnancy Category: B (tentative). See Pregnancy Code inside back cover.
Animal studies: No birth defects reported in mouse, rat or rabbit studies.
Human studies: Information from adequate studies of pregnant women is not available.
Avoid this drug during the last 3 months. Use it during the first 6 months only if clearly needed. Ask physician for guidance.

Advisability of Use if Breast-Feeding
Presence of this drug in breast milk: Unknown.
Avoid drug or refrain from nursing.

Habit-Forming Potential: None.

Effects of Overdosage: Drowsiness, nausea, vomiting, diarrhea.

Possible Effects of Long-Term Use: None reported.

Suggested Periodic Examinations While Taking This Drug   (at physician's discretion)
Complete blood cell counts, liver and kidney function tests, complete eye examinations if vision is altered in any way.

▷ **While Taking This Drug, Observe the Following**
Foods: No restrictions.
Beverages: No restrictions. May be taken with milk.
▷   *Alcohol*: Use with caution. The irritant action of alcohol on the stomach lining, added to the irritant action of this drug in sensitive individuals, can increase the risk of stomach ulceration and/or bleeding.
Tobacco Smoking: No interactions expected.
▷   *Other Drugs*
Ketoprofen may *increase* the effects of
   • acetaminophen (Tylenol, etc.), and increase the risk of kidney damage; avoid prolonged use of this combination.
   • anticoagulants (Coumadin, etc.), and increase the risk of bleeding; monitor prothrombin time, adjust dose accordingly.

Ketoprofen *taken concurrently* with the following drugs may increase the risk of bleeding; avoid these combinations:

- aspirin.
- dipyridamole (Persantine).
- indomethacin (Indocin).
- sulfinpyrazone (Anturane).
- valproic acid (Depakene).

▷ *Driving, Hazardous Activities*: This drug may cause drowsiness or dizziness. Restrict activities as necessary.

Aviation Note: The use of this drug *may be a disqualification* for piloting. Consult a designated Aviation Medical Examiner.

Exposure to Sun: This drug can cause photosensitivity (see Glossary). Avoid excessive exposure to sun until tolerance has been determined.

LABETALOL
(la BET a lohl)

Introduced: 1978

Class: Antihypertensive, Alpha- and Beta-Adrenergic Blocker

Prescription: USA: Yes
Canada: Yes

Controlled Drug: USA: No
Canada: No

Available as Generic: No

Brand Names: Normodyne, Trandate

BENEFITS versus RISKS	
Possible Benefits	*Possible Risks*
EFFECTIVE, WELL-TOLERATED ANTIHYPERTENSIVE in mild to moderate high blood pressure	CONGESTIVE HEART FAILURE in advanced heart disease
	Worsening of angina in coronary heart disease (if drug is abruptly withdrawn)
	Masking of low blood sugar (hypoglycemia) in drug-treated diabetes

▷ **Principal Uses**

As a Single Drug Product: The treatment of mild to moderately severe high blood pressure. May be used alone or concurrently with other antihypertensive drugs, such as diuretics.

How This Drug Works: By blocking certain actions of the sympathetic nervous system, this drug

- reduces the rate and contraction force of the heart, thus lowering the ejection pressure of blood leaving the heart.

- reduces the degree of contraction of blood vessel walls, resulting in their relaxation and expansion and consequent lowering of blood pressure.

Available Dosage Forms and Strengths
Injection — 5 mg per ml
Tablets — 100 mg, 200 mg, 300 mg

▷ **Usual Adult Dosage Range:**   Initially, 100 mg twice daily, 12 hours apart; the dose may be increased by 100 mg twice daily every 2 to 3 days as required to reduce blood pressure. The usual maintenance dose is 200 to 400 mg twice daily. The total dose should not exceed 2400 mg/24 hours, given as 800 mg 3 times daily. **Note: Actual dosage and administration schedule must be determined by the physician for each patient individually.**

▷ **Dosing Instructions:**   Take at the same times each day, preferably following the morning and evening meals. The tablet may be crushed for administration. Do not discontinue this drug abruptly.

Usual Duration of Use: Continual use on a regular schedule for 10 to 14 days is usually necessary to determine this drug's effectiveness in lowering blood pressure. The long-term use (months to years) of this drug will be determined by the course of your blood pressure over time and your response to the overall treatment program (weight reduction, salt restriction, smoking cessation, etc.).

▷ **This Drug Should Not Be Taken If**
- you have had an allergic reaction to it previously.
- you have active bronchial asthma.
- you have congestive heart failure.
- you have an abnormally slow heart rate or a serious form of heart block.

▷ **Inform Your Physician Before Taking This Drug If**
- you have had an adverse reaction to any "beta-blocker" drug in the past (see Drug Class, Section Four).
- you have a history of serious heart disease, with or without episodes of heart failure.
- you have a history of hay fever (allergic rhinitis), asthma, chronic bronchitis or emphysema.
- you have a history of overactive thyroid function (hyperthyroidism).
- you have a history of low blood sugar (hypoglycemia).
- you have impaired liver or kidney function.
- you have diabetes or myasthenia gravis.
- you are currently taking any form of digitalis, quinidine or reserpine, or any "calcium-blocker" drug (see Drug Class, Section Four).
- you plan to have surgery under general anesthesia in the near future.

Possible Side-Effects   (natural, expected and unavoidable drug actions)
Lethargy and fatigability (11%), light-headedness in upright position (see orthostatic hypotension in Glossary).

▷ **Possible Adverse Effects**   (unusual, unexpected and infrequent reactions)
If any of the following develop, consult your physician promptly.

Mild Adverse Effects
   Allergic Reactions: Skin rash, itching.
   Headache, drowsiness, dizziness (20%), scalp tingling (during early treatment).
   Indigestion, nausea, diarrhea.
   Joint and muscle discomfort, fluid retention (edema).
   Impaired sexual function.

Serious Adverse Effects
   Chest pain, shortness of breath, precipitation of congestive heart failure.
   Induction of bronchial asthma (in asthmatic individuals).
   Liver damage with jaundice (rare).
   Difficult urination (urinary bladder retention).

CAUTION

1. ***Do not discontinue this drug suddenly*** without the knowledge and guidance of your physician. Carry a notation on your person that you are taking this drug.
2. Consult your physician or pharmacist before using nasal decongestants usually present in over-the-counter cold preparations and nose drops. These can cause sudden increases in blood pressure when taken concurrently with beta-blocker drugs.
3. Report the development of any tendency to emotional depression.

Precautions for Use

By Infants and Children: Safety and effectiveness for use by those under 12 years of age have not been established. However, if this drug is used, observe for the development of low blood sugar (hypoglycemia) during periods of reduced food intake.

By Those over 60 Years of Age: Proceed *cautiously* with all antihypertensive drugs. Unacceptably high blood pressure should be reduced without creating the risks associated with excessively low blood pressure. Start treatment with small doses, and monitor the blood pressure response frequently. Sudden, rapid and excessive reduction of blood pressure can predispose to stroke or heart attack. Observe for dizziness, unsteadiness, tendency to fall, confusion, hallucinations, depression or urinary frequency.

▷ **Advisability of Use During Pregnancy**

Pregnancy Category: C (tentative). See Pregnancy Code inside back cover.
   Animal studies: No significant increase in birth defects found in rats or rabbits; some increase in fetal deaths reported.
   Human studies: Information from adequate studies of pregnant women is not available.
   Use this drug only if clearly needed. Ask physician for guidance.

Advisability of Use if Breast-Feeding

Presence of this drug in breast milk: Yes, in very small amounts.
Avoid drug or refrain from nursing.

Habit-Forming Potential: None.

Effects of Overdosage: Weakness, slow pulse, low blood pressure, fainting, cold and sweaty skin, congestive heart failure, possible coma and convulsions.

Possible Effects of Long-Term Use: Reduced heart reserve and eventual heart failure in susceptible individuals with advanced heart disease.

Suggested Periodic Examinations While Taking This Drug   (at physician's discretion)
Measurements of blood pressure, evaluation of heart function.

▷ **While Taking This Drug, Observe the Following**
Foods: No restrictions. Avoid excessive salt intake.
Beverages: No restrictions. May be taken with milk.
▷ *Alcohol*: Use with caution until the combined effect has been determined. Alcohol may exaggerate this drug's ability to lower blood pressure and may increase its mild sedative effect.
Tobacco Smoking: Nicotine may reduce this drug's effectiveness in treating high blood pressure. In addition, high doses of this drug may potentiate the constriction of the bronchial tubes caused by regular smoking.
▷ *Other Drugs*
Labetalol may *increase* the effects of
• other antihypertensive drugs and cause excessive lowering of blood pressure. Dosage adjustments may be necessary.
Labetalol *taken concurrently* with
• clonidine (Catapres) requires close monitoring for rebound high blood pressure if clonidine is withdrawn while labetalol is still being taken.
• insulin requires close monitoring to avoid undetected hypoglycemia (see Glossary).
▷ *Driving, Hazardous Activities*: Use caution until the full extent of fatigue, dizziness and blood pressure change has been determined.
Aviation Note: The use of this drug *is a disqualification* for piloting. Consult a designated Aviation Medical Examiner.
Exposure to Sun: No restrictions.
Exposure to Heat: Caution advised. Hot environments can lower the blood pressure and exaggerate the effects of this drug.
Exposure to Cold: Caution advised. Cold environments can enhance the circulatory deficiency in the extremities that may occur with some beta-blocker drugs. The elderly should take precautions to prevent hypothermia (see Glossary).
Heavy Exercise or Exertion: It is advisable to avoid exertion that produces light-headedness, excessive fatigue or muscle cramping. The use of this drug may intensify the hypertensive response to isometric exercise.
Occurrence of Unrelated Illness: The fever that accompanies systemic infections can lower the blood pressure and require adjustment of dosage.

Illnesses that cause nausea or vomiting may interrupt the regular dosage schedule. Ask your physician for guidance.

Discontinuation: It is advisable to avoid sudden discontinuation of this drug in all situations. If possible, gradual reduction of dose over a period of 2 to 3 weeks is recommended. Ask your physician for specific guidance.

LEVODOPA
(lee voh DOH pa)

Introduced: 1967

Class: Antiparkinsonism

Prescription: USA: Yes
Canada: Yes

Controlled Drug: USA: No
Canada: No

Available as Generic: USA: Yes
Canada: No

Brand Names: Dopar, Larodopa, ✿Prolopa [CD], Sinemet [CD]

BENEFITS versus RISKS	
Possible Benefits	*Possible Risks*
EFFECTIVE RELIEF OF SYMPTOMS IN 80% OF CASES OF IDIOPATHIC PARKINSON'S DISEASE	Emotional depression, confusion, abnormal thinking and behavior
	Abnormal involuntary movements
	Heart rhythm disturbance
	Urinary bladder retention
	Induction of peptic ulcer (rare)
	Blood cell abnormalities: hemolytic anemia reduced white blood cell count (both rare)

▷ **Principal Uses**

As a Single Drug Product: Used exclusively to treat the major types of Parkinson's disease: paralysis agitans ("shaking palsy" of unknown cause), the type that follows encephalitis, the parkinsonism that develops with aging (associated with hardening of the brain arteries), and the forms of parkinsonism that follow poisoning by carbon monoxide or manganese.

As a Combination Drug Product [CD]: This drug is available in combination with carbidopa, a chemical that prevents the decomposition of levodopa before it reaches its site of action in the brain. The addition of carbidopa reduces the amount of levodopa required by 75%. This combination is more effective in smaller doses and reduces the frequency and severity of adverse effects.

How This Drug Works: Not completely established. Present thinking is that levodopa enters the brain tissue and is converted to dopamine. After sufficient dosage, this corrects the deficiency of dopamine (that is thought to be the cause of parkinsonism) and restores a more normal balance of the chemicals responsible for transmission of nerve impulses in appropriate control centers of the brain.

Available Dosage Forms and Strengths
Capsules — 100 mg, 250 mg, 500 mg
Tablets — 100 mg, 250 mg, 500 mg

▷ **Usual Adult Dosage Range:** Initially, 250 mg 2 to 4 times/day. The dose may be increased cautiously by increments of 100 to 750 mg at 3- to 7-day intervals as needed and tolerated. The total dosage should not exceed 8000 mg/24 hours. If the combination drug Sinemet is used, the total levodopa requirement will be considerably less. **Note: Actual dosage and administration schedule must be determined by the physician for each patient individually.**

▷ **Dosing Instructions:** Preferably taken with or following carbohydrate foods to reduce stomach irritation; when possible, do not take this drug concurrently with high protein foods. The tablet may be crushed for administration.

Usual Duration of Use: Continual use on a regular schedule for 3 to 6 weeks is usually necessary to determine this drug's effectiveness in relieving the major symptoms of parkinsonism. The determination of maximal effectiveness may require continual use for 6 months. Long-term use (months to years) requires supervision and periodic evaluation by your physician; dosage adjustments will be necessary and unavoidable during the course of the disorder.

▷ **This Drug Should Not Be Taken If**
- you are allergic to any of the drugs bearing the brand names listed.
- you have narrow-angle glaucoma (inadequately controlled).
- you are taking, or have taken within the past 14 days, any monoamine oxidase (MAO) inhibitor drug (see Drug Class, Section Four).

▷ **Inform Your Physician Before Taking This Drug If**
- you have diabetes, epilepsy, heart disease, high blood pressure or chronic lung disease.
- you have impaired liver or kidney function.
- you have a history of peptic ulcer disease or malignant melanoma.
- you plan to have surgery under general anesthesia in the near future.

Possible Side-Effects (natural, expected and unavoidable drug actions)
Fatigue, lethargy, altered taste, offensive body odor, orthostatic hypotension (see Glossary).
Pink to red coloration of urine, turning black on exposure to air (of no significance).

▷ **Possible Adverse Effects** (unusual, unexpected and infrequent reactions)
If any of the following develop, consult your physician promptly.
Mild Adverse Effects
Allergic Reactions: Skin rash, itching.

Headache, dizziness, numbness, unsteadiness, insomnia, nightmares, blurred vision, double vision.

Loss of appetite, nausea, vomiting, dry mouth, difficult swallowing, excessive gas, diarrhea, constipation.

Loss of hair (rare).

Serious Adverse Effects

Idiosyncratic Reactions: Hemolytic anemia (see Glossary).

Confusion, delusions, hallucinations, agitation, paranoia, depression, psychotic episodes, seizures.

Abnormal involuntary movements of the head, face and extremities.

Disturbances of heart rhythm, high blood pressure (rare).

Development of peptic ulcer, gastrointestinal bleeding.

Urinary bladder retention, prolonged and painful erection of the penis.

Abnormally low white blood cell count—lowered resistance to infection, fever, sore throat.

▷ **Adverse Effects That May Mimic Natural Diseases or Disorders**

Mental reactions may resemble idiopathic psychosis.

Natural Diseases or Disorders That May Be Activated by This Drug

Latent peptic ulcer.

CAUTION
1. To reduce the high frequency of serious adverse effects, it is advisable to begin treatment with small doses, and to increase dosage gradually until the desired response is achieved.
2. As improvement occurs, avoid excessive and hurried activity (which often causes falls and injury).

Precautions for Use

By Infants and Children: This drug can cause precocious puberty when taken by the prepubertal boy. Observe closely for hypersexual behavior and for premature growth of the genital organs.

By Those over 60 Years of Age: Treatment should begin with half of the usual adult dose; dosage increases should be made cautiously in small increments as needed and tolerated. Observe for the possible development of significant behavioral changes: depression or inappropriate elation, acute confusion, agitation, paranoia, dementia, nightmares and hallucinations. Abnormal involuntary movements may also occur.

▷ **Advisability of Use During Pregnancy**

Pregnancy Category: C (tentative). See Pregnancy Code inside back cover.

Animal studies: Significant birth defects reported in rodent studies.

Human studies: Information from adequate studies of pregnant women is not available.

Avoid use of drug during the first 3 months. Use only if clearly needed during the last 6 months.

Advisability of Use if Breast-Feeding

Presence of this drug in breast milk: Yes.

Avoid drug or refrain from nursing.

Habit-Forming Potential: None.

Effects of Overdosage: Muscle twitching, spastic closure of eyelids, nausea, vomiting, diarrhea, weakness, fainting, confusion, agitation, hallucinations.

Possible Effects of Long-Term Use: Development of abnormal involuntary movements involving the head, face, mouth and extremities. These may be reversible and may gradually subside as the drug is withdrawn.

Suggested Periodic Examinations While Taking This Drug (at physician's discretion)

Complete blood cell counts; measurements of internal eye pressure; blood pressure measurements in lying, sitting and standing positions.

▷ **While Taking This Drug, Observe the Following**

Foods: No restrictions. Insofar as possible, do not take concurrently with protein foods; proteins compete for absorption.

Nutritional Support: If taken alone (without carbidopa), monitor for the development of peripheral neuritis and take small supplements of pyridoxine (vitamin B-6) if needed: 10 mg or less; larger doses can decrease the effectiveness of levodopa. If taken in combination with carbidopa (Sinemet), supplemental pyridoxine is not required.

Beverages: No restrictions. May be taken with milk.

▷ *Alcohol*: No interactions expected.

Tobacco Smoking: No interactions expected.

Marijuana Smoking: Increased fatigue and lethargy; possible accentuation of orthostatic hypotension (see Glossary).

▷ *Other Drugs*

Levodopa *taken concurrently* with

- monoamine oxidase (MAO) inhibitor drugs (see Drug Class, Section Four) may cause a dangerous rise in blood pressure and body temperature. Do not use these drugs concurrently.

The following drugs may *decrease* the effects of levodopa

- papaverine (Cerespan, Pavabid, Vasospan, etc.).
- phenytoin (Dilantin, etc.).
- pyridoxine (vitamin B-6).

▷ *Driving, Hazardous Activities*: This drug may cause dizziness, impaired vision and orthostatic hypotension. Restrict activities as necessary.

Aviation Note: Parkinson's disease *is a disqualification* for piloting. Consult a designated Aviation Medical Examiner.

Exposure to Sun: No restrictions.

Exposure to Heat: Use caution. This drug can cause flushing and excessive sweating and predispose to heat exhaustion.

Occurrence of Unrelated Illness: Suspicious dark-colored skin lesions should be evaluated carefully to exclude the possibility of malignant melanoma. During the course of any intercurrent infection, monitor the white blood cell count carefully for normal response.

LITHIUM
(LITH i um)

Introduced: 1949

Prescription: USA: Yes
Canada: Yes

Available as Generic: USA: Yes
Canada: No

Class: Antidepressant, Antimanic

Controlled Drug: USA: No
Canada: No

Brand Names: ❦Carbolith, Cibalith-S, Eskalith, ❦Lithane, ❦Lithizine, Lithobid, Lithonate, Lithotabs

---

BENEFITS versus RISKS

Possible Benefits	*Possible Risks*
RAPID REVERSAL OF ACUTE MANIA in 80% of users	VERY NARROW MARGIN BETWEEN TREATMENT AND TOXIC BLOOD LEVELS
STABILIZATION OF MOOD in 60% to 70% of users with manic-depressive disorder	POTENTIALLY FATAL TOXICITY with inadequate monitoring
Prevention of recurrent depression in "responders"	Infrequent induction of diabetes mellitus, hypothyroidism
	Diabetes insipiduslike syndrome (excessive dilute urine without sugar)

▷ **Principal Uses**

As a Single Drug Product: Used primarily in the management of manic-depressive disorders. While its principal use is the prompt correction of acute mania, it is also used to stabilize these disorders by reducing the frequency and severity of recurrent manic-depressive mood swings. It is also beneficial in treating the depression phase of these disorders in individuals who do not experience the manic phase. Additional uses (experimental) include the prevention of cluster headaches and the stimulation of production of white blood cells.

How This Drug Works: Not completely established. It is thought that lithium may act to correct chemical imbalances in certain nerve impulse transmitters (dopamine and norepinephrine) that influence emotional status and behavior.

Available Dosage Forms and Strengths

Capsules — 150 mg, 300 mg
Syrup — 8 mEq per 5 ml teaspoonful
Tablets — 300 mg
Tablets, prolonged-action — 300 mg, 450 mg

▷ **Usual Adult Dosage Range:** First day: 300 mg taken 3 times, 6 hours apart; second day and thereafter: increase dose to 1200 mg/24 hours and later to 1800 mg/24 hours if needed and tolerated. The usual maintenance dose is 600 to 1200 mg/24 hours taken in 3 divided doses. The total daily dosage should not exceed 3600 mg. **Note: Actual dosage and administration schedule must be determined by the physician for each patient individually.**

▷ **Dosing Instructions:**   May be taken after meals to reduce stomach irritation. The capsules may be opened and the regular tablets may be crushed for administration; the prolonged-action tablets should be swallowed whole and not altered.

Usual Duration of Use: Continual use on a regular schedule for 1 to 3 weeks is usually necessary to determine this drug's effectiveness in correcting acute mania; several months of continual treatment may be required to correct depression. Long-term use (months to years) requires supervision and periodic evaluation by your physician.

▷ **This Drug Should Not Be Taken If**
- you have had an allergic reaction to any dosage form of it previously.
- you have uncontrolled diabetes or uncorrected hypothyroidism.
- you are breast-feeding.
- you will be unable to comply with the need for regular monitoring of lithium blood levels.

▷ **Inform Your Physician Before Taking This Drug If**
- you have a history of a schizopheniclike thought disorder.
- you have any type of organic brain disease, or a history of grand mal epilepsy.
- you have diabetes, heart disease, hypothyroidism or impaired kidney function.
- you are on a salt-restricted diet.
- you are pregnant or planning pregnancy.
- you are taking any diuretic drug or a cortisonelike steroid preparation.

Possible Side-Effects   (natural, expected and unavoidable drug actions)
Increased thirst and urine volume may occur in 60% of initial users and in 20% of long-term maintenance users. Weight gain may occur in first few months of use. Drowsiness and lethargy may occur in sensitive individuals.

▷ **Possible Adverse Effects**   (unusual, unexpected and infrequent reactions)
If any of the following develop, consult your physician promptly.
Mild Adverse Effects
Allergic Reactions: Skin rashes, generalized itching.
Skin dryness, loss of hair.
Headache, dullness, dizziness, weakness, blurred vision, ringing in ears, fine hand tremor, unsteadiness.
Metallic taste, loss of appetite, stomach irritation, nausea, vomiting, diarrhea.
Serious Adverse Effects
"Blackout" spells, confusion, stupor, slurred speech, spasmodic movements of extremities, epilepticlike seizures.

Loss of bladder or rectal control.

Diabetes insipiduslike syndrome: loss of kidney concentrating power, excessive dilute urine.

Sexual impotence (uncommon).

▷ **Adverse Effects That May Mimic Natural Diseases or Disorders**

Painful discoloration and coldness of the hands and feet may resemble Raynaud's syndrome.

Natural Diseases or Disorders That May Be Activated by This Drug

Diabetes mellitus may be worsened. Psoriasis may be intensified. Myasthenia gravis may be induced (1 case).

CAUTION

1. This drug has a very narrow margin of safe use. The blood level of drug required to be effective is quite close to the level that can cause toxic effects. Periodic measurements of blood lithium levels are mandatory for appropriate adjustments of dosage. Follow instructions exactly regarding drug dosage and periodic blood examinations.
2. Lithium should be discontinued at the first signs of toxicity: drowsiness, sluggishness, muscle twitching, vomiting or diarrhea.
3. The major causes of lithium toxicity are
   - accidental overdose (sometimes due to inadequate monitoring of blood levels).
   - impaired kidney function.
   - salt restriction.
   - inadequate fluid intake, dehydration.
   - concurrent use of diuretics.
   - intercurrent illness.
   - childbirth (rapid decrease in kidney clearance of lithium).
   - initiation of treatment with a new drug.
4. Over-the-counter preparations that contain iodides (some cough products and vitamin-mineral supplements) should be avoided because of the added antithyroid effect when taken with lithium.

Precautions for Use

By Infants and Children: Safety and effectiveness for use by those under 12 years of age have not been established. Follow physician's instructions exactly.

By Those over 60 Years of Age: Initial and maintenance doses should be smaller than standard doses for younger adults; treatment should start with a "test" dose of 75 to 150 mg daily. Observe closely for early indications of toxic effects, especially if on a low-salt diet and using diuretics. Parkinsonian reactions (abnormal gait and movements) occur with greater frequency; coma can develop without warning symptoms.

▷ **Advisability of Use During Pregnancy**

Pregnancy Category: D (tentative). See Pregnancy Code inside back cover.

Animal studies: Cleft palate reported in mice; eye, ear and palate defects reported in rats.

Human studies: Information from adequate studies of pregnant women is not available. However, cardiovascular defects and goiter in newborn infants (of mothers using lithium) have been reported. If the infant's blood level of lithium approaches the toxic range before delivery, the newborn may suffer the "floppy infant" syndrome: weakness, lethargy, unresponsiveness, low body temperature, weak cry and poor feeding ability.

Avoid use of drug during the first 3 months. Use only if clearly necessary during the last 6 months. Monitor mother's blood lithium levels carefully to avoid possible toxicity.

Advisability of Use if Breast-Feeding
Presence of this drug in breast milk: Yes, in significant amounts.
Avoid drug or refrain from nursing.

Habit-Forming Potential: None.

Effects of Overdosage: Drowsiness, weakness, lack of coordination, nausea, vomiting, diarrhea, muscle spasms, blurred vision, dizziness, staggering gait, slurred speech, confusion, stupor, coma, seizures.

Possible Effects of Long-Term Use: Hypothyroidism (5%), goiter, reduced sugar tolerance, diabetes insipiduslike syndrome, serious kidney damage.

Suggested Periodic Examinations While Taking This Drug (at physician's discretion)
Regular determinations of blood lithium levels are absolutely essential to the safe and effective use of this drug.
Periodic evaluation of thyroid gland size and function.
Complete blood cell counts; kidney function tests.

▷ **While Taking This Drug, Observe the Following**
Foods: Maintain a normal diet; **do not** restrict your use of salt.
Beverages: No restrictions. Drink at least 2.5 to 3 quarts of liquids/24 hours. This drug may be taken with milk.
▷ *Alcohol*: Use with caution until the combined effects have been determined. Avoid alcohol completely if any symptoms of lithium toxicity develop.
Tobacco Smoking: No interactions expected.
Marijuana Smoking: Possible increase in apathy, lethargy, drowsiness or sluggishness; accentuation of lithium-induced tremor; possible increased risk of precipitating psychotic behavior.
▷ *Other Drugs*
Lithium *taken concurrently* with
• carbamazepine (Tegretol) or with
• chlorpromazine (Thorazine, etc.) or with
• haloperidol (Haldol) is usually well tolerated; however, it may cause a severe neurotoxic reaction in susceptible individuals. These combinations should be used very cautiously.
• diazepam (Valium) may cause hypothermia.

The following drugs may *increase* the effects of lithium
- indomethacin (Indocin).
- piroxicam (Feldene).
- thiazide diuretics (see Drug Class, Section Four).

The following drugs may *decrease* the effects of lithium
- sodium bicarbonate.
- theophylline (Theo-Dur, etc.) and related drugs.

▷ *Driving, Hazardous Activities*: This drug may impair mental alertness, judgment, physical coordination and reaction time. Restrict activities as necessary.

Aviation Note: The use of this drug *is a disqualification* for piloting. Consult a designated Aviation Medical Examiner.

Exposure to Sun: No restrictions.

Exposure to Heat: Excessive sweating can cause significant depletion of salt and water and resultant lithium toxicity. Avoid sauna baths.

Occurrence of Unrelated Illness: Any illness that causes fever, sweating, vomiting or diarrhea can result in significant alterations of blood and tissue lithium concentrations. Close monitoring of your physical condition and blood lithium levels is necessary to prevent serious toxicity.

Discontinuation: Sudden discontinuation does not cause withdrawal symptoms. Avoid premature discontinuation; some individuals may require continual treatment for up to a year to achieve maximal response. Discontinuation by "responders" may result in recurrence of either mania or depression. Lithium should be discontinued if symptoms of brain toxicity appear or if an uncorrectable diabetes insipiduslike syndrome develops.

LOPERAMIDE
(loh PER a mide)

Introduced: 1977

Prescription: USA: Yes
Canada: Yes

Available as Generic: No

Brand Names: Imodium

Class: Antidiarrheal

Controlled Drug: USA: No
Canada: No

BENEFITS versus RISKS	
Possible Benefits	*Possible Risks*
EFFECTIVE RELIEF OF INTESTINAL CRAMPING AND DIARRHEA	Drowsiness
	Constipation
	Induction of toxic megacolon

▷ **Principal Uses**

As a Single Drug Product: Used primarily for the control of cramping and diarrhea associated with acute gastroenteritis and chronic enteritis and colitis. Also used to reduce the volume of discharge from ileostomies.

How This Drug Works: Not completely established. It is thought that this drug acts directly on the nerve supply of the gastrointestinal tract to reduce its motility and propulsive contractions, thus relieving cramping and diarrhea.

Available Dosage Forms and Strengths
Capsules — 2 mg
Liquid — 1 mg per 5 ml teaspoonful

▷ **Usual Adult Dosage Range:**   For acute diarrhea: 4 mg initially, then 2 mg after each unformed stool until diarrhea is controlled. For chronic diarrhea: 4 to 8 mg/day in divided doses, taken 8 to 12 hours apart. The total daily dosage should not exceed 16 mg. **Note: Actual dosage and administration schedule must be determined by the physician for each patient individually.**

▷ **Dosing Instructions:**   May be taken on an empty stomach or with food if stomach irritation occurs. The capsule may be opened for administration.

Usual Duration of Use: Continual use on a regular schedule for 48 hours is usually necessary to determine this drug's effectiveness in controlling acute diarrhea; continual use for 10 days may be needed to evaluate its effectiveness in controlling chronic diarrhea. If diarrhea persists, consult your physician.

▷ **This Drug Should Not Be Taken If**
- you have had an allergic reaction to it previously.
- it is prescribed for a child under 2 years of age.

▷ **Inform Your Physician Before Taking This Drug If**
- you have a history of liver disease or impaired liver function.
- you have regional enteritis or ulcerative colitis.

Possible Side-Effects   (natural, expected and unavoidable drug actions)
Drowsiness, constipation.

▷ **Possible Adverse Effects**   (unusual, unexpected and infrequent reactions)
If any of the following develop, consult your physician promptly.
Mild Adverse Effects
Allergic Reactions: Skin rash.
Fatigue, dizziness.
Reduced appetite, dry mouth, nausea, vomiting, stomach pain, bloating.
Serious Adverse Effects
"Toxic megacolon" (distended, immobile colon with fluid retention) may develop while treating acute ulcerative colitis.

CAUTION
1. Do not exceed recommended doses.
2. If used to treat chronic diarrhea, report promptly any development of bloating, abdominal distension, nausea, vomiting, constipation or abdominal pain.

Precautions for Use
By Infants and Children: Do not use in those under 2 years of age. Follow physician's instructions exactly regarding dosage. Observe for drowsiness, irritability, personality changes and altered behavior.
By Those over 60 Years of Age: Start treatment with small doses. You may be more sensitive to the sedative and constipating effects of this drug.

▷ **Advisability of Use During Pregnancy**
Pregnancy Category: B (tentative). See Pregnancy Code inside back cover.
Animal studies: No birth defects found in rat and rabbit studies.
Human studies: Information from adequate studies of pregnant women is not available.
Use sparingly and only if clearly needed. Ask physician for guidance.

Advisability of Use if Breast-Feeding
Presence of this drug in breast milk: Unknown.
Avoid drug or refrain from nursing.

Habit-Forming Potential: None.

Effects of Overdosage: Drowsiness, lethargy, depression, dry mouth.

Possible Effects of Long-Term Use: None identified.

Suggested Periodic Examinations While Taking This Drug   (at physician's discretion)
None required.

▷ **While Taking This Drug, Observe the Following**
Foods: No restrictions. Follow prescribed diet.
Beverages: No restrictions. May be taken with milk.
▷   *Alcohol*: Use with caution until combined effects have been determined. This drug may increase the depressant action of alcohol on the brain.
Tobacco Smoking: No interactions expected.
▷   *Other Drugs*: No significant drug interactions reported.
▷   *Driving, Hazardous Activities*: This drug may cause drowsiness or dizziness. Restrict activities as necessary.
Aviation Note: The use of this drug *is a disqualification* for piloting. Consult a designated Aviation Medical Examiner.
Exposure to Sun: No restrictions.

LORAZEPAM ✗

(lor AZ e pam)

Introduced: 1971

Class: Mild Tranquilizer, Benzodiazepines

Prescription: USA: Yes
Canada: Yes

Controlled Drug: USA: C-IV*
Canada: No

Available as Generic: USA: Yes
Canada: No

Brand Names: ✹Apo-Lorazepam, Ativan, ✹Novolorazepam

BENEFITS versus RISKS

Possible Benefits	*Possible Risks*
RELIEF OF ANXIETY AND NERVOUS TENSION in 70% to 80% of users	Habit-forming potential with prolonged use
Wide margin of safety with therapeutic doses	Minor impairment of mental functions
Very few drug interactions	

▷ **Principal Uses**

As a Single Drug Product: Used primarily to provide short-term relief of mild to moderate anxiety. While it is less sedative than the barbiturates, it is also used at bedtime to produce a calming effect that permits natural sleep.

How This Drug Works: It is thought that this drug produces a calming effect by enhancing the action of the nerve transmitter gamma-aminobutyric acid (GABA), which in turn blocks the arousal of higher brain centers.

Available Dosage Forms and Strengths

Injection — 2 mg per ml, 4 mg per ml
Tablets — 0.5 mg, 1 mg, 2 mg

▷ **Usual Adult Dosage Range:** 1 to 10 mg/24 hours. For anxiety: 2 to 3 mg, 2 or 3 times/day. For insomnia: 2 to 4 mg at bedtime. The total daily dose should not exceed 10 mg. **Note: Actual dosage and administration schedule must be determined by the physician for each patient individually.**

▷ **Dosing Instructions:** May be taken on empty stomach or with food or milk. The tablet may be crushed for administration. Do not discontinue this drug abruptly if taken for more than 4 weeks.

Usual Duration of Use: Continual use on a regular schedule for 3 to 5 days is usually necessary to determine this drug's effectiveness in relieving mod-

---

*See Schedules of Controlled Drugs inside back cover.

erate anxiety. Limit continual use to 1 to 3 weeks. Avoid uninterrupted and prolonged use.

▷ **This Drug Should Not Be Taken If**
- you have had an allergic reaction to any dosage form of it previously.
- you have acute narrow-angle glaucoma.
- it is prescribed for a child under 12 years of age.

▷ **Inform Your Physician Before Taking This Drug If**
- you are allergic to any benzodiazepine drug (see Drug Class, Section Four).
- you have a history of alcoholism or drug abuse.
- you are pregnant or planning pregnancy.
- you have impaired liver or kidney function.
- you have a history of serious depression or mental disorder.
- you have any of the following: asthma, emphysema, epilepsy, myasthenia gravis.

Possible Side-Effects   (natural, expected and unavoidable drug actions)
Drowsiness, lethargy, unsteadiness, "hangover" effects on the day following bedtime use.

▷ **Possible Adverse Effects**   (unusual, unexpected and infrequent reactions)
If any of the following develop, consult your physician promptly.
Mild Adverse Effects
Allergic Reactions: Skin rash.
Dizziness (6%), fainting, blurred vision, double vision, slurred speech, headache, sweating, nausea, indigestion.
Serious Adverse Effects
Disorientation, emotional depression, agitation, disturbed sleep, periodic amnesia.

CAUTION
1. This drug should not be discontinued abruptly if it has been taken continually for more than 4 weeks.
2. The concurrent use of some over-the-counter drug products that contain antihistamines (allergy and cold preparations, sleep aids) can cause excessive sedation in sensitive individuals.
3. If this drug is taken at bedtime as a hypnotic, significant impairment of intellectual and motor functions may persist into the following day; avoid hazardous activities and the use of alcohol.

Precautions for Use
By Infants and Children: Safety and effectiveness for use by those under 12 years of age have not been established. This drug should not be used in the hyperactive or psychotic child of any age. Observe for excessive sedation and incoordination.
By Those over 60 Years of Age: It is advisable to use smaller doses at longer intervals to avoid overdosage. Observe for the possible development of lethargy, indifference, fatigue, weakness, unsteadiness, disturbing

dreams, nightmares and paradoxical reactions of excitement, agitation, anger, hostility and rage.

▷ **Advisability of Use During Pregnancy**

Pregnancy Category: C (tentative). See Pregnancy Code inside back cover.

Animal studies: Skeletal and eye defects reported in rabbits.

Human studies: Information from adequate studies of pregnant women is not available. No birth defects have been reported with the use of this drug.

Avoid drug completely during the first 3 months; avoid during the last 6 months if possible. Frequent use in late pregnancy may cause the "floppy infant" syndrome in the newborn: weakness, lethargy, unresponsiveness, depressed breathing, low body temperature.

Advisability of Use if Breast-Feeding

Presence of this drug in breast milk: Yes, in small amounts.

Monitor nursing infant closely and discontinue drug or nursing if adverse effects develop.

Habit-Forming Potential: This drug can produce psychological and/or physical dependence (see Glossary) if used in large doses for an extended period of time.

Effects of Overdosage: Marked drowsiness, weakness, feeling of drunkenness, staggering gait, tremor, stupor progressing to deep sleep or coma.

Possible Effects of Long-Term Use: Psychological and/or physical dependence.

Suggested Periodic Examinations While Taking This Drug   (at physician's discretion)

Complete blood cell counts and liver function tests during long-term use. (Other drugs of this class are known to cause blood cell and liver function disorders rarely.)

▷ **While Taking This Drug, Observe the Following**

Foods: No restrictions.

Beverages: Avoid excessive intake of caffeine-containing beverages: coffee, tea, cola. May be taken with milk.

▷ *Alcohol:* Use with extreme caution until the combined effect is determined. Alcohol may increase the absorption of this drug and add to its depressant effects on the brain. It is advisable to avoid alcohol completely—throughout the day and night—if it is necessary to drive or to engage in any hazardous activity.

Tobacco Smoking: Heavy smoking may reduce the calming action of this drug.

Marijuana Smoking: Increased sedation and significant impairment of intellectual and physical performance.

▷ *Other Drugs*

Lorazepam may *increase* the effects of

• other sedatives, hypnotics, tranquilizers, anticonvulsants and narcotic drugs; excessive sedation may result.

▷ *Driving, Hazardous Activities:* This drug can impair mental alertness, judgment, physical coordination and reaction time. Avoid hazardous activities accordingly.

Aviation Note: The use of this drug *is a disqualification* for piloting. Consult a designated Aviation Medical Examiner.

Exposure to Sun: No restrictions.

Exposure to Heat: Use caution until the effect of excessive perspiration is determined. Because of reduced urine volume, this drug may accumulate in the body and produce effects of overdosage.

Discontinuation: Avoid sudden discontinuation if this drug has been taken for over 4 weeks without interruption. Dosage should be tapered gradually to prevent a withdrawal syndrome that could include depression, confusion, hallucinations, tremor, seizures, muscle cramping, sweating and vomiting.

MAGALDRATE
(MAG al drayt)

Other Names: Antacid

Introduced: 1960

Class: Antacids

Prescription: USA: No
    Canada: No

Controlled Drug: USA: No
    Canada: No

Available as Generic: No

Brand Names: Lowsium, Riopan

BENEFITS versus RISKS

Possible Benefits	*Possible Risks*
EFFECTIVE NEUTRALIZATION OF STOMACH ACIDS (short-term)	EXCESSIVE LOSS OF BODY PHOSPHORUS (with prolonged use)
EFFECTIVE RELIEF OF HEARTBURN, SOUR STOMACH AND ACID INDIGESTION	Significant drug interactions

---

▷ **Principal Uses**

As a Single Drug Product: Used primarily to provide symptomatic relief in the treatment of peptic ulcer disease, gastritis, esophagitis, hiatal hernia and conditions associated with the production of excessive stomach acid.

How This Drug Works: By neutralizing some of the hydrochloric acid in the stomach, this drug reduces the degree of acidity and thus lessens the irritating effect of digestive juices on inflamed or ulcerated tissues. By reducing the action of the digestive enzyme pepsin, this drug is thought to create a more favorable environment for the healing of peptic ulcer.

Available Dosage Forms and Strengths
Oral suspensions — 480 mg per 5 ml teaspoonful, 540 mg per 5 ml
                  teaspoonful
    Tablets — 480 mg
Tablets, chewable — 480 mg

▷ **Usual Adult Dosage Range:**   Suspension: 1 to 2 teaspoonsful between meals and at bedtime; the total daily dose should not exceed 20 teaspoonsful. Tablets: 480 to 960 mg between meals and at bedtime; the total daily dose should not exceed 9600 mg. **Note: For long-term use, actual dosage and administration schedule must be determined by the physician for each patient individually.**

▷ **Dosing Instructions:**   Best taken between meals and at bedtime. When used on a regular basis for continuous effect, as in the treatment of peptic ulcer, it is most effective when taken 1 to 3 hours after eating. May be followed by a sip of water. Shake the suspension well before measuring the dose. Chewable tablets should be chewed thoroughly before swallowing.

Usual Duration of Use: Continual use on a regular schedule should not exceed 2 weeks without your physician's guidance. When used to promote healing of peptic ulcer, antacid medication should be continued for 4 to 6 weeks after all symptoms of ulcer activity have disappeared.

▷ **This Drug Should Not Be Taken If**
   • you have a known allergy or sensitivity to any of its components.

▷ **Inform Your Physician Before Taking This Drug If**
   • you have chronic constipation or diarrhea.
   • you have impaired kidney function.
   • you are taking any form of anticoagulant, digitalis or tetracycline antibiotic.

Possible Side-Effects   (natural, expected and unavoidable drug actions)
   Depletion of body phosphorus (with prolonged use).

▷ **Possible Adverse Effects**   (unusual, unexpected and infrequent reactions)
   If any of the following develop, consult your physician promptly.
   Mild Adverse Effects
   None reported.
   Serious Adverse Effects
   With large doses or prolonged use: abnormally high blood levels of magnesium, causing mood and mental changes, fatigue, weakness, dizziness and irregular heartbeats.

CAUTION
   1. Do not take *any antacid* regularly for more than 2 weeks without your physician's guidance.
   2. If symptoms requiring the use of antacids persist, consult your physician for definitive diagnosis and appropriate treatment.

3. If frequent and continual use of antacids is necessary, it is advisable to use aluminum and/or magnesium preparations (such as this one); they are less absorbable than calcium and sodium antacids.
4. Do not exceed the maximal daily dose stated on the product label.
5. Do not swallow chewable tablets and wafers whole. These preparations must be thoroughly sucked or chewed before swallowing, and preferably followed by a small amount of water or milk. Antacid tablets designed for chewing can cause intestinal obstruction if swallowed whole.
6. Shake all liquid preparations of antacids well before measuring the dose.

Precautions for Use

By Infants and Children: Ask physician for guidance.

By Those over 60 Years of Age: If you develop constipation with the use of this antacid, consult your physician or pharmacist for guidance. Do not allow this condition to go uncorrected.

▷ Advisability of Use During Pregnancy

Pregnancy Category: C (tentative). See Pregnancy Code inside back cover.

Animal studies: No information available.

Human studies: Information from adequate studies of pregnant women is not available. Some studies indicate the possibility of fetal damage from antacids containing *magnesium*; this antacid does contain magnesium. (Read the labels on all antacid products carefully to determine their exact composition.)

Avoid this drug during the first 3 months. If clearly needed, use it sparingly and in small doses during the last 6 months.

Advisability of Use if Breast-Feeding

Presence of this drug in breast milk: Unknown.

Monitor nursing infant closely and discontinue drug or nursing if adverse effects develop.

Habit-Forming Potential: None.

Effects of Overdosage: Possible constipation or diarrhea, depending upon individual sensitivity.

Possible Effects of Long-Term Use: Decreased levels of blood phosphates, resulting in loss of calcium and phosphate from bone with weakening of bone structure (osteomalacia).

Suggested Periodic Examinations While Taking This Drug   (at physician's discretion)

Measurements of blood calcium and phosphorus levels (with long-term use).

▷ While Taking This Drug, Observe the Following

Foods: Follow the diet prescribed by your physican. Maintain regular intake of high-phosphate foods such as meats, poultry, fish, eggs, dairy products and cereals.

Beverages: No restrictions. Tablets may be taken with milk.
▷ *Alcohol*: No interactions expected. However, alcoholic beverages may increase stomach acidity and thus increase antacid requirements.
Tobacco Smoking: No interactions expected. However, nicotine may increase stomach acidity and thus increase antacid requirements.
▷ *Other Drugs*
Magaldrate may *decrease* the effects of
- oral anticoagulants (Coumadin, etc.).
- beta-adrenergic blocking drugs (see Drug Class, Section Four).
- chloroquine (Aralen).
- diflunisal (Dolobid).
- digoxin (Lanoxin).
- iron preparations.
- nitrofurantoin (Furadantin, etc.).
- penicillamine (Cuprimine, Depen).
- phenothiazines (Thorazine, etc., see Drug Class, Section Four).
- sodium polystyrene sulfonate (Kayexalate).
- tetracyclines (see Drug Class, Section Four).

Note: Allow at least 1 to 2 hours between doses of antacids and the preceding medications.
▷ *Driving, Hazardous Activities*: No precautions or restrictions.
Aviation Note: No restrictions.
Exposure to Sun: No restrictions.

MAGNESIUM CARBONATE
(mag NEEZ ee um KAR boh nayt)

Other Names: Antacid

Class: Antacids

Prescription: USA: No
Canada: No

Controlled Drug: USA: No
Canada: No

Available as Generic: Yes

Brand Names: Algicon [CD], Alkets [CD], Bisodol Powder [CD], Di-Gel Tablets [CD], Gaviscon Liquid [CD], Marblen [CD]

Note: This drug is not marketed as a single drug product. It is available in combination with other antacids; the more widely used combinations containing this drug are listed here. For additional information regarding this drug, see the Drug Profile of Magaldrate, a magnesium-containing antacid with actions and characteristics representative of this drug class.

MAGNESIUM HYDROXIDE
(mag NEEZ ee um hi DROX ide)

Other Names: Antacid

Introduced: 1873   **Class:** Antacids

Prescription: USA: No   **Controlled Drug:** USA: No
    Canada: No   Canada: No

Available as Generic: Yes

Brand Names: Aludrox [CD], ♣Amphojel Plus [CD], ♣Amphojel 500 [CD], Ascriptin Preparations [CD], Bisodol Tablets [CD], Camalox [CD], Delcid [CD], Di-Gel Advanced Formula [CD], Di-Gel Liquid [CD], Di-Gel Tablets [CD], ♣Diovol [CD], ♣Diovol Ex [CD], Gelusil Preparations [CD], Kolantyl [CD], Maalox No.1 & No.2 [CD], Maalox Plus [CD], Maalox TC [CD], Magnatril [CD], Milk of Magnesia, Mylanta Preparations [CD], ♣Neutralca-S [CD], Silain-Gel [CD], ♣Univol Suspension [CD], ♣Univol Tablets [CD], Vanquish [CD], WinGel [CD]

BENEFITS versus RISKS

Possible Benefits

EFFECTIVE NEUTRALIZATION
  OF STOMACH ACIDS (short-
  term)
EFFECTIVE RELIEF OF
  HEARTBURN, SOUR STOMACH
  AND ACID INDIGESTION

Possible Risks

EXCESSIVE LOSS OF BODY
  PHOSPHORUS (with prolonged
  use)
Significant drug interactions

▷ **Principal Uses**

As a Single Drug Product: Used primarily to provide symptomatic relief in the treatment of peptic ulcer disease, gastritis, esophagitis, hiatal hernia and conditions associated with the production of excessive stomach acid. This drug is also used as a mild laxative (in larger doses).

As a Combination Drug Product [CD]: Antacids of different chemical composition are often combined to reduce unwanted side-effects of each other. For example, the laxative effects of magnesium antacids can correct the constipating effects of aluminum hydroxide—hence their frequent combination in popular antacid products. Antacids are sometimes combined with drugs that cause stomach irritation, such as aspirin and related compounds, to make such drugs less irritating.

How This Drug Works: By neutralizing some of the hydrochloric acid in the stomach, this drug reduces the degree of acidity and thus lessens the irritating effect of digestive juices on inflamed or ulcerated tissues. By reducing the action of the digestive enzyme pepsin, this drug is thought to create a more favorable environment for the healing of peptic ulcer.

Available Dosage Forms: Concentrates; gels; liquids; powders; suspensions; tablets; tablets, chewable; wafers

▷ **Usual Adult Dosage Range:**   Suspension: 1 to 4 teaspoonsful (depending on strength of product) between meals and at bedtime; the total daily dose should not exceed 16 teaspoonsful. Tablets: 1 to 4 tablets (depending on strength of product) between meals and at bedtime; the total daily dose should not exceed 16 tablets. **Note: For long-term use, actual dosage and administration schedule must be determined by the physician for each patient individually.**

▷ **Dosing Instructions:**   Best taken between meals and at bedtime. When used on a regular basis for continuous effect, as in the treatment of peptic ulcer, it is most effective when taken 1 to 3 hours after eating. May be followed by a sip of water. Shake the suspension well before measuring the dose. Chewable tablets should be chewed thoroughly before swallowing.

 Usual Duration of Use: Continual use on a regular schedule should not exceed 2 weeks without your physician's guidance. When used to promote healing of peptic ulcer, antacid medication should be continued for 4 to 6 weeks after all symptoms of ulcer activity have disappeared.

▷ **This Drug Should Not Be Taken If**
 • you have a known allergy or sensitivity to any of its components.

▷ **Inform Your Physician Before Taking This Drug If**
 • you have chronic constipation or diarrhea.
 • you have impaired kidney function.
 • you are taking any form of anticoagulant, digitalis or tetracycline antibiotic.

 Possible Side-Effects   (natural, expected and unavoidable drug actions)
 Laxative effect (with large doses).
 Depletion of body phosphorus (with prolonged use).

▷ **Possible Adverse Effects**   (unusual, unexpected and infrequent reactions)
 If any of the following develop, consult your physician promptly.
 Mild Adverse Effects
 Nausea, vomiting, stomach cramping.
 Serious Adverse Effects
 With large doses or prolonged use: abnormally high blood levels of magnesium, causing mood and mental changes, fatigue, weakness, dizziness and irregular heartbeats.

CAUTION
 1. Do not take *any antacid* regularly for more than 2 weeks without your physician's guidance.
 2. If symptoms requiring the use of antacids persist, consult your physician for definitive diagnosis and appropriate treatment.
 3. If frequent and continual use of antacids is necessary, it is advisable to use aluminum and/or magnesium preparations (such as this one); they are less absorbable than calcium and sodium antacids.
 4. Do not exceed the maximal daily dose stated on the product label.
 5. Do not swallow chewable tablets and wafers whole. These preparations must be thoroughly sucked or chewed before swallowing, and prefer-

ably followed by a small amount of water or milk. Antacid tablets designed for chewing can cause intestinal obstruction if swallowed whole.

6. Shake all liquid preparations of antacids well before measuring the dose.

Precautions for Use

By Infants and Children: Ask physician for guidance.

By Those over 60 Years of Age: If you develop diarrhea with the use of this antacid, consult your physician or pharmacist for guidance. Do not allow this condition to go uncorrected.

▷ **Advisability of Use During Pregnancy**

Pregnancy Category: C (tentative). See Pregnancy Code inside back cover.

Animal studies: No information available.

Human studies: Information from adequate studies of pregnant women is not available. Some studies indicate the possibility of fetal damage from antacids containing *magnesium*; this antacid does contain magnesium. (Read the labels on all antacid products carefully to determine their exact composition.)

Avoid this drug during the first 3 months. If clearly needed, use it sparingly and in small doses during the last 6 months.

Advisability of Use if Breast-Feeding

Presence of this drug in breast milk: Unknown.

Monitor nursing infant closely and discontinue drug or nursing if adverse effects develop.

Habit-Forming Potential: None.

Effects of Overdosage: Possible nausea, vomiting, abdominal cramping and diarrhea, depending upon individual sensitivity.

Possible Effects of Long-Term Use: Decreased levels of blood phosphates resulting in loss of calcium and phosphate from bone with weakening of bone structure (osteomalacia).

Suggested Periodic Examinations While Taking This Drug   (at physician's discretion)

Measurements of blood calcium and phosphorus levels (with long-term use).

▷ **While Taking This Drug, Observe the Following**

Foods: Follow the diet prescribed by your physican. Maintain regular intake of high-phosphate foods such as meats, poultry, fish, eggs, dairy products and cereals.

Beverages: No restrictions. Tablets may be taken with milk.

▷   *Alcohol*: No interactions expected. However, alcoholic beverages may increase stomach acidity and thus increase antacid requirements.

Tobacco Smoking: No interactions expected. However, nicotine may increase stomach acidity and thus increase antacid requirements.

▷ *Other Drugs*
Magnesium hydroxide may *decrease* the effects of
- oral anticoagulants (Coumadin, etc.).
- digoxin (Lanoxin).
- iron preparations.
- nitrofurantoin (Furadantin, etc.).
- penicillamine (Cuprimine, Depen).
- sodium polystyrene sulfonate (Kayexalate).
- tetracyclines (see Drug Class, Section Four).

Note: Allow at least 1 to 2 hours between doses of antacids and the preceding medications.

▷ *Driving, Hazardous Activities*: No precautions or restrictions.
Aviation Note: No restrictions.
Exposure to Sun: No restrictions.

MAGNESIUM TRISILICATE
(mag NEEZ ee um tri SIL i kayt)

Other Names: Antacid

Introduced: 1936	**Class:** Antacids
Prescription: USA: No Canada: No	**Controlled Drug:** USA: No Canada: No

Available as Generic: Yes

Brand Names: Gaviscon Tablets [CD], Gaviscon-2 Tablets [CD], Magnatril [CD]

Note: This drug is not marketed as a single drug product. It is available in combination with other antacids; the more widely used combinations containing this drug are listed here. For additional information regarding this drug, see the Drug Profile of Magnesium Hydroxide, a magnesium antacid with actions and characteristics representative of this drug class.

MAPROTILINE
(ma PROH ti leen)

Introduced: 1974	**Class:** Antidepressant
Prescription: USA: Yes Canada: Yes	**Controlled Drug:** USA: No Canada: No

Available as Generic: No

Brand Names: Ludiomil

```
┌─────────────────────────────────────────────────────────────────┐
│                     BENEFITS versus RISKS                         │
│                                                                   │
│       Possible Benefits              Possible Risks               │
│   EFFECTIVE RELIEF OF ALL       ADVERSE BEHAVIORAL                 │
│     TYPES OF DEPRESSION            EFFECTS: Confusion,             │
│                                    disorientation, hallucinations │
│                                 CONVERSION OF DEPRESSION           │
│                                    TO MANIA in manic-depressive    │
│                                    disorders                       │
│                                 Irregular heart rhythms            │
│                                 Rare liver toxicity with jaundice  │
└─────────────────────────────────────────────────────────────────┘
```

▷ **Principal Uses**

As a Single Drug Product: To relieve the symptoms associated with spontaneous (endogenous) depression and with reactive depressions, and to initiate the restoration of normal mood. This drug should be used only when a diagnosis of true depression of significant degree has been established. It should not be used to treat mild and transient despondency that may be associated with many life situations in the absence of a bona fide affective illness.

How This Drug Works: It is thought that this drug relieves depression by slowly restoring the nerve impulse transmitter norepinephrine to normal levels within brain tissue.

Available Dosage Forms and Strengths

Tablets — 10 mg (in Canada), 25 mg, 50 mg, 75 mg

▷ **Usual Adult Dosage Range:** Initially 25 mg 3 times daily. Dose may be increased cautiously as needed and tolerated by 10 to 25 mg daily at intervals of 1 week. Usual maintenance dose is 50 to 100 mg/24 hours. The total daily dose should not exceed 150 mg. When the optimal requirement is determined, it may be taken at bedtime as one dose. **Note: Actual dosage and administration schedule must be determined by the physician for each patient individually.**

▷ **Dosing Instructions:** May be taken without regard to meals. Tablet may be crushed for administration.

Usual Duration of Use: Some benefit may be apparent within 1 to 2 weeks, but adequate response may require continual use for 4 to 6 weeks or longer. Long-term use should not exceed 6 months without evaluation regarding the need for continuation of the drug.

▷ **This Drug Should Not Be Taken If**
- you have had an allergic reaction to it previously.
- you are taking or have taken within the past 14 days any monoamine oxidase (MAO) inhibitor drug (see Drug Class, Section Four).
- you are recovering from a recent heart attack.

▷ **Inform Your Physician Before Taking This Drug If**
- you are allergic or overly sensitive to any tricyclic antidepressant (see Drug Class, Section Four).
- you have a history of any of the following: alcoholism, asthma, epilepsy, glaucoma, heart disease, paranoia, prostate gland enlargement, schizophrenia or overactive thyroid function.
- you have impaired liver function.
- you plan to have surgery under general anesthesia in the near future.

Possible Side-Effects (natural, expected and unavoidable drug actions)
Drowsiness, blurred vision, dry mouth, constipation, impaired urination.

▷ **Possible Adverse Effects** (unusual, unexpected and infrequent reactions)
If any of the following develop, consult your physician promptly.
Mild Adverse Effects
Allergic Reactions: Skin rash, itching.
Insomnia, nervousness, palpitations, dizziness, unsteadiness, tremors, fainting, weakness.
Nausea, vomiting, acid indigestion, diarrhea.
Increased sweating.
Serious Adverse Effects
Behavioral effects: anxiety, confusion, hallucinations.
Aggravation of paranoid psychosis and schizophrenia.
Aggravation of seizure disorders (epilepsy).
Liver toxicity with jaundice (see Glossary).

▷ **Adverse Effects That May Mimic Natural Diseases or Disorders**
The development of jaundice may suggest viral hepatitis.

Natural Diseases or Disorders That May Be Activated by This Drug
Latent epilepsy, glaucoma, prostatism (see Glossary).

CAUTION
1. Dosage must be adjusted for each person individually. Report for follow-up evaluation and laboratory tests as directed by your physician.
2. Observe for early indications of toxicity: confusion, agitation, rapid heartbeat.
3. It is advisable to withhold this drug if electroconvulsive therapy (ECT, "shock" treatment) is to be used to treat your depression.

Precautions for Use
By Infants and Children: Safety and effectiveness for use by those under 18 years of age have not been established.
By Those over 60 Years of Age: During the first 2 weeks of treatment, observe for the development of confusion, agitation, forgetfulness, disorientation, delusions and hallucinations. Reduction of dosage or discontinuation may be necessary. Unsteadiness may predispose to falling and injury. This drug can increase the degree of impaired urination associated with prostate gland enlargement (prostatism).

▷ **Advisability of Use During Pregnancy**
Pregnancy Category: B (tentative). See Pregnancy Code inside back cover.
Animal studies: No birth defects found in mouse, rat or rabbit studies.
Human studies: Information from adequate studies of pregnant women is not available.
Avoid use of drug during first 3 months. Use during the last 6 months only if clearly needed.

Advisability of Use if Breast-Feeding
Presence of this drug in breast milk: Yes.
Monitor nursing infant closely for drowsiness or failure to feed properly; discontinue drug or nursing if adverse effects develop.

Habit-Forming Potential: None.

Effects of Overdosage: Confusion, hallucinations, marked drowsiness, heart palpitations, dilated pupils, tremors, stupor, deep sleep, coma, convulsions.

Suggested Periodic Examinations While Taking This Drug   (at physician's discretion)
Complete blood cell counts, liver function tests, serial blood pressure readings and electrocardiograms.

▷ **While Taking This Drug, Observe the Following**
Foods: No restrictions.
Beverages: No restrictions. May be taken with milk.
▷ *Alcohol*: Avoid completely. This drug can markedly increase the intoxicating effects of alcohol and accentuate its depressant action on brain function.
Tobacco Smoking: No interactions expected.
Marijuana Smoking: Increased drowsiness and dryness of mouth; possible reduced effectiveness of this drug.
▷ *Other Drugs*
Maprotiline may *increase* the effects of
• atropinelike drugs (see Drug Class, Section Four).
• all drugs with sedative effects, and cause excessive sedation.
Maprotiline may *decrease* the effects of
• clonidine (Catapres).
• guanethidine (Ismelin).
• methyldopa (Aldomet).
• reserpine (Serpasil, Ser-Ap-Es, etc.).
Maprotiline *taken concurrently* with
• amphetaminelike drugs may cause severe high blood pressure and/or high fever (see Drug Class, Section Four).
• antiseizure drugs requires careful monitoring for change in seizure patterns; dosage adjustments may be necessary.
• ethchlorvynol (Placidyl) may cause delirium; avoid concurrent use.

- monoamine oxidase (MAO) inhibitor drugs may cause high fever, delirium and convulsions (see Drug Class, Section Four).
- thyroid preparations may impair heart rhythm and function.

Ask physician for guidance regarding adjustment of thyroid dose.

The following drugs may *decrease* the effects of maprotiline

- estrogens.
- oral contraceptives.

▷ *Driving, Hazardous Activities*: This drug may impair mental alertness, judgment, physical coordination and reaction time. Avoid hazardous activities.

Aviation Note: The use of this drug *is a disqualification* for piloting. Consult a designated Aviation Medical Examiner.

Exposure to Sun: Use caution until sensitivity to sun has been determined. This drug may cause photosensitivity (see Glossary).

Exposure to Heat: This drug can inhibit sweating and impair the body's adaptation to hot environments, increasing the risk of heat stroke. Avoid saunas.

Exposure to Cold: The elderly should use caution and avoid conditions conducive to hypothermia (see Glossary).

Discontinuation: It is advisable to discontinue this drug gradually. Abrupt withdrawal after long-term use may cause headache, malaise and nausea.

MECLIZINE
(MEK li zeen)

Other Names: Meclozine

Introduced: 1951

Class: Antinausea, Antivertigo, Antihistamines

Prescription: USA: Varies
Canada: Yes

Controlled Drug: USA: No
Canada: No

Available as Generic: USA: Yes
Canada: No

Brand Names: Antivert, ❧Bonamine, Bonine, Ru-Vert-M

BENEFITS versus RISKS

Possible Benefits	*Possible Risks*
EFFECTIVE PREVENTION OF MOTION SICKNESS	Mild sedation
Moderately effective relief of nausea and vertigo	Mild atropinelike effects

---

▷ **Principal Uses**

As a Single Drug Product: Used primarily to control dizziness and vertigo associated with disorders of the inner ear. Also used to prevent or relieve the nausea, vomiting and dizziness characteristic of motion sickness.

As a Combination Drug Product [CD]: This drug is available in Canada in combination with niacin (nicotinic acid), which is added because of its ability to dilate blood vessels and (theoretically) improve circulation.

How This Drug Works: Not completely established. It is thought that this drug reduces the sensitivity of the nerve pathways connecting the organ of equilibrium in the inner ear with the vomiting center in the brain; this prevents or reduces the occurrence of nausea, vomiting and vertigo.

Available Dosage Forms and Strengths
Tablets — 12.5 mg, 25 mg, 50 mg
Tablets, chewable — 25 mg

▷ **Usual Adult Dosage Range:**   12.5 to 25 mg, once or twice daily as needed for vertigo. For motion sickness: 25 to 50 mg taken 1 hour before travel; repeat once daily if needed. Total daily dosage should not exceed 100 mg. **Note: Actual dosage and administration schedule must be determined by the physician for each patient individually.**

▷ **Dosing Instructions:**   May be taken without regard to food. The regular tablet may be crushed for administration.

Usual Duration of Use: Continual use on a regular schedule for 2 to 4 days is usually necessary to determine this drug's effectiveness in relieving vertigo or preventing motion sickness. Duration of use should not exceed 5 days if this drug is not effective.

▷ **This Drug Should Not Be Taken If**
  • you have had an allergic reaction to it previously.
  • you are taking, or have taken within the past 14 days, any monoamine oxidase (MAO) inhibitor drug (see Drug Class, Section Four).
  • you are, or think you may be, pregnant.

▷ **Inform Your Physician Before Taking This Drug If**
  • you have had an unfavorable response to any antihistamine drug in the past.
  • you have any of the following: asthma, epilepsy, glaucoma, peptic ulcer disease, prostate gland enlargement.

Possible Side-Effects   (natural, expected and unavoidable drug actions)
Mild drowsiness, lethargy, impaired concentration, dry mouth, constipation.

▷ **Possible Adverse Effects**   (unusual, unexpected and infrequent reactions)
  If any of the following develop, consult your physician promptly.
  Mild Adverse Effects
  Allergic Reactions: No significant reactions identified.
  Blurred vision.

Serious Adverse Effects
Possible increase in prostatism (see Glossary).

Natural Diseases or Disorders That May Be Activated by This Drug
Latent epilepsy, glaucoma, prostatism.

CAUTION
1. Discontinue this drug 5 days before diagnostic skin testing for allergies.
2. Avoid this drug completely in children with flulike infections or chicken pox. Although a cause-and-effect relationship has not been established, this drug may contribute to the development of Reye syndrome (see Glossary) in susceptible children.

Precautions for Use
By Infants and Children: Safety and effectiveness for use by those under 12 years of age have not been established. See *CAUTION*.
By Those over 60 Years of Age: Observe for increased susceptibility to drowsiness, dizziness and impaired thinking, judgment and memory; the antihistamine-sedative effect can cause a hypoactive syndrome that may be mistaken for emotional depression or senility.

▷ **Advisability of Use During Pregnancy**
Pregnancy Category: C (tentative). See Pregnancy Code inside back cover.
Animal studies: Significant birth defects reported in mouse, rat and ferret studies.
Human studies: Information from studies of pregnant women is inconclusive. No increase in birth defects was reported in 2076 exposures in 2 studies; 12 cleft lips or palates were reported in 3333 exposures in another study.
Avoid this drug completely during the first 3 months. Use it during the last 6 months only if clearly needed. **Note:** This drug is *contraindicated* during pregnancy by one manufacturer.

Advisability of Use if Breast-Feeding
Presence of this drug in breast milk: Unknown.
Avoid drug or refrain from nursing.

Habit-Forming Potential: None.

Effects of Overdosage: Marked drowsiness, confusion, unsteadiness, tremors, stupor progressing to coma; in children: excitement, hallucinations, overactivity, seizures.

Possible Effects of Long-Term Use: Development of tolerance and loss of effectiveness.

Suggested Periodic Examinations While Taking This Drug (at physician's discretion)
None required.

▷ **While Taking This Drug, Observe the Following**
Foods: No restrictions.
Beverages: No restrictions. May be taken with milk.

▷   *Alcohol*: Use with extreme caution until the combined effects have been determined. The combination of alcohol and antihistamines can cause rapid and marked sedation.

Tobacco Smoking: No interactions expected.

▷   *Other Drugs*

Meclizine may *increase* the effects of

- all other drugs with atropinelike effects.
- all other drugs with sedative effects.

The following drugs may *increase* the effects of meclizine

- monoamine oxidase (MAO) inhibitor drugs may prolong its atropinelike effects (see Drug Class, Section Four).

▷   *Driving, Hazardous Activities*: This drug may impair mental alertness, judgment, physical coordination and reaction time. Restrict activities as necessary.

Aviation Note: The use of this drug *is a disqualification* for piloting. Consult a designated Aviation Medical Examiner.

Exposure to Sun: No restrictions.

MECLOFENAMATE
(me kloh fen AM ayt)

Introduced: 1977

Class: Mild Analgesic, Anti-inflammatory

Prescription: USA: Yes
Canada: Yes

Controlled Drug: USA: No
Canada: No

Available as Generic: No

Brand Names: Meclomen

BENEFITS versus RISKS	
Possible Benefits	*Possible Risks*
EFFECTIVE RELIEF OF MILD TO MODERATE PAIN AND INFLAMMATION	Gastrointestinal pain, ulceration, bleeding (rare)
	Rare liver or kidney damage
	Rare fluid retention
	Rare bone marrow depression

▷ **Principal Uses**

As a Single Drug Product: Used primarily to relieve mild to moderately severe pain and inflammation associated with acute and chronic rheumatoid arthritis and osteoarthritis.

How This Drug Works: Not completely established. It is thought that this drug reduces the tissue concentrations of prostaglandins (and related compounds), chemicals involved in the production of inflammation and pain.

Available Dosage Forms and Strengths
Capsules — 50 mg, 100 mg

▷ **Usual Adult Dosage Range:**   200 to 400 mg daily, in 3 or 4 divided doses. Total daily dosage should not exceed 400 mg. **Note: Actual dosage and administration schedule must be determined by the physician for each patient individually.**

▷ **Dosing Instructions:**   Take with food or milk to prevent stomach irritation. Take with a full glass of water and remain upright (do not lie down) for 30 minutes. The capsule may be opened for administration.

Usual Duration of Use: Continual use on a regular schedule for 2 to 3 weeks is usually necessary to determine this drug's effectiveness in relieving the discomfort of arthritis. Long-term use (months to years) requires supervision and periodic evaluation by your physician.

▷ **This Drug Should Not Be Taken If**
  • you have had an allergic reaction to it previously.
  • you are subject to asthma or nasal polyps caused by aspirin.
  • you have active peptic ulcer disease, regional enteritis, ulcerative colitis or any form of gastrointestinal bleeding.
  • you have a bleeding disorder or a blood cell disorder.
  • you have severe impairment of kidney function.

▷ **Inform Your Physician Before Taking This Drug If**
  • you are allergic to aspirin or to other aspirin substitutes.
  • you have a history of peptic ulcer disease, regional enteritis or ulcerative colitis.
  • you have a history of any type of bleeding disorder.
  • you have impaired liver or kidney function.
  • you have high blood pressure or a history of heart failure.
  • you are taking any of the following: acetaminophen, aspirin or other aspirin substitutes, anticoagulants, oral antidiabetic drugs or cortisone-like drugs.

Possible Side-Effects   (natural, expected and unavoidable drug actions)
Ringing in ears, fluid retention.

▷ **Possible Adverse Effects**   (unusual, unexpected and infrequent reactions)
If any of the following develop, consult your physician promptly.
Mild Adverse Effects
Allergic Reactions: Skin rash, hives, itching.
Headache, dizziness, altered or blurred vision, depression.
Mouth sores, indigestion, nausea, vomiting (11%), diarrhea (10% to 33%).
Serious Adverse Effects
Allergic Reactions: Severe skin reactions, drug fever (see Glossary).
Active peptic ulcer, with or without bleeding.
Liver damage with jaundice (see Glossary).
Kidney damage with painful urination, bloody urine, reduced urine formation.

Rare bone marrow depression (see Glossary)—fatigue, weakness, fever, sore throat, abnormal bleeding or bruising.

Possible Delayed Adverse Effects
Mild anemia due to "silent" blood loss from the stomach (less than that caused by aspirin).

▷ **Adverse Effects That May Mimic Natural Diseases or Disorders**
Liver reaction may suggest viral hepatitis.

Natural Diseases or Disorders That May Be Activated by This Drug
Peptic ulcer disease, ulcerative colitis.

CAUTION
1. Dosage should always be limited to the smallest amount that produces reasonable improvement.
2. This drug may mask early indications of infection. Inform your physician if you think you are developing an infection of any kind.

Precautions for Use
By Infants and Children: Safety and effectiveness for use by those under 14 years of age have not been established.
By Those over 60 Years of Age: Small doses are advisable until tolerance is determined. Observe for any indications of liver or kidney toxicity, fluid retention, dizziness, confusion, impaired memory, stomach bleeding or diarrhea.

▷ **Advisability of Use During Pregnancy**
Pregnancy Category: B (tentative). See Pregnancy Code inside back cover.
Animal studies: Some minor birth defects reported in rodents.
Human studies: Information from adequate studies of pregnant women is not available.
Avoid this drug during the first and last 3 months. Use it during the second 3 months only if clearly needed. Ask physician for guidance.
The manufacturer does not recommend the use of this drug during pregnancy.

Advisability of Use if Breast-Feeding
Presence of this drug in breast milk: Unknown.
Avoid drug or refrain from nursing.

Habit-Forming Potential: None.

Effects of Overdosage: Drowsiness, nausea, vomiting, diarrhea, marked agitation, irrational behavior, seizures.

Possible Effects of Long-Term Use: None identified.

Suggested Periodic Examinations While Taking This Drug   (at physician's discretion)
Complete blood cell counts, liver and kidney function tests, complete eye examinations if vision is altered in any way.

▷ **While Taking This Drug, Observe the Following**
Foods: No restrictions.

Beverages: No restrictions. May be taken with milk.
▷ *Alcohol*: Use with caution. The irritant action of alcohol on the stomach lining, added to the irritant action of this drug in sensitive individuals, can increase the risk of stomach ulceration and/or bleeding.
Tobacco Smoking: No interactions expected.
▷ *Other Drugs*
Meclofenamate may *increase* the effects of
• acetaminophen (Tylenol, etc.), and increase the risk of kidney damage; avoid prolonged use of this combination.
• anticoagulants (Coumadin, etc.), and increase the risk of bleeding; monitor prothrombin time, adjust dose accordingly.
Meclofenamate *taken concurrently* with the following drugs may increase the risk of bleeding; avoid these combinations:
• aspirin.
• dipyridamole (Persantine).
• sulfinpyrazone (Anturane).
• valproic acid (Depakene).
▷ *Driving, Hazardous Activities*: This drug may cause dizziness or altered vision. Restrict activities as necessary.
Aviation Note: The use of this drug *may be a disqualification* for piloting. Consult a designated Aviation Medical Examiner.
Exposure to Sun: No restrictions.

MEDROXYPROGESTERONE
(me DROX ee proh JESS te rohn)

Introduced: 1959

Class: Female Sex Hormones, Progestins

Prescription: USA: Yes
Canada: Yes

Controlled Drug: USA: No
Canada: No

Available as Generic: No

Brand Names: Amen, Curretab, Provera

BENEFITS versus RISKS

Possible Benefits	*Possible Risks*
EFFECTIVE TREATMENT OF ABSENT OR ABNORMAL MENSTRUATION due to hormone imbalance	Thrombophlebitis (rare)
	Pulmonary embolism (rare)
	Liver reaction with jaundice (rare)
	Drug-induced birth defects
EFFECTIVE CONTRACEPTION when given by injection	
Useful adjunctive therapy in selected cases of uterine and kidney cancer	

▷ **Principal Uses**

As a Single Drug Product: Used primarily to initiate and regulate menstruation and to correct abnormal patterns of menstrual bleeding caused by hormonal imbalance (and not by organic disease). The injectable form of this drug is a very effective contraceptive (but is not approved for this use in the USA).

How This Drug Works: By inducing and maintaining a lining in the uterus that resembles pregnancy, this drug can prevent uterine bleeding until it is withdrawn. By suppressing the release of the pituitary gland hormone that induces ovulation, and by stimulating the secretion of mucus by the uterine cervix (to resist the passage of sperm), this drug can prevent pregnancy.

Available Dosage Forms and Strengths

Tablets — 2.5 mg, 5 mg, 10 mg, 100 mg

▷ **Usual Adult Dosage Range:**   To initiate menstruation: 5 to 10 mg/day for 5 to 10 days, started at any time; to correct abnormal bleeding: 5 to 10 mg/day for 5 to 10 days, started on the sixteenth or twenty-first day of the menstrual cycle. Withdrawal bleeding usually begins within 3 to 7 days after stopping the drug. **Note: Actual dosage and administration schedule must be determined by the physician for each patient individually.**

▷ **Dosing Instructions:**   Take on an empty stomach or with food to prevent nausea. The tablet may be crushed for administration.

Usual Duration of Use: Continual use on a regular schedule for 2 or 3 menstrual cycles is usually necessary to determine this drug's effectiveness in correcting abnormal patterns of menstrual bleeding.

▷ **This Drug Should Not Be Taken If**

- you have had an allergic reaction to it previously.
- you are pregnant.
- you have seriously impaired liver function.
- you have a history of cancer of the breast or reproductive organs.
- you have a history of thrombophlebitis, embolism or stroke.
- you have abnormal and unexplained vaginal bleeding.

▷ **Inform Your Physician Before Taking This Drug If**

- you have impaired kidney function.
- you have any of the following disorders: asthma, diabetes, emotional depression, epilepsy, heart disease, migraine headaches.

Possible Side-Effects   (natural, expected and unavoidable drug actions)

Fluid retention, weight gain, changes in menstrual timing and flow, spotting between periods.

▷ **Possible Adverse Effects**   (unusual, unexpected and infrequent reactions)

If any of the following develop, consult your physician promptly.

Mild Adverse Effects
Allergic Reactions: Skin rash, hives, itching.
Fatigue, weakness, nausea.
Acne, excessive hair growth, breast tenderness, milk formation.

Serious Adverse Effects
Liver toxicity with jaundice (see Glossary): yellow eyes and skin, dark-colored urine, light-colored stools.
Thrombophlebitis (inflammation of a vein with blood clot formation): pain or tenderness in thigh or leg, with or without swelling of the foot, ankle or leg.
Pulmonary embolism (movement of blood clot to lung): sudden shortness of breath, chest pain, cough, bloody sputum.
Stroke (blood clot in the brain): sudden headache, blackouts, sudden weakness or paralysis of any part of the body, severe dizziness, double vision, slurred speech, inability to speak.
Retinal thrombosis (blood clot in principal blood vessel to the eye): sudden impairment or loss of vision.

▷ **Adverse Effects That May Mimic Natural Diseases or Disorders**
Liver toxicity may suggest viral hepatitis.

CAUTION
1. There is an increased risk of birth defects in children whose mothers take this drug during the first 4 months of pregnancy.
2. Inform your physician promptly if you think you may be pregnant.
3. This drug should not be used as a test for pregnancy.

Precautions for Use
By Infants and Children: Not used in this age group.
By Those over 60 Years of Age: Used selectively as adjunctive therapy in treating cancer of the breast, uterus and kidney. Observe for excessive fluid retention.

▷ **Advisability of Use During Pregnancy**
Pregnancy Category: X. See Pregnancy Code inside back cover.
Animal studies: Genital defects reported in rat and rabbit studies; masculinization of the female rodent fetus; various defects in chick embryo and rabbit.
Human studies: Masculinization of the female genitals: enlargement of the clitoris, fusion of the labia. Increased risk of heart, nervous system and limb defects also reported.
Avoid this drug completely during entire pregnancy.

Advisability of Use if Breast-Feeding
Presence of this drug in breast milk: Yes.
Avoid drug or refrain from nursing.

Habit-Forming Potential: None.

Effects of Overdosage: Nausea, vomiting, fluid retention, breast enlargement and discomfort, abnormal vaginal bleeding.

Possible Effects of Long-Term Use: None reported in humans.

Suggested Periodic Examinations While Taking This Drug   (at physician's discretion)
>   Regular examinations (every 6 to 12 months) of the breasts and reproductive organs (pelvic examination of the uterus and ovaries, including Pap smear).

▷ **While Taking This Drug, Observe the Following**
>   *Foods*: No restrictions.
>   *Beverages*: No restrictions.
▷   *Alcohol*: No interactions expected.
>   *Tobacco Smoking*: It is advisable to smoke lightly or not at all.
▷   *Other Drugs*
>   The following drugs may *decrease* the effects of medroxyprogesterone
>   • rifampin (Rifadin, Rimactane, etc.) may hasten its elimination.
▷   *Driving, Hazardous Activities*: Usually no restrictions. Consult your physician for assessment of individual risk and for guidance regarding specific restrictions.
>   *Aviation Note*: The use of this drug *may be a disqualification* for piloting. Consult a designated Aviation Medical Examiner.
>   *Exposure to Sun*: No restrictions.

MEPERIDINE ✄
(me PER i deen)

Other Names: Pethidine

Introduced: 1939	**Class:** Strong Analgesic, Opioids
Prescription: USA: Yes	**Controlled Drug:** USA: C-II*
Canada: Yes	Canada: <N>

Available as Generic: Yes

Brand Names: Demerol, Demerol (APAP) [CD], Pethadol

BENEFITS versus RISKS

Possible Benefits	*Possible Risks*
EFFECTIVE RELIEF OF MODERATE TO SEVERE PAIN	POTENTIAL FOR HABIT FORMATION (DEPENDENCE)
	Weakness, fainting
	Disorientation, hallucinations
	Interference with urination

---

*See Schedules of Controlled Drugs inside back cover.

▷ **Principal Uses**

As a Single Drug Product: This potent analgesic is used by mouth or injection to relieve moderate to severe pain of any cause.

As a Combination Drug Product [CD]: This drug is available in combination with acetaminophen (APAP) to create a dosage form that utilizes two pain relievers, one of which also reduces fever.

How This Drug Works: Acting primarily as a depressant of certain brain functions, this drug suppresses the perception of pain and calms the emotional response to pain.

Available Dosage Forms and Strengths

Injections — 10 mg per ml, 25 mg per ml, 50 mg per ml, 75 mg per ml, 100 mg per ml, 400 mg per ml

Syrup — 50 mg per 5 ml teaspoonful

Tablets — 50 mg, 100 mg

▷ **Usual Adult Dosage Range:** Taken by mouth: 50 to 150 mg/3 to 4 hours as needed to relieve pain; the usual dose is 100 mg. The total daily dosage should not exceed 900 mg. **Note: Actual dosage and administration schedule must be determined by the physician for each patient individually.**

▷ **Dosing Instructions:** May be taken with or following food to reduce stomach irritation or nausea. The tablet may be crushed for administration. The syrup may be diluted in 4 ounces of water to reduce the numbing effect on the tongue and mouth tissues.

Usual Duration of Use: As required to control pain. Continual use should not exceed 5 to 7 days without interruption and reassessment of need.

▷ **This Drug Should Not Be Taken If**
- you have had an allergic reaction to any dosage form of it previously.
- you are having an acute attack of asthma.
- you are taking, or have taken within the past 14 days, any monoamine oxidase (MAO) inhibitor drug (see Drug Class, Section Four).

▷ **Inform Your Physician Before Taking This Drug If**
- you have a history of drug abuse or alcoholism.
- you have impaired liver or kidney function.
- you have a history of asthma, epilepsy or glaucoma.
- you are taking any other drugs that have a sedative effect.
- you plan to have surgery under general anesthesia in the near future.

Possible Side-Effects (natural, expected and unavoidable drug actions)
Drowsiness, light-headedness, weakness, euphoria, dry mouth, urinary retention, constipation.

▷ **Possible Adverse Effects** (unusual, unexpected and infrequent reactions)
If any of the following develop, consult your physician promptly.
Mild Adverse Effects
Allergic Reactions: Skin rash, hives, itching.

Headache, dizziness, impaired concentration, sensation of drunkenness, confusion, depression, blurred or double vision.

Facial flushing, sweating, heart palpitation.

Nausea, vomiting.

Serious Adverse Effects

Drop in blood pressure, causing severe weakness and fainting.

Disorientation, hallucinations, unstable gait, tremor, muscle twitching.

▷ **Adverse Effects That May Mimic Natural Diseases or Disorders**

Paradoxical behavioral disturbances may suggest psychotic disorder.

CAUTION

1. If you have asthma, chronic bronchitis or emphysema, the excessive use of this drug may cause significant respiratory difficulty, thickening of bronchial secretions and suppression of coughing.
2. The concurrent use of this drug with atropinelike drugs can increase the risk of urinary retention and reduced intestinal function.
3. Do not take this drug following acute head injury.

Precautions for Use

By Infants and Children: Do not use this drug in infants under 1 year of age because of their vulnerability to life-threatening respiratory depression.

By Those over 60 Years of Age: Use small doses initially and increase dosage as needed and tolerated. Limit use to short-term treatment only if possible. There may be increased susceptibility to the development of drowsiness, dizziness, unsteadiness, falling, urinary retention and constipation (often leading to fecal impaction).

▷ **Advisability of Use During Pregnancy**

Pregnancy Category: C (tentative). See Pregnancy Code inside back cover.

Animal studies: Significant birth defects reported in hamster studies.

Human studies: Information from adequate studies of pregnant women is not available. However, no significant increase in birth defects was found in 1100 exposures to this drug.

Avoid during the first 3 months. Use sparingly and in small doses during the last 6 months only if clearly needed.

Advisability of Use if Breast-Feeding

Presence of this drug in breast milk: Yes.

Avoid drug or refrain from nursing.

Habit-Forming Potential: This drug can cause psychological and physical dependence (see Glossary).

Effects of Overdosage: Marked drowsiness, confusion, tremors, convulsions, stupor progressing to coma.

Possible Effects of Long-Term Use: Psychological and physical dependence, chronic constipation.

Suggested Periodic Examinations While Taking This Drug (at physician's discretion)

None.

▷ **While Taking This Drug, Observe the Following**
   Foods: No restrictions.
   Beverages: No restrictions. May be taken with milk.
▷ *Alcohol*: Use extreme caution until the combined effects have been determined. Opioid analgesics can intensify the intoxicating effects of alcohol, and alcohol can intensify the depressant effects of opioids on brain function, breathing and circulation. Alcohol is best avoided.
   Tobacco Smoking: No interactions expected.
   Marijuana Smoking: Increase in drowsiness and pain relief; impairment of mental and physical performance.
▷ *Other Drugs*
   Meperidine may *increase* the effects of
   • other drugs with sedative effects.
   • atropinelike drugs, and increase the risk of constipation and urinary retention.
   Meperidine *taken concurrently* with
   • monoamine oxidase (MAO) inhibitor drugs (see Drug Class, Section Four) can cause the equivalent of an acute narcotic overdose: unconsciousness; severe depression of breathing, heart action and circulation. A variation of this reaction can be excitability, convulsions, high fever and rapid heart action.
   • phenothiazines (see Drug Class, Section Four) can cause excessive and prolonged depression of brain functions, breathing and circulation.
▷ *Driving, Hazardous Activities*: This drug can impair mental alertness, judgment, reaction time and physical coordination. Avoid hazardous activities.
   Aviation Note: The use of this drug *is a disqualification* for piloting. Consult a designated Aviation Medical Examiner.
   Exposure to Sun: No restrictions.
   Discontinuation: It is advisable to limit this drug to short-term use. If it is necessary to use it for extended periods of time, discontinuation should be gradual to minimize possible effects of withdrawal.

METAPROTERENOL
(met a proh TER e nohl)

Other Names: Orciprenaline

Introduced: 1964   **Class:** Antiasthmatic, Bronchodilator

Prescription: USA: Yes   **Controlled Drug:** USA: No
   Canada: Yes   Canada: No

Available as Generic: No

Brand Names: Alupent, Metaprel

```
┌─────────────────────────────────────────────────────────────────┐
│                     BENEFITS versus RISKS                         │
│                                                                   │
│      Possible Benefits                  Possible Risks            │
│  VERY EFFECTIVE RELIEF OF        Increased blood pressure         │
│     BRONCHOSPASM                 Fine hand tremor                 │
│                                  Irregular heart rhythm (with     │
│                                      excessive use)               │
└─────────────────────────────────────────────────────────────────┘
```

▷ **Principal Uses**

As a Single Drug Product: To relieve acute bronchial asthma and to reduce the frequency and severity of chronic, recurrent asthmatic attacks; also used to relieve reversible bronchospasm associated with chronic bronchitis and emphysema.

How This Drug Works: By stimulating certain sympathetic nerve terminals, this drug acts to dilate those bronchial tubes that are in sustained constriction, thereby increasing the size of the airway and improving the ability to breathe.

Available Dosage Forms and Strengths

Powder for inhalation — 0.65 mg/inhalation
Solution for nebulization — 0.6%, 5%
Syrup — 10 mg per 5 ml teaspoonful
Tablets — 10 mg, 20 mg

▷ **Usual Adult Dosage Range:**   Inhaler: 2 or 3 inhalations/3 to 4 hours; do not exceed 12 inhalations/day. Hand nebulizer: 5 to 15 inhalations/4 hours; do not exceed 40 inhalations/day. Syrup and tablets: 20 mg/6 to 8 hours. **Note: Actual dosage and administration schedule must be determined by the physician for each patient individually.**

▷ **Dosing Instructions:**   May be taken on empty stomach or with food or milk. Tablets should not be crushed for administration. For aerosol and nebulizer, follow the written instructions carefully. Do not overuse.

Usual Duration of Use: According to individual requirements. Do not use beyond the time necessary to terminate episodes of asthma.

▷ **This Drug Should Not Be Taken If**
  • you have had an allergic reaction to any dosage form of it previously.
  • you currently have an irregular heart rhythm.
  • you are taking, or have taken within the past 2 weeks, any monoamine oxidase (MAO) inhibitor drug (see Drug Class, Section Four).

▷ **Inform Your Physician Before Taking This Drug If**
  • you are overly sensitive to other drugs that stimulate the sympathetic nervous system.
  • you are currently using epinephrine (Adrenalin, Primatene Mist, etc.) to relieve asthmatic breathing.

- you have any type of heart or circulatory disorder, especially high blood pressure or coronary heart disease.
- you have diabetes or an overactive thyroid gland (hyperthyroidism).
- you are taking any form of digitalis or any stimulant drug.

Possible Side-Effects   (natural, expected and unavoidable drug actions)
Aerosol—dryness or irritation of mouth or throat, altered taste. Tablet—nervousness, palpitation.

▷ **Possible Adverse Effects**   (unusual, unexpected and infrequent reactions)
  If any of the following develop, consult your physician promptly.
  Mild Adverse Effects
  Headache, dizziness, restlessness, insomnia, fine tremor of hands.
  Rapid, pounding heartbeat; increased sweating; muscle cramps in arms and legs.
  Nausea, heartburn, vomiting.
  Serious Adverse Effects
  Rapid or irregular heart rhythm, intensification of angina, increased blood pressure.

Natural Diseases or Disorders That May Be Activated By This Drug
Latent coronary artery disease, diabetes or high blood pressure.

CAUTION
  1. Concurrent use of this drug by aerosol inhalation with beclomethasone aerosol (Beclovent, Vanceril) may increase the risk of toxicity due to fluorocarbon propellants. It is advisable to use this aerosol 20 to 30 minutes *before* beclomethasone aerosol. This will reduce the risk of toxicity and will enhance the penetration of beclomethasone.
  2. *Avoid excessive use of aerosol inhalation.* The excessive or prolonged use of this drug by inhalation can reduce its effectiveness and cause serious heart rhythm disturbances, including cardiac arrest.
  3. Do not use this drug concurrently with epinephrine. These two drugs may be used alternately if an interval of 4 hours is allowed between doses.
  4. If you do not respond to your usually effective dose, ask your physician for guidance. Do not increase the size or frequency of the dose without your physician's approval.

Precautions for Use
  By Infants and Children: Safety and effectiveness of use of the aerosol and nebulized solution have not been established for children under 12 years of age. Safety and effectiveness of use of the syrup and tablet have not been established for children under 6 years of age.
  By Those over 60 Years of Age: Avoid excessive and continual use. If acute asthma is not relieved promptly, other drugs will have to be tried. Observe for the development of nervousness, palpitations, irregular heart rhythm and muscle tremors. Use with extreme caution if you have hardening of the arteries, heart disease or high blood pressure.

▷ **Advisability of Use During Pregnancy**

Pregnancy Category: C (tentative). See Pregnancy Code inside back cover.
Animal studies: Significant birth defects reported in rabbit studies.
Human studies: Information from adequate studies of pregnant women is not available.
Avoid use during first 3 months. Use during the last 6 months only if clearly needed.

Advisability of Use if Breast-Feeding

Presence of this drug in breast milk: Unknown.
Avoid drug or refrain from nursing.

Habit-Forming Potential: None.

Effects of Overdosage: Nervousness, palpitation, rapid heart rate, sweating, headache, tremor, vomiting, chest pain.

Possible Effects of Long-Term Use: Loss of effectiveness. See *CAUTION* category.

Suggested Periodic Examinations While Taking This Drug   (at physician's discretion)

Blood pressure measurements, evaluation of heart status.

▷ **While Taking This Drug, Observe the Following**

Foods: No restrictions.
Beverages: Avoid excessive use of caffeine-containing beverages: coffee, tea, cola, chocolate.

▷   *Alcohol*: No interactions expected.

Tobacco Smoking: No interactions expected.

▷   *Other Drugs*

Metaproterenol *taken concurrently* with

  • monoamine oxidase (MAO) inhibitor drugs may cause excessive increase in blood pressure and undesirable heart stimulation.

▷   *Driving, Hazardous Activities*: Usually no restrictions. Use caution if excessive nervousness or dizziness occurs.

Aviation Note: The use of this drug *is a disqualification* for piloting. Consult a designated Aviation Medical Examiner.

Exposure to Sun: No restrictions.

Heavy Exercise or Exertion: Use caution. Excessive exercise can induce asthma in sensitive individuals.

METHADONE
(METH a dohn)

Introduced: 1948

Prescription: USA: Yes

Available as Generic: Yes

Brand Names: Dolophine

Class: Strong Analgesic, Opioids

Controlled Drug: USA: C-II*

BENEFITS versus RISKS	
Possible Benefits	*Possible Risks*
EFFECTIVE RELIEF OF MODERATE TO SEVERE PAIN	POTENTIAL FOR HABIT FORMATION (DEPENDENCE) Weakness, fainting Disorientation, hallucinations Interference with urination

▷ **Principal Uses**

As a Single Drug Product: This potent analgesic is used by mouth or injection to relieve moderate to severe pain of any cause. Its primary use today is to provide an appropriate substitute for heroin in treatment programs for drug addiction.

How This Drug Works: Acting primarily as a depressant of certain brain functions, this drug suppresses the perception of pain and calms the emotional response to pain.

Available Dosage Forms and Strengths

    Concentrate — 10 mg per ml
    Injection — 10 mg per ml
    Oral solution — 5 mg per 5 ml teaspoonful (8% alcohol), 10 mg per 5 ml teaspoonful (8% alcohol)
    Tablets — 5 mg, 10 mg
Tablets, dispersible — 40 mg

▷ **Usual Adult Dosage Range:** Taken by mouth: 2.5 to 10 mg/3 to 4 hours as needed to relieve pain. The total daily dosage should not exceed 80 mg. (Dosage schedules for maintenance treatment during heroin withdrawal must be individualized.) **Note: Actual dosage and administration schedule must be determined by the physician for each patient individually.**

▷ **Dosing Instructions:** May be taken with or following food to reduce stomach irritation or nausea. The tablet may be crushed for administration. The concentrate must be diluted in 3 ounces (or more) of water before swallowing.

Usual Duration of Use: As required to control pain. Continual use should not exceed 5 to 7 days without interruption and reassessment of need.

*See Schedules of Controlled Drugs inside back cover.

▷ **This Drug Should Not Be Taken If**
- you have had an allergic reaction to any dosage form of it previously.
- you are having an acute attack of asthma.

▷ **Inform Your Physician Before Taking This Drug If**
- you have a history of drug abuse or alcoholism.
- you have impaired liver or kidney function.
- you have a history of asthma or other chronic lung disease.
- you are taking any other drugs that have a sedative effect.
- you are taking, or have taken within the past 14 days, any monoamine oxidase (MAO) inhibitor drug (see Drug Class, Section Four).
- you plan to have surgery under general anesthesia in the near future.

Possible Side-Effects   (natural, expected and unavoidable drug actions)
Drowsiness, light-headedness, weakness, euphoria, dry mouth, urinary retention, constipation.

▷ **Possible Adverse Effects**   (unusual, unexpected and infrequent reactions)
If any of the following develop, consult your physician promptly.
Mild Adverse Effects
Allergic Reactions: Skin rash, hives, itching.
Headache, dizziness, impaired concentration, sensation of drunkenness, confusion, depression, blurred or double vision.
Facial flushing, sweating, heart palpitation.
Nausea, vomiting.
Serious Adverse Effects
Drop in blood pressure, causing severe weakness and fainting.
Disorientation, hallucinations, unstable gait, tremor, muscle twitching.

▷ **Adverse Effects That May Mimic Natural Diseases or Disorders**
Paradoxical behavioral disturbances may suggest psychotic disorder.

CAUTION
1. If you have asthma, chronic bronchitis or emphysema, the excessive use of this drug may cause significant respiratory difficulty, thickening of bronchial secretions and suppression of coughing.
2. The concurrent use of this drug with atropinelike drugs can increase the risk of urinary retention and reduced intestinal function.
3. Do not take this drug following acute head injury.

Precautions for Use
By Infants and Children: Do not use this drug in infants under 1 year of age because of their vulnerability to life-threatening respiratory depression.
By Those over 60 Years of Age: Use small doses initially and increase dosage as needed and tolerated. Limit use to short-term treatment only if possible. There may be increased susceptibility to the development of drowsiness, dizziness, unsteadiness, falling, urinary retention and constipation (often leading to fecal impaction).

▷ **Advisability of Use During Pregnancy**
Pregnancy Category: C (tentative). See Pregnancy Code inside back cover.
Animal studies: Significant birth defects reported in mice and hamster studies.
Human studies: Information from adequate studies of pregnant women is not available.
Avoid during the first 3 months. Use sparingly and in small doses during the last 6 months only if clearly needed.

Advisability of Use if Breast-Feeding
Presence of this drug in breast milk: Yes.
Avoid drug or refrain from nursing.

Habit-Forming Potential: This drug can cause psychological and physical dependence (see Glossary).

Effects of Overdosage: Marked drowsiness, confusion, tremors, convulsions, stupor progressing to coma.

Possible Effects of Long-Term Use: Psychological and physical dependence, chronic constipation.

Suggested Periodic Examinations While Taking This Drug (at physician's discretion)
None.

▷ **While Taking This Drug, Observe the Following**
Foods: No restrictions.
Beverages: No restrictions. May be taken with milk.
▷ *Alcohol*: Use extreme caution until the combined effects have been determined. Opioid analgesics can intensify the intoxicating effects of alcohol, and alcohol can intensify the depressant effects of opioids on brain function, breathing and circulation. Alcohol is best avoided.
Tobacco Smoking: No interactions expected.
Marijuana Smoking: Increase in drowsiness and pain relief; impairment of mental and physical performance.
▷ *Other Drugs*
Methadone may *increase* the effects of
• other drugs with sedative effects, and cause excessive sedation.
Methadone *taken concurrently* with
• monoamine oxidase (MAO) inhibitor drugs (see Drug Class, Section Four) requires cautious observation for indications of nervous system toxicity.
The following drugs may *decrease* the effects of methadone
• phenytoin (Dilantin, etc.).
• rifampin (Rifadin, Rimactane, etc.).
▷ *Driving, Hazardous Activities*: This drug can impair mental alertness, judgment, reaction time and physical coordination. Avoid hazardous activities.
Aviation Note: The use of this drug *is a disqualification* for piloting. Consult a designated Aviation Medical Examiner.

Exposure to Sun: No restrictions.

Discontinuation: It is advisable to limit this drug to short-term use. If it is necessary to use it for extended periods of time, discontinuation should be gradual to minimize possible effects of withdrawal (stomach cramps, tearing eyes, nasal discharge, chills and tremors.

METHOCARBAMOL
(meth oh KAR ba mohl)

Introduced: 1957

Prescription: USA: Yes
Canada: No

Available as Generic: USA: Yes
Canada: No

Class: Muscle Relaxant

Controlled Drug: USA: No
Canada: No

Brand Names: Robaxin, Robaxin-750, Robaxisal [CD], ✚Robaxisal-C [CD]

BENEFITS versus RISKS	
Possible Benefits	*Possible Risks*
Mild to moderate relief of discomfort due to spasm of voluntary muscles	White blood cell reduction (rare) Drowsiness, weakness Blurred or double vision

▷ **Principal Uses**

As a Single Drug Product: Used primarily to relieve the pain and stiffness associated with spasm of voluntary muscles, such as that resulting from accidental injury of musculoskeletal structures. It is often necessary to supplement the use of this drug with other treatment measures, such as rest, support and physiotherapy.

As a Combination Drug Product [CD]: It is combined with aspirin (and with codeine in Canada) to enhance its effectiveness in relieving discomfort. Aspirin and codeine are effective analgesics and may be necessary to control the pain that is not relieved by methocarbamol alone.

How This Drug Works: Not completely established. It is thought that this drug may relieve muscle spasm and pain by blocking the transmission of nerve impulses over reflex pathways and/or by producing a sedative effect that decreases the perception of pain.

Available Dosage Forms and Strengths
Injection — 100 mg per ml
Tablets — 500 mg, 750 mg

▷ **Usual Adult Dosage Range:** Initially, 1500 mg 4 times/day for the first 2 to 3 days; for maintenance, 750 to 1000 mg 4 times/day, or 1500 mg 3 times/day. The total daily dose should not exceed 8000 mg. **Actual dos-**

age and administration schedule must be determined by the physician for each patient individually.

▷ **Dosing Instructions:**   Take either on empty stomach or with food to prevent stomach irritation. The tablet may be crushed for administration.

Usual Duration of Use: Continual use on a regular schedule for 2 to 3 days is usually necessary to determine this drug's effectiveness in relieving the discomfort of muscle spasm. Evaluate need for continued use after periods of 7 to 10 days.

▷ **This Drug Should Not Be Taken If**
- you have had an allergic reaction to it previously.
- you have active liver disease.

▷ **Inform Your Physician Before Taking This Drug If**
- you have experienced any unfavorable reactions to muscle relaxants in the past.
- you have epilepsy or myasthenia gravis.
- you have a history of liver or kidney disease.

Possible Side-Effects   (natural, expected and unavoidable drug actions)
Drowsiness, light-headedness, weakness.
Brown, black, green or blue discoloration of the urine (of no significance).

▷ **Possible Adverse Effects**   (unusual, unexpected and infrequent reactions)
If any of the following develop, consult your physician promptly.
Mild Adverse Effects
Allergic Reactions: Skin rash, hives, itching, fever.
Headache, dizziness, faintness, unsteadiness, blurred or double vision, red eyes, congested nose.
Indigestion, heartburn, nausea, vomiting.
Serious Adverse Effects
Abnormally low white blood cell count: fever, sore throat, infections.

CAUTION
All muscle relaxants cause some degree of sedation. Use caution if other sedatives, tranquilizers or pain relievers are taken concurrently with this drug.

Precautions for Use
By Infants and Children: Dosage is based on the child's age and weight. Consult your physician for exact dosage schedule.
By Those over 60 Years of Age: Small doses are advisable initially. You may be more susceptible to the development of drowsiness, dizziness, weakness, unsteadiness and falling.

▷ **Advisability of Use During Pregnancy**
Pregnancy Category: C (tentative). See Pregnancy Code inside back cover.
Animal studies: No data available.

Human studies: Information from adequate studies of pregnant women is not available.

Avoid drug if possible; use only if clearly needed.

Advisability of Use if Breast-Feeding
Presence of this drug in breast milk: Yes, in small amounts.
Avoid drug or refrain from nursing.

Habit-Forming Potential: None.

Effects of Overdosage: Nausea, vomiting, diarrhea, headache, drowsiness, dizziness, marked weakness, impaired coordination, sense of paralysis of arms and legs, rapid and weak pulse, shallow breathing, cold and sweaty skin.

Possible Effects of Long-Term Use: None reported.

Suggested Periodic Examinations While Taking This Drug   (at physician's discretion)
Complete blood cell counts.

▷ **While Taking This Drug, Observe the Following**
Foods: No restrictions.
Beverages: No restrictions. May be taken with milk.
▷ *Alcohol*: Use with caution until the combined effect has been determined. This drug may add to the depressant action of alcohol on the brain.
Tobacco Smoking: No interactions expected.
Marijuana Smoking: Moderate to marked drowsiness, muscle weakness, incoordination, accentuation of orthostatic hypotension (see Glossary).
▷ *Other Drugs*
Methocarbamol may *increase* the effects of
• all other drugs with sedative effects and cause excessive sedation.
▷ *Driving, Hazardous Activities*: This drug may cause drowsiness, light-headedness or dizziness in susceptible individuals. Avoid hazardous activities if these drug effects occur.
Aviation Note: The use of this drug *is a disqualification* for piloting. Consult a designated Aviation Medical Examiner.
Exposure to Sun: No restrictions.

METHOTREXATE
(meth oh TREX ayt)

Other Names: Amethopterin, MTX

Introduced: 1948

Class: Anticancer drugs, Antipsoriasis

Prescription: USA: Yes
Canada: Yes

Controlled Drug: USA: No
Canada: No

Available as Generic: Yes

Brand Names: Folex, Mexate

```
┌─────────────────────────────────────────────────────────────────┐
│                     BENEFITS versus RISKS                         │
│                                                                   │
│         Possible Benefits              Possible Risks             │
│  EFFECTIVE TREATMENT OF           GASTROINTESTINAL                 │
│     SOME CASES OF SEVERE            ULCERATION AND BLEEDING        │
│     DISABLING PSORIASIS           MOUTH AND THROAT                 │
│  EFFECTIVE TREATMENT OF             ULCERATON                      │
│     CERTAIN ADULT AND             SEVERE BONE MARROW               │
│     CHILDHOOD CANCERS               DEPRESSION                     │
│  PREVENTION OF REJECTION OF       DAMAGE TO LUNGS, LIVER AND       │
│     BONE MARROW TRANS-              KIDNEYS                        │
│     PLANTS                        Loss of hair                    │
│  Helpful adjunctive therapy in                                    │
│     rheumatoid arthritis and related                              │
│     disorders                                                     │
└─────────────────────────────────────────────────────────────────┘
```

▷ **Principal Uses**

As a Single Drug Product: This very potent drug is used to treat (1) severe and widespread forms of disabling psoriasis that have failed to respond to all standard treatment procedures; (2) various types of both adult and childhood cancer. In addition, it is used to prevent rejection of transplanted bone marrow. More recently, it is being used experimentally in the treatment of connective tissue disorders such as rheumatoid arthritis, scleroderma and related conditions.

How This Drug Works: By interfering with the normal utilization of folic acid in tissue cell reproduction, this drug retards abnormally rapid tissue growth (as in psoriasis and cancer).

Available Dosage Forms and Strengths

Injections — 2.5 mg per ml, 25 mg per ml

Injections (preservative-free) — 25 mg per ml

Tablets — 2.5 mg

▷ **Usual Adult Dosage Range:** For psoriasis (alternate schedules): (1) 10 to 50 mg once/week; (2) 2.5 to 5 mg/12 hours for 3 doses, or every 8 hours for 4 doses, once a week up to a maximum of 30 mg/week; (3) 2.5 mg/day for 5 days, followed by 2 days without drug, with gradual increase in dosage to a maximum of 6.25 mg/day. **Note: Actual dosage and administration schedule must be determined by the physician for each patient individually.**

▷ **Dosing Instructions:** May be taken with food to reduce stomach irritation. Drink at least 2 to 3 quarts of liquids daily. The tablet may be crushed for administration.

Usual Duration of Use: Continual use on a regular schedule for several weeks is usually necessary to determine this drug's effectiveness in reducing the severity and extent of psoriasis. After a favorable response has been achieved, the dosage should be reduced to the smallest amount that will maintain acceptable improvement. Long-term use (months to years) requires supervision and periodic evaluation by your physician.

▷ **This Drug Should Not Be Taken If**
- you have had an allergic reaction to it previously.
- you currently have, or have had a recent exposure to, either chicken pox or shingles (herpes zoster).
- you are pregnant or planning pregnancy in the near future, and you are taking this drug to treat psoriasis or rheumatoid arthritis.
- you have active liver disease, peptic ulcer, regional enteritis or ulcerative colitis.
- you currently have a blood cell or bone marrow disorder.

▷ **Inform Your Physician Before Taking This Drug If**
- you have a chronic infection of any kind.
- you have impaired liver or kidney function.
- you have a history of bone marrow impairment of any kind, especially drug-induced bone marrow depression.
- you have a history of gout, peptic ulcer disease, regional enteritis or ulcerative colitis.

Possible Side-Effects   (natural, expected and unavoidable drug actions)
The following are due to the pharmacological actions of this drug. **Report such developments to your physician promptly.**
Sores on the lips, in the mouth or throat; vomiting; intestinal cramping; diarrhea (may be bloody); painful urination; bloody urine.
Reduced resistance to infection, fatigue, weakness, fever, abnormal bleeding or bruising (bone marrow depression).

▷ **Possible Adverse Effects**   (unusual, unexpected and infrequent reactions)
If any of the following develop, consult your physician promptly.
Mild Adverse Effects
Allergic Reactions: Skin rash, hives, itching.
Headache, drowsiness, blurred vision.
Loss of appetite, nausea, vomiting.
Loss of hair, loss of skin pigmentation, acne.
Altered menstrual pattern.
Serious Adverse Effects
Allergic Reactions: Drug-induced pneumonia: cough, chest pain, shortness of breath.
Nervous system toxicity: speech disturbances, paralysis, seizures.
Liver toxicity with jaundice (see Glossary).
Kidney toxicity: reduced urine volume, kidney failure.

Possible Delayed Adverse Effects
Some reports suggest that methotrexate therapy may contribute to the later development of secondary cancers. Other studies have not confirmed this.

CAUTION
1. This drug has a high potential for serious toxicity. Its use must be

monitored carefully and continually by a physician who is skilled in its proper administration.

2. Appropriate laboratory examinations, performed before and during the use of this drug, are mandatory. Comply fully with your physician's instructions regarding periodic studies.

3. Women with potential for pregnancy should have a pregnancy test before taking this drug and should use an effective form of contraception during its use and for 8 weeks following its discontinuation.

4. Administration of live virus vaccines should be avoided during use of this drug. Because immune functions are suppressed by this drug, live virus vaccines could actually produce infection rather than stimulate an immune response.

Precautions for Use
By Those over 60 Years of Age: Careful evaluation of kidney function should be made before starting treatment and during the entire course of therapy.

▷ **Advisability of Use During Pregnancy**
Pregnancy Category: D (tentative). See Pregnancy Code inside back cover.
Animal studies: Skull and facial defects reported in mice.
Human studies: This drug is known to cause fetal deaths and birth defects. Its use during pregnancy to treat psoriasis or rheumatoid arthritis cannot be justified. If its use during pregnancy is deemed necessary to treat a responsive type of cancer, it should be avoided during the first 3 months if possible.

Advisability of Use if Breast-Feeding
Presence of this drug in breast milk: Yes.
Avoid drug or refrain from nursing.

Habit-Forming Potential: None.

Effects of Overdosage: The side-effects and adverse effects listed previously develop earlier and with greater severity.

Possible Effects of Long-Term Use: Liver fibrosis and cirrhosis occur in 3% to 5% of long-term users (35 to 49 months).

Suggested Periodic Examinations While Taking This Drug (at physician's discretion)
Complete blood cell counts, liver and kidney function tests, blood uric acid levels, chest X-ray examinations.

▷ **While Taking This Drug, Observe the Following**
Foods: Avoid highly seasoned foods that could be irritating. Between courses of treatment, eat liberally of the following foods: beef, chicken, lamb and pork liver, asparagus, navy beans, kale and spinach.
Beverages: No restrictions. This drug may be taken with milk.
▷   *Alcohol*: Avoid completely.
Tobacco Smoking: No interactions expected.

▷   *Other Drugs*
    Methotrexate may *decrease* the effects of
    • digoxin (Lanoxin).
    • phenytoin (Dilantin).
    The following drugs may *increase* the effects of methotrexate and enhance
    its toxicity
    • aspirin and other salicylates.
    • probenecid (Benemid).
▷ *Driving, Hazardous Activities*: This drug may cause drowsiness, dizziness or
    blurred vision. Restrict activities as necessary.
    Aviation Note: The use of this drug *is a disqualification* for piloting. Consult a
    designated Aviation Medical Examiner.
    Exposure to Sun: Use caution until skin sensitivity has been determined. This
    drug can cause photosensitivity. Avoid ultraviolet lamps.

METHYCLOTHIAZIDE
(METH ee kloh THI a zide)

Introduced: 1960

Class: Antihypertensive, Diuretic,
Thiazides

Prescription: USA: Yes
Canada: Yes

Controlled Drug: USA: No
Canada: No

Available as Generic: USA: Yes
Canada: No

Brand Names: Aquatensen, Diutensen [CD], Diutensen-R [CD], ♣Duretic,
Enduron, Enduronyl [CD], Enduronyl Forte [CD]

BENEFITS versus RISKS

Possible Benefits	*Possible Risks*
EFFECTIVE, WELL-TOLERATED DIURETIC	Loss of body potassium
POSSIBLY EFFECTIVE IN MILD HYPERTENSION	Increased blood sugar
ENHANCES EFFECTIVENESS OF OTHER ANTIHYPERTENSIVES	Increased blood uric acid
Beneficial in treatment of diabetes insipidus	Increased blood calcium
	Rare blood cell disorders

▷ **Principal Uses**
    As a Single Drug Product: Thiazide diuretics are used primarily to (1)
    increase the volume of urine (diuresis) to correct the excessive fluid
    retention associated with congestive heart failure and certain types of
    liver and kidney disease; and (2) initiate treatment for high blood
    pressure (hypertension). They are often the first drugs tried in treating

mild to moderate hypertension. Less frequent uses include the treatment of diabetes insipidus and the prevention of kidney stones that contain calcium.

As a Combination Drug Product [CD]: When this drug is used alone to treat hypertension, it is referred to as a "step 1" antihypertensive. Should it fail to reduce the blood pressure adequately, a "step 2" antihypertensive drug is added to be taken concurrently with the step 1 drug. These drugs may be combined into one drug product. Thiazides are available in combination with beta-blockers, hydralazine, methyldopa, reserpine and other diuretics to increase their effectiveness in treating hypertension.

How This Drug Works: By increasing the elimination of salt and water from the body (through increased urine production), this drug reduces the volume of fluid in the blood and body tissues and lowers the sodium content throughout the body. By relaxing the walls of smaller arteries and allowing them to expand, this drug increases the total capacity of the arterial system. The combined effect of these two actions (reduced blood volume in expanded space) results in lowering of blood pressure.

Available Dosage Forms and Strengths
   Tablets — 2.5 mg, 5 mg

▷ **Usual Adult Dosage Range:**   As antihypertensive: 2.5 to 5 mg/day initially; 2.5 to 10 mg/day for maintenance. As diuretic: 2.5 to 10 mg/day initially; the smallest effective dose should be determined. The total daily dose should not exceed 10 mg. **Note: Actual dosage and administration schedule must be determined by the physician for each patient individually.**

▷ **Dosing Instructions:**   May be taken with or following meals to reduce stomach irritation. Best taken in the morning to avoid nighttime urination. The tablet may be crushed for administration.

Usual Duration of Use: Continual use on a regular schedule for 2 to 3 weeks is usually necessary to determine this drug's effectiveness in lowering high blood pressure. Long-term use (months to years) requires periodic evaluation of response and possible dosage adjustment. Use as a diuretic should be intermittent with "drug holidays" (no drug taken) to reduce the risk of sodium and potassium imbalance.

▷ **This Drug Should Not Be Taken If**
   • you have had an allergic reaction to any dosage form of it previously.

▷ **Inform Your Physician Before Taking This Drug If**
   • you are allergic to any form of "sulfa" drug.
   • you are pregnant or planning pregnancy.
   • you have a history of kidney or liver disease.
   • you have diabetes, gout or lupus erythematosus.

- you are taking any form of cortisone, digitalis, oral antidiabetic drug or insulin.
- you plan to have surgery under general anesthesia in the near future.

Possible Side-Effects   (natural, expected and unavoidable drug actions)
Light-headedness on arising from sitting or lying position (see orthostatic hypotension in Glossary).
Increase in blood sugar level, affecting control of diabetes.
Increase in blood uric acid level, affecting control of gout.
Decrease in blood potassium level, causing muscle weakness and cramping.

▷ **Possible Adverse Effects**   (unusual, unexpected and infrequent reactions)
If any of the following develop, consult your physician promptly.
Mild Adverse Effects
Allergic Reactions: Skin rashes, hives, drug fever.
Headache, dizziness, blurred or yellow vision.
Reduced appetite, indigestion, nausea, vomiting, diarrhea.
Serious Adverse Effects
Allergic Reactions: Hepatitis with jaundice (see Glossary), anaphylactic reaction (see Glossary), severe skin reactions.
Inflammation of the pancreas—severe abdominal pain.
Bone marrow depression (see Glossary)—fatigue, weakness, fever, sore throat, abnormal bleeding or bruising.

▷ **Adverse Effects That May Mimic Natural Diseases or Disorders**
Liver reaction may suggest viral hepatitis.

Natural Diseases or Disorders That May Be Activated by This Drug
Diabetes, gout, systemic lupus erythematosus.

CAUTION
1. Do not exceed recommended doses. Increased dosage can cause excessive loss of sodium and potassium, with resultant loss of appetite, nausea, fatigue, weakness, confusion and tingling in the extremities.
2. If you are also taking a digitalis preparation (digitoxin, digoxin), ensure an adequate intake of high-potassium foods to prevent potassium deficiency—a potential cause of digitalis toxicity. (See Table of High Potassium Foods in Section Six).

Precautions for Use
By Infants and Children: Avoid overdosage that could cause serious dehydration. Significant potassium loss can occur within the first 2 weeks of drug use.
By Those over 60 Years of Age: Small doses are advisable until your individual response has been determined. You may be more susceptible to the development of impaired thinking, orthostatic hypotension, potassium loss and blood sugar increase. Overdosage and extended use of this drug can cause excessive loss of body water, thickening (increased viscosity) of the blood and an increased tendency for the blood to clot—predispos-

ing to stroke, heart attack or thrombophlebitis (vein inflammation with blood clot).

▷ **Advisability of Use During Pregnancy**
Pregnancy Category: D (tentative). See Pregnancy Code inside back cover.
Animal studies: No information available.
Human studies: Information from adequate studies of pregnant women is not available.
This drug should not be used during pregnancy unless a very serious complication occurs for which this drug is significantly beneficial. Ask physician for guidance.

Advisability of Use if Breast-Feeding
Presence of this drug in breast milk: Yes, in small amounts.
Avoid drug or refrain from nursing.

Habit-Forming Potential: None.

Effects of Overdosage: Dry mouth, thirst, lethargy, weakness, muscle cramping, nausea, vomiting, drowsiness progressing to stupor or coma.

Possible Effects of Long-Term Use: Impaired balance of water, salt and potassium in blood and body tissues. Development of diabetes in predisposed individuals. Pathological changes in parathyroid glands with increased blood calcium levels and decreased blood phosphate levels.

Suggested Periodic Examinations While Taking This Drug (at physician's discretion)
Complete blood cell counts, measurements of blood levels of sodium, potassium, chloride, sugar and uric acid.
Kidney and liver function tests.

▷ **While Taking This Drug, Observe the Following**
Foods: Consult your physician regarding the advisability of eating foods rich in potassium. If so advised, see the Table of High Potassium Foods in Section Six. Follow physician's advice regarding the use of salt.
Beverages: No restrictions. This drug may be taken with milk.
▷ *Alcohol*: Use with caution until the combined effects have been determined. Alcohol may exaggerate the blood-pressure-lowering effects of this drug and cause orthostatic hypotension.
Tobacco Smoking: No interactions expected. Follow physician's advice.
▷ *Other Drugs*
Methyclothiazide may *increase* the effects of
• other antihypertensive drugs; dosage adjustments may be necessary to prevent excessive lowering of blood pressure.
• lithium, and cause lithium toxicity.
Methyclothiazide may *decrease* the effects of
• oral antidiabetic drugs (sulfonylureas); dosage adjustments may be necessary for proper control of blood sugar.

Methyclothiazide *taken concurrently* with
- digitalis preparations (digitoxin, digoxin) requires very careful monitoring and dosage adjustments to prevent fluctuations of blood potassium levels and serious disturbances of heart rhythm.

The following drugs may *decrease* the effects of methyclothiazide
- cholestyramine (Cuemid, Questran) may interfere with its absorption.
- colestipol (Colestid) may interfere with its absorption.

Take cholestyramine and colestipol 1 hour before any oral diuretic.

▷ *Driving, Hazardous Activities*: Use caution until the possible occurrence of orthostatic hypotension, dizziness or impaired vision has been determined.

Aviation Note: The use of this drug *may be a disqualification* for piloting. Consult a designated Aviation Medical Examiner.

Exposure to Sun: Use caution until sensitivity has been determined. This drug can cause photosensitivity (see Glossary).

Exposure to Heat: Avoid excessive perspiring, which could cause additional loss of salt and water from the body.

Heavy Exercise or Exertion: Avoid exertion that produces light-headedness, excessive fatigue or muscle cramping. Isometric exercises—the "overload" technique for strengthening individual muscles—can raise blood pressure significantly. Ask physician for guidance regarding participation in this form of exercise.

Occurrence of Unrelated Illness: Illnesses that cause vomiting or diarrhea can produce a serious imbalance of important body chemistry. Consult your physician for guidance.

Discontinuation: This drug should not be stopped abruptly following long-term use; serious thiazide-withdrawal fluid retention (edema) can develop after sudden withdrawal. The dose should be reduced gradually. It may be advisable to discontinue this drug 5 to 7 days before major surgery. Ask your physician, surgeon and/or anesthesiologist for guidance regarding dosage adjustment or drug withdrawal.

METHYLDOPA
(meth il DOH pa)

Other Names: Alpha-Methyldopa

Introduced: 1963   **Class:** Antihypertensive

Prescription: USA: Yes   **Controlled Drug:** USA: No
Canada: Yes   Canada: No

Available as Generic: Yes

Brand Names: Aldochlor-150/250 [CD], Aldomet, Aldoril-15/25 [CD], Aldoril D30/D50 [CD], ♣Apo-Methazide [CD], ♣Apo-Methyldopa, ♣Dopamet, ♣Medimet-250, ♣Novodoparil [CD], ♣Novomedopa, ♣PMS Dopazide [CD]

```
                  BENEFITS versus RISKS

        Possible Benefits              Possible Risks
EFFECTIVE STEP-2 OR -3          LIVER TOXICITY (may be severe)
  ANTIHYPERTENSIVE IN 66%       Mental depression
  OF CASES OF MILD TO           Water retention
  SEVERE HYPERTENSION when      Hemolytic anemia (less than 1%)
  used adjunctively with other  Drug fever
  drugs                         Blood cell disorders (rare)
Symptomatic relief in cases of
  Raynaud's disease
```

▷ **Principal Uses**

   As a Single Drug Product: Used as a "step 2" or "step 3" medication in conjunction with other antihypertensive drugs in the treatment of moderate to severe high blood pressure.

   As a Combination Drug Product [CD]: This drug is available in combination with chlorothiazide and with hydrochlorothiazide, mild diuretics that represent "step 1" antihypertensive drugs. Combinations of "step 1" and "step 2" drugs are more effective and more convenient for long-term use.

How This Drug Works: By decreasing the activity of the vasomotor center in the brain, this drug reduces the ability of the sympathetic nervous system to maintain the degree of blood vessel constriction that is responsible for blood pressure elevation. This change results in relaxation of blood vessel walls and lowering of blood pressure.

Available Dosage Forms and Strengths
   Injection — 250 mg per 5 ml
   Oral suspension — 250 mg per 5 ml teaspoonful (1% alcohol)
   Tablets — 125 mg, 250 mg, 500 mg

▷ **Usual Adult Dosage Range:**   Initially, 250 mg 2 or 3 times/day for 2 days; increase dose as needed and tolerated. For maintenance, 500 to 2000 mg/day in 2 to 4 divided doses. The total daily dose should not exceed 3000 mg. **Note: Actual dosage and administration schedule must be determined by the physician for each patient individually.**

▷ **Dosing Instructions:**   May be taken without regard to meals. The tablet may be crushed for administration.

Usual Duration of Use: Continual use on a regular schedule for 2 to 4 weeks is usually necessary to determine this drug's effectiveness in controlling high blood pressure. Long-term use (months to years) requires supervision and periodic evaluation by your physician.

▷ **This Drug Should Not Be Taken If**
   • you have had an allergic reaction to it previously.
   • you have active liver disease.
   • you have a mild and uncomplicated case of hypertension.

▷ **Inform Your Physician Before Taking This Drug If**
- you have a history of liver disease or impaired liver function.
- you have a history of mental depression or porphyria.
- you are taking any monoamine oxidase (MAO) inhibitor drugs, phenothiazines or tricyclic antidepressant drugs (see Drug Classes, Section Four).
- you plan to have surgery under general anesthesia in the near future.

Possible Side-Effects   (natural, expected and unavoidable drug actions)
Drowsiness, lethargy and weakness; these may occur during the first few weeks and then subside.
Light-headedness in upright position (see orthostatic hypotension in Glossary).
Nasal stuffiness, dry mouth.

▷ **Possible Adverse Effects**   (unusual, unexpected and infrequent reactions)
If any of the following develop, consult your physician promptly.
Mild Adverse Effects
Allergic Reactions: Skin rash, joint and muscle discomfort, fever.
Headache, dizziness.
Irritation of tongue, nausea, vomiting, diarrhea.
Water retention, weight gain, breast enlargement, milk production, impaired sex drive and performance.
Serious Adverse Effects
Allergic Reactions: Hepatitis with jaundice (see Glossary).
Idiosyncratic Reactions: Episodes of high fever (not due to infection), 1% of users.
Bone marrow depression (see Glossary): fatigue, weakness, fever, sore throat, abnormal bleeding or bruising.
Inflammation of the pancreas: abdominal pain, fever, nausea, vomiting.
Parkinson-like disorders (see Glossary).
Behavioral changes: depression, confusion, nightmares.

▷ **Adverse Effects That May Mimic Natural Diseases or Disorders**
Liver toxicity may suggest viral hepatitis.
Idiosyncratic fever may suggest a viral flulike infection.
Abnormal involuntary movements of extremities may suggest Huntington's disease.

Natural Diseases or Disorders That May Be Activated by This Drug
Porphyria, latent coronary artery insufficiency, lupus erythematosuslike syndrome.

CAUTION
1. If this drug is used as the sole agent, the blood pressure may be very erratic. Observe for the development of tolerance and loss of effectiveness.
2. This drug is most effective when combined with a diuretic.
3. Avoid concurrent use with other drugs known to depress bone marrow function.
4. Report the development of any tendency to emotional depression.

Precautions for Use

By Infants and Children: Observe for the development of hemolytic anemia, abnormal liver function, excessive sedation and nightmares.

By Those over 60 Years of Age: The basic rule in treating hypertension after 60 is to proceed cautiously. Unacceptably high blood pressure should be reduced without creating risks associated with excessively low blood pressure. Sudden, rapid and excessive reduction of blood pressure can predispose to stroke or heart attack. Adverse effects are common: drowsiness (50%), depression (10%), forgetfulness, reduced mental acuity, nasal congestion, dry mouth, hallucinations. This drug can cause parkinsonism or intensify existing parkinsonism.

▷ **Advisability of Use During Pregnancy**

Pregnancy Category: B (tentative). See Pregnancy Code inside back cover.

Animal studies: No birth defects reported in mice, rats or rabbits.

Human studies: Information from adequate studies of pregnant women is not available.

Use this drug only if clearly needed. Use the minimal effective dose.

Advisability of Use if Breast-Feeding

Presence of this drug in breast milk: Yes.

If drug is necessary, monitor infant for drowsiness and inadequate feeding.

Habit-Forming Potential: None.

Effects of Overdosage: Marked drowsiness, weakness, confusion, nausea, vomiting, stupor progressing to coma.

Possible Effects of Long-Term Use: Water retention (if not taken with a diuretic). Development of hemolytic anemia (see Glossary).

Suggested Periodic Examinations While Taking This Drug (at physician's discretion)

Complete blood cell counts, liver function tests.

▷ **While Taking This Drug, Observe the Following**

Foods: Avoid excessive salt. When possible, avoid high-protein foods at the time this drug is taken; this drug competes with proteins for absorption.

Beverages: No restrictions. May be taken with milk.

▷ *Alcohol*: Use with extreme caution until the combined effects have been determined. This combination can cause marked sedation and exaggerated drop in blood pressure.

Tobacco Smoking: No interactions expected.

▷ *Other Drugs*

Methyldopa may *increase* the effects of

• tolbutamide (Orinase), and cause excessive hypoglycemia.

• other drugs with sedative effects, and cause excessive sedation.

Methyldopa *taken concurrently* with

• beta-blocker drugs may rarely cause hypertensive reactions (see Drug Class, Section Four).

• haloperidol (Haldol) may cause dementia, disorientation and abnormal behavior.

- monoamine oxidase (MAO) inhibitor drugs may cause hallucinations and hypertension (see Drug Class, Section Four).
- phenothiazines may cause hypertension (see Drug Class, Section Four).

The following drugs may *decrease* the effects of methyldopa

- tricyclic antidepressants (see Drug Class, Section Four).

▷ *Driving, Hazardous Activities*: This drug may cause drowsiness and fatigue. Restrict activities as necessary.

Aviation Note: The use of this drug *may be a disqualification* for piloting. Consult a designated Aviation Medical Examiner.

Exposure to Sun: No restrictions.

Heavy Exercise or Exertion: Use caution. Excessive physical activity may increase the possibility of orthostatic hypotension. Isometric exercises—the "overload" technique for strengthening individual muscles—can raise blood pressure significantly. Ask your physician for guidance.

Discontinuation: It may be advisable to discontinue this drug 5 to 7 days before surgery under general anesthesia. Consult your surgeon and/or anesthesiologist regarding dosage adjustment or withdrawal of this drug prior to surgery.

METHYLPHENIDATE
(meth il FEN i dayt)

Introduced: 1956

Class: Stimulant, Amphetaminelike Drugs

Prescription: USA: Yes
Canada: Yes

Controlled Drug: USA: C-II*
Canada: <C>

Available as Generic: USA: Yes
Canada: No

Brand Names: Ritalin, Ritalin-SR

BENEFITS versus RISKS

Possible Benefits	*Possible Risks*
EFFECTIVE CONTROL OF NARCOLEPSY	POTENTIAL FOR SERIOUS PSYCHOLOGICAL DEPENDENCE
USEFUL AS ADJUNCTIVE TREATMENT IN THE ATTENTION DEFICIT DISORDERS OF CHILDHOOD	SUPPRESSION OF GROWTH IN CHILDHOOD
Useful in treatment of mild to moderate depression	Abnormal behavior
Useful in some cases of emotional withdrawal in the elderly	Rare blood cell disorders

---

*See Schedules of Controlled Drugs inside back cover.

▷ **Principal Uses**

As a Single Drug Product: Used primarily to treat (1) narcolepsy, recurrent spells of uncontrollable drowsiness and sleep; and (2) attention-deficit disorders of childhood, formerly known as the hyperactive child syndrome, minimal brain damage and minimal brain dysfunction. Additional uses include the treatment of mild to moderate depression, and the management of apathetic and withdrawal states in the elderly.

How This Drug Works: Not completely established. It is thought that this drug may increase the release of the nerve impulse transmitter norepinephrine. The resulting stimulation of brain function improves alertness and concentration, and increases learning ability and attention span. The primary action that calms the overactive child is not known.

Available Dosage Forms and Strengths
Tablets — 5 mg, 10 mg, 20 mg
Tablets, prolonged action — 20 mg

▷ **Usual Adult Dosage Range:** 5 to 20 mg 2 or 3 times/day. **Note: Actual dosage and administration schedule must be determined by the physician for each patient individually.**

▷ **Dosing Instructions:** Take tablet 30 to 45 minutes before meals. The regular tablet may be crushed for administration; the prolonged action tablet should be taken whole, not crushed.

Usual Duration of Use: Continual use on a regular schedule for 3 to 4 weeks is usually necessary to determine this drug's effectiveness in controlling the symptoms of narcolepsy or improving the behavior of attention-deficit children. Long-term use (months to years) requires supervision and periodic evaluation by your physician.

▷ **This Drug Should Not Be Taken If**
- you have had an allergic reaction to it previously.
- you have glaucoma (inadequately treated).
- you are experiencing a period of severe anxiety, nervous tension or emotional depression.

▷ **Inform Your Physician Before Taking This Drug If**
- you have high blood pressure, angina or epilepsy.
- you are taking, or have taken within the past 14 days, any monoamine oxidase (MAO) inhibitor drug (see Drug Class, Section Four).

Possible Side-Effects (natural, expected and unavoidable drug actions)
Nervousness, insomnia.

▷ **Possible Adverse Effects** (unusual, unexpected and infrequent reactions)
If any of the following develop, consult your physician promptly.

Mild Adverse Effects
   Allergic Reactions: Skin rash, hives, drug fever, joint pains.
   Headache, dizziness, rapid and forceful heart palpitation.
   Reduced appetite, nausea, abdominal discomfort.
Serious Adverse Effects
   Allergic Reactions: Severe skin reactions, extensive bruising due to allergic
      destruction of blood platelets (see Glossary).
   Idiosyncratic Reactions: Abnormal patterns of behavior.
   Abnormally low red blood cell and white blood cell counts.

Natural Diseases or Disorders That May Be Activated by This Drug
   Latent epilepsy.

CAUTION
   1. Careful dosage adjustments on an individual basis are mandatory.
   2. Paradoxical reactions (see Glossary) can occur, causing aggravation of
       initial symptoms for which this drug was prescribed.

Precautions for Use
   By Infants and Children: Safety and effectiveness for use by those under 6
      years of age have not been established. If this drug is not benefical in
      managing an attention deficit disorder after a trial of one month, it
      should be discontinued. During long-term use, monitor the child for nor-
      mal growth and development.
   By Those over 60 Years of Age: Start with small doses to determine your toler-
      ance for this drug. You may be more susceptible to the development of
      nervousness, agitation, insomnia, high blood pressure, angina or disturb-
      ance of heart rhythm.

▷ Advisability of Use During Pregnancy
   Pregnancy Category: B (tentative). See Pregnancy Code inside back cover.
      Animal studies: No birth defects found in mouse studies.
      Human studies: Information from adequate studies of pregnant women is
      not available.
   Use this drug only if clearly needed. Ask physician for guidance.

Advisability of Use if Breast-Feeding
   Presence of this drug in breast milk: Unknown.
   Avoid drug or refrain from nursing.

Habit-Forming Potential: This drug can produce tolerance and cause serious
   psychological dependence (see Glossary), a potentially dangerous characteristic of amphetaminelike drugs (see Drug Class, Section Four).

Effects of Overdosage: Headache, vomiting, agitation, tremors, muscle
   twitching, dry mouth, sweating, fever, confusion, hallucinations,
   seizures, coma.

Possible Effects of Long-Term Use: Suppression of growth (in weight and/or
   height) has been reported in children during long-term use of this drug.

Suggested Periodic Examinations While Taking This Drug   (at physician's discretion)

Complete blood cell counts, blood pressure measurements.

▷ **While Taking This Drug, Observe the Following**

Foods: Avoid foods rich in tyramine (see Glossary); this drug in combination with tyramine may cause an excessive rise in blood pressure.

Beverages: Avoid beverages prepared from meat or meat extracts. This drug may be taken with milk.

▷ *Alcohol*: Avoid beer, Chianti wines and vermouth.

Tobacco Smoking: No interactions expected.

▷ *Other Drugs*

Methylphenidate may *increase* the effects of

- tricyclic antidepressants, and enhance their toxic effects (see Drug Class, Section Four).

Methylphenidate may *decrease* the effects of

- guanethidine (Ismelin), and impair its ability to lower blood pressure.

Methylphenidate *taken concurrently* with

- anticonvulsants may cause a significant change in the pattern of epileptic seizures; dosage adjustments may be necessary for proper control.
- monoamine oxidase (MAO) inhibitor drugs (see Drug Class, Section Four) may cause a significant rise in blood pressure. Avoid the concurrent use of these drugs.

▷ *Driving, Hazardous Activities*: This drug may cause dizziness or drowsiness. Restrict activities as necessary.

Aviation Note: The use of this drug *is a disqualification* for piloting. Consult a designated Aviation Medical Examiner.

Exposure to Sun: No restrictions.

Discontinuation: If it has been necessary to use this drug for an extended period of time, do not discontinue it abruptly. Careful supervision is necessary during withdrawal to prevent severe depression and erratic behavior.

METHYLPREDNISOLONE
(meth il pred NIS oh lohn)

Introduced: 1957

Class: Cortisonelike Drugs

Prescription: USA: Yes
 Canada: Yes

Controlled Drug: USA: No
 Canada: No

Available as Generic: USA: Yes
 Canada: No

Brand Names: Medrol, Medrol Enpak

BENEFITS versus RISKS

Possible Benefits

EFFECTIVE RELIEF OF
SYMPTOMS IN A WIDE
VARIETY OF INFLAMMATORY
AND ALLERGIC DISORDERS
EFFECTIVE IMMUNO-
SUPPRESSION in selected
benign and malignant disorders

Possible Risks

Short-term use (up to 10 days) is
usually well tolerated. Long-term
use (exceeding 2 weeks) is
associated with many possible
adverse effects:
ALTERED MOOD AND
PERSONALITY
CATARACTS, GLAUCOMA
HYPERTENSION
OSTEOPOROSIS
ASEPTIC BONE NECROSIS
INCREASED SUSCEPTIBILITY TO
INFECTIONS
(See Possible Adverse Effects and
Possible Effects of Long-Term
Use)

▷ **Principal Uses**

As a Single Drug Product: This potent drug of the cortisone class is used in
the treatment of a wide variety of allergic and inflammatory conditions.
It is used most commonly in the management of serious skin disorders,
asthma, regional enteritis, ulcerative colitis and all types of major rheumatic disorders including bursitis, tendinitis and most forms of arthritis.

How This Drug Works: Not fully established. It is thought that this drug's
anti-inflammatory effect is due to its ability to inhibit the normal defensive functions of certain white blood cells. Its immunosuppressant effect
is attributed to a reduced production of lymphocytes and antibodies.

Available Dosage Forms and Strengths
Ointment — 0.25%, 1%
Retention enema — 40 mg/bottle
Tablets — 2 mg, 4 mg, 8 mg, 16 mg, 24 mg, 32 mg

▷ **Usual Adult Dosage Range:**   4 to 48 mg daily as a single dose or in divided
doses. **Note: Actual dosage and administration schedule must be determined by the physician for each patient individually.**

▷ **Dosing Instructions:**   Take with or following food to prevent stomach irritation, preferably in the morning. The tablet may be crushed for administration.

Usual Duration of Use: For acute disorders: 4 to 10 days. For chronic disorders: according to individual requirements. The duration of use should
not exceed the time necessary to obtain adequate symptomatic relief in
acute self-limiting conditions, or the time required to stabilize a chronic
condition and permit gradual withdrawal. Because of its intermediate

duration of action, this drug is appropriate for alternate-day administration.

▷ **This Drug Should Not Be Taken If**
- you have had an allergic reaction to any dosage form of it previously.
- you have active peptic ulcer disease.
- you have an active infection of the eye caused by the herpes simplex virus.
- you have active tuberculosis.

▷ **Inform Your Physician Before Taking This Drug If**
- you have had an unfavorable reaction to any cortisonelike drug in the past.
- you have a history of peptic ulcer disease, thrombophlebitis or tuberculosis.
- you have any of the following: diabetes, glaucoma, high blood pressure, deficient thyroid function or myasthenia gravis.
- you plan to have surgery of any kind in the near future.

Possible Side-Effects   (natural, expected and unavoidable drug actions)
Increased appetite, weight gain, retention of salt and water, excretion of potassium, increased susceptibility to infection.

▷ **Possible Adverse Effects**   (unusual, unexpected and infrequent reactions)
If any of the following develop, consult your physician promptly.
Mild Adverse Effects
Allergic Reactions: Skin rash.
Headache, dizziness, insomnia.
Acid indigestion, abdominal distension.
Muscle cramping and weakness.
Irregular or altered menstruation.
Acne, excessive growth of facial hair.
Serious Adverse Effects
Mental and emotional disturbances of serious magnitude.
Reactivation of latent tuberculosis.
Development of peptic ulcer.
Increased blood pressure.
Development of inflammation of the pancreas.
Thrombophlebitis (inflammation of a vein with the formation of blood clot)—pain or tenderness in thigh or leg, with or without swelling of the foot, ankle or leg.
Pulmonary embolism (movement of a blood clot to the lung)—sudden shortness of breath, pain in the chest, coughing, bloody sputum.

▷ **Adverse Effects That May Mimic Natural Diseases or Disorders**
Pattern of symptoms and signs resembling Cushing's syndrome.

Natural Diseases or Disorders That May Be Activated by This Drug
Latent diabetes, glaucoma, peptic ulcer disease, tuberculosis.

CAUTION
1. It is advisable to carry a card of personal identification with a notation that you are taking this drug, if your course of treatment is to exceed 1 week.
2. Do not discontinue this drug abruptly if you are using it for long-term treatment.
3. If vaccination against measles, rabies, smallpox or yellow fever is required, discontinue this drug 72 hours before vaccination and do not resume it for at least 14 days after vaccination.

Precautions for Use

By Infants and Children: Avoid prolonged use if possible. During long-term use, observe for suppression of normal growth and the possibility of increased intracranial pressure. Following long-term use, the child may be at risk for adrenal gland deficiency during stress for as long as 18 months after cessation of this drug.

By Those over 60 Years of Age: Cortisonelike drugs should be used very sparingly after 60 and only when the disorder under treatment is unresponsive to adequate trials of unrelated drugs. Avoid prolonged use of this drug. Continual use (even in small doses) can increase the severity of diabetes, enhance fluid retention, raise blood pressure, weaken resistance to infection, induce stomach ulcer and accelerate the development of cataract and osteoporosis.

▷ **Advisability of Use During Pregnancy**

Pregnancy Category: C (tentative). See Pregnancy Code inside back cover.

Animal studies: Birth defects reported in mice, rats and rabbits.

Human studies: Information from adequate studies of pregnant women is not available.

Avoid completely during the first 3 months. Limit use during the last 6 months as much as possible. If used, examine infant for possible deficiency of adrenal gland function.

Advisability of Use if Breast-Feeding

Presence of this drug in breast milk: Yes.

Avoid drug or refrain from nursing.

Habit-Forming Potential: Use of this drug to suppress symptoms over an extended period of time may produce a state of functional dependence (see Glossary). In the treatment of conditions like asthma and rheumatoid arthritis, it is advisable to keep the dose as small as possible and to attempt drug withdrawal after periods of reasonable improvement. Such procedures may reduce the degree of "steroid rebound"—the return of symptoms as the drug is withdrawn.

Effects of Overdosage: Fatigue, muscle weakness, stomach irritation, acid indigestion, excessive sweating, facial flushing, fluid retention, swelling of extremities, increased blood pressure.

Possible Effects of Long-Term Use: Increased blood sugar (possible diabetes), increased fat deposits on the trunk of the body ("buffalo hump"), rounding of the face ("moon face"), thinning and fragility of skin, loss of texture and strength of bones (osteoporosis, aseptic necrosis), cataracts, glaucoma, retarded growth and development in children.

Suggested Periodic Examinations While Taking This Drug (at physician's discretion)

Measurements of blood pressure, blood sugar and potassium levels.

Complete eye examinations at regular intervals.

Chest X-ray if history of tuberculosis.

Determination of the rate of development of the growing child to detect retardation of normal growth.

▷ **While Taking This Drug, Observe the Following**

Foods: No interactions expected. Ask physician regarding need to restrict salt intake or to eat potassium-rich foods. During long-term use of this drug, it is advisable to eat a high-protein diet.

Nutritional Support: During long-term use, take a vitamin D supplement. During wound repair, take a zinc supplement.

Beverages: No restrictions. Drink all forms of milk liberally.

▷ *Alcohol*: No interactions expected. Use caution if you are prone to peptic ulcer disease.

Tobacco Smoking: Nicotine increases the blood levels of naturally produced cortisone and related hormones. Heavy smoking may add to the expected actions of this drug and requires close observation for excessive effects.

Marijuana Smoking: May cause additional impairment of immunity.

▷ *Other Drugs*

Methylprednisolone may *decrease* the effects of
- isoniazid (INH, Niconyl, etc.).
- salicylates (aspirin, sodium salicylate, etc.).

Methylprednisolone *taken concurrently* with
- oral anticoagulants may either increase or decrease their effectiveness; consult physician regarding the need for prothrombin time testing and dosage adjustment.

The following drugs may *decrease* the effects of methylprednisolone
- antacids may reduce its absorption.
- barbiturates (Amytal, Butisol, phenobarbital, etc.).
- phenytoin (Dilantin, etc.).
- rifampin (Rifadin, Rimactane, etc.).

▷ *Driving, Hazardous Activities*: Usually no restrictions. Be alert to the rare occurrence of dizziness.

Aviation Note: The use of this drug *may be a disqualification* for piloting. Consult a designated Aviation Medical Examiner.

Exposure to Sun: No restrictions.

Occurrence of Unrelated Illness: This drug may decrease natural resistance to infection. Inform your physician if you develop an infection of any kind. It may also reduce your body's ability to respond to the stress of acute illness, injury or surgery. Keep your physician fully informed of any significant changes in your state of health.

Discontinuation: If you have been taking this drug for an extended period of time, do not discontinue it abruptly. Ask physician for guidance regarding gradual withdrawal. For a period of 2 years after discontinuing this drug, it is essential in the event of illness, injury or surgery that you inform attending medical personnel that you have used this drug in the past. The period of impaired response to stress following the use of cortisonelike drugs may last for 1 to 2 years.

METOCLOPRAMIDE
(met oh kloh PRA mide)

Introduced: 1973

Class: Gastrointestinal Stimulant, Antivomiting Agent

Prescription: USA: Yes
Canada: Yes

Controlled Drug: USA: No
Canada: No

Available as Generic: No

Brand Names: ✦Emex, ✦Maxeran, Reglan

BENEFITS versus RISKS

Possible Benefits	*Possible Risks*
EFFECTIVE STOMACH STIMULANT FOR CORRECTING DELAYED EMPTYING	Sedation and fatigue (10%)
	Parkinson-like reactions (see Glossary), 1 in 500
Symptomatic relief in reflux esophagitis	Tardive dyskinesia (see Glossary), rare
Relief of nausea and vomiting associated with migrane headache	

▷ **Principal Uses**

As a Single Drug Product: Used primarily to stimulate contractions of the stomach and thereby facilitate timely emptying of the stomach in disorders such as (1) the stomach retention (gastroparesis) associated with diabetes; (2) acid reflux from the stomach into the esophagus (esophagitis); (3) the nausea and vomiting associated with migraine headaches; and (4) the nausea and vomiting induced by anticancer drugs.

How This Drug Works: Not completely established. It is thought that this drug inhibits relaxation of the stomach muscles and enhances the stimulation of the parasympathetic nervous system that is responsible for stomach muscle contractions. This action accelerates emptying of the stomach into the intestine.

Available Dosage Forms and Strengths
    Injection — 5 mg per ml
      Syrup — 5 mg per 5 ml teaspoonful
    Tablets — 10 mg

▷ **Usual Adult Dosage Range:** 10 to 15 mg 4 times/day. The total daily dose should not exceed 0.5 mg per kilogram of body weight. **Note: Actual dosage and administration schedule must be determined by the physician for each patient individually.**

▷ **Dosing Instructions:** Take tablet or syrup 30 minutes before each meal and at bedtime. The tablet may be crushed for administration.

Usual Duration of Use: Continual use on a regular schedule for 5 to 7 days is usually necessary to determine this drug's effectiveness in accelerating stomach emptying and relieving symptoms of heartburn, fullness and belching. Long-term use (months to years) requires supervision and periodic evaluation by your physician.

▷ **This Drug Should Not Be Taken If**
- you have had an allergic reaction to it previously.
- you have a seizure disorder of any kind.
- you have active gastrointestinal bleeding.
- you have a pheochromocytoma (adrenalin-producing tumor).

▷ **Inform Your Physician Before Taking This Drug If**
- you are allergic or overly sensitive to procaine or procainamide.
- you have impaired liver or kidney function.
- you have Parkinson's disease.
- you are taking any atropinelike drugs, antipsychotic drugs or opioid analgesics (see Drug Classes, Section Four).

Possible Side-Effects (natural, expected and unavoidable drug actions)
Drowsiness and lethargy (10%), breast tenderness and swelling, milk production.

▷ **Possible Adverse Effects** (unusual, unexpected and infrequent reactions)
If any of the following develop, consult your physician promptly.
Mild Adverse Effects
Allergic Reactions: Skin rash.
Headache, dizziness, restlessness, depression, insomnia.
Dry mouth, nausea, diarrhea, constipation.
Altered menstrual pattern.
Serious Adverse Effects
Parkinson-like reactions (see Glossary).
Tardive dyskinesia (see Glossary).

Precautions for Use
By Infants and Children: Observe for the early development of Parkinson-like reactions soon after starting treatment. Use the smallest effective dose to minimize such reactions.
By Those over 60 Years of Age: Parkinson-like reactions and tardive dyskine-

sias are more likely to occur with the use of high doses over an extended period of time. Determine the smallest effective dose and use this only when clearly needed.

▷ **Advisability of Use During Pregnancy**
Pregnancy Category: B (tentative). See Pregnancy Code inside back cover.
Animal studies: No birth defects found due to this drug.
Human studies: Information from adequate studies of pregnant women is not available.
Use this drug only if clearly needed.

Advisability of Use if Breast-Feeding
Presence of this drug in breast milk: Yes.
Avoid drug or refrain from nursing.

Habit-Forming Potential: None.

Effects of Overdosage: Marked drowsiness, confusion, muscle spasms, jerking movements of head and face, tremors, shuffling gait.

Possible Effects of Long-Term Use: Parkinson-like reactions may appear within several months of use. Tardive dyskinesias usually occur after a year of continual use; they may persist after this drug is discontinued.

Suggested Periodic Examinations While Taking This Drug   (at physician's discretion)
During long-term use, observe for the development of fine, wormlike movements on the surface of the tongue; these may be the first indications of an emerging tardive dyskinesia.

▷ **While Taking This Drug, Observe the Following**
Foods: No restrictions.
Beverages: No restrictions. May be taken with milk.
▷ *Alcohol*: Use with extreme caution. Combined effects can result in excessive sedation and marked intoxication. Alcohol is best avoided.
Tobacco Smoking: No interactions expected.
▷ *Other Drugs*
Metoclopramide may *decrease* the effects of
• cimetidine (Tagamet).
• digoxin (slow-dissolving dosage forms), and reduce its effectiveness.
Metoclopramide *taken concurrently* with
• major antipsychotic drugs (phenothiazines, thiothixenes, haloperidol, etc.) may increase the risk of developing Parkinson-like reactions.
The following drugs may *decrease* the effects of metoclopramide
• atropinelike drugs.
• opioid analgesics (see Drug Class, Section Four).
▷ *Driving, Hazardous Activities*: This drug may cause drowsiness and dizziness. Restrict activities as necessary.
Aviation Note: The use of this drug *may be a disqualification* for piloting. Consult a designated Aviation Medical Examiner.
Exposure to Sun: No restrictions.

METOLAZONE
(me TOHL a zohn)

Introduced: 1974

Class: Antihypertensive, Diuretic, Sulfonamides

Prescription: USA: Yes
Canada: Yes

Controlled Drug: USA: No
Canada: No

Available as Generic: USA: No
Canada: No

Brand Names: Diulo, Zaroxolyn

BENEFITS versus RISKS

Possible Benefits	*Possible Risks*
EFFECTIVE, WELL-TOLERATED DIURETIC	Loss of body potassium
	Increased blood sugar
POSSIBLY EFFECTIVE IN MILD HYPERTENSION	Increased blood uric acid
	Rare liver damage, jaundice
ENHANCES EFFECTIVENESS OF OTHER ANTIHYPERTENSIVES	Rare blood cell disorder: abnormally low white blood cell count

---

▷ **Principal Uses**

As a Single Drug Product: Diuretics of this class are used primarily to (1) increase the volume of urine (diuresis) to correct the excessive fluid retention associated with congestive heart failure and certain types of liver and kidney disease; and (2) initiate treatment for high blood pressure (hypertension). They are often the first drugs tried ("step 1") in treating mild to moderate hypertension.

How This Drug Works: By increasing the elimination of salt and water from the body (through increased urine production), this drug reduces the volume of fluid in the blood and body tissues and lowers the sodium content throughout the body. By relaxing the walls of smaller arteries and allowing them to expand, this drug increases the total capacity of the arterial system. The combined effect of these two actions (reduced blood volume in expanded space) results in lowering of blood pressure.

Available Dosage Forms and Strengths
Tablets — 2.5 mg, 5 mg, 10 mg

▷ **Usual Adult Dosage Range:** As antihypertensive: 2.5 to 5 mg/day initially; 2.5 to 10 mg/day for maintenance. As diuretic: 2.5 to 10 mg/day initially; the smallest effective dose should be determined. The total daily dose should not exceed 20 mg. **Note: Actual dosage and administration schedule must be determined by the physician for each patient individually.**

▷ **Dosing Instructions:**   May be taken with or following food to reduce stomach irritation. Best taken as one dose in the morning to avoid nighttime urination. The tablet may be crushed for administration.

Usual Duration of Use: Continual use on a regular schedule for 2 to 3 weeks is usually necessary to determine this drug's effectiveness in lowering high blood pressure. Long-term use (months to years) requires periodic evaluation of response and possible dosage adjustment. Use as a diuretic should be intermittent with "drug holidays" (no drug taken) to reduce the risk of sodium and potassium imbalance.

▷ **This Drug Should Not Be Taken If**
  • you have had an allergic reaction to it previously.

▷ **Inform Your Physician Before Taking This Drug If**
  • you are allergic to any form of "sulfa" drug.
  • you are pregnant or planning pregnancy.
  • you have a history of kidney or liver disease.
  • you have diabetes, gout or lupus erythematosus.
  • you are taking any form of cortisone, digitalis, oral antidiabetic drug or insulin.
  • you plan to have surgery under general anesthesia in the near future.

Possible Side-Effects   (natural, expected and unavoidable drug actions)
  Light-headedness on arising from sitting or lying position (see orthostatic hypotension in Glossary).
  Increase in blood sugar level, affecting control of diabetes.
  Increase in blood uric acid level, affecting control of gout.
  Decrease in blood potassium level, causing muscle weakness and cramping.

▷ **Possible Adverse Effects**   (unusual, unexpected and infrequent reactions)
  If any of the following develop, consult your physician promptly.
  Mild Adverse Effects
  Allergic Reactions: Skin rashes, hives.
  Headache, dizziness, blurred vision.
  Reduced appetite, indigestion, nausea, vomiting, diarrhea.
  Serious Adverse Effects
  Allergic Reactions: Hepatitis with jaundice (see Glossary).
  Idiosyncratic Reactions: Muscle pains and cramping, seizures, collapse.
  Acute gout attacks (in susceptible individuals).
  Acute to chronic muscle disorders (due to potassium loss).
  Abnormally low white blood cell count: fever, sore throat, infections.

▷ **Adverse Effects That May Mimic Natural Diseases or Disorders**
  Liver reaction may suggest viral hepatitis.

Natural Diseases or Disorders That May Be Activated by This Drug
  Diabetes, gout, systemic lupus erythematosus (questionable).

CAUTION
  1. Do not exceed recommended doses. Increased dosage can cause exces-

sive loss of sodium and potassium, with resultant loss of appetite, nausea, fatigue, weakness, confusion and tingling in the extremities.

2. If you are also taking a digitalis preparation (digitoxin, digoxin), ensure an adequate intake of high-potassium foods to prevent potassium deficiency—a potential cause of digitalis toxicity. (See Table of High Potassium Foods in Section Six).

Precautions for Use

By Infants and Children: Safety and effectiveness for use by those under 12 years of age have not been established. Avoid overdosage that could cause serious dehydration. Significant potassium loss can occur within the first 2 weeks of drug use.

By Those over 60 Years of Age: Small doses are advisable until your individual response has been determined. You may be more susceptible to the development of impaired thinking, orthostatic hypotension, potassium loss and blood sugar increase. Overdosage and extended use of this drug can cause excessive loss of body water, thickening (increased viscosity) of the blood and an increased tendency for the blood to clot—predisposing to stroke, heart attack or thrombophlebitis (vein inflammation with blood clot).

▷ Advisability of Use During Pregnancy

Pregnancy Category: D (tentative). See Pregnancy Code inside back cover.

Animal studies: No birth defects reported in mouse, rat or rabbit studies.

Human studies: Information from adequate studies of pregnant women is not available.

This drug should not be used during pregnancy unless a very serious complication occurs for which this drug is significantly beneficial. Ask physician for guidance.

Advisability of Use if Breast-Feeding

Presence of this drug in breast milk: Yes.

Avoid drug if possible. If use is necessary, monitor nursing infant closely and discontinue drug or nursing if adverse effects develop.

Habit-Forming Potential: None.

Effects of Overdosage: Dry mouth, thirst, lethargy, weakness, muscle cramping, nausea, vomiting, drowsiness progressing to stupor or coma.

Possible Effects of Long-Term Use: Impaired balance of water, salt and potassium in blood and body tissues. Development of diabetes in predisposed individuals. Pathological changes in parathyroid glands (with increased blood calcium levels and decreased blood phosphate levels) have been reported with the long-term use of thiazide diuretics, a class chemically related to this diuretic.

Suggested Periodic Examinations While Taking This Drug   (at physician's discretion)

Complete blood cell counts, measurements of blood levels of sodium, potassium, chloride, sugar and uric acid.

Kidney and liver function tests.

▷ **While Taking This Drug, Observe the Following**

Foods: Consult your physician regarding the advisability of eating foods rich in potassium. If so advised, see the Table of High Potassium Foods in Section Six. Follow physician's advice regarding the use of salt.

Beverages: No restrictions. This drug may be taken with milk.

▷ *Alcohol*: Use with caution until the combined effects have been determined. Alcohol may exaggerate the blood-pressure-lowering effects of this drug and cause orthostatic hypotension.

Tobacco Smoking: No interactions expected. Follow physician's advice.

▷ *Other Drugs*

Metolazone may *increase* the effects of
- other antihypertensive drugs; dosage adjustments may be necessary to prevent excessive lowering of blood pressure.
- lithium, and cause lithium toxicity.

Metolazone may *decrease* the effects of
- oral antidiabetic drugs (sulfonylureas); dosage adjustments may be necessary for proper control of blood sugar.

Metolazone *taken concurrently* with
- digitalis preparations (digitoxin, digoxin) requires very careful monitoring and dosage adjustments to prevent fluctuations of blood potassium levels and serious disturbances of heart rhythm.

The following drugs may *decrease* the effects of metolazone
- cholestyramine (Cuemid, Questran) may interfere with its absorption.
- colestipol (Colestid) may interfere with its absorption.

Take cholestyramine and colestipol 1 hour before any oral diuretic.

▷ *Driving, Hazardous Activities*: Use caution until the possible occurrence of orthostatic hypotension, dizziness or impaired vision has been determined.

Aviation Note: The use of this drug *may be a disqualification* for piloting. Consult a designated Aviation Medical Examiner.

Exposure to Sun: Use caution until sensitivity has been determined. This drug may cause photosensitivity (see Glossary).

Exposure to Heat: Avoid excessive perspiring, which could cause additional loss of salt and water from the body.

Heavy Exercise or Exertion: Avoid exertion that produces light-headedness, excessive fatigue or muscle cramping. Isometric exercises—the "overload" technique for strengthening individual muscles—can raise blood pressure significantly. Ask physician for guidance regarding participation in this form of exercise.

Occurrence of Unrelated Illness: Illnesses that cause vomiting or diarrhea can produce a serious imbalance of important body chemistry. Consult your physician for guidance.

Discontinuation: This drug should not be stopped abruptly following long-term use; serious diuretic-withdrawal fluid retention (edema) can develop after sudden discontinuation. The dose should be reduced gradually. It may be advisable to discontinue this drug 5 to 7 days before major surgery. Ask your physician, surgeon and/or anesthesiologist for guidance regarding dosage adjustment or drug withdrawal.

METOPROLOL
(me TOH proh lohl)

Introduced: 1974

Class: Antihypertensive, Beta-Adrenergic Blocker

Prescription: USA: Yes
Canada: Yes

Controlled Drug: USA: No
Canada: No

Available as Generic: No

Brand Names: ✤Apo-Metoprolol, ✤Betaloc, Lopressor, Lopressor HCT [CD]

BENEFITS versus RISKS

Possible Benefits	*Possible Risks*
EFFECTIVE, WELL-TOLERATED ANTIHYPERTENSIVE in mild to moderate high blood pressure	CONGESTIVE HEART FAILURE in advanced heart disease
	Worsening of angina in coronary heart disease (abrupt withdrawal)
	Masking of low blood sugar (hypoglycemia) in drug-treated diabetes
	Provocation of asthma (with high doses)

▷ **Principal Uses**
   As a Single Drug Product: The treatment of mild to moderately severe high blood pressure. May be used alone or concurrently with other antihypertensive drugs, such as diuretics. Also used to reduce the risk of recurrent heart attack.

How This Drug Works: By blocking certain actions of the sympathetic nervous system, this drug
   • reduces the rate the contraction force of the heart, thus lowering the ejection pressure of the blood leaving the heart.
   • reduces the degree of contraction of blood vessel walls, resulting in their relaxation and expansion and consequent lowering of blood pressure.
   • prolongs the conduction time of nerve impulses through the heart, of benefit in the management of certain heart rhythm disorders.

Available Dosage Forms and Strengths
   Injection — 1 mg per ml
   Tablets — 50 mg, 100 mg

▷ **Usual Adult Dosage Range:** Initially, 50 mg twice daily (12 hours apart). The dose may be increased gradually at intervals of 7 to 10 days as needed and tolerated, up to 300 mg/day. For maintenance, 100 mg twice/day. The total daily dose should not exceed 450 mg. **Note: Actual dosage and administration schedule must be determined by the physician for each patient individually.**

▷ **Dosing Instructions:** May be taken without regard to eating. The tablet may be crushed for administration. Do not discontinue this drug abruptly.

Usual Duration of Use: Continual use on a regular schedule for 10 to 14 days is usually necessary to determine this drug's effectiveness in lowering blood pressure. The long-term use of this drug (months to years) will be determined by the course of your blood pressure over time and your response to the overall treatment program (weight reduction, salt restriction, smoking cessation, etc.).

▷ **This Drug Should Not Be Taken If**
- you have had an allergic reaction to it previously.
- you have congestive heart failure.
- you have an abnormally slow heart rate or a serious form of heart block.
- you are taking, or have taken within the past 14 days, any monoamine oxidase (MAO) inhibitor drug (see Drug Class, Section Four).

▷ **Inform Your Physician Before Taking This Drug If**
- you have had an adverse reaction to any "beta-blocker" drug in the past (see Drug Class, Section Four).
- you have a history of serious heart disease, with or without episodes of heart failure.
- you have a history of hay fever (allergic rhinitis), asthma, chronic bronchitis or emphysema.
- you have a history of overactive thyroid function (hyperthyroidism).
- you have a history of low blood sugar (hypoglycemia).
- you have impaired liver or kidney function.
- you have diabetes or myasthenia gravis.
- you are currently taking any form of digitalis, quinidine or reserpine, or any "calcium-blocker" drug (see Drug Class, Section Four).
- you plan to have surgery under general anesthesia in the near future.

Possible Side-Effects (natural, expected and unavoidable drug actions)
Lethargy and fatigability (10%), cold extremities, slow heart rate (15%), light-headedness in upright position (see orthostatic hypotension in Glossary).

▷ **Possible Adverse Effects** (unusual, unexpected and infrequent reactions)
If any of the following develop, consult your physician promptly.
Mild Adverse Effects
Allergic Reactions: Skin rash, itching.
Headache, dizziness (10%), insomnia, abnormal dreams.
Indigestion, nausea, vomiting, constipation, diarrhea.
Joint and muscle discomfort, fluid retention (edema).
Serious Adverse Effects
Mental depression (5%), anxiety, impotence (rare).
Chest pain, shortness of breath, precipitation of congestive heart failure.
Induction of bronchial asthma (in asthmatic individuals).

CAUTION
1. ***Do not discontinue this drug suddenly*** without the knowledge and guidance of your physician. Carry a notation on your person that you are taking this drug.
2. Consult your physician or pharmacist before using nasal decongestants usually present in over-the-counter cold preparations and nose drops. These can cause sudden increases in blood pressure when taken concurrently with beta-blocker drugs.
3. Report the development of any tendency to emotional depression.

Precautions for Use
By Infants and Children: Safety and effectiveness for use by those under 12 years of age have not been established. However, if this drug is used, observe for the development of low blood sugar (hypoglycemia) during periods of reduced food intake.
By Those over 60 Years of Age: Proceed *cautiously* with all antihypertensive drugs. Unacceptably high blood pressure should be reduced without creating the risks associated with excessively low blood pressure. Start treatment with small doses, and monitor the blood pressure response frequently. Sudden, rapid and excessive reduction of blood pressure can predispose to stroke or heart attack. Observe for dizziness, unsteadiness, tendency to fall, confusion, hallucinations, depression or urinary frequency.

▷ **Advisability of Use During Pregnancy**
Pregnancy Category: B (tentative). See Pregnancy Code inside back cover.
Animal studies: No significant increase in birth defects due to this drug.
Human studies: Information from adequate studies of pregnant women is not available.
Use this drug only if clearly needed. Ask physician for guidance.

Advisability of Use if Breast-Feeding
Presence of this drug in breast milk: Yes, in large amounts.
Avoid drug or refrain from nursing.

Habit-Forming Potential: None.

Effects of Overdosage: Weakness, slow pulse, low blood pressure, fainting, cold and sweaty skin, congestive heart failure, possible coma and convulsions.

Possible Effects of Long-Term Use: Reduced heart reserve and eventual heart failure in susceptible individuals with advanced heart disease.

Suggested Periodic Examinations While Taking This Drug   (at physician's discretion)
Measurements of blood pressure, evaluation of heart function.

▷ **While Taking This Drug, Observe the Following**
Foods: No restrictions. Avoid excessive salt intake.
Beverages: No restrictions. May be taken with milk.

▷ *Alcohol:* Use with caution until the combined effect has been determined. Alcohol may exaggerate this drug's ability to lower the blood pressure and may increase its mild sedative effect.

Tobacco Smoking: Nicotine may reduce this drug's effectiveness in treating high blood pressure. In addition, high doses of this drug may potentiate the constriction of the bronchial tubes caused by regular smoking.

▷ *Other Drugs*

Metoprolol may *increase* the effects of

- other antihypertensive drugs, and cause excessive lowering of the blood pressure. Dosage adjustments may be necessary.
- reserpine (Ser-Ap-Es, etc.), and cause sedation, depression, slowing of the heart rate and lowering of the blood pressure.
- verapamil (Calan, Isoptin), and cause excessive depression of heart function; monitor this combination closely.

Metoprolol *taken concurrently* with

- clonidine (Catapres) requires close monitoring for rebound high blood pressure if clonidine is withdrawn while metoprolol is still being taken.
- insulin requires close monitoring to avoid undetected hypoglycemia (see Glossary).

The following drugs may *increase* the effects of metoprolol

- cimetidine (Tagamet).
- methimazole (Tapazole).
- oral contraceptives.
- propylthiouracil (Propacil).

The following drugs may *decrease* the effects of metoprolol

- barbiturates (phenobarbital, etc.).
- indomethacin (Indocin), and possibly other "aspirin substitutes," may impair metoprolol's antihypertensive effect.
- rifampin (Rifadin, Rimactane).

▷ *Driving, Hazardous Activities:* Use caution until the full extent of drowsiness, lethargy and blood pressure change has been determined.

Aviation Note: The use of this drug *is a disqualification* for piloting. Consult a designated Aviation Medical Examiner.

Exposure to Sun: No restrictions.

Exposure to Heat: Caution advised. Hot environments can lower the blood pressure and exaggerate the effects of this drug.

Exposure to Cold: Caution advised. Cold environments can enhance the circulatory deficiency in the extremities that may occur with this drug. The elderly should take precautions to prevent hypothermia (see Glossary).

Heavy Exercise or Exertion: It is advisable to avoid exertion that produces light-headedness, excessive fatigue or muscle cramping. The use of this drug may intensify the hypertensive response to isometric exercise.

Occurrence of Unrelated Illness: The fever that accompanies systemic infections can lower the blood pressure and require adjustment of dosage.

Illnesses that cause nausea or vomiting may interrupt the regular dosage schedule. Ask your physician for guidance.

Discontinuation: It is advisable to avoid sudden discontinuation of this drug in all situations. If possible, gradual reduction of dose over a period of 2 to 3 weeks is recommended. Ask your physician for specific guidance.

METRONIDAZOLE
(me troh NI da zohl)

Introduced: 1960

Prescription: USA: Yes
Canada: Yes

Class: Anti-infective

Controlled Drug: USA: No
Canada: No

Available as Generic: Yes

Brand Names: ♣Apo-Metronidazole, Flagyl, Metizole, Metryl, ♣Neo-Tric, ♣Novonidazole, ♣PMS-Metronidazole, Protostat

---

BENEFITS versus RISKS

Possible Benefits	*Possible Risks*
EFFECTIVE TREATMENT FOR TRICHOMONAS INFECTIONS, AMEBIC DYSENTERY AND GIARDIASIS	Superinfection with yeast organisms
	Peripheral neuropathy (see Glossary)
Effective treatment for some anaerobic bacterial infections	Abnormally low white blood cell count (transient)
	Aggravation of epilepsy

▷ **Principal Uses**

As a Single Drug Product: Used primarily to treat trichomonas infections of the vaginal canal and cervix and of the male urethra. It is also used to treat amebic dysentery, giardia infections of the intestine and serious infections caused by certain strains of anaerobic bacteria.

How This Drug Works: By interacting with DNA, this drug destroys essential components of the nucleus that are necessary for the cell life and growth of infecting organisms.

Available Dosage Forms and Strengths
Injection — 500 mg per 100 ml
Tablets — 250 mg, 500 mg

▷ **Usual Adult Dosage Range:** Varies with infection to be treated.
For trichomoniasis: One-day course—2 grams as a single dose; or 1 gram for 2 doses 12 hours apart. Seven-day course—250 mg 3 times/day for 7 consecutive days. (The 7-day course is preferred.)
For amebiasis: 500 to 750 mg 3 times/day for 5 to 10 consecutive days.
For giardiasis: 2 grams once/day for 3 days; or 250 to 500 mg 3 times/day for 5 to 7 days.

The total daily dosage should not exceed 4 grams (4000 mg).
Note: Actual dosage and administration schedule must be determined by the physician for each patient individually.

▷ **Dosing Instructions:**   May be taken with or following food to reduce stomach irritation. The tablet may be crushed for administration.

Usual Duration of Use: Continual use on a regular schedule as outlined is necessary to ensure this drug's effectiveness. Do not repeat the course of treatment without your physician's approval.

▷ **This Drug Should Not Be Taken If**
  • you have had an allergic reaction to it previously.
  • you currently have a bone marrow or blood cell disorder.
  • you have any type of central nervous system disorder, including epilepsy.

▷ **Inform Your Physician Before Taking This Drug If**
  • you have a history of any type of blood cell disorder, especially one induced by drugs.
  • you have impaired liver or kidney function.
  • you are pregnant or breast-feeding.

Possible Side-Effects   (natural, expected and unavoidable drug actions)
  A sharp, metallic, unpleasant taste.
  Dark discoloration of the urine (of no significance).
  Superinfection (see Glossary) by yeast organisms in the mouth or vagina.

▷ **Possible Adverse Effects**   (unusual, unexpected and infrequent reactions)
  If any of the following develop, consult your physician promptly.
  Mild Adverse Effects
  Allergic Reactions: Skin rash, hives, flushing, itching.
  Headache, dizziness, incoordination, unsteadiness.
  Loss of appetite, nausea, vomiting, abdominal cramps, diarrhea.
  Irritation of mouth and tongue, possibly due to yeast infection.
  Serious Adverse Effects
  Idiosyncratic Reactions: Abnormal behavior, confusion, depression.
  Peripheral neuropathy (see Glossary).
  Abnormally low white blood cell count (transient): fever, sore throat, infections.

Possible Delayed Adverse Effects
  Studies have shown that this drug can cause cancer in mice and possibly in rats. There is no evidence to date that this drug causes cancer in man when used in the dosages specified earlier. Follow your physician's instructions exactly. Avoid unnecessary or prolonged use.

▷ **Adverse Effects That May Mimic Natural Diseases or Disorders**
  Behavioral changes may suggest spontaneous psychosis.

Natural Diseases or Disorders That May Be Activated by This Drug
  Latent yeast infections.

CAUTION

1. Troublesome and persistent diarrhea can develop in sensitive individuals. If diarrhea persists for more than 24 hours, discontinue this drug and consult with your physician.
2. Discontinue this drug immediately if you develop any indications of toxic effects on the brain or nervous system: confusion, irritability, dizziness, incoordination, unsteady stance or gait, muscle jerking or twitching, numbness or weakness in the extremities.

Precautions for Use

By Infants and Children: Avoid use in those with a history of bone marrow or blood cell disorders.

By Those over 60 Years of Age: Natural changes in the skin may predispose to yeast infections in the genital and anal regions. Report the development of rashes and itching promptly.

▷ **Advisability of Use During Pregnancy**

Pregnancy Category: X (tentative). See Pregnancy Code inside back cover.

Animal studies: No birth defects reported in rat studies. However, this drug is known to cause cancer in mice and possibly in rats.

Human studies: No increase in birth defects reported in 206 exposures to this drug during the first 3 months. However, information from adequate studies of pregnant women is not available.

The manufacturer advises against the use of this drug during the first 3 months. Use during the last 6 months is not advised unless it is absolutely essential to the mother's health.

Advisability of Use if Breast-Feeding

Presence of this drug in breast milk: Yes.

Avoid drug or refrain from nursing.

Habit-Forming Potential: None.

Effects of Overdosage: Weakness, stomach irritation, nausea, vomiting, confusion, disorientation.

Possible Effects of Long-Term Use: None reported. Avoid long-term use.

Suggested Periodic Examinations While Taking This Drug   (at physician's discretion)

Complete blood cell counts.

▷ **While Taking This Drug, Observe the Following**

Foods: No restrictions.

Beverages: No restrictions. May be taken with milk.

▷   *Alcohol*: Use caution until combined effects have been determined. A disulfiramlike reaction has been reported (see Glossary).

Tobacco Smoking: No interactions expected.

▷   *Other Drugs*

Metronidazole may *increase* the effects of

- warfarin (Coumadin, etc.), and cause abnormal bleeding. The prothrombin time should be monitored closely, especially during the first 10 days of concurrent use.

Metronidazole *taken concurrently* with

- disulfiram (Antabuse) may cause severe emotional and behavioral disturbances.

▷ *Driving, Hazardous Activities*: This drug may cause dizziness or incoordination. Restrict activities as necessary.

Aviation Note: The use of this drug *may be a disqualification* for piloting. Consult a designated Aviation Medical Examiner.

Exposure to Sun: No restrictions.

MEXILETINE
(mex IL e teen)

Introduced: 1973

Prescription: USA: Yes
Canada: Yes

Available as Generic: No

Brand Names: Mexitil

Class: Antiarrhythmic

Controlled Drug: USA: No
Canada: No

BENEFITS versus RISKS

Possible Benefits	*Possible Risks*
EFFECTIVE TREATMENT IN 30% OF SELECTED HEART RHYTHM DISORDERS	NARROW TREATMENT RANGE FREQUENT ADVERSE EFFECTS (up to 40% of users) WORSENING OF SOME ARRHYTHMIAS Rare seizures, liver injury and reduced white blood cell count

---

▷ **Principal Uses**

As a Single Drug Product: This drug is classified as a Class 1B agent, similar to lidocaine in its actions. It is used primarily to correct and prevent the recurrence of (1) abnormally rapid heart rates (tachycardia) that arise in the ventricles (lower heart chambers); and (2) premature beats arising in the ventricles.

How This Drug Works: By slowing the transmission of electrical impulses throughout the conduction system of the heart, this drug assists in restoring normal heart rate and rhythm in selected types of arrhythmia.

Available Dosage Forms and Strengths
Capsules — 150 mg, 200 mg, 250 mg

▷ **Usual Adult Dosage Range:** Initiate treatment with 200 mg/8 hours. At intervals of 2 to 3 days, increase dose by 50 to 100 mg as needed and tolerated.

The total daily dosage should not exceed 1200 mg. Measurement of drug blood levels is advised (when available) to determine the optimal dose and schedule. **Note: Actual dosage and administration schedule must be determined by the physician for each patient individually.**

▷ **Dosing Instructions:** Take with food or antacid to reduce stomach irritation. Take at same times each day to obtain uniform results. The capsule may be opened for administration.

Usual Duration of Use: Continual use on a regular schedule for 1 to 2 weeks is usually necessary to determine this drug's effectiveness in correcting or preventing responsive rhythm disorders. Long-term use requires supervision and periodic evaluation by your physician.

▷ **This Drug Should Not Be Taken If**
- you have had an allergic reaction to it previously.
- you have second-degree or third-degree heart block (determined by electrocardiogram), uncorrected by a pacemaker.

▷ **Inform Your Physician Before Taking This Drug If**
- you have had any unfavorable reactions to other antiarrhythmic drugs in the past.
- you have a history of heart disease of any kind, especially "heart block" or heart failure.
- you have impaired liver function.
- you have a seizure disorder of any kind.
- you are taking any form of digitalis, a potassium supplement or any diuretic drug that can cause excessive loss of body potassium (ask physician).

Possible Side-Effects (natural, expected and unavoidable drug actions)
Nervousness (11%), light-headedness (10%).

▷ **Possible Adverse Effects** (unusual, unexpected and infrequent reactions)
If any of the following develop, consult your physician promptly.
Mild Adverse Effects
Allergic Reactions: Skin rash (4%).
Headache (7%), dizziness (26%), visual disturbance (7%), fatigue (3%), weakness (5%), tremor (13%).
Loss of appetite, indigestion, nausea (39%), vomiting, constipation (4%), diarrhea (5%), abdominal pain (1%).
Serious Adverse Effects
Idiosyncratic Reactions: Depression, confusion, amnesia, hallucinations, seizures (all rare).
Drug-induced heart rhythm disorders (1%), shortness of breath (5%), palpitations (7%), chest pain (7%), swelling of feet.
Sexual impotence, urinary retention.
Liver damage with jaundice (see Glossary).
Abnormally low white blood cell and blood platelet counts (rare): fever, sore throat, abnormal bleeding or bruising.

▷ **Adverse Effects That May Mimic Natural Diseases or Disorders**
Liver toxicity may suggest viral hepatitis.

Natural Diseases or Disorders That May Be Activated by This Drug
Latent epilepsy.

CAUTION
1. Thorough evaluation of your heart function (including electrocardiograms) is necessary prior to using this drug.
2. Periodic evaluation of your heart function is necessary to determine your response to this drug. Some individuals may experience worsening of their heart rhythm disorder and/or deterioration of heart function. Close monitoring of heart rate, rhythm and overall performance is essential.
3. Dosage must be adjusted carefully for each individual. Do not change your dosage without the knowledge and supervision of your physician.
4. Do not take any other antiarrhythmic drug while taking this drug unless you are directed to do so by your physician.
5. Carry a card of personal identification with the notation that you are taking this drug. Inform all attending medical personnel that you are taking this drug, especially if you require surgery of any kind.

Precautions for Use
By Infants and Children: Safety and effectiveness for use by those under 12 years of age have not been established. Initial use of this drug requires hospitalization and supervision by a qualified cardiologist.
By Those over 60 Years of Age: Reduced liver function may require reduction in dosage. Observe carefully for light-headedness, dizziness, unsteadiness and tendency to fall.

▷ **Advisability of Use During Pregnancy**
Pregnancy Category: C (tentative). See Pregnancy Code inside back cover.
Animal studies: No birth defects reported in mice, rats or rabbits. However, an increased rate of fetal resorption was found.
Human studies: Information from adequate studies of pregnant women is not available.
Avoid during first 3 months. Use this drug only if clearly needed. Ask physician for guidance.

Advisability of Use if Breast-Feeding
Presence of this drug in breast milk: Yes.
Avoid drug or refrain from nursing.

Habit-Forming Potential: None.

Effects of Overdosage: Impaired urination, constipation, marked drop in blood pressure, abnormal heart rhythms, congestive heart failure, dizziness, incoordination, seizures.

Possible Effects of Long-Term Use: None reported.

Suggested Periodic Examinations While Taking This Drug (at physician's discretion)
Electrocardiograms, complete blood cell counts, liver function tests.

▷ **While Taking This Drug, Observe the Following**
Foods: No restrictions. Ask physician regarding need for salt restriction.
Beverages: No restrictions. May be taken with milk.

▷ *Alcohol*: Use caution until the combined effects have been determined. Alcohol can increase the blood-pressure-lowering effects of this drug.
Tobacco Smoking: Nicotine can cause irritability of the heart and reduce the effectiveness of this drug. Follow physician's advice regarding smoking.

▷ *Other Drugs*
Mexiletine may *increase* the effects of
• antihypertensive drugs, and cause excessive lowering of blood pressure.
• beta-blocker drugs (see Drug Class, Section Four).
The following drugs may *decrease* the effects of mexiletine
• phenytoin (Dilantin, etc.).
• rifampin (Rifadin, Rimactane).

▷ *Driving, Hazardous Activities*: This drug may cause weakness, dizziness or blurred vision. Restrict activities as necessary.
Aviation Note: The use of this drug *may be a disqualification* for piloting. Consult a designated Aviation Medical Examiner.
Exposure to Sun: No restrictions.
Occurrence of Unrelated Illness: Disorders that cause vomiting, diarrhea or dehydration can affect this drug's action adversely. Report such developments promptly.
Discontinuation: This drug should not be discontinued abruptly following long-term use. Ask your physician for guidance regarding gradual dose reduction.

MINOCYCLINE
(min oh SI kleen)

Introduced: 1970

Prescription: USA: Yes
Canada: Yes

Available as Generic: No

Brand Names: Minocin

Class: Antibiotic, Tetracyclines

Controlled Drug: USA: No
Canada: No

BENEFITS versus RISKS

Possible Benefits	*Possible Risks*
EFFECTIVE TREATMENT OF INFECTIONS due to susceptible microorganisms	Allergic reactions
	Drug-induced colitis
	Drug-induced dizziness and unsteadiness
	Fungal superinfections

▷ **Principal Uses**

As a Single Drug Product: This member of the tetracycline drug class is used primarily to treat (1) a broad range of infections caused by susceptible bacteria and protozoa, and (2) severe, resistant pustular acne.

How This Drug Works: This drug prevents the growth and multiplication of susceptible bacteria by interfering with their formation of essential proteins.

Available Dosage Forms and Strengths

Capsules — 50 mg, 100 mg
Oral suspension — 50 mg per 5 ml teaspoonful (5% alcohol)
Tablets, film coated — 50 mg, 100 mg

▷ **Usual Adult Dosage Range:** Initially, 200 mg; then 100 mg/12 hours or 50 mg/6 hours. The total daily dosage should not exceed 350 mg the first day or 200 mg thereafter. **Note: Actual dosage and administration schedule must be determined by the physician for each patient individually.**

▷ **Dosing Instructions:** May be taken without regard to food. Take at same time each day, with a full glass of water or milk. Take the full course prescribed. The tablet may be crushed and the capsule may be opened for administration.

Usual Duration of Use: The time required to control the infection and be free of fever and symptoms for 48 hours. This varies with the nature of the infection.

▷ **This Drug Should Not Be Taken If**
- you are allergic to any tetracycline drug (see Drug Class, Section Four).
- you are pregnant or breast-feeding.

▷ **Inform Your Physician Before Taking This Drug If**
- it is prescribed for a child under 8 years of age.
- you have a history of liver or kidney disease.
- you have systemic lupus erythematosus.
- you are taking any penicillin drug.
- you are taking any anticoagulant drug.
- you plan to have surgery under general anesthesia in the near future.

Possible Side-Effects (natural, expected and unavoidable drug actions)
Superinfections (see Glossary), often due to yeast organisms. These can

occur in the mouth, intestinal tract, rectum and/or vagina, resulting in rectal and vaginal itching.

▷ **Possible Adverse Effects**   (unusual, unexpected and infrequent reactions)
If any of the following develop, consult your physician promptly.
Mild Adverse Effects
Allergic Reactions: Skin rash, hives, itching of hands and feet, swelling of face or extremities.
Marked dizziness, unsteadiness, incoordination (usually occurs during the first 3 days).
Pigmentation of skin.
Loss of appetite, stomach irritation, nausea, vomiting, diarrhea.
Irritation of mouth or tongue, "black tongue," sore throat, abdominal cramping or pain.
Serious Adverse Effects
Allergic Reactions: Anaphylactic reaction (see Glossary), asthma, fever, swollen joints, abnormal bleeding or bruising.
Permanent discoloration and/or malformation of teeth when taken under 8 years of age, including unborn child and infant.

Natural Diseases or Disorders That May Be Activated by This Drug
Systemic lupus erythematosus.

CAUTION
1. Antacids, dairy products and preparations containing aluminum, bismuth, calcium, iron, magnesium or zinc can prevent adequate absorption of this drug and reduce its effectiveness significantly.
2. Troublesome and persistent diarrhea can develop in sensitive individuals. If diarrhea persists for more than 24 hours, discontinue this drug and consult your physician.
3. If surgery under general anesthesia is required while taking this drug, the choice of anesthetic agent must be considered carefully to prevent serious kidney damage.

Precautions for Use
By Infants and Children: If possible, tetracyclines should not be given to children under 8 years of age because of the risk of permanent discoloration and deformity of the teeth. Rarely, young infants may develop increased intracranial pressure within the first 4 days of receiving this drug. Tetracyclines may inhibit normal bone growth and development.
By Those over 60 Years of Age: Dosage must be carefully individualized and based upon determinations of kidney function. Natural skin changes may predispose to severe and prolonged itching reactions in the genital and anal regions.

▷ **Advisability of Use During Pregnancy**
Pregnancy Category: D (tentative). See Pregnancy Code inside back cover.
Animal studies: Tetracycline causes limb defects in rats, rabbits and chickens.
Human studies: Information from studies of pregnant women indicates

that this drug can cause impaired development and discoloration of teeth and other developmental defects.

It is advisable to avoid this drug completely during entire pregnancy.

Advisability of Use if Breast-Feeding
Presence of this drug in breast milk: Yes.
Avoid drug or refrain from nursing.

Habit-Forming Potential: None.

Effects of Overdosage: Dizziness, nausea, vomiting, diarrhea.

Possible Effects of Long-Term Use: Superinfections; rarely, impairment of bone marrow, liver or kidney function.

Suggested Periodic Examinations While Taking This Drug   (at physician's discretion)
Complete blood cell counts, liver and kidney function tests.
During extended use, sputum and stool examinations may detect early superinfection due to yeast organisms.

▷ **While Taking This Drug, Observe the Following**
Foods: No restrictions.
Beverages: No restrictions.
▷   *Alcohol*: No interactions expected. However, it is best avoided if you have active liver disease.
Tobacco Smoking: No interactions expected.
▷   *Other Drugs*
Tetracyclines may *increase* the effects of
• oral anticoagulants, and make it necessary to reduce their dosage.
• digoxin (Lanoxin), and cause digitalis toxicity.
• lithium (Eskalith, Lithane, etc.), and increase the risk of lithium toxicity.
Tetracyclines may *decrease* the effects of
• oral contraceptives, and impair their effectiveness in preventing pregnancy.
• penicillins, and impair their effectiveness in treating infections.
Tetracyclines *taken concurrently* with
• methoxyflurane anesthesia may impair kidney function.
The following drugs may *decrease* the effects of tetracyclines
• antacids (aluminum and magnesium preparations, sodium bicarbonate, etc.) may reduce drug absorption.
• iron and mineral preparations may reduce drug absorption.
▷   *Driving, Hazardous Activities*: This drug may cause marked dizziness or incoordination. Restrict activities as necessary.
Aviation Note: The use of this drug *may be a disqualification* for piloting. Consult a designated Aviation Medical Examiner.
Exposure to Sun: Use caution until sensitivity has been determined. Some tetracyclines can cause photosensitivity (see Glossary).

MINOXIDIL
(min OX i dil)

Introduced: 1972

Prescription: USA: Yes
Canada: Yes

Available as Generic: No

Brand Names: Loniten

Class: Antihypertensive

Controlled Drug: USA: No
Canada: No

BENEFITS versus RISKS

Possible Benefits	*Possible Risks*
A POTENT, LONG-ACTING ANTIHYPERTENSIVE	EXCESSIVE HAIR GROWTH (80% of users)
EFFECTIVE IN 75% OF CASES OF SEVERE HYPERTENSION	SALT AND WATER RETENTION
EFFECTIVE IN ACCELERATED AND MALIGNANT HYPERTENSION	Excessively rapid heart rate
	Aggravation of angina

▷ **Principal Uses**

As a Single Drug Product: Currently the use of this drug is limited to the treatment of severe high blood pressure that cannot be controlled by conventional therapy. Investigations are under way to determine the value of this drug when used in lotions and ointments to treat scalp baldness. These dosage forms are experimental and not available to the public at the time of writing.

How This Drug Works: By causing direct relaxation of the constricted muscles within the walls of small arteries throughout the body, this drug permits expansion of the arteries with resultant lowering of blood pressure.

Available Dosage Forms and Strengths

Tablets — 2.5 mg, 10 mg

▷ **Usual Adult Dosage Range:** Initially, 5 mg/24 hours in one dose. Gradually increase dose to 10 mg, 20 mg, then 40 mg/24 hours, taken in 1 or 2 divided doses daily, as needed and tolerated. The usual maintenance dose is 10 to 40 mg/24 hours. The total daily dosage should not exceed 50 mg. **Note: Actual dosage and administration schedule must be determined by the physician for each patient individually.**

▷ **Dosing Instructions:** May be taken with or following food to prevent nausea. Take at the same time each day. The tablet may be crushed for administration.

Usual Duration of Use: Continual use on a regular schedule for 3 to 7 days is usually necessary to determine this drug's effectiveness in controlling severe hypertension. Long-term use (months to years) requires supervision and periodic evaluation by your physician.

▷ **This Drug Should Not Be Taken If**
  • you have had an allergic reaction to it previously.
  • you are known to have a pheochromocytoma (an adrenalin-producing tumor).
  • you have pulmonary hypertension due to mitral valve stenosis.

▷ **Inform Your Physician Before Taking This Drug If**
  • you are pregnant or planning pregnancy.
  • you have a history of coronary artery disease or impaired heart function.
  • you have a history of stroke or impaired brain circulation.
  • you have impaired liver or kidney function.

Possible Side-Effects   (natural, expected and unavoidable drug actions)
  Increased heart rate, fluid retention with weight gain (7%), excessive hair growth on face, arms, legs and back (80%).

▷ **Possible Adverse Effects**   (unusual, unexpected and infrequent reactions)
  If any of the following develop, consult your physician promptly.
  Mild Adverse Effects
  Allergic Reactions: Skin rash (less than 1%).
  Nausea, increased thirst.
  Breast tenderness (less than 1%).
  Serious Adverse Effects
  Idiosyncratic Reactions: Fluid formation around the heart (pericardial effusion) (3%).
  Development of angina pectoris; development of high blood pressure in the lung circulation (pulmonary hypertension).

Natural Diseases or Disorders That May Be Activated by This Drug
  Latent coronary artery disease with symptomatic angina.

CAUTION
  1. The long-term use of this drug usually requires the concurrent use of an effective diuretic to counteract salt and water retention.
  2. The long-term use of this drug often requires the concurrent use of a beta-blocker drug to control excessive acceleration of the heart rate.
  3. It is best to avoid the concurrent use of this drug and guanethidine; the combination can cause severe orthostatic hypotension (see Glossary).
  4. Consult your physician regarding the advisability of using a "no salt added" diet.

Precautions for Use
  By Infants and Children: Dosage schedules should be determined by a qualified pediatrician. Monitor closely for salt and water retention.
  By Those over 60 Years of Age: This drug must be used very cautiously by this age group. Start treatment with small doses and limit the total daily dose to 75 mg. Headache, palpitation and rapid heart rate due to this drug are more common in this age group and can mimic acute anxiety states. Observe for dizziness, unsteadiness, fainting and falling.

▷ **Advisability of Use During Pregnancy**
Pregnancy Category: C (tentative). See Pregnancy Code inside back cover.
Animal studies: No birth defects reported in rats or rabbits. However, studies did reveal decreased fertility and increased fetal deaths.
Human studies: Information from adequate studies of pregnant women is not available.
Avoid during the first 3 months. Use only if clearly needed during the last 6 months.

Advisability of Use if Breast-Feeding
Presence of this drug in breast milk: Unknown.
Avoid drug or refrain from nursing.

Habit-Forming Potential: None.

Effects of Overdosage: Headache, dizziness, weakness, nausea, marked low blood pressure, weak and rapid pulse, loss of consciousness.

Possible Effects of Long-Term Use: Excessive growth of hair occurs in 80% of users after 1 to 2 months. This may be accompanied by darkening of the skin and coarsening of facial features.

Suggested Periodic Examinations While Taking This Drug (at physician's discretion)
Body weight measurement for insidious gain due to water retention.
Electrocardiographic and echocardiographic heart examinations.

▷ **While Taking This Drug, Observe the Following**
Foods: Avoid excessive salt and heavily salted foods.
Beverages: No restrictions. May be taken with milk.
▷ *Alcohol*: Use with extreme caution until combined effects have been determined. Alcohol can exaggerate the blood-pressure-lowering effects of this drug.
Tobacco Smoking: Best avoided. Nicotine can contribute significantly to the development of angina in susceptible individuals.
▷ *Other Drugs*
Minoxidil may *increase* the effects of
• all other antihypertensive drugs; careful dosage adjustments are mandatory.
Minoxidil *taken concurrently* with
• guanethidine (Ismelin, Esimil) may cause severe orthostatic hypotension; avoid this combination.
▷ *Driving, Hazardous Activities*: This drug may cause dizziness and fatigue. Restrict activities as necessary.
Aviation Note: The use of this drug *is a disqualification* for piloting. Consult a designated Aviation Medical Examiner.
Exposure to Sun: No restrictions.
Discontinuation: This drug should not be stopped abruptly. If it is to be discontinued, consult your physician regarding gradual reduction in dosage and appropriate replacement with other drugs.

MOLINDONE
(moh LIN dohn)

Introduced: 1971

Prescription: USA: Yes

Available as Generic: No

Brand Names: Moban

Class: Strong Tranquilizer, Antipsychotic

Controlled Drug: USA: No

BENEFITS versus RISKS

Possible Benefits	*Possible Risks*
EFFECTIVE TREATMENT OF SOME CASES OF ACUTE AND CHRONIC SCHIZOPHRENIA	NARROW TREATMENT MARGIN SERIOUS TOXIC EFFECTS ON BRAIN:
May be effective in schizophrenia that has not responded to other drugs	PARKINSON-LIKE REACTIONS SEVERE RESTLESSNESS ABNORMAL INVOLUNTARY MOVEMENTS TARDIVE DYSKINESIAS (see Glossary)
	Liver toxicity, jaundice
	Atropinelike side-effects

▷ **Principal Uses**

As a Single Drug Product: Used primarily in the management of acute and chronic schizophrenia to control thought disorder, disorientation, hallucinations, perceptual distortions and hostility. It is sometimes effective in chronic schizophrenic individuals who have not responded to other antipsychotic drugs.

How This Drug Works: Not completely established. It is thought that by decreasing dopamine activity in the reticular activating system of the brain, this drug improves distorted patterns of thinking and behavior.

Available Dosage Forms and Strengths

Concentrate — 20 mg per ml

Tablets — 5 mg, 10 mg, 25 mg, 50 mg, 100 mg

▷ **Usual Adult Dosage Range:** Initially, 50 to 75 mg/day in 3 or 4 divided doses; dose may be increased gradually in 3 to 4 days to 100 mg/day as needed and tolerated. For maintenance: mild psychosis—5 to 15 mg, 3 or 4 times/day; moderate psychosis—10 to 25 mg, 3 or 4 times/day; severe psychosis—up to 225 mg/day, in 3 or 4 divided doses. The total daily dosage should not exceed 225 mg. **Note: Actual dosage and administration schedule must be determined by the physician for each patient individually.**

▷ **Dosing Instructions:**   Take with food or milk to reduce stomach irritation. The liquid concentrate may be diluted with water, milk, fruit juice or carbonated beverages. The tablet may be crushed for administration.

Usual Duration of Use: Continual use on a regular schedule for 3 to 6 weeks is usually necessary to determine this drug's effectiveness in controlling the features of schizophrenia. Long-term use (months to years) requires supervision and periodic evaluation by your physician.

▷ **This Drug Should Not Be Taken If**
   • you have had an allergic reaction to it previously.
   • you have acute alcoholic intoxication.

▷ **Inform Your Physician Before Taking This Drug If**
   • you are taking any drugs that have sedative effects.
   • you use alcohol excessively.
   • you have any type of seizure disorder.
   • you have any type of glaucoma.
   • you have Parkinson's disease or an enlarged prostate gland.
   • you have impaired liver or kidney function.
   • you have a history of breast cancer.

Possible Side-Effects   (natural, expected and unavoidable drug actions)
   Drowsiness, dry mouth, nasal congestion, constipation, impaired urination.
   Parkinson-like reactions (see Glossary).

▷ **Possible Adverse Effects**   (unusual, unexpected and infrequent reactions)
   If any of the following develop, consult your physician promptly.
   Mild Adverse Effects
   Allergic Reactions: Skin rash.
   Headache, dizziness, blurred vision, lethargy, unsteadiness, insomnia, depression, euphoria, ringing in ears.
   Rapid heartbeat, low blood pressure, fainting.
   Loss of appetite, indigestion, nausea.
   Breast engorgement, milk production, altered menstrual patterns, increased libido.
   Serious Adverse Effects
   Allergic Reactions: Liver reaction with jaundice.
   Spasms of face and neck muscles, abnormal involuntary movements of extremities, severe restlessness.
   Development of tardive dyskinesias (see Glossary).
   Neuroleptic malignant syndrome: high fever, fast heart rate, difficult breathing, severe muscle rigidity, loss of bladder control, seizures.

▷ **Adverse Effects That May Mimic Natural Diseases or Disorders**
   Parkinson-like reactions may be mistaken for naturally occurring Parkinson's disease.
   Liver reactions may suggest viral hepatitis.

CAUTION
1. This drug may alter the pattern of epileptic seizures and require dosage adjustments of anticonvulsant drugs.
2. Obtain prompt evaluation of any change or disturbance of vision.
3. There is a very narrow margin between the effective therapeutic dose and the dose that can cause Parkinson-like reactions. Inform your physician promptly if suggestive symptoms develop.

Precautions for Use

By Infants and Children: Safety and effectiveness for use by those under 12 years of age have not been established.

By Those over 60 Years of Age: Start treatment with small doses. This drug can aggravate an existing prostatism (see Glossary). You may be more susceptible to the development of Parkinson-like reactions or tardive dyskinesia. Report any suggestive symptoms promptly.

▷ **Advisability of Use During Pregnancy**

Pregnancy Category: B (tentative). See Pregnancy Code inside back cover.

Animal studies: No birth defects reported in mice, rats or rabbits.

Human studies: Information from adequate studies of pregnant women is not available.

Because of its inherent toxicity for brain tissue, avoid use during pregnancy if possible.

Advisability of Use if Breast-Feeding

Presence of this drug in breast milk: Unknown.

Avoid drug or refrain from nursing.

Habit-Forming Potential: None.

Effects of Overdosage: Marked drowsiness, weakness, tremor, agitation, impaired stance and gait, stupor progressing to coma, possible seizures.

Possible Effects of Long-Term Use: Development of tardive dyskinesias.

Suggested Periodic Examinations While Taking This Drug   (at physician's discretion)

Complete blood cell counts, liver function tests.

▷ **While Taking This Drug, Observe the Following**

Foods: No restrictions.

Beverages: No restrictions. May be taken with milk.

▷   *Alcohol*: Avoid completely. Alcohol can increase the sedative action of this drug and enhance its depressant effects on brain function. Also, this drug can increase the intoxicating effects of alcohol.

Tobacco Smoking: No interactions expected.

▷   *Other Drugs*

Molindone may *increase* the effects of

- all drugs containing atropine or having atropinelike effects (see Drug Class, Section Four).
- all drugs with sedative effects, and cause excessive sedation.

Molindone *taken concurrently* with
- antiepileptic drugs (anticonvulsants) may require close monitoring for changes in seizure patterns and need for dosage adjustments.

▷ *Driving, Hazardous Activities*: This drug may cause dizziness and drowsiness. Restrict activities as necessary.

Aviation Note: The use of this drug *is a disqualification* for piloting. Consult a designated Aviation Medical Examiner.

Exposure to Sun: No restrictions.

Exposure to Heat: Use caution and avoid excessive heat as much as possible. This drug may impair the regulation of body temperature and increase the risk of heat stroke.

Discontinuation: Do not stop taking this drug suddenly after long-term use. Ask your physician for guidance regarding gradual dosage reduction and withdrawal.

NADOLOL
(nay DOH lohl)

Introduced: 1976

Class: Antianginal, Antihypertensive, Beta-Adrenergic Blocker

Prescription: USA: Yes
Canada: Yes

Controlled Drug: USA: No
Canada: No

Available as Generic: No

Brand Names: Corgard, Corzide [CD]

BENEFITS versus RISKS	
Possible Benefits	*Possible Risks*
EFFECTIVE, WELL-TOLERATED ANTIHYPERTENSIVE in mild to moderate high blood pressure EFFECTIVE ANTIANGINAL DRUG IN CLASSICAL CORONARY ARTERY DISEASE with moderate to severe angina	CONGESTIVE HEART FAILURE in advanced heart disease Provocation of asthma (in predisposed individuals) Masking of hypoglycemia in drug-dependent diabetes Worsening of angina following abrupt withdrawal

▷ **Principal Uses**

As a Single Drug Product: This "beta-blocker" drug is used primarily to (1) treat moderately high blood pressure, and (2) contribute to the management of coronary artery disease by preventing attacks of effort-induced angina. (This drug is contraindicated in Prinzmetal's vasospastic angina.)

As a Combination Drug Product [CD]: This drug is available in combination with bendroflumethiazide, a mild diuretic "step 1" antihypertensive drug. This combination product is more effective and more convenient for long-term use.

How This Drug Works: By blocking certain actions of the sympathetic nervous system, this drug

- reduces the rate and contraction force of the heart, thus lowering the oxygen requirement of the heart muscle and reducing the ejection pressure of the blood leaving the heart; these actions reduce the frequency of angina and lower blood pressure.
- reduces the degree of contraction of blood vessel walls, resulting in their relaxation and expansion and consequent lowering of blood pressure.
- prolongs the conduction time of nerve impulses through the heart, of benefit in the management of certain heart rhythm disorders.

Available Dosage Forms and Strengths
Tablets — 40 mg, 80 mg, 120 mg, 160 mg

▷ **Usual Adult Dosage Range:**   For hypertension: Initially, 40 mg daily in one dose; this may be increased gradually as needed and tolerated, up to 640 mg/24 hours. The usual maintenance dose is 80 to 320 mg/24 hours. The total daily dosage should not exceed 640 mg. For angina: Initially, 40 mg daily in one dose; increase gradually at intervals of 3 to 7 days up to 240 mg/24 hours. The usual maintenance dose is 80 to 240 mg/24 hours. The total daily dose should not exceed 240 mg. **Note: Actual dosage and administration schedule must be determined by the physician for each patient individually.**

▷ **Dosing Instructions:**   May be taken without regard to eating. The tablet may be crushed for administration. Do not discontinue this drug abruptly.

Usual Duration of Use: Continual use on a regular schedule for 10 to 14 days is usually necessary to determine this drug's effectiveness in lowering blood pressure and preventing effort-induced angina. The long-term use of this drug (months to years) will be determined by the course of your blood pressure and angina over time and your response to the overall treatment program (weight reduction, salt restriction, smoking cessation, etc.).

▷ **This Drug Should Not Be Taken If**
- you have had an allergic reaction to it previously.
- you have congestive heart failure.
- you have an abnormally slow heart rate or a serious form of heart block.
- you are subject to bronchial asthma.
- you are presently experiencing seasonal hay fever.
- you are taking, or have taken within the past 14 days, any monoamine oxidase (MAO) inhibitor drug (see Drug Class, Section Four).

▷ **Inform Your Physician Before Taking This Drug If**
- you have had an adverse reaction to any "beta-blocker" drug in the past (see Drug Class, Section Four).

- you have a history of serious heart disease, with or without episodes of heart failure.
- you have a history of hay fever (allergic rhinitis), asthma, chronic bronchitis or emphysema.
- you have a history of overactive thyroid function (hyperthyroidism).
- you have a history of low blood sugar (hypoglycemia).
- you have impaired liver or kidney function.
- you have diabetes or myasthenia gravis.
- you are currently taking any form of digitalis, quinidine or reserpine, or any "calcium-blocker" drug (see Drug Class, Section Four).
- you plan to have surgery under general anesthesia in the near future.

Possible Side-Effects (natural, expected and unavoidable drug actions)
Lethargy and fatigability, cold extremities, slow heart rate, light-headedness in upright position (see orthostatic hypotension in Glossary).

▷ **Possible Adverse Effects** (unusual, unexpected and infrequent reactions)
If any of the following develop, consult your physician promptly.
Mild Adverse Effects
Allergic Reactions: Skin rash, itching, drug fever.
Headache, dizziness, insomnia, vivid dreaming, visual disturbances, ringing in ears, slurred speech.
Indigestion, nausea, vomiting, diarrhea, abdominal pain.
Numbness and tingling of extremities.
Serious Adverse Effects
Allergic Reactions: Facial swelling.
Chest pain, shortness of breath, precipitation of congestive heart failure.
Intensification of heart block.
Induction of bronchial asthma (in asthmatic individuals).
Masking of warning indications of acute hypoglycemia in drug-treated diabetes.
Decreased libido, sexual impotence (rare).

▷ **Adverse Effects That May Mimic Natural Diseases or Disorders**
Impaired circulation to the extremities may resemble Raynaud's phenomenon.

Natural Diseases or Disorders That May Be Activated by This Drug
Bronchial asthma, Prinzmetal's variant (vasospastic) angina, latent Raynaud's disease, myasthenia gravis (questionable).

CAUTION
1. *Do not discontinue this drug suddenly* without the knowledge and guidance of your physician. Carry a notation on your person that you are taking this drug.
2. Consult your physician or pharmacist before using nasal decongestants usually present in over-the-counter cold preparations and nose drops. These can cause sudden increases in blood pressure when taken concurrently with beta-blocker drugs.
3. Report the development of any tendency to emotional depression.

Precautions for Use

By Infants and Children: Safety and effectiveness for use by those under 12 years of age have not been established. However, if this drug is used, observe for the development of low blood sugar (hypoglycemia) during periods of reduced food intake.

By Those over 60 Years of Age: Proceed *cautiously* with all antihypertensive drugs. Unacceptably high blood pressure should be reduced without creating the risks associated with excessively low blood pressure. Start treatment with small doses, and monitor the blood pressure response frequently. Sudden, rapid and excessive reduction of blood pressure can predispose to stroke or heart attack. Observe for dizziness, unsteadiness, tendency to fall, confusion, hallucinations, depression or urinary frequency.

▷ **Advisability of Use During Pregnancy**

Pregnancy Category: C (tentative). See Pregnancy Code inside back cover.

Animal studies: No significant increase in birth defects due to this drug, but embryotoxicity reported in rabbits.

Human studies: Information from adequate studies of pregnant women is not available.

Avoid use during the first 3 months if possible. Use this drug only if clearly needed. Ask physician for guidance.

Advisability of Use if Breast-Feeding

Presence of this drug in breast milk: Yes, in large amounts.

Avoid drug or refrain from nursing.

Habit-Forming Potential: None.

Effects of Overdosage: Weakness, slow pulse, low blood pressure, fainting, cold and sweaty skin, congestive heart failure, possible coma and convulsions.

Possible Effects of Long-Term Use: Reduced heart reserve and eventual heart failure in susceptible individuals with advanced heart disease.

Suggested Periodic Examinations While Taking This Drug   (at physician's discretion)

Measurements of blood pressure, evaluation of heart function.

▷ **While Taking This Drug, Observe the Following**

Foods: No restrictions. Avoid excessive salt intake.

Beverages: No restrictions. May be taken with milk.

▷   *Alcohol*: Use with caution until the combined effect has been determined. Alcohol may exaggerate this drug's ability to lower blood pressure and may increase its mild sedative effect.

Tobacco Smoking: Nicotine may reduce this drug's effectiveness in treating high blood pressure and angina. In addition, high doses of this drug may potentiate the constriction of the bronchial tubes caused by regular smoking.

▷   *Other Drugs*
Nadolol may *increase* the effects of
- other antihypertensive drugs, and cause excessive lowering of blood pressure. Dosage adjustments may be necessary.
- reserpine (Ser-Ap-Es, etc.), and cause sedation, depression, slowing of the heart rate and lowering of blood pressure.
- verapamil (Calan, Isoptin), and cause excessive depression of heart function; monitor this combination closely.

Nadolol may *decrease* the effects of
- theophyllines (Aminophyllin, Theo-Dur, etc.), and reduce their effectiveness in treating asthma.

Nadolol *taken concurrently* with
- clonidine (Catapres) requires close monitoring for rebound high blood pressure if clonidine is withdrawn while nadolol is still being taken.
- insulin requires close monitoring to avoid undetected hypoglycemia (see Glossary).

The following drugs may *decrease* the effects of nadolol
- indomethacin (Indocin), and possibly other "aspirin substitutes," may impair nadolol's antihypertensive effect.

▷   *Driving, Hazardous Activities*: Use caution until the full extent of drowsiness, lethargy and blood pressure change has been determined.

Aviation Note: The use of this drug *is a disqualification* for piloting. Consult a designated Aviation Medical Examiner.

Exposure to Sun: No restrictions.

Exposure to Heat: Caution advised. Hot environments can lower the blood pressure and exaggerate the effects of this drug.

Exposure to Cold: Caution advised. Cold environments can enhance the circulatory deficiency in the extremities that may occur with this drug. The elderly should take precautions to prevent hypothermia (see Glossary).

Heavy Exercise or Exertion: It is advisable to avoid exertion that produces light-headedness, excessive fatigue or muscle cramping. The use of this drug may intensify the hypertensive response to isometric exercise.

Occurrence of Unrelated Illness: The fever that accompanies systemic infections can lower the blood pressure and require adjustment of dosage. Illnesses that cause nausea or vomiting may interrupt the regular dosage schedule. Ask your physician for guidance.

Discontinuation: It is advisable to avoid sudden discontinuation of this drug in all situations. If possible, gradual reduction of dose over a period of 2 to 3 weeks is recommended. Ask your physician for specific guidance.

NAPROXEN
(na PROX en)

Introduced: 1974

Class: Mild Analgesic, Anti-inflammatory

Prescription: USA: Yes
Canada: Yes

Controlled Drug: USA: No
Canada: No

Available as Generic: No

Brand Names: Anaprox, ✚Apo-Naproxen, Naprosyn, ✚Naxen, ✚Novonaprox

---

BENEFITS versus RISKS

Possible Benefits	*Possible Risks*
EFFECTIVE RELIEF OF MILD TO MODERATE PAIN AND INFLAMMATION	Gastrointestinal pain, ulceration, bleeding (rare)
	Drug-induced hepatitis with jaundice (rare)
	Rare kidney damage
	Mild fluid retention
	Reduced white blood cell and platelet counts

▷ **Principal Uses**

As a Single Drug Product: Used primarily to relieve mild to moderately severe pain associated with (1) musculoskeletal injuries; (2) acute and chronic gout, rheumatoid arthritis and osteoarthritis; (3) dental, obstetrical and orthopedic surgery; and (4) menstrual cramps. It is also used to prevent and relieve migrainelike headaches.

How This Drug Works: Not completely established. It is thought that this drug reduces the tissue concentrations of prostaglandins (and related compounds), chemicals involved in the production of inflammation and pain.

Available Dosage Forms and Strengths

Tablets — 250 mg, 275 mg, 375 mg, 500 mg

▷ **Usual Adult Dosage Range**

As analgesic: initially, 500 mg; then 250 mg every 6 to 8 hours as needed.

As antiarthritic: 250, 375 or 500 mg twice/day, 12 hours apart.

As antigout: initially, 750 mg; then 250 mg/8 hrs until acute attack is relieved.

For menstrual pain: initially, 500 mg; then 250 mg every 6 to 8 hours as needed.

The total daily dosage should not exceed 1250 mg.

Note: Actual dosage and administration schedule must be determined by the physician for each patient individually.

▷ **Dosing Instructions:** Take either on an empty stomach or with food or milk to prevent stomach irritation. Take with a full glass of water and remain upright (do not lie down) for 30 minutes. The tablet may be crushed for administration.

Usual Duration of Use: Continual use on a regular schedule for 1 to 2 weeks is usually necessary to determine this drug's effectiveness in relieving the discomfort of arthritis. Long-term use requires supervision and periodic evaluation by the physician.

▷ **This Drug Should Not Be Taken If**
- you have had an allergic reaction to it previously.
- you are subject to asthma or nasal polyps caused by aspirin.
- you have active peptic ulcer disease or any form of gastrointestinal bleeding.
- you have a bleeding disorder or a blood cell disorder.
- you have active liver disease.
- you have severe impairment of kidney function.

▷ **Inform Your Physician Before Taking This Drug If**
- you are allergic to aspirin or to other aspirin substitutes.
- you have a history of peptic ulcer disease or any type of bleeding disorder.
- you have impaired liver or kidney function.
- you have high blood pressure or a history of heart failure.
- you are taking any of the following: acetaminophen, aspirin or other aspirin substitutes, anticoagulants, oral antidiabetic drugs.

Possible Side-Effects   (natural, expected and unavoidable drug actions)
Fluid retention (weight gain), prolongation of bleeding time.

▷ **Possible Adverse Effects**   (unusual, unexpected and infrequent reactions)
If any of the following develop, consult your physician promptly.
Mild Adverse Effects
Allergic Reactions: Skin rash, hives, itching, localized swellings, spontaneous bruising.
Headache, dizziness, altered or blurred vision, ringing in the ears, drowsiness, fatigue, inability to concentrate.
Mouth sores, indigestion, nausea, vomiting, abdominal pain, diarrhea.
Serious Adverse Effects
Active peptic ulcer, stomach or intestinal bleeding, diverticulitis.
Liver damage with jaundice (see Glossary).
Kidney damage with painful urination, bloody urine, reduced urine formation.
Visual disturbances due to corneal changes, lens opacities, retinal changes.
Impaired hearing.
Reduction of white blood cell and/or platelet counts.

Possible Delayed Adverse Effects
Mild anemia due to "silent" blood loss from the stomach (less than that caused by aspirin).

▷ **Adverse Effects That May Mimic Natural Diseases or Disorders**
Liver reaction may suggest viral hepatitis.

Natural Diseases or Disorders That May Be Activated by This Drug
Peptic ulcer disease, ulcerative colitis.

CAUTION
1. Dosage should always be limited to the smallest amount that produces reasonable improvement.
2. This drug may mask early indications of infection. Inform your physician if you think you are developing an infection of any kind.

Precautions for Use
By Infants and Children: Indications and dosage recommendations for use by those under 12 years of age have not been established.
By Those over 60 Years of Age: Small doses are advisable until tolerance is determined. Observe for any indications of liver or kidney toxicity, fluid retention, dizziness, confusion, impaired memory, stomach bleeding or constipation.

▷ **Advisability of Use During Pregnancy**
Pregnancy Category: B (tentative). See Pregnancy Code inside back cover.
Animal studies: No birth defects reported in mice, rats or rabbits.
Human studies: Information from adequate studies of pregnant women is not available.
Avoid this drug during the last 3 months. Use it during the first 6 months only if clearly needed. Ask physician for guidance.

Advisability of Use if Breast-Feeding
Presence of this drug in breast milk: Yes, in minute amounts.
Avoid drug or refrain from nursing.

Habit-Forming Potential: None.

Effects of Overdosage: Possible drowsiness, dizziness, ringing in the ears, nausea, vomiting, indigestion.

Possible Effects of Long-Term Use: Eye changes such as opacities in the cornea or lens, retinal changes in the macular area. Kidney damage.

Suggested Periodic Examinations While Taking This Drug   (at physician's discretion)
Complete blood cell counts, liver and kidney function tests.
Complete eye examinations if vision is altered in any way.
Hearing examinations if ringing in the ears or hearing loss develops.

▷ **While Taking This Drug, Observe the Following**
Foods: No restrictions.
Beverages: No restrictions. May be taken with milk.
▷ *Alcohol*: Use with caution. The irritant action of alcohol on the stomach lining, added to the irritant action of this drug in sensitive individuals, can increase the risk of stomach ulceration and/or bleeding.
Tobacco Smoking: No interactions expected.

▷   *Other Drugs*

Naproxen may *increase* the effects of

- acetaminophen (Tylenol, etc.), and increase the risk of kidney damage; avoid prolonged use of this combination.
- anticoagulants (Coumadin, etc.), and increase the risk of bleeding; monitor prothrombin time and adjust dose accordingly.

Naproxen *taken concurrently* with the following drugs may increase the risk of bleeding; avoid these combinations:

- aspirin.
- dipyridamole (Persantine).
- indomethacin (Indocin).
- sulfinpyrazone (Anturane).
- valproic acid (Depakene).

▷   *Driving, Hazardous Activities*: This drug may cause drowsiness or dizziness. Restrict activities as necessary.

Aviation Note: The use of this drug *may be a disqualification* for piloting. Consult a designated Aviation Medical Examiner.

Exposure to Sun: No restrictions.

NIFEDIPINE
(ni FED i peen)

Introduced: 1972

Class: Antianginal, Calcium Channel Blocker

Prescription: USA: Yes
Canada: Yes

Controlled Drug: USA: No
Canada: No

Available as Generic: No

Brand Names: Adalat, Procardia

BENEFITS versus RISKS	
Possible Benefits	*Possible Risks*
EFFECTIVE PREVENTION OF BOTH MAJOR TYPES OF ANGINA	Rare increase in angina upon starting treatment
	Rare precipitation of congestive heart failure
	Very rare drug-induced hepatitis

▷ **Principal Uses**

As a Single Drug Product: Used primarily to treat (1) angina pectoris due to coronary artery spasm (Prinzmetal's variant angina) that occurs spontaneously and is not associated with exertion; and (2) classical angina-of-effort (due to atherosclerotic disease of the coronary arteries) in individuals who have not responded to or cannot tolerate the nitrates and "beta-blocker" drugs customarily used to treat this disorder.

How This Drug Works: Not completely established. It is thought that by blocking the normal passage of calcium through certain cell walls (which is necessary for the function of nerve and muscle tissue), this drug slows the spread of electrical activity through the conduction system of the heart and inhibits the contraction of coronary arteries and peripheral arterioles. As a result of these combined effects, this drug

- prevents spontaneous spasm of the coronary arteries (Prinzmetal's type of angina).
- reduces the rate and contraction force of the heart during exertion, thus lowering the oxygen requirement of the heart muscle; this reduces the occurrence of effort-induced angina (classical angina pectoris).
- reduces the degree of contraction of peripheral arterial walls, resulting in their relaxation and consequent lowering of blood pressure. This further reduces the workload of the heart during exertion and contributes to the prevention of angina.

Available Dosage Forms and Strengths
Capsules — 10 mg

▷ **Usual Adult Dosage Range:**   Initially, 10 mg 3 times daily. Dose may be increased gradually at 7- to 14-day intervals (as needed and tolerated) up to 30 mg 3 or 4 times/day. The usual maintenance dose is 10 to 20 mg 3 times/day. The total daily dosage should not exceed 180 mg. **Note: Actual dosage and administration schedule must be determined by the physician for each patient individually.**

▷ **Dosing Instructions:**   May be taken with or following food to reduce stomach irritation. The capsule should be swallowed whole (not altered).

Usual Duration of Use: Continual use on a regular schedule for 2 to 4 weeks is usually necessary to determine this drug's effectiveness in reducing the frequency and severity of angina. For long-term use (months to years), determine the smallest effective dose. Supervision and periodic evaluation by your physician are essential.

▷ **This Drug Should Not Be Taken If**
- you have had an allergic reaction to it previously.
- you have active liver disease.
- you have low blood pressure—systolic pressure below 90.

▷ **Inform Your Physician Before Taking This Drug If**
- you have had an unfavorable response to any "calcium blocker" drug in the past.
- you are currently taking any form of digitalis or a "beta-blocker" drug (see Drug Class, Section Four).
- you are taking any drugs that lower blood pressure.
- you have a history of congestive heart failure, heart attack or stroke.
- you are subject to disturbances of heart rhythm.
- you have impaired liver or kidney function.
- you have diabetes.
- you have a history of drug-induced liver damage.

Possible Side-Effects   (natural, expected and unavoidable drug actions)
Low blood pressure, rapid heart rate, swelling of the feet and ankles (7%), flushing and sensation of warmth (25%), sweating.

▷ **Possible Adverse Effects**   (unusual, unexpected and infrequent reactions)
If any of the following develop, consult your physician promptly.
Mild Adverse Effects
Allergic Reactions: Skin rash, hives, itching, fever.
Headache (23%), dizziness (27%), weakness (12%), nervousness (7%), blurred vision.
Palpitation (7%), shortness of breath, wheezing (6%), cough.
Heartburn (11%), nausea, cramps, diarrhea (2%).
Tremors, muscle cramps (8%).
Serious Adverse Effects
Allergic Reactions: Drug-induced hepatitis (very rare).
Idiosyncratic Reactions: Joint stiffness and inflammation.
Increased frequency or severity of angina on initiation of treatment or following an increase in dose.
Marked drop in blood pressure with fainting.
Impaired sexual function.

▷ **Adverse Effects That May Mimic Natural Diseases or Disorders**
An allergic rash and swelling of the legs may resemble erysipelas.
Drug-induced hepatitis may suggest viral hepatitis.

CAUTION
1. Be sure to inform all physicians and dentists you consult that you are taking this drug. Note the use of this drug on your card of personal identification.
2. You may use nitroglycerin and other nitrate drugs as needed to relieve acute episodes of angina pain. However, if you detect that your angina attacks are becoming more frequent or intense, notify your physician promptly.

Precautions for Use
By Infants and Children: Safety and effectiveness for use by those under 12 years of age have not been established.
By Those over 60 Years of Age: You may be more susceptible to the development of weakness, dizziness, fainting and falling. Take necessary precautions to prevent injury. Report promptly any changes in your pattern of thirst and urination.

▷ **Advisability of Use During Pregnancy**
Pregnancy Category: C (tentative). See Pregnancy Code inside back cover.
Animal studies: Embryo and fetal deaths reported in mice, rats and rabbits; birth defects reported in rats.
Human studies: Information from adequate studies of pregnant women is not available.
Avoid this drug during the first 3 months. Use during the last 6 months only if clearly needed. Ask physician for guidance.

Advisability of Use if Breast-Feeding
Presence of this drug in breast milk: Unknown.
Avoid drug or refrain from nursing.

Habit-Forming Potential: None.

Effects of Overdosage: Weakness, light-headedness, fainting, fast pulse, low
blood pressure, shortness of breath, flushed and warm skin, tremors.

Possible Effects of Long-Term Use: None reported.

Suggested Periodic Examinations While Taking This Drug   (at physician's
discretion)
Evaluations of heart function, including electrocardiograms; measurements of blood pressure in supine, sitting and standing positions.

▷ **While Taking This Drug, Observe the Following**
Foods: No restrictions. Avoid excessive salt intake.
Beverages: No restrictions. May be taken with milk.
▷ *Alcohol*: Use with caution until combined effects have been determined.
Alcohol may exaggerate the drop in blood pressure experienced by some
individuals.
Tobacco Smoking: Nicotine may reduce the effectiveness of this drug. Follow
your physician's advice regarding smoking.
Marijuana Smoking: Possible reduced effectiveness of this drug; mild to
moderate increase in angina; possible changes in electrocardiogram,
confusing interpretation.
▷ *Other Drugs*
Nifedipine *taken concurrently* with
• "beta-blocker" drugs or digitalis preparations (see Drug Classes, Section
Four) may affect heart rate and rhythm adversely. Careful monitoring by
your physician is necessary if these drugs are taken concurrently.
The following drugs may *increase* the effects of nifedipine
• cimetidine (Tagamet).
▷ *Driving, Hazardous Activities*: Usually no restrictions. This drug may cause
drowsiness or dizziness. Restrict activities as necessary.
Aviation Note: Coronary artery disease *is a disqualification* for piloting. Consult a designated Aviation Medical Examiner.
Exposure to Sun: No restrictions.
Exposure to Heat: Caution advised. Hot environments can exaggerate the
blood-pressure-lowering effects of this drug. Observe for light-headedness or weakness.
Heavy Exercise or Exertion: This drug may improve your ability to be more
active without resulting angina pain. Use caution and avoid excessive
exercise that could impair heart function in the absence of warning pain.
Discontinuation: Do not discontinue this drug abruptly. Consult your physician regarding gradual withdrawal. Observe for the possible development of rebound angina.

NITROFURANTOIN
(ni troh fyur AN toin)

Introduced: 1953

Prescription: USA: Yes
Canada: Yes

Available as Generic: Yes

Class: Urinary Anti-infective

Controlled Drug: USA: No
Canada: No

Brand Names: ♣Apo-Nitrofurantoin, Furadantin, Furalan, Furantoin, Macrodantin, ♣Nephronex, ♣Novofuran

---

BENEFITS versus RISKS

Possible Benefits	*Possible Risks*
EFFECTIVE TREATMENT OF SOME URINARY TRACT INFECTIONS	ALLERGIC REACTIONS: Anaphylaxis Rashes, hives Repetitive asthma Lung inflammation Drug-induced hepatitis Peripheral neuropathy (see Glossary) Blood cell disorders: Hemolytic anemia (see Glossary) Reduced white blood cell count Superinfections

---

▷ **Principal Uses**

As a Single Drug Product: Because this drug is concentrated in the urine and attains only low levels in the blood, its use is limited to the prevention or treatment of infections in the urinary tract.

How This Drug Works: Not completely established. It is thought that by interfering with some bacterial enzyme systems, this drug is bacteriostatic (growth retarding) in low to moderate concentrations and bactericidal (killing) in high concentrations.

Available Dosage Forms and Strengths

Capsules — 25 mg, 50 mg, 100 mg
Oral suspension — 25 mg per 5 ml teaspoonful
Tablets — 50 mg, 100 mg

▷ **Usual Adult Dosage Range:** For treatment of active infections: 50 to 100 mg/6 hrs. For prevention: 50 to 100 mg once/day at bedtime. The total daily dosage should not exceed 600 mg. **Note: Actual dosage and administration schedule must be determined by the physician for each patient individually.**

▷ **Dosing Instructions:** Preferably taken with or following food to facilitate absorption and reduce stomach irritation. The tablet may be crushed and the capsule opened for administration, but this drug can stain the teeth yellow on contact.

Usual Duration of Use: Continual use on a regular schedule for 7 to 10 days is usually necessary to determine this drug's effectiveness in curing urinary tract infections. Long-term use for prevention (months to years) requires supervision and periodic evaluation by your physician.

▷ **This Drug Should Not Be Taken If**
  • you have had an allergic reaction to it previously.
  • you have severely impaired kidney function.
  • you have active liver disease.
  • you are in the last month of pregnancy.

▷ **Inform Your Physician Before Taking This Drug If**
  • you are allergic to any nitrofuran drug.
  • you have impaired liver or kidney function.
  • you have a deficiency of glucose-6-phosphate dehydrogenase in your red blood cells.
  • you have chronic anemia or diabetes.

Possible Side-Effects   (natural, expected and unavoidable drug actions)
  Superinfections (see Glossary) in the urinary tract.
  Brown discoloration of the urine, of no significance.

▷ **Possible Adverse Effects**   (unusual, unexpected and infrequent reactions)
  If any of the following develop, consult your physician promptly.
  Mild Adverse Effects
  Allergic Reactions: Skin rashes, hives, localized swellings, itching, fever.
  Headache, dizziness, drowsiness, burning and tearing of eyes, impaired color vision, muscle aching, loss of hair.
  Loss of appetite, nausea, vomiting, diarrhea, abdominal cramping.
  Serious Adverse Effects
  Allergic Reactions: Anaphylaxis (see Glossary), interstitial pneumonitis (lung inflammation), asthma, hepatitis.
  Idiosyncratic Reactions: Hemolytic anemia (see Glossary).
  Peripheral neuropathy (see Glossary).
  Blood cell disorders: reduced red and white blood cell counts.

▷ **Adverse Effects That May Mimic Natural Diseases or Disorders**
  Allergic pneumonitis may suggest an infectious pneumonia.
  Allergic hepatitis may suggest viral hepatitis.

Natural Diseases or Disorders That May Be Activated by This Drug
  Latent asthma.

CAUTION
  Troublesome and persistent diarrhea can develop in sensitive individuals. If diarrhea persists for more than 24 hours, discontinue this drug and consult your physician.

Precautions for Use
  By Infants and Children: This drug should not be used in infants under 1

month of age. Observe closely for the possible development of increased intracranial pressure.

By Those over 60 Years of Age: Dosage must be carefully individualized on the basis of kidney function. This age group is more susceptible to skin rashes, nausea, vomiting and constipation.

▷ **Advisability of Use During Pregnancy**

Pregnancy Category: C (tentative). See Pregnancy Code inside back cover.

Animal studies: No information available.

Human studies: No significant increase in birth defects reported in 590 exposures. Information from adequate studies of pregnant women is not available.

Avoid use of drug during the last few weeks of pregnancy. Use otherwise only if clearly needed. Ask your physician for guidance.

Advisability of Use if Breast-Feeding

Presence of this drug in breast milk: Yes, in small amounts.

Avoid drug or refrain from nursing.

Habit-Forming Potential: None.

Effects of Overdosage: Nausea, vomiting, diarrhea.

Possible Effects of Long-Term Use: Allergic reactions in lungs or liver, peripheral neuropathy, superinfections within the urinary tract.

Suggested Periodic Examinations While Taking This Drug   (at physician's discretion)

Complete blood cell counts, liver function tests, X-ray examinations of lungs during long-term use.

▷ **While Taking This Drug, Observe the Following**

Foods: No restrictions. Eat liberally of the following foods: beef, chicken, lamb and pork liver, asparagus, navy beans (good sources of folic acid).

Beverages: No restrictions. May be taken with milk.

▷ *Alcohol*: Use with extreme caution until the combined effects have been determined. This drug, in combination with alcohol, may cause a disulfiramlike reaction (see Glossary) in sensitive individuals.

Tobacco Smoking: No interactions expected.

▷ *Other Drugs*

The following drugs may *decrease* the effects of nitrofurantoin

• antacids that contain magnesium can prevent the absorption of nitrofurantoin and reduce its effectiveness.

▷ *Driving, Hazardous Activities*: This drug may cause dizziness. Restrict activities as necessary.

Aviation Note: The use of this drug *may be a disqualification* for piloting. Consult a designated Aviation Medical Examiner.

Exposure to Sun: No restrictions.

NITROGLYCERIN
(ni troh GLIS er in)

Introduced: 1847

Prescription: USA: Yes
Canada: No

Class: Antianginal, Nitrates

Controlled Drug: USA: No
Canada: No

Available as Generic: Yes

Brand Names: Nitro-Bid, Nitrodisc, Nitro-Dur, Nitrogard, ♣Nitrogard-SR, Nitroglyn, Nitrol, Nitrolingual Spray, Nitrong, ♣Nitrostabilin, Nitrostat, Transderm-Nitro, ♣Tridil

---

BENEFITS versus RISKS

Possible Benefits	*Possible Risks*
EFFECTIVE RELIEF AND PREVENTION OF ANGINA EFFECTIVE ADJUNCTIVE TREATMENT IN SELECTED CASES OF CONGESTIVE HEART FAILURE	Orthostatic hypotension (see Glossary) with and without fainting Skin rash (rare) Altered hemoglobin with large doses (very rare)

▷ **Principal Uses**

As a Single Drug Product: Used primarily in the treatment of symptomatic coronary artery disease. The rapid-action forms are used to relieve acute attacks of anginal pain at their onset. The sustained-action forms are used to prevent the development of angina.

How This Drug Works: By direct action on the muscles in blood vessel walls, this drug relaxes and dilates both arteries and veins. Its beneficial effects in the management of angina are due to two mechanisms of action: (1) dilation of narrowed coronary arteries; (2) dilation of veins in the general circulation, with consequent reduction of the volume and pressure of blood entering the heart. The net effects are improved blood supply to the heart muscle and reduced workload for the heart. Both actions reduce the frequency and severity of angina.

Available Dosage Forms and Strengths

Canisters, sublingual spray — 13.8 grams (200 doses)
Capsules, prolonged action — 2.5 mg, 6.5 mg, 9 mg
Ointment — 2%
Tablets, buccal — 1 mg, 2 mg, 3 mg
Tablets, prolonged action — 2.6 mg, 6.5 mg, 9 mg
Tablets, sublingual — 0.15 mg, 0.3 mg, 0.4 mg, 0.6 mg
Transdermal systems — 2.5 mg, 5 mg, 7.5 mg, 10 mg, 15 mg

▷ **Usual Adult Dosage Range:** According to dosage form:

Sublingual spray—1 metered spray (0.4 mg) under tongue/3 to 5 minutes, up to 3 doses within 15 minutes, to relieve acute angina. To prevent angina, 1 spray taken 5 to 10 minutes before exertion.

Sublingual tablets—0.15 to 0.6 mg dissolved under tongue at 5-minute intervals to relieve acute angina.

Prolonged action tablets—1.3 to 6.5 mg at 8- to 12-hour intervals to prevent angina.

Prolonged action capsules—2.5 to 9 mg at 8- to 12-hour intervals to prevent angina.

Ointment—2.5 to 5 cm (1 to 2 inches, 15 to 30 mg) applied in a thin, even layer of uniform size to hairless skin at 3- to 4-hour intervals to prevent angina.

Buccal tablets—1 to 2 mg/4 to 5 hours placed between cheek and gum.

Transdermal patches—5 sq cm to 30 sq cm patch applied to hairless skin once/24 hrs to prevent angina.

Note: Actual dosage and administration schedule must be determined by the physician for each patient individually.

▷ **Dosing Instructions:** Dosage forms to be swallowed are best taken when stomach is empty (1 hour before or 2 hours after eating) to obtain maximal blood levels. Tablets should not be crushed for administration. Capsules may be opened, but the contents should not be crushed or chewed before swallowing.

Usual Duration of Use: Continual use on a regular schedule for 3 to 5 days is usually necessary to determine this drug's effectiveness in preventing and relieving acute anginal attacks. Individual dosage adjustments will be necessary for optimal results. Long-term use (months to years) requires supervision and periodic evaluation by your physician.

▷ **This Drug Should Not Be Taken If**
  • you have had an allergic reaction to it previously.
  • you are severely anemic.
  • you have closed-angle glaucoma (inadequately treated).

▷ **Inform Your Physician Before Taking This Drug If**
  • you have had an unfavorable response to other nitrate drugs in the past.
  • you have low blood pressure.
  • you have any form of glaucoma.

Possible Side-Effects (natural, expected and unavoidable drug actions)
  Flushing of face, headaches (50%), orthostatic hypotension (see Glossary), rapid heart rate, palpitation.

▷ **Possible Adverse Effects** (unusual, unexpected and infrequent reactions)
  If any of the following develop, consult your physician promptly.
  Mild Adverse Effects
  Allergic Reactions: Skin rash.
  Throbbing headaches (may be severe and persistent), dizziness, fainting.
  Nausea, vomiting.
  Serious Adverse Effects
  Allergic Reactions: Severe skin reactions with peeling.
  Idiosyncratic Reactions: Methemoglobinemia (very rare).

▷ **Adverse Effects That May Mimic Natural Diseases or Disorders**
Hypotensive spells (sudden drops in blood pressure) due to this drug may be mistaken for late-onset epilepsy.

CAUTION
1. This drug can provoke migraine headaches in susceptible individuals.
2. In the presence of impaired brain circulation (cerebral arteriosclerosis), this drug can cause transient ischemic attacks—periods of temporary speech impairment, paralysis, numbness, etc.
3. The development of tolerance to long-acting forms of nitrates will render the sublingual tablets ineffective for the relief of acute angina. Sensitivity to the drug's antianginal effect is restored after one week of abstinence from the long-acting forms.
4. Many over-the-counter (OTC) drug products for allergies, colds and coughs contain drugs that may counteract the desired effects of this drug. Ask your physician or pharmacist for guidance before using any such medications.

Precautions for Use
By Infants and Children: Limited usefulness and experience in this age group. Dosage schedules not established.
By Those over 60 Years of Age: Begin treatment with small doses and increase dose cautiously as needed and tolerated. You may be more susceptible to the development of flushing, throbbing headache, dizziness, "blackout" spells, fainting and falling.

▷ **Advisability of Use During Pregnancy**
Pregnancy Category: C (tentative). See Pregnancy Code inside back cover.
Animal studies: No information available.
Human studies: Information from adequate studies of pregnant women is not available.
Use this drug only if clearly needed. Ask physician for guidance.

Advisability of Use if Breast-Feeding
Presence of this drug in breast milk: Unknown.
Monitor nursing infant closely and discontinue drug or nursing if adverse effects develop.

Habit-Forming Potential: None.

Effects of Overdosage: Throbbing headache, dizziness, marked flushing, nausea, vomiting, abdominal cramps, confusion, delirium, paralysis, seizures, circulatory collapse.

Possible Effects of Long-Term Use: The development of tolerance (see Glossary) and the temporary loss of effectiveness.

Suggested Periodic Examinations While Taking This Drug   (at physician's discretion)
Measurements of blood pressure and internal eye pressures.
Evaluation of hemoglobin.

▷ **While Taking This Drug, Observe the Following**

Foods: No restrictions.

Beverages: No restrictions. May be taken with milk.

▷ *Alcohol*: Use extreme caution until the combined effects have been determined. Avoid alcohol completely in the presence of any side-effects or adverse effects from nitroglycerin. Never use alcohol in the presence of a nitroglycerin headache.

Tobacco Smoking: Nicotine can reduce the effectiveness of this drug. Follow your physician's advice regarding smoking.

Marijuana Smoking: Possible reduced effectiveness of this drug; mild to moderate increase in angina; possible changes in the electrocardiogram, confusing interpretation.

▷ *Other Drugs*

Nitroglycerin *taken concurrently* with

- antihypertensive drugs may cause excessive lowering of blood pressure. Careful dosage adjustments may be necessary.

The following drugs may *increase* the effects of nitroglycerin

- aspirin, in analgesic doses (500 mg or more).

▷ *Driving, Hazardous Activities*: Usually no restrictions. This drug may cause dizziness or faintness. Restrict activities as necessary.

Aviation Note: Coronary artery disease *is a disqualification* for piloting. Consult a designated Aviation Medical Examiner.

Exposure to Sun: No restrictions.

Exposure to Heat: Use caution. Hot environments can cause significant lowering of blood pressure.

Exposure to Cold: Cold environments can increase the need for this drug and limit its effectiveness.

Heavy Exercise or Exertion: This drug can increase your tolerance for exercise. Use good judgment regarding excessive exertion in the absence of anginal pain.

Discontinuation: Do not stop this drug abruptly after long-term use. It is advisable to reduce the dose (of the prolonged-action dosage forms) gradually over a period of 4 to 6 weeks. Observe for rebound angina.

Special Storage Instructions: For sublingual tablets, to prevent loss of strength

- keep tablets in the original glass container.
- do not transfer tablets to a plastic or metallic container (such as a pillbox).
- do not place absorbent cotton, paper (such as the prescription label), or other material inside the container.
- do not store other drugs in the same container.
- close the container tightly immediately after each use.
- store at room temperature.

ORAL CONTRACEPTIVES
(or al kon tra SEP tivs)

Other Names: Estrogens/Progestins

Introduced: 1956

Class: Female Sex Hormones

Prescription: USA: Yes
Canada: Yes

Controlled Drug: USA: No
Canada: No

Available as Generic: USA: No
Canada: No

Brand Names: Brevicon, Demulen, Enovid, Enovid-E, Loestrin, Lo/Ovral, Micronor*, Modicon, Nordette, Norinyl, Norinyl 2, Norlestrin, Nor-Q.D.*, Ortho-Novum, Ortho-Novum 2, Ovcon, Ovral, Ovrette*, Ovulen, Tri-Norinyl, Triphasil

---

BENEFITS versus RISKS

Possible Benefits	*Possible Risks*
HIGHLY EFFECTIVE FOR CONTRACEPTIVE PROTECTION	SERIOUS, LIFE-THREATENING THROMBOEMBOLIC DISORDERS in susceptible individuals
Moderately effective as adjunctive treatment in management of excessive menses and endometriosis	Hypertension
	Fluid retention
	Intensification of migrainelike headaches
	Intensification of fibrocystic breast changes
	Accelerated growth of uterine fibroid tumors
	Drug-induced hepatitis with jaundice
	Benign liver tumors (rare)

▷ **Principal Uses**

As a Single Drug Product: The "Mini-Pill" contains only one component—a progestin. This has been shown to be slightly less effective than the combination of estrogen and progestin in preventing pregnancy.

As a Combination Drug Product [CD]: Most oral contraceptives consist of a combination of a type of estrogen and a type of progestin. These products are the most effective form of contraception available. While used primarily to prevent pregnancy, they are sometimes used to treat menstrual irregularity, excessively heavy menstrual flow and endometriosis.

How This Drug Works: When the combination of an estrogen and a progestin is taken in sufficient dosage and on a regular basis, the blood and tissue

---

*"Mini-Pill" type, contains progestin only.

levels of these hormones increase to resemble those that occur during pregnancy. This results in suppression of the two pituitary gland hormones that normally produce ovulation (the formation and release of an egg by the ovary). In addition, these drugs may (1) alter the cervical mucus so that it resists the passage of sperm, and (2) alter the lining of the uterus so that it resists implantation of the egg (if ovulation occurs).

Available Dosage Forms and Strengths

Tablets — several combinations of synthetic estrogens and progestins in varying strengths; see the package label of the brand prescribed.

▷ **Usual Adult Dosage Range:** Initiate treatment with the first tablet on the fifth day after the onset of menstruation. Follow with 1 tablet daily (taken at the same time each day) for 21 consecutive days. Resume treatment on the eighth day following the last tablet taken during the preceding cycle. The schedule is to take the drug daily for 3 weeks and to omit it for 1 week. For the Mini-Pill (progestin only), initiate treatment on the first day of menstruation and take 1 tablet daily, every day, throughout the year (no interruption). **Note: Actual dosage and administration schedule must be determined by the physician for each patient individually.**

▷ **Dosing Instructions:** May be taken with or after food to reduce stomach irritation. To ensure regular (every day) use and uniform blood levels, it is advisable to take the tablet at the same time daily. The tablets may be crushed for administration.

Usual Duration of Use: According to individual needs and circumstances. Long-term use (months to years) requires supervision and periodic evaluation by your physician every 6 months.

▷ **This Drug Should Not Be Taken If**
- you have had a significant allergic reaction to any dosage form of it previously.
- you have a history of thrombophlebitis, embolism, heart attack or stroke.
- you have breast cancer.
- you have active liver disease, seriously impaired liver function or a history of liver tumor.
- you have abnormal and unexplained vaginal bleeding.
- you have sickle cell disease.
- you are pregnant.

▷ **Inform Your Physician Before Taking This Drug If**
- you have had an unfavorable reaction to any oral contraceptive previously.
- you have a history of cancer of the breast or reproductive organs.
- you have any of the following conditions: fibrocystic breast changes, fibroid tumors of the uterus, endometriosis, migrainelike headaches, epilepsy, asthma, heart disease, high blood pressure, gallbladder disease, diabetes or porphyria.

- you smoke tobacco on a regular basis.
- you plan to have surgery in the near future.

Possible Side-Effects   (natural, expected and unavoidable drug actions)
Fluid retention, weight gain, "breakthrough" bleeding (spotting in middle of menstrual cycle), altered menstrual pattern, lack of menstruation (during and following cessation of drug), increased susceptibility to yeast infection of the genital tissues.

▷ **Possible Adverse Effects**   (unusual, unexpected and infrequent reactions)
If any of the following develop, consult your physician promptly.
Mild Adverse Effects
Allergic Reactions: Skin rash, hives, itching.
Headache, nervous tension, irritability, accentuation of migraine headaches.
Nausea, vomiting, bloating, diarrhea.
Breast enlargement, tenderness, milk production.
Tannish pigmentation of the face.
Reduced tolerance to contact lenses.
Impaired color vision: blue tinge to objects, blue halo around lights.
Serious Adverse Effects
Allergic Reactions: Erythema multiforme and nodosum (skin reactions), loss of scalp hair.
Idiosyncratic Reactions: Joint and muscle pains.
Emotional depression, rise in blood pressure (in susceptible individuals).
Eye changes: optic neuritis, retinal thrombosis, altered curvature of the cornea, cataracts.
Gallbladder disease, benign liver tumors, jaundice, rise in blood sugar.
Erosion of uterine cervix, enlargement of uterine fibroid tumors, cystitis-like syndrome.
Thrombophlebitis (inflammation of a vein with formation of blood clot)—pain or tenderness in thigh or leg, with or without swelling of foot or leg.
Pulmonary embolism (movement of blood clot to lung)—sudden shortness of breath, pain in chest, coughing, bloody sputum.
Stroke (blood clot in brain)—headaches, blackout, sudden weakness or paralysis of any part of the body, severe dizziness, altered vision, slurred speech, inability to speak.
Heart attack (blood clot in coronary artery)—sudden pain in chest, neck, jaw or arm; weakness; sweating; nausea.
Mesenteric thrombosis—blood clot in abdominal artery.

Possible Delayed Adverse Effects
Estrogens taken during pregnancy can predispose the female child to the later development of cancer of the vagina or cervix following puberty.

▷ **Adverse Effects That May Mimic Natural Diseases or Disorders**
Liver reactions may suggest viral hepatitis.

Natural Diseases or Disorders That May Be Activated by This Drug
Latent hypertension, diabetes mellitus, acute intermittent porphyria, lupus erythematosuslike syndrome.

CAUTION
1. The incidence of serious adverse effects due to the use of these drugs is very low. However, any unusual development should be reported and evaluated promptly.
2. Studies indicate that women over 30 years of age who smoke and use oral contraceptives are at significantly greater risk of having a serious cardiovascular event than are nonusers.
3. The risk of thromboembolism increases with the amount of estrogen in the product and with the age of the user. Low-estrogen combinations are advised.
4. It is advisable to discontinue these drugs 1 month prior to elective surgery to reduce the risk of postsurgical thromboembolism.
5. Investigate promptly any alteration or disturbance of vision that occurs during the use of these drugs.
6. Investigate promptly the nature of recurrent, persistent or severe headaches that develop while taking these drugs.
7. Observe for significant change of mood. Discontinue this drug if depression develops.
8. Certain commonly used drugs may reduce the effectiveness of oral contraceptives. Some of these are listed in the category of *Other Drugs*.
9. Diarrhea lasting more than a few hours (and occurring during the days the drug is taken) can prevent adequate absorption of these drugs and impair their effectiveness as contraceptives.
10. If 2 consecutive menstrual periods are missed, consult your physician regarding the advisability of performing a pregnancy test. Do not continue to use these drugs until your pregnancy status is determined.

▷ **Advisability of Use During Pregnancy**
Pregnancy Category: X. See Pregnancy Code inside back cover.
Animal studies: Genital defects reported in mice and guinea pigs; cleft palate reported in rodents.
Human studies: Information from studies of pregnant women indicates that estrogens can masculinize the female fetus. In addition, limb defects and heart malformations have been reported.
It is now known that estrogens taken during pregnancy can predispose the female child to the development of cancer of the vagina or cervix following puberty.
Avoid these drugs completely during entire pregnancy.

Advisability of Use if Breast-Feeding
Presence of these drugs in breast milk: Yes, in minute amounts.
These drugs may suppress milk formation if started early following delivery.

Breast-feeding is considered to be safe during the use of oral contraceptives.

Habit-Forming Potential: None.

Effects of Overdosage: Headache, drowsiness, nausea, vomiting, fluid retention, abnormal vaginal bleeding, breast enlargement and discomfort.

Possible Effects of Long-Term Use: High blood pressure, gallbladder disease with stones, accelerated growth of uterine fibroid tumors, absent menstruation and impaired fertility after discontinuation of drug.

Suggested Periodic Examinations While Taking This Drug (at physician's discretion)

Regular (every 6 months) evaluation of the breasts and pelvic organs, including Pap smears. Liver function tests as indicated.

▷ **While Taking This Drug, Observe the Following**

Foods: Avoid excessive use of salt if fluid retention occurs.

Beverages: No restrictions. May be taken with milk.

▷   *Alcohol*: No interactions expected.

Tobacco Smoking: Recent studies indicate that heavy smoking (15 or more cigarettes daily) in association with the use of oral contraceptives significantly increases the risk of heart attack (coronary thrombosis). Heavy smoking should be considered a contraindication to the use of oral contraceptives.

▷   *Other Drugs*

Oral contraceptives may *increase* the effects of

- some benzodiazepines, and cause excessive sedation.
- metoprolol (Lopressor), and cause excessive beta-blocker effects.
- prednisolone and prednisone, and cause excessive cortisonelike effects.
- theophyllines, and increase the risk of toxic effects.

Oral contraceptives *taken concurrently* with

- antidiabetic drugs may cause unpredictable fluctuations of blood sugar.
- tricyclic antidepressants (Elavil, Sinequan, etc.) may enhance their adverse effects and reduce their antidepressant effectiveness.
- troleandomycin (TAO) may increase the incidence of liver toxicity and jaundice.
- warfarin (Coumadin) may cause unpredictable alterations of prothrombin activity.

The following drugs may *decrease* the effects of oral contraceptives (and impair their effectiveness)

- barbiturates (phenobarbital, etc.; see Drug Class, Section Four).
- carbamazepine (Tegretol).
- griseofulvin (Fulvicin, etc.).
- penicillins (ampicillin, penicillin V).
- phenytoin (Dilantin).
- primidone (Mysoline).

- rifampin (Rifadin, Rimactane).
- tetracyclines (see Drug Class, Section Four).

▷ *Driving, Hazardous Activities*: Usually no restrictions. Consult your physician for assessment of individual risk and for guidance regarding specific restrictions.

Aviation Note: Usually no restrictions. However, it is advisable to observe for the rare occurrence of disturbed vision and to restrict activities accordingly. Consult a designated Aviation Medical Examiner.

Exposure to Sun: Use caution until full effect is known. These drugs can cause photosensitivity (see Glossary).

Discontinuation: Do not discontinue this drug if "breakthrough" bleeding occurs. If spotting or bleeding continues, consult your physician. A preparation with a higher estrogen content may be required. Remember: Omitting this drug for only 1 day may allow pregnancy to occur. It is advisable to avoid pregnancy for 3 to 6 months after discontinuing these drugs; aborted fetuses from women who became pregnant within 6 months after discontinuation reveal significantly increased chromosome abnormalities.

OXAZEPAM
(ox AZ e pam)

Introduced: 1965

Prescription: USA: Yes
Canada: Yes

Available as Generic: USA: No
Canada: Yes

Class: Mild Tranquilizer, Benzodiazepines

Controlled Drug: USA: C-IV*
Canada: No

Brand Names: ♣Apo-Oxazepam, ♣Oxpam, Serax, ♣Zapex

BENEFITS versus RISKS	
Possible Benefits	*Possible Risks*
RELIEF OF ANXIETY AND NERVOUS TENSION in 70% to 80% of users	Habit-forming potential with prolonged use
Wide margin of safety with therapeutic doses	Minor impairment of mental functions
Very few drug interactions	Very rare jaundice
	Very rare blood cell disorders

▷ **Principal Uses**

As a Single Drug Product: Used primarily to (1) provide short-term relief of mild to moderate anxiety; (2) relieve the symptoms of acute alcohol

*See Schedules of Controlled Drugs inside back cover.

withdrawal: agitation, tremors, hallucinations, incipient delirium tremens.

How This Drug Works: It is thought that this drug produces a calming effect by enhancing the action of the nerve transmitter gamma-aminobutyric acid (GABA), which in turn blocks the arousal of higher brain centers.

Available Dosage Forms and Strengths
Capsules — 10 mg, 15 mg, 30 mg
Tablets — 15 mg

▷ **Usual Adult Dosage Range:**   30 to 120 mg/24 hours, in 3 or 4 divided doses. The total daily dosage should not exceed 180 mg. **Note: Actual dosage and administration schedule must be determined by the physician for each patient individually.**

▷ **Dosing Instructions:**   May be taken on empty stomach or with food or milk as needed to prevent stomach irritation. The tablet may be crushed and the capsule may be opened for administration. Do not discontinue this drug abruptly if taken for more than 4 weeks.

Usual Duration of Use: Continual use on a regular schedule for 3 to 5 days is usually necessary to determine this drug's effectiveness in relieving moderate anxiety. Limit continual use to 1 to 3 weeks. Avoid uninterrupted and prolonged use.

▷ **This Drug Should Not Be Taken If**
  • you have had an allergic reaction to any dosage form of it previously.
  • you have acute narrow-angle glaucoma.
  • it is prescribed for a child under 6 years of age.

▷ **Inform Your Physician Before Taking This Drug If**
  • you are allergic to any benzodiazepine drug (see Drug Class, Section Four).
  • you have a history of alcoholism or drug abuse.
  • you are pregnant or planning pregnancy.
  • you have impaired liver or kidney function.
  • you have a history of serious depression or mental disorder.
  • you have any of the following: asthma, emphysema, epilepsy, myasthenia gravis.
  • you are taking any drugs with sedative effects.

Possible Side-Effects   (natural, expected and unavoidable drug actions)
Drowsiness, lethargy, unsteadiness, "hangover" effects on the day following bedtime use.

▷ **Possible Adverse Effects**   (unusual, unexpected and infrequent reactions)
  If any of the following develop, consult your physician promptly.
  Mild Adverse Effects
  Allergic Reactions: Skin rashes, hives.

Dizziness, fainting, blurred vision, double vision, slurred speech, sweating, nausea, menstrual irregularity.

Serious Adverse Effects

Allergic Reactions: Liver reaction with jaundice (see Glossary).

Abnormally low white blood cells: fever, sore throat, infections.

Paradoxical responses of excitement, agitation, anger, rage.

▷ **Adverse Effects That May Mimic Natural Diseases or Disorders**

Liver reaction with jaundice may suggest viral hepatitis.

CAUTION

1. This drug should not be discontinued abruptly if it has been taken continually for more than 4 weeks.
2. The concurrent use of some over-the-counter drug products that contain antihistamines (allergy and cold preparations, sleep aids) can cause excessive sedation in sensitive individuals.

Precautions for Use

By Infants and Children: Safety and effectiveness for use by those under 6 years of age have not been established. This drug should not be used in the hyperactive or psychotic child of any age. Observe for excessive sedation and incoordination.

By Those over 60 Years of Age: It is advisable to use smaller doses at longer intervals to avoid overdosage. Observe for the possible development of lethargy, indifference, fatigue, weakness, unsteadiness, disturbing dreams, nightmares and paradoxical reactions of excitement, agitation, anger, hostility and rage.

▷ **Advisability of Use During Pregnancy**

Pregnancy Category: C (tentative). See Pregnancy Code inside back cover.

Animal studies: No birth defects found in mice, rats or rabbits.

Human studies: Information from adequate studies of pregnant women is not available. No birth defects have been reported with the use of this drug. However, available information regarding the use of other drugs of this class (benzodiazepines) is conflicting and inconclusive. Some studies found an increase in serious birth defects associated with the use of 2 benzodiazepines. Other studies have found no significant increase in birth defects.

Frequent use in late pregnancy can cause the "floppy infant" syndrome in the newborn: weakness, lethargy, unresponsiveness, depressed breathing, low body temperature. Avoid use during entire pregnancy if possible.

Advisability of Use if Breast-Feeding

Presence of this drug in breast milk: Yes.

Avoid drug or refrain from nursing.

Habit-Forming Potential: This drug can produce psychological and/or physical dependence (see Glossary) if used in large doses for an extended period of time.

Effects of Overdosage: Marked drowsiness, weakness, feeling of drunkenness, staggering gait, tremor, stupor progressing to deep sleep or coma.

Possible Effects of Long-Term Use: Psychological and/or physical dependence, rare blood cell disorders.

Suggested Periodic Examinations While Taking This Drug   (at physician's discretion)
Complete blood cell counts during long-term use.
Liver function tests.

▷ **While Taking This Drug, Observe the Following**
Foods: No restrictions.
Beverages: Avoid excessive intake of caffeine-containing beverages: coffee, tea, cola. May be taken with milk.
▷   *Alcohol*: Use with extreme caution until the combined effect is determined. Alcohol may increase the depressant effects of this drug on the brain. It is advisable to avoid alcohol completely—throughout the day and night—if it is necessary to drive or to engage in any hazardous activity.
Tobacco Smoking: Heavy smoking may reduce the calming action of this drug.
Marijuana Smoking: Increased sedation and significant impairment of intellectual and physical performance.
▷   *Other Drugs*
Oxazepam may *increase* the effects of
• digoxin (Lanoxin), and cause digoxin toxicity.
• phenytoin (Dilantin), and cause phenytoin toxicity.
Oxazepam may *decrease* the effects of
• levodopa (Sinemet, etc.), and reduce its effectiveness in treating Parkinson's disease.
The following drugs may *decrease* the effects of oxazepam
• oral contraceptives.
• theophylline (aminophylline, Theo-Dur, etc.).
▷   *Driving, Hazardous Activities*: This drug can impair mental alertness, judgment, physical coordination and reaction time. Avoid hazardous activities accordingly.
Aviation Note: The use of this drug *is a disqualification* for piloting. Consult a designated Aviation Medical Examiner.
Exposure to Sun: No restrictions.
Exposure to Heat: Use caution until the effect of excessive perspiration is determined. Because of reduced urine volume, this drug may accumulate in the body and produce effects of overdosage.

Discontinuation: Avoid sudden discontinuation if this drug has been taken for over 4 weeks without interruption. Dosage should be tapered gradually to prevent a withdrawal syndrome that could include depression, confusion, hallucinations, tremor, seizures, muscle cramping, sweating and vomiting.

OXYCODONE ✖
(ox ee KOH dohn)

Introduced: 1950

Prescription: USA: Yes
Canada: Yes

Available as Generic: USA: Yes
Canada: No

Class: Analgesic, Narcotic

Controlled Drug: USA: C-II*
Canada: <N>

Brand Names: ♣Oxycocet [CD], ♣Oxycodan [CD], Percocet✗ [CD], ♣Percocet-Demi [CD], Percodan [CD], Percodan-Demi [CD], ♣Supeudol, Tylox [CD]

BENEFITS versus RISKS	
Possible Benefits	*Possible Risks*
EFFECTIVE RELIEF OF MODERATE TO SEVERE PAIN	POTENTIAL FOR HABIT FORMATION (DEPENDENCE) Sedative effects Mild allergic reactions (infrequent) Nausea, constipation

▷ **Principal Uses**

As a Single Drug Product: Used primarily in tablet and suppository form (Canada) to relieve moderate to severe pain.

As a Combination Drug Product [CD]: Oxycodone is available in combinations with acetaminophen and with aspirin. These milder pain relievers are added to enhance the analgesic effect and to reduce fever when present.

How This Drug Works: Acting primarily as a depressant of certain brain functions, this drug suppresses the perception of pain and calms the emotional response to pain.

Available Dosage Forms and Strengths

Solution — 5 mg per 5 ml teaspoonful
Suppositories — 10 mg, 20 mg (Canada)
Tablets — 5 mg, 10 mg (Canada)
Tablets — 2.44 mg, 4.88 mg (in combination drugs)

*See Schedules of Controlled Drugs inside back cover.

▷ **Usual Adult Dosage Range:**   5 mg/3 to 6 hours as needed. May be increased to 10 mg/4 hours if needed for severe pain. The total daily dosage should not exceed 60 mg. **Note: Actual dosage and administration schedule must be determined by the physician for each patient individually.**

▷ **Dosing Instructions:**   May be taken with or following food to reduce stomach irritation or nausea. The tablet may be crushed for administration.

Usual Duration of Use: As required to control pain. Continual use should not exceed 5 to 7 days without interruption and reassessment of need.

▷ **This Drug Should Not Be Taken If**
- you have had an allergic reaction to any dosage form of it previously.
- you are having an acute attack of asthma.

▷ **Inform Your Physician Before Taking This Drug If**
- you have had an unfavorable reaction to any narcotic drug in the past.
- you have a history of drug abuse or alcoholism.
- you have chronic lung disease with impaired breathing.
- you have impaired liver or kidney function.
- you have gallbladder disease, a seizure disorder or an underactive thyroid gland.
- you have difficulty emptying the urinary bladder.
- you are taking any other drugs that have a sedative effect.
- you plan to have surgery under general anesthesia in the near future.

Possible Side-Effects   (natural, expected and unavoidable drug actions)
Drowsiness, light-headedness, dry mouth, urinary retention, constipation.

▷ **Possible Adverse Effects**   (unusual, unexpected and infrequent reactions)
If any of the following develop, consult your physician promptly.
Mild Adverse Effects
Allergic Reactions: Skin rash, hives, itching.
Idiosyncratic Reactions: Skin rash and itching when combined with dairy products (milk or cheese).
Dizziness, impaired concentration, sensation of drunkenness, confusion, depression, blurred or double vision.
Nausea, vomiting.
Serious Adverse Effects
Impaired breathing: use with caution in chronic lung disease.

CAUTION
1. If you have asthma, chronic bronchitis or emphysema, the excessive use of this drug may cause significant respiratory difficulty, thickening of bronchial secretions and suppression of coughing.
2. The concurrent use of this drug with atropinelike drugs can increase the risk of urinary retention and reduced intestinal function.
3. Do not take this drug following acute head injury.

Precautions for Use
By Infants and Children: Do not use this drug in children under 2 years of age because of their vulnerability to life-threatening respiratory depression.

By Those over 60 Years of Age: Use small doses initially and increase dosage as needed and tolerated. Limit use to short-term treatment only. There may be increased susceptibility to the development of drowsiness, dizziness, unsteadiness, falling, urinary retention and constipation (often leading to fecal impaction).

▷ **Advisability of Use During Pregnancy**
Pregnancy Category: C (tentative). See Pregnancy Code inside back cover.
Animal studies: No information available.
Human studies: Information from adequate studies of pregnant women is not available. Oxycodone taken repeatedly during the last few weeks before delivery may cause withdrawal symptoms in the newborn infant.
Use this drug only if clearly needed and in small, infrequent doses.

Advisability of Use if Breast-Feeding
Presence of this drug in breast milk: Unknown.
Avoid drug or refrain from nursing.

Habit-Forming Potential: Psychological and/or physical dependence can develop with use of large doses for an extended period of time.

Effects of Overdosage: Drowsiness, restlessness, agitation, nausea, vomiting, dry mouth, vertigo, weakness, lethargy, stupor, coma, seizures.

Possible Effects of Long-Term Use: Psychological and physical dependence, chronic constipation.

Suggested Periodic Examinations While Taking This Drug (at physician's discretion)
None.

▷ **While Taking This Drug, Observe the Following**
Foods: No restrictions.
Beverages: No restrictions. May be taken with milk.
▷ *Alcohol*: Use extreme caution until the combined effects have been determined. Oxycodone can intensify the intoxicating effects of alcohol, and alcohol can intensify the depressant effects of oxycodone on brain function, breathing and circulation.
Tobacco Smoking: No interactions expected.
Marijuana Smoking: Increase in drowsiness and pain relief; impairment of mental and physical performance.
▷ *Other Drugs*
Oxycodone may *increase* the effects of
• other drugs with sedative effects.
• atropinelike drugs, and increase the risk of constipation and urinary retention.
▷ *Driving, Hazardous Activities*: This drug can impair mental alertness, judgment, reaction time and physical coordination. Avoid hazardous activities accordingly.
Aviation Note: The use of this drug *is a disqualification* for piloting. Consult a designated Aviation Medical Examiner.

Exposure to Sun: No restrictions.

Discontinuation: It is advisable to limit this drug to short-term use. If it is necessary to use it for extended periods of time, discontinuation should be gradual to minimize possible effects of withdrawal.

OXYMETAZOLINE
(ox ee met AZ oh leen)

Introduced: 1964

Class: Decongestant

Prescription: USA: No
Canada: No

Controlled Drug: USA: No
Canada: No

Available as Generic: USA: Yes
Canada: No

Brand Names: Afrin, Dristan Long Lasting, Duration, 4-Way Long Acting Nasal Spray, ♣Nafrine, Neo-Synephrine 12 Hour, ♣Oculclear, Sinex Long Lasting

---

BENEFITS versus RISKS

Possible Benefits	*Possible Risks*
EFFECTIVE, LONG-LASTING DECONGESTION OF NASAL AND SINUS TISSUES EFFECTIVE DECONGESTION OF INFLAMED EYES	"REBOUND" CONGESTION WITH EXCESSIVE USE Mild irritation of ocular or nasal tissues Systemic effects (via absorption with excessive use): nervousness, insomnia, hypertension

---

▷ **Principal Uses**

As a Single Drug Product: Used primarily as a decongestant nose drop or spray to relieve swelling and congestion of the nasal membranes due to colds or allergy. It is also used as an eye drop to relieve inflammation and swelling of the conjunctival membranes ("red eyes") due to allergy or chemical irritation.

How This Drug Works: By contracting the walls of arterioles and thus reducing their size, this drug decreases the volume of blood in the tissues, resulting in shrinkage of tissue mass (decongestion). This expands the nasal airway and enlarges the openings into the sinuses and eustachian tubes. The same action on the conjunctival vessels in the eye results in clearing of the capillary congestion (redness) and swelling.

Available Dosage Forms and Strengths

Drops, eye — 0.025%
Drops, nose — 0.05%

Drops, pediatric — 0.025%
Spray, nose — 0.05%

▷ **Usual Adult Dosage Range:**   Eye drops: 1 or 2 drops in affected eye/6 to 8 hours. Nose drops and spray: 2 or 3 drops or sprays into each nostril twice/day, morning and evening, 12 hours apart. For long-term use, consult your physician.

▷ **Dosing Instructions:**   Do not exceed the recommended doses. The nasal spray is more effective than the drops and is less likely to cause systemic absorption.

Usual Duration of Use: Continual use on a regular schedule for 3 to 5 days is usually necessary to determine this drug's effectiveness in relieving eye and nasal congestion. If there is no significant improvement after 1 week of use, consult your physician for further evaluation.

▷ **This Drug Should Not Be Taken If**
- you have had an allergic reaction to it previously.
- for the eye drops: you have untreated narrow-angle glaucoma or an active eye infection.

▷ **Inform Your Physician Before Taking This Drug If**
- you have high blood pressure or heart disease.
- you have diabetes or an overactive thyroid gland (hyperthyroidism).
- you are taking any beta-blocker drug (see Drug Class, Section Four).
- you are taking, or have taken within the past 14 days, any monoamine oxidase (MAO) inhibitor drug (see Drug Class, Section Four).

Possible Side-Effects   (natural, expected and unavoidable drug actions)
Dryness or irritation of the nose, nervousness, insomnia.

▷ **Possible Adverse Effects**   (unusual, unexpected and infrequent reactions)
  If any of the following develop, consult your physician promptly.
  Mild Adverse Effects
  Headache, light-headedness, burning or stinging of the nose, heart palpitation, tremors.
  Serious Adverse Effects
  None reported.

CAUTION
1. Too frequent use, or extended use, of nose drops or sprays containing this drug may cause a secondary rebound congestion resulting in a form of functional dependence (see Glossary).
2. Many over-the-counter drug products for allergies, colds and coughs contain drugs that may interact unfavorably with this drug. Ask your physician or pharmacist for guidance before using such medications.

Precautions for Use
  By Infants and Children: Children may be especially susceptible to systemic absorption of this drug. Avoid excessive use.

By Those over 60 Years of Age: Use small doses until your tolerance has been determined. Observe for possible nervousness, insomnia or palpitation.

▷ **Advisability of Use During Pregnancy**
   Pregnancy Category: C (tentative). See Pregnancy Code inside back cover.
   Animal studies: No information available.
   Human studies: Information from adequate studies of pregnant women is not available.
   Limit use to small, infrequent doses.

Advisability of Use if Breast-Feeding
   Presence of this drug in breast milk: Unknown.
   Monitor nursing infant closely and discontinue drug or nursing if adverse effects develop.

Habit-Forming Potential: Frequent or excessive use may cause functional dependence (see Glossary).

Effects of Overdosage: Headache, restlessness, anxiety, agitation, palpitation, sweating.

Possible Effects of Long-Term Use: Secondary rebound congestion and chemical irritation of nasal tissues.

Suggested Periodic Examinations While Taking This Drug   (at physician's discretion)
   None required.

▷ **While Taking This Drug, Observe the Following**
   Foods: No restrictions.
   Beverages: Heavy use of coffee or tea may add to the nervousness or insomnia experienced by sensitive individuals.
▷ *Alcohol*: No interactions expected.
   Tobacco Smoking: No interactions expected.
▷ *Other Drugs*
   Oxymetazoline **taken concurrently** with
   • beta-blocker drugs or monoamine oxidase (MAO) inhibitor drugs may cause dangerous elevations of blood pressure. Observe for headache or palpitation.
▷ *Driving, Hazardous Activities*: No restrictions.
   Aviation Note: The use of this drug **may be a disqualification** for piloting. Consult a designated Aviation Medical Examiner.
   Exposure to Sun: No restrictions.

PENICILLIN V ✗
(pen i SIL in VEE)

Introduced: 1953

Prescription: USA: Yes
Canada: Yes

Available as Generic: USA: Yes
Canada: Yes

Class: Antibiotic, Penicillins

Controlled Drug: USA: No
Canada: No

Brand Names: ♣Apo-Penicillin VK, Betapen-VK, Ledercillin VK, ♣Nadopen-V, ♣Novopen-VK, Penapar VK, ♣Pen-Vee, Pen-Vee K, Pfizerpen VK, ♣PVF, ♣PVF K, Repen-VK, Robicillin VK, SK-Penicillin VK, Uticillin VK, V-Cillin K, ♣VC-K 500, Veetids

---

BENEFITS versus RISKS

Possible Benefits	*Possible Risks*
EFFECTIVE TREATMENT OF INFECTIONS due to susceptible microorganisms	ALLERGIC REACTIONS, mild to severe, in 3% of the general population and 15% of allergic individuals
	Superinfections (yeast)
	Drug-induced colitis

▷ **Principal Uses**

As a Single Drug Product: This type of penicillin is used primarily to treat responsive infections of the upper and lower respiratory tract, the middle ear and the skin. Equally important uses are the prevention of rheumatic fever and the prevention of bacterial endocarditis in individuals with valvular heart disease.

How This Drug Works: This drug destroys susceptible infecting bacteria by interfering with their ability to produce new protective cell walls as they multiply and grow.

Available Dosage Forms and Strengths

Oral solution — 125 mg per 5 ml, 250 mg per 5-ml teaspoonful
Tablets — 125 mg, 250 mg, 500 mg

▷ **Usual Adult Dosage Range:** Dosage is based upon the results of sensitivity testing of the causative organism, the severity of the infection and the response of the patient. Depending upon the specific infection, the dosage range is 125 to 500 mg/6 to 8 hours. For the prevention of bacterial endocarditis: 2 grams (2000 mg) taken 30 to 60 minutes before the procedure, followed by 500 mg/6 hours for 8 doses. The total daily dosage should not exceed 7 grams (7000 mg). **Note: Actual dosage and administration schedule must be determined by the physician for each patient individually.**

▷ **Dosing Instructions:**   May be taken on an empty stomach or with food or milk. Absorption may be slightly faster if taken when stomach is empty. The tablet may be crushed for administration.

Usual Duration of Use: For all streptococcal infections—not less than 10 consecutive days (without interruption) to reduce the possibility of developing rheumatic fever or glomerulonephritis. For all other infections—as long as necessary to eradicate the infection.

▷ **This Drug Should Not Be Taken If**
   • you have had an allergic reaction to any dosage form of it previously.
   • you are certain you are allergic to *any* form of penicillin.

▷ **Inform Your Physician Before Taking This Drug If**
   • you suspect you may be allergic to penicillin or you have a history of a previous "reaction" of any type to penicillin.
   • you are allergic to any cephalosporin antibiotic (Ancef, Anspor, Ceclor, Ceporan, Ceporex, Kafocin, Keflex, Keflin, Kefzol, Loridine, Ultracef, Velosef; see Drug Class, Section Four).
   • you are allergic by nature (hay fever, asthma, hives, eczema).

Possible Side-Effects   (natural, expected and unavoidable drug actions)
Superinfections (see Glossary), often due to yeast organisms.

▷ **Possible Adverse Effects**   (unusual, unexpected and infrequent reactions)
If any of the following develop, consult your physician promptly.
Mild Adverse Effects
Allergic Reactions: Skin rashes, hives, itching.
Irritations of mouth and tongue, "black tongue," nausea, vomiting, mild diarrhea, dizziness (rare).
Serious Adverse Effects
Allergic Reactions: Anaphylactic reaction (see Glossary), severe skin reactions, drug fever, swollen painful joints, sore throat, abnormal bleeding or bruising.
Drug-induced colitis.

CAUTION
   1.   Take the exact dose and the full course prescribed.
   2.   This drug should not be used concurrently with antibiotics like erythromycin or tetracycline.

Precautions for Use
By Infants and Children: Observe the allergic child closely for evidence of a developing allergy to penicillin. This drug may cause diarrhea, which sometimes necessitates discontinuation.
By Those over 60 Years of Age: Natural changes in the skin may predispose to prolonged itching reactions in the genital and anal regions. Report such reactions promptly.

▷ **Advisability of Use During Pregnancy**
Pregnancy Category: B (tentative). See Pregnancy Code inside back cover.

Animal studies: Birth defects of the limbs reported in mice. (Not confirmed in other studies.)

Human studies: Information from adequate studies of pregnant women indicates no increased risk of birth defects in 3546 pregnancies exposed to penicillin derivatives.

This drug is considered safe for use during any period of pregnancy.

Advisability of Use if Breast-Feeding
Presence of this drug in breast milk: Yes.

The nursing infant may be sensitized to penicillin. Avoid drug if possible or refrain from nursing.

Habit-Forming Potential: None.

Effects of Overdosage: Possible nausea, vomiting and/or diarrhea.

Possible Effects of Long-Term Use: Superinfections, often due to yeast organisms.

Suggested Periodic Examinations While Taking This Drug   (at physician's discretion)
Complete blood cell counts, kidney function tests.

▷ **While Taking This Drug, Observe the Following**
   Foods: No restrictions.
   Beverages: No restrictions. May be taken with milk.
▷ *Alcohol*: No interactions expected.
   Tobacco Smoking: No interactions expected.
▷ *Other Drugs*
   Penicillin V may *decrease* the effects of
   • oral contraceptives in some women, and impair their effectiveness in preventing pregnancy.
   The following drugs may *decrease* the effects of penicillin V
   • antacids may reduce the absorption of penicillin V.
   • chloramphenicol (Chloromycetin).
   • erythromycin (Erythrocin, E-Mycin, etc.).
   • tetracyclines (Achromycin, Declomycin, Minocin, etc.). (See Drug Class, Section Four.)
▷ *Driving, Hazardous Activities*: Usually no restrictions. Be alert to the rare occurrence of dizziness and/or nausea, and restrict activities accordingly.
   Aviation Note: The use of this drug *may be a disqualification* for piloting. Consult a designated Aviation Medical Examiner.
   Exposure to Sun: No restrictions.
   Special Storage Instructions: Oral solutions should be refrigerated.
   Observe the Following Expiration Times: Do not take the oral solution of this drug if older than 7 days when kept at room temperature or 14 days when kept refrigerated.

PENTAZOCINE
(pen TAZ oh seen)

Introduced: 1967

Prescription: USA: Yes
Canada: Yes

Available as Generic: USA: No
Canada: No

Class: Analgesic, Narcotic

Controlled Drug: USA: C-IV*
Canada: <N>

Brand Names: Talacen [CD], Talwin, Talwin Compound [CD], ✿Talwin Compound-50 [CD], Talwin Nx [CD]

BENEFITS versus RISKS

Possible Benefits	*Possible Risks*
EFFECTIVE RELIEF OF MODERATE TO SEVERE PAIN	POTENTIAL FOR HABIT FORMATION (DEPENDENCE)
	Sedative effects
	Mental and behavioral disturbances
	Low blood pressure, fainting
	Nausea, constipation

▷ **Principal Uses**

As a Single Drug Product: Used exclusively to relieve acute or chronic pain of moderate to severe degree from any cause.

As a Combination Drug Product [CD]: Pentazocine is available in combinations with acetaminophen and with aspirin. These milder pain relievers are added to enhance the analgesic effect and to reduce fever when present. In the USA the tablet form of pentazocine also contains naloxone (Talwin Nx), a narcotic antagonist that renders the drug ineffective if abused.

How This Drug Works: Acting primarily as a depressant of certain brain functions, this drug suppresses the perception of pain and calms the emotional response to pain.

Available Dosage Forms and Strengths

Injection — 30 mg per ml
Tablets — 50 mg (Canada)
Tablets — 50 mg with 0.5 mg of naloxone (USA)

▷ **Usual Adult Dosage Range:** 50 mg/3 to 4 hours as needed. May be increased to 100 mg/4 hours if needed for severe pain. The total daily dosage should not exceed 600 mg. **Note: Actual dosage and administration schedule must be determined by the physician for each patient individually.**

*See Schedules of Controlled Drugs inside back cover.

▷ **Dosing Instructions:** May be taken with or following food to reduce stomach irritation or nausea. The tablet may be crushed for administration.

Usual Duration of Use: As required to control pain. Continual use should not exceed 5 to 7 days without interruption and reassessment of need.

▷ **This Drug Should Not Be Taken If**
- you have had an allergic reaction to any dosage form of it previously.
- you are having an acute attack of asthma.

▷ **Inform Your Physician Before Taking This Drug If**
- you have had an unfavorable reaction to any narcotic drug in the past.
- you have a history of drug abuse or alcoholism.
- you have chronic lung disease with impaired breathing.
- you have impaired liver or kidney function.
- you have gallbladder disease, a seizure disorder or an underactive thyroid gland.
- you have difficulty emptying the urinary bladder.
- you are taking any other drugs that have a sedative effect.
- you plan to have surgery under general anesthesia in the near future.

Possible Side-Effects (natural, expected and unavoidable drug actions)
Drowsiness, light-headedness, weakness, urinary retention, constipation.

▷ **Possible Adverse Effects** (unusual, unexpected and infrequent reactions)
If any of the following develop, consult your physician promptly.
Mild Adverse Effects
Allergic Reactions: Skin rash, hives, itching, swelling of face.
Headache, dizziness, impaired concentration, sensation of drunkenness, blurred or double vision, flushing, sweating.
Nausea, vomiting, indigestion, diarrhea.
Serious Adverse Effects
Marked drop in blood pressure, possible fainting.
Impaired breathing: use with caution in chronic lung disease.
Mental and behavioral disturbances, hallucinations, tremor.
Bone marrow depression (see Glossary) of a mild and reversible nature (rare).
Aggravation of prostatism (see Glossary).

CAUTION
1. The use of this drug with atropinelike drugs may increase the risk of urinary retention and reduced intestinal function.
2. Do not take this drug following acute head injury.

Precautions for Use
By Infants and Children: Safety and effectiveness for use by those under 12 years of age have not been established.
By Those over 60 Years of Age: Use small doses initially and increase dosage as needed and tolerated. Limit use to short-term treatment only. There may be increased susceptibility to the development of drowsiness, dizziness, unsteadiness, falling, urinary retention and constipation.

▷ **Advisability of Use During Pregnancy**
    Pregnancy Category: C (tentative). See Pregnancy Code inside back cover.
    Animal studies: Significant birth defects reported in hamsters.
    Human studies: Information from adequate studies of pregnant women is
       not available. Pentazocine taken repeatedly during the last few weeks
       before delivery may cause withdrawal symptoms in the newborn infant.
       Avoid this drug during the first 3 months. Use only if clearly needed and in
       small, infrequent doses during the last 6 months.

Advisability of Use if Breast-Feeding
    Presence of this drug in breast milk: Unknown.
    Avoid drug or refrain from nursing.

Habit-Forming Potential: Psychological and/or physical dependence can
    develop with use of large doses for an extended period of time.

Effects of Overdosage: Anxiety, disturbed thoughts, hallucinations, progres-
    sive drowsiness, stupor, depressed breathing.

Possible Effects of Long-Term Use: Psychological and physical dependence,
    chronic constipation.

Suggested Periodic Examinations While Taking This Drug (at physician's
    discretion)
    Complete blood cell counts, if used for an extended period of time.

▷ **While Taking This Drug, Observe the Following**
    Foods: No restrictions.
    Beverages: No restrictions. May be taken with milk.
▷ *Alcohol*: Use extreme caution until the combined effects have been deter-
       mined. Pentazocine can intensify the intoxicating effects of alcohol, and
       alcohol can intensify the depressant effects of pentazocine on brain
       function, breathing and circulation.
    Tobacco Smoking: Heavy smoking may reduce the effectiveness of
       pentazocine and make larger doses necessary.
    Marijuana Smoking: Increase in drowsiness and pain relief; impairment of
       mental and physical performance.
▷ *Other Drugs*
    Pentazocine may *increase* the effects of
    • other drugs with sedative effects.
    • atropinelike drugs, and increase the risk of constipation and urinary
       retention.
▷ *Driving, Hazardous Activities*: This drug can impair mental alertness, judg-
       ment, reaction time and physical coordination. Avoid hazardous activi-
       ties accordingly.
    Aviation Note: The use of this drug *is a disqualification* for piloting. Consult a
       designated Aviation Medical Examiner.
    Exposure to Sun: No restrictions.
    Discontinuation: It is advisable to limit this drug to short-term use. If it is
       necessary to use it for extended periods of time, discontinuation should
       be gradual to minimize possible effects of withdrawal.

PENTOXIFYLLINE
(pen tox I fi leen)

Other Names: Oxpentifylline

Introduced: 1972

Prescription: USA: Yes
Canada: Yes

Available as Generic: No

Brand Names: Trental

Class: Blood Flow Agent, Xanthines

Controlled Drug: USA: No
Canada: No

BENEFITS versus RISKS	
Possible Benefits	*Possible Risks*
IMPROVED BLOOD FLOW IN PERIPHERAL ARTERIAL DISEASE	Reduced blood pressure, angina, abnormal heart rhythms (in susceptible individuals)
REDUCTION OF INTERMITTENT CLAUDICATION PAIN	Indigestion, nausea, vomiting Dizziness, flushing

▷ **Principal Uses**

As a Single Drug Product: Used primarily (as adjunctive treatment) in the management of peripheral obstructive arterial disease to improve arterial blood flow and reduce the frequency and severity of muscle pain due to intermittent claudication.

How This Drug Works: This drug is thought to improve blood flow through the microcirculation and to increase the oxygen supply to working muscles by way of three mechanisms: (1) reduction of blood viscosity due to decreased levels of fibrinogen in the blood; (2) increased flexibility of the red blood cells (carrying oxygen) due to an increase in cyclic AMP (enzyme) within red blood cells; this permits easier passage through the minute blood vessels of the microcirculation; and (3) prevention of red blood cell and platelet aggregation.

Available Dosage Forms and Strengths

Tablets, prolonged action — 400 mg

▷ **Usual Adult Dosage Range:** 400 mg 3 times/day. If adverse nervous system or gastrointestinal effects occur, reduce the dose to 400 mg twice/day. **Note: Actual dosage and administration schedule must be determined by the physician for each patient individually.**

▷ **Dosing Instructions:** Take with or following food to reduce stomach irritation. Swallow the tablet whole without breaking, crushing or chewing.

Usual Duration of Use: Continual use on a regular schedule for 8 weeks is usually necessary to determine this drug's effectiveness in preventing or delaying the pains of intermittent claudication associated with walking. Long-term use (months to years) requires supervision and periodic evaluation by your physician.

▷ **This Drug Should Not Be Taken If**
- you have had an allergic reaction to it previously.

▷ **Inform Your Physician Before Taking This Drug If**
- you are allergic to other xanthine drugs: caffeine, theophylline, theobromine.
- you have impaired kidney function.
- you have low blood pressure, impaired brain circulation or coronary artery disease.
- you smoke tobacco.
- you are taking any antihypertensive drugs.

Possible Side-Effects   (natural, expected and unavoidable drug actions)
Usually none with recommended doses.

▷ **Possible Adverse Effects**   (unusual, unexpected and infrequent reactions)
If any of the following develop, consult your physician promptly.
Mild Adverse Effects
Allergic Reactions: Skin rash.
Headache (1.2%), dizziness (1.9%), tremor.
Indigestion (2.8%), nausea (2.2%), vomiting (1.2%).
Serious Adverse Effects
Development of angina or heart rhythm disorders in the presence of coronary artery disease.

CAUTION
Use this drug with caution in the presence of impaired circulation within the brain (cerebral arteriosclerosis) or coronary artery disease. If any related symptoms develop, consult your physician for prompt evaluation.

Precautions for Use
By Infants and Children: Safety and effectiveness for use by those under 18 years of age have not been established. Use by this age group is not anticipated.
By Those over 60 Years of Age: You may be more susceptible to the adverse effects listed. Observe closely for any indications of dizziness or chest pain and report these promptly.

▷ **Advisability of Use During Pregnancy**
Pregnancy Category: C (tentative). See Pregnancy Code inside back cover.
Animal studies: Increased fetal resorptions reported in rats, but no birth defects found in rats or rabbits.

Human studies: Information from adequate studies of pregnant women is not available.

Avoid use during the first 3 months. Use otherwise only if clearly needed.

Advisability of Use if Breast-Feeding
Presence of this drug in breast milk: Unknown.
Avoid drug or refrain from nursing.

Habit-Forming Potential: None.

Effects of Overdosage: Drowsiness, flushing, faintness, excitement, seizures.

Possible Effects of Long-Term Use: None reported.

Suggested Periodic Examinations While Taking This Drug   (at physician's discretion)
Blood pressure measurements, evaluation of heart status.

▷ **While Taking This Drug, Observe the Following**
Foods: No restrictions.
Beverages: No restrictions. May be taken with milk.
▷ *Alcohol*: Use caution until the combined effects have been determined. Alcohol may increase the blood-pressure-lowering effect of this drug.
Tobacco Smoking: Nicotine constricts arteries and will impair the effectiveness of this drug significantly. Avoid all use of tobacco.
▷ *Other Drugs*
Pentoxifylline may *increase* the effects of
• antihypertensive drugs, and cause excessive lowering of blood pressure.
• warfarin (Coumadin, etc.), and increase the possibility of unwanted bleeding; monitor prothrombin times as appropriate.
▷ *Driving, Hazardous Activities*: This drug may cause drowsiness or dizziness. Restrict activities as necessary.
Aviation Note: The use of this drug *may be a disqualification* for piloting. Consult a designated Aviation Medical Examiner.
Exposure to Sun: No restrictions.

PERPHENAZINE
(per FEN a zeen)

Introduced: 1957

Class: Strong Tranquilizer, Phenothiazines

Prescription: USA: Yes
Canada: Yes

Controlled Drug: USA: No
Canada: No

Available as Generic: USA: No
Canada: Yes

Brand Names: ♣Apo-Perphenazine, Etrafon [CD], ♣Phenazine, ♣PMS Levazine, Triavil [CD], Trilafon

```
┌─────────────────────────────────────────────────────────────────┐
│                      BENEFITS versus RISKS                        │
│                                                                   │
│      Possible Benefits                    Possible Risks          │
│  EFFECTIVE CONTROL OF ACUTE       SERIOUS TOXIC EFFECTS ON        │
│    MENTAL DISORDERS in the          BRAIN with long-term use      │
│    majority of patients           Liver damage with jaundice      │
│  Beneficial effects on thinking, mood  (infrequent)               │
│    and behavior                   Rare blood cell disorders:      │
│  Relief of anxiety and tension      hemolytic anemia              │
│  Moderately effective control of    abnormally low white blood cell│
│    nausea and vomiting              and platelet counts           │
└─────────────────────────────────────────────────────────────────┘
```

▷ **Principal Uses**

As a Single Drug Product: This antipsychotic drug is used primarily to treat acute and chronic psychotic disorders such as agitated depression, schizophrenia and similar states of mental dysfunction. It may be used as a tranquilizer in the management of agitated and disruptive behavior in the absence of true psychosis. Less frequently, it may be used to relieve severe nausea or vomiting.

As a Combination Drug Product [CD]: This drug is available in combination with amitriptyline, an effective antidepressant. In some cases of severe agitated depression, the combination of a specific antipsychotic drug and a specific antidepressant drug will be more effective than either drug used alone.

How This Drug Works: Not completely established. Present theory is that by inhibiting the action of dopamine, this drug acts to correct an imbalance of nerve impulse transmissions that is thought to be responsible for certain mental disorders.

Available Dosage Forms and Strengths
Concentrate — 16 mg per 5-ml teaspoonful
Injection — 5 mg per ml
Tablets — 2 mg, 4 mg, 8 mg, 16 mg
Tablets, prolonged action — 8 mg

▷ **Usual Adult Dosage Range:**   Initially 2 to 16 mg 2 to 4 times daily. Dose may be increased by 4 mg at 3- to 4-day intervals as needed and tolerated. Usual dosage range is 8 to 24 mg daily. The total daily dosage should not exceed 64 mg. **Note: Actual dosage and administration schedule must be determined by the physician for each patient individually.**

▷ **Dosing Instructions:**   May be taken with or following meals to reduce stomach irritation. The regular tablets may be crushed for administration; the prolonged-action tablets should be taken whole, not broken, crushed or chewed.

Usual Duration of Use: Continual use on a regular schedule for several weeks is usually necessary to determine this drug's effectiveness in controlling psychotic disorders. If it is not significantly beneficial within 6 weeks, it should be discontinued. Long-term use (months to years) requires periodic evaluation of response, appropriate dosage adjustment and consideration of continued need.

▷ **This Drug Should Not Be Taken If**
- you are allergic to any of the drugs bearing the brand names listed.
- you have active liver disease.
- you have cancer of the breast.
- you have a current blood cell or bone marrow disorder.

▷ **Inform Your Physician Before Taking This Drug If**
- you are allergic or abnormally sensitive to any phenothiazine drug (see Drug Class, Section Four).
- you have impaired liver or kidney function.
- you have any type of seizure disorder.
- you have diabetes, glaucoma or heart disease.
- you have a history of lupus erythematosus.
- you are taking any drug with sedative effects.
- you plan to have surgery under general or spinal anesthesia in the near future.

Possible Side-Effects (natural, expected and unavoidable drug actions.
Drowsiness (usually during the first 2 weeks), orthostatic hypotension (see Glossary), blurred vision, dry mouth, nasal congestion, constipation, impaired urination.
Pink or purple coloration of urine, of no significance.

▷ **Possible Adverse Effects** (unusual, unexpected and infrequent reactions)
If any of the following develop, consult your physician promptly.
Mild Adverse Effects
Allergic Reactions: Skin rash, hives, low-grade fever.
Lowering of body temperature, especially in the elderly. (See Hypothermia in Glossary).
Increased appetite and weight gain.
Breast fullness, tenderness, milk production, menstrual irregularity.
Dizziness, weakness, agitation, insomnia, impaired day and night vision.
Chronic constipation, fecal impaction.
Serious Adverse Effects
Allergic Reactions: Hepatitis with jaundice (see Glossary), severe skin reactions, anaphylactic reaction (see Glossary).
Idiosyncratic Reactions: High fever.
Depression, disorientation, seizures, deposits in cornea, lens and retina.
Rapid heart rate, heart rhythm disorders.
Blood cell disorders: hemolytic anemia, reduced white blood cell and blood platelet counts.
Nervous system reactions: Parkinson-like disorders (see Glossary), severe restlessness, muscle spasms involving the face and neck, tardive dyskinesia (see Glossary).

▷ **Adverse Effects That May Mimic Natural Diseases or Disorders**
Nervous system reactions may suggest true Parkinson's disease.

Liver reactions may suggest viral hepatitis.
Reactions resembling systemic lupus erythematosus can occur.

Natural Diseases or Disorders That May Be Activated by This Drug
Latent epilepsy, glaucoma, diabetes mellitus, prostatism (see Glossary).

CAUTION
1. Many over-the-counter medications (see OTC Drugs in Glossary) for allergies, colds and coughs contain drugs that can interact unfavorably with this drug. Ask your physician or pharmacist for guidance before using any such medications.
2. Antacids that contain aluminum and/or magnesium can prevent the absorption of this drug and reduce its effectiveness.
3. Obtain prompt evaluation of any change or disturbance of vision.

Precautions for Use
By Infants and Children: Use of this drug is not recommended in children under 12 years of age. Do not use this drug in the presence of symptoms suggestive of Reye syndrome (see Glossary). Children with acute infectious diseases (flulike infections, chicken pox, measles, etc.) are more prone to develop muscular spasms of the face, back and extremities when this drug is given to control nausea or vomiting.

By Those over 60 Years of Age: Small doses are advisable until individual response has been determined. You may be more susceptible to the development of drowsiness, lethargy, constipation, lowering of body temperature (hypothermia) and orthostatic hypotension (see Glossary). This drug can enhance existing prostatism (see Glossary). You may also be more susceptible to the development of Parkinson-like reactions and/or tardive dyskinesia (see discussion of these terms in Glossary). These reactions must be recognized early since they may become unresponsive to treatment and irreversible.

▷ Advisability of Use During Pregnancy
Pregnancy Category: C (tentative). See Pregnancy Code inside back cover.
Animal studies: Cleft palate reported in mouse and rat studies.
Human studies: No increase in birth defects reported in 166 exposures. Information from adequate studies of pregnant women is not available.
Avoid drug during the first 3 months; avoid during the last month because of possible effects on the newborn infant.

Advisability of Use if Breast-Feeding
Presence of this drug in breast milk: Yes, in minute amounts.
Monitor nursing infant closely and discontinue drug or nursing if adverse effects develop.

Habit-Forming Potential: None.

Effects of Overdosage: Marked drowsiness, weakness, tremor, agitation, unsteadiness, deep sleep, coma, convulsions.

Possible Effects of Long-Term Use: Opacities in the cornea or lens of the eye, pigmentation of the retina. Tardive dyskinesia (see Glossary).

Suggested Periodic Examinations While Taking This Drug (at physician's discretion)

Complete blood cell counts, especially between the fourth and tenth weeks of treatment.

Liver function tests, electrocardiograms.

Complete eye examinations—eye structures and vision.

Careful inspection of the tongue for early evidence of fine, involuntary, wavelike movements that could indicate the beginning of tardive dyskinesia.

▷ **While Taking This Drug, Observe the Following**

Foods: No restrictions.

Nutritional Support: A riboflavin (vitamin B-2) supplement should be taken with long-term use.

Beverages: No restrictions. May be taken with milk.

▷   *Alcohol:* Avoid completely. Alcohol can increase the sedative action of phenothiazines and accentuate their depressant effects on brain function and blood pressure. Phenothiazines can increase the intoxicating effects of alcohol.

Tobacco Smoking: Possible reduction of drowsiness from drug.

Marijuana Smoking: Moderate increase in drowsiness; accentuation of orthostatic hypotension; increased risk of precipitating latent psychoses, confusing the interpretation of mental status and drug responses.

▷   *Other Drugs*

Perphenazine may ***increase*** the effects of

- all sedative drugs, especially meperidine (Demerol), and cause excessive sedation.
- all atropinelike drugs, and cause nervous system toxicity.

Perphenazine may ***decrease*** the effects of

- guanethidine (Ismelin, Esimil), and reduce its effectiveness in lowering blood pressure.

Perphenazine ***taken concurrently*** with

- lithium (Lithobid, Lithotabs) may impair the effectiveness of lithium and cause nervous system toxicity.

The following drugs may ***decrease*** the effects of perphenazine

- antacids containing aluminum and/or magnesium.
- barbiturates (see Drug Class, Section Four).
- benztropine (Cogentin).
- disulfiram (Antabuse).
- trihexyphenidyl (Artane).

▷   *Driving, Hazardous Activities:* This drug can impair mental alertness, judgment and physical coordination. Avoid hazardous activities.

Aviation Note: The use of this drug ***is a disqualification*** for piloting. Consult a designated Aviation Medical Examiner.

Exposure to Sun: Use caution until sensitivity has been determined. Some phenothiazines can cause photosensitivity (see Glossary).

Exposure to Heat: Use caution and avoid excessive heat as much as possible.

This drug may impair the regulation of body temperature and increase the risk of heat stroke.

Exposure to Cold: Use caution and dress warmly. This drug can increase the risk of hypothermia in the elderly.

Discontinuation: After a period of long-term use, do not discontinue this drug suddenly. Gradual withdrawal over 2 to 3 weeks under physician supervision is recommended. Do not discontinue this drug without your physician's knowledge and approval. The relapse rate of schizophrenia after discontinuation is 50% to 60%.

PHENAZOPYRIDINE
(fen az oh PEER i deen)

Introduced: 1927

Class: Urinary Analgesic

Prescription: USA: Varies
Canada: No

Controlled Drug: USA: No
Canada: No

Available as Generic: USA: Yes
Canada: No

Brand Names: Azo Gantanol [CD], Azo Gantrisin [CD], ♣Phenazo, Pyridium, Pyridium Plus [CD], ♣Pyronium, Thiosulfil-A [CD], Urobiotic-250 [CD], ♣Uro Gantanol [CD]

BENEFITS versus RISKS

Possible Benefits	*Possible Risks*
EFFECTIVE RELIEF OF URINARY URGENCY AND DISCOMFORT	DRUG-INDUCED HEPATITIS (rare) Hemolytic anemia (rare)

▷ **Principal Uses**

As a Single Drug Product: Used exclusively in the treatment of lower urinary tract infections and irritations to relieve the urgency to urinate and the discomfort that accompanies the passage of urine (as in cystitis, urethritis and prostatitis).

As a Combination Drug Product [CD]: This drug is available in combinations with several anti-infective drugs that are commonly used to treat urinary tract infections. Each combination product provides a drug to eradicate the infection and a drug to relieve the discomfort during the early period of treatment.

How This Drug Works: Not completely established. By its direct local anesthetic effect on the tissues lining the lower urinary tract, this drug provides symptomatic relief of pain, burning, pressure and the sense of urgency to void.

Available Dosage Forms and Strengths
Tablets — 100 mg, 200 mg

▷ **Usual Adult Dosage Range:**   100 to 200 mg 3 or 4 times/day, as needed and tolerated. **Note: Actual dosage and administration schedule must be determined by the physician for each patient individually.**

▷ **Dosing Instructions:**   Take with or after food to reduce stomach irritation. The tablet should be taken whole, not broken or crushed for administration.

Usual Duration of Use: Continual use on a regular schedule for 12 to 24 hours is usually necessary to determine this drug's effectiveness in relieving urinary urgency and discomfort. This drug is intended for short-term use; do not continue to take it after the bladder disorder has been corrected.

▷ **This Drug Should Not Be Taken If**
  • you have had an allergic reaction to it previously.
  • you have active liver disease.

▷ **Inform Your Physician Before Taking This Drug If**
  • you have a history of liver or kidney disease.
  • you have had a drug-induced blood cell disorder in the past.

Possible Side-Effects   (natural, expected and unavoidable drug actions)
Reddish-orange discoloration of the urine (of no significance).

▷ **Possible Adverse Effects**   (unusual, unexpected and infrequent reactions)
  If any of the following develop, consult your physician promptly.
  Mild Adverse Effects
  Allergic Reactions: Skin rash.
  Headache, dizziness, indigestion, abdominal cramping.
  Serious Adverse Effects
  Allergic Reactions: Drug-induced hepatitis, with or without jaundice (see Glossary).
  Idiosyncratic Reactions: Hemolytic anemia (see Glossary) in sensitive individuals; this is more likely to occur in the presence of impaired kidney function.

▷ **Adverse Effects That May Mimic Natural Diseases or Disorders**
  Liver reaction may suggest viral hepatitis.

CAUTION
  It is important to understand that this drug is only an analgesic, and that its action is limited to the relief of symptoms. It has no curative effect on the underlying condition that is responsible for the symptoms. Consult your physician regarding the need for specific anti-infective therapy.

Precautions for Use
  By Infants and Children: Consult your physician regarding appropriate dosage. Limit use to the time required for adequate relief of symptoms.

By Those over 60 Years of Age: The natural decline in kidney function that occurs after 60 may require that you use smaller doses. Observe for the development of a yellowish coloration of the eyes or skin—an indication of excessive drug accumulation. If this occurs, consult your physician.

▷ **Advisability of Use During Pregnancy**

Pregnancy Category: B (tentative). See Pregnancy Code inside back cover.
Animal studies: No birth defects found.
Human studies: Information from studies of pregnant women indicates no increase in birth defects in 1109 exposures to this drug.
Limit use to small doses for short periods of time. Ask your physician for guidance.

Advisability of Use if Breast-Feeding
Presence of this drug in breast milk: Unknown.
Avoid drug or refrain from nursing.

Habit-Forming Potential: None.

Effects of Overdosage: Nausea, vomiting, abdominal discomfort, skin discoloration, hemolytic anemia (in susceptible individuals), altered hemoglobin resulting in weakness and shortness of breath.

Possible Effects of Long-Term Use: Orange-yellow discoloration of the skin; hemolytic anemia.

Suggested Periodic Examinations While Taking This Drug   (at physician's discretion)
None for short-term use; red blood cell counts and liver-function tests during long-term use.

▷ **While Taking This Drug, Observe the Following**

Foods: No restrictions.
Beverages: No restrictions.
▷ *Alcohol*: No interactions expected.
Tobacco Smoking: No interactions expected.
▷ *Other Drugs*: No significant interactions with other drugs have been reported.
▷ *Driving, Hazardous Activities*: Usually no restrictions. This drug may cause dizziness. Restrict activities as necessary.
Aviation Note: The use of this drug *may be a disqualification* for piloting. Consult a designated Aviation Medical Examiner.
Exposure to Sun: No restrictions.

PHENELZINE
(FEN el zeen)

Introduced: 1961

Prescription: USA: Yes
Canada: Yes

Available as Generic: No

Brand Names: Nardil

Class: Antidepressant, MAO
Inhibitor

Controlled Drug: USA: No
Canada: No

BENEFITS versus RISKS

Possible Benefits	*Possible Risks*
EFFECTIVE RELIEF OF REACTIVE, NEUROTIC, ATYPICAL DEPRESSIONS with associated anxiety or phobia Beneficial in some depressions that are not responsive to other treatments	DANGEROUS INTERACTIONS WITH MANY DRUGS AND FOODS CONDUCIVE TO HYPERTENSIVE CRISIS DISORDERED HEART RATE AND RHYTHM Drug-induced hepatitis (rare) Mental changes: agitation, confusion, impaired memory, hypomania

---

▷ **Principal Uses**

As a Single Drug Product: This potent MAO inhibitor drug is used exclusively to treat severe situational (reactive or neurotic) depression, atypical depression, and (though less effective) severe endogenous depression. Because of the supervision required during its use and its potential for serious adverse effects, this drug is usually reserved to treat depressions that have not responded satisfactorily to other antidepressant therapy.

How This Drug Works: Not completely established. It is thought that by inhibiting the action of a certain enzyme (monoamine oxidase) in brain tissue, this drug produces an increase of those nerve impulse transmitters that maintain normal mood and emotional stability.

Available Dosage Forms and Strengths
Tablets — 15 mg

▷ **Usual Adult Dosage Range:** Initially, 15 mg 3 times/day; increase rapidly up to 60 mg/day, as needed and tolerated, until improvement is apparent. For maintenance, reduce dose gradually over several weeks to the smallest dose that will maintain optimal improvement; this may be as low as 15 mg daily or every other day. The total daily dosage should not exceed

90 mg. **Note: Actual dosage and administration schedule must be determined by the physician for each patient individually.**

▷ **Dosing Instructions:**   May be taken on an empty stomach or with food. Do not take this drug in the late evening; it can interfere with sleep. The tablet may be crushed for administration.

Usual Duration of Use: Continual use on a regular schedule for 3 to 4 weeks is usually necessary to determine this drug's effectiveness in relieving depression. Once the optimal maintenance dose has been determined, it may be continued indefinitely. Long-term use (months to years) requires supervision and periodic evaluation by your physician.

▷ **This Drug Should Not Be Taken If**
- you have had an allergic reaction to it previously.
- you have advanced heart disease.
- you have active liver disease or impaired liver function.
- you have an adrenalin-producing tumor (pheochromocytoma).
- you are taking any of the following drugs: another MAO inhibitor, a tricyclic antidepressant, carbamazepine (see Drug Classes, Section Four).

▷ **Inform Your Physician Before Taking This Drug If**
- you have high blood pressure.
- you have had a stroke, or you have impaired circulation to the brain.
- you have coronary heart disease.
- you have frequent or severe headaches.
- you have diabetes, epilepsy, schizophrenia or an overactive thyroid gland (hyperthyroidism).
- you have impaired kidney function.
- you plan to have surgery under general or spinal anesthesia in the near future.

Possible Side-Effects   (natural, expected and unavoidable drug actions)
Insomnia if taken in the evening. Orthostatic hypotension (see Glossary). Fluid retention (swelling of feet and ankles).

▷ **Possible Adverse Effects**   (unusual, unexpected and infrequent reactions)
If any of the following develop, consult your physician promptly.
Mild Adverse Effects
Allergic Reactions: Skin rash.
Headache, dizziness, drowsiness, weakness, agitation, confusion, impaired memory, tremors, muscle twitching, blurred vision, impaired red-green color vision.
Dry mouth, increased appetite, indigestion, constipation.
Serious Adverse Effects
Drug-induced hepatitis with jaundice (see Glossary).
Hypertensive crisis: rapid and extreme rise in blood pressure, severe throbbing headache, palpitation, nausea, vomiting, sweating, risk of brain hemorrhage.

Unusual excitement or nervousness.
Disturbances of heart rate and rhythm.
Reduced sexual potency.

▷ **Adverse Effects That May Mimic Natural Diseases or Disorders**
Drug-induced hepatitis may suggest viral hepatitis.

Natural Diseases or Disorders That May Be Activated by This Drug
Latent epilepsy, schizophrenia.
This drug may convert a depression into the manic phase of a manic-depressive disorder.

CAUTION
1. Careful dosage adjustment is mandatory. Determine the lowest effective dose and do not exceed it.
2. The development of a severe headache or palpitation may indicate a dangerous elevation of blood pressure. Discontinue this drug immediately and consult your physician.
3. This drug may suppress anginal pain that would normally serve as a warning of excessive demand on the heart.
4. This drug may increase the possibility of hypoglycemic reactions if used concurrently with insulin or oral antidiabetic drugs (sulfonylureas, see Drug Class, Section Four). It may also delay recovery from hypoglycemia.
5. This drug can alter the threshold for convulsions in anyone with epilepsy or a seizure disorder. Dosages of anticonvulsant drugs may require adjustment.
6. This drug should be discontinued 2 weeks before elective surgery under general or spinal anesthesia. Consult your surgeon or anesthesiologist.
7. Many over-the-counter drug products contain ingredients that can cause serious interactions if taken concurrently with this drug. Avoid use of the following: cold and sinus medications, nasal decongestants, hay fever preparations, asthma inhalants, appetite and weight control products, "pep" pills. Consult your physician or pharmacist regarding their safe use with this drug.
8. It is advisable to carry a card of personal identification with the notation that you are taking this drug. Notify all medical personnel that may attend you that you are taking this drug.

Precautions for Use
By Infants and Children: Safety and effectiveness for use by those under 16 years of age have not been established.
By Those over 60 Years of Age: This drug is not recommended for use by anyone over 60. However, if poor response to other treatment justifies consideration of a trial of this drug, it is inadvisable to use it in the presence of high blood pressure, hardening of the arteries, impaired circula-

tion within the brain or coronary artery disease. This drug will intensify existing prostatism (see Glossary). Fluid retention is more prominent in this age group.

▷ **Advisability of Use During Pregnancy**
Pregnancy Category: C (tentative). See Pregnancy Code inside back cover.
Animal studies: No information available.
Human studies: Information from adequate studies of pregnant women is not available. Birth defects have been reported with the use of this drug. Avoid this drug completely if possible. Ask your physician for guidance.

Advisability of Use if Breast-Feeding
Presence of this drug in breast milk: Probably yes.
Avoid drug or refrain from nursing.

Habit-Forming Potential: None.

Effects of Overdosage: Overstimulation, agitation, anxiety, restlessness, insomnia, confusion, delirium, hallucinations, seizures, high fever, circulatory collapse, coma.

Possible Effects of Long-Term Use: The conversion of mental depression into a state of hypomania: excessive mental and physical activity, excitement, agitation, loud and rapid talking, delusional thinking.

Suggested Periodic Examinations While Taking This Drug   (at physician's discretion)
Blood pressure measurements in lying, sitting and standing positions.
Complete blood cell counts, liver function tests.

▷ **While Taking This Drug, Observe the Following**
Foods: ***All tyramine-rich foods should be avoided completely.*** See Tyramine in the Glossary for a compete list of foods and beverages to avoid while taking this drug.
Beverages: Limit coffee, tea and cola beverages to one serving daily. See Tyramine in the Glossary.
▷   *Alcohol*: Use extreme caution until the combined effects have been determined. Alcohol can increase the depressant effects of this drug on brain function.
Tobacco Smoking: No interactions expected.
▷   *Other Drugs*
Phenelzine may *increase* the effects of
• amphetamine and related drugs.
• appetite suppressants.
• all drugs with stimulant effects on the nervous system, and cause excessive rise in blood pressure.
• all drugs with sedative effects, and cause excessive sedation.
• insulin.
• sulfonylureas (see Drug Class, Section Four).

Phenelzine *taken concurrently* with

- carbamazepine (Tegretol) may cause severe toxic reactions.
- levodopa (Dopar, Sinemet) may cause a dangerous rise in blood pressure.
- meperidine (Demerol) may cause high fever, seizures and coma.
- methyldopa (Aldomet) may cause a dangerous rise in blood pressure.
- methylphenidate (Ritalin) may cause severe headache, weakness and numbness in the extremities.
- tricyclic antidepressants may cause severe toxic reactions including high fever, delirium, tremor, seizures and coma.

Note: Consult your physician before taking *any other drugs* while taking phenelzine.

▷   *Driving, Hazardous Activities*: This drug may cause dizziness, drowsiness and blurred vision. Restrict activities as necessary.

Aviation Note: The use of this drug *is a disqualification* for piloting. Consult a designated Aviation Medical Examiner.

Exposure to Sun: No restrictions.

Occurrence of Unrelated Illness: Because of the very serious and life-threatening interactions that can occur between this drug and many others, it is mandatory that you inform each physician and dentist you consult that you are taking this drug.

Discontinuation: If this drug is not effective after 4 weeks of continual use, it should be discontinued. If it is effective, continue to take it in proper dosage until advised to stop. Do not discontinue it abruptly. If another antidepressant is to be tried, a drug-free waiting period of 14 days must elapse between the discontinuation of this drug and initiation of the new one. All precautions regarding the avoidance of tyramine-rich foods and other drugs must be observed during this 14-day period.

PHENOBARBITAL ⚕
(fee noh BAR bi tawl)

Other Names: Phenobarbitone

Introduced: 1912

Class: Sedative, Anticonvulsant, Barbiturates

Prescription: USA: Yes
Canada: Yes

Controlled Drug: USA: C-IV*
Canada: <C>

Available as Generic: Yes

Brand Names: Barbita, Belladenal [CD], Belladenal-S [CD], Bellergal [CD], Bellergal-S [CD], ✦Gardenal, Luminal, Sedadrope, SK-Phenobarbital, Solfoton

*See Schedules of Controlled Drugs inside back cover.

BENEFITS versus RISKS

Possible Benefits	*Possible Risks*
EFFECTIVE CONTROL OF TONIC-CLONIC SEIZURES AND ALL TYPES OF PARTIAL SEIZURES	POTENTIAL FOR DEPENDENCE LIFE-THREATENING TOXICITY WITH OVERDOSAGE
EFFECTIVE CONTROL OF FEBRILE SEIZURES OF CHILDHOOD	Drug-induced hepatitis Rare blood cell disorders:
Effective relief of anxiety and nervous tension	abnormally low red cell, white cell and platelet counts

---

▷ **Principal Uses**

As a Single Drug Product: This barbiturate drug has two primary uses: (1) as a mild sedative to relieve anxiety, nervous tension and insomnia; and (2) as an anticonvulsant to control grand mal epilepsy and all types of partial seizures. It is also used to control febrile seizures of childhood.

As a Combination Drug Product [CD]: This drug is available in many combinations with derivatives of belladonna, an antispasmodic commonly used to treat functional disorders of the gastrointestinal tract. It is also available in combination with bronchodilators for the treatment of asthma, and with ergotamine for the treatment of headaches.

How This Drug Works: Not completely established. It is thought that by impeding the transfer of sodium and potassium across cell membranes, this drug selectively blocks the transmission of nerve impulses. This could serve to produce a sedative effect and to suppress the spread of nerve impulses that are responsible for epileptic seizures.

Available Dosage Forms and Strengths

Capsules — 16 mg
Capsules, prolonged action — 65 mg
Drops — 16 mg per ml
Elixir — 20 mg per 5-ml teaspoonful
Liquid — 15 mg per 5-ml teaspoonful
Tablets — 8 mg, 15 mg, 16 mg, 30 mg, 32 mg, 65 mg, 100 mg

▷ **Usual Adult Dosage Range:** As sedative: 15 to 30 mg 2 to 4 times/day. As hypnotic: 100 to 200 mg at bedtime. As anticonvulsant: 100 to 200 mg given as a single dose at bedtime. The total daily dosage should not exceed 600 mg. **Note: Actual dosage and administration schedule must be determined by the physician for each patient individually.**

▷ **Dosing Instructions:** May be taken with or after food to reduce stomach irritation. Regular tablets may be crushed and capsules opened for administration. Prolonged-action dosage forms should be swallowed whole without alteration.

Usual Duration of Use: Continual use on a regular schedule for 3 to 5 days is usually necessary to determine this drug's effectiveness in relieving anxiety and tension, and for 4 to 6 weeks to determine its ability to control seizures. If used to treat anxiety-tension states, its use should not exceed 4 weeks without reappraisal of continued need. Long-term use for seizure control (months to years) requires supervision and periodic evaluation by your physician.

▷ **This Drug Should Not Be Taken If**
- you have had an allergic reaction to it previously.
- you are subject to acute intermittent porphyria (see Glossary).

▷ **Inform Your Physician Before Taking This Drug If**
- you are allergic or overly sensitive to any barbiturate drug (see Drug Class, Section Four).
- you are pregnant or planning pregnancy.
- you have a history of alcohol or drug abuse.
- you are taking any drugs with sedative effects.
- you have any type of seizure disorder.
- you have myasthenia gravis.
- you have impaired liver, kidney or thyroid gland function.
- you plan to have surgery under general anesthesia in the near future.

Possible Side-Effects   (natural, expected and unavoidable drug actions)
Drowsiness, impaired concentration, mental and physical sluggishness.

▷ **Possible Adverse Effects**   (unusual, unexpected and infrequent reactions)
If any of the following develop, consult your physician promptly.
Mild Adverse Effects
Allergic Reactions: Skin rashes, hives, localized swellings of face, drug fever (see Glossary).
Dizziness, unsteadiness, impaired vision, double vision.
Nausea, vomiting, diarrhea.
Shoulder-hand syndrome: pain and stiffness in the shoulder, pain and swelling in the hand.
Serious Adverse Effects
Allergic Reactions: Drug-induced hepatitis with jaundice (see Glossary).
Idiosyncratic Reactions: Paradoxical excitement and delirium (instead of sedation).
Mental depression, abnormal involuntary movements.
Blood cell disorders: deficiencies of all blood cell types causing fatigue, weakness, fever, sore throat, abnormal bleeding or bruising.

▷ **Adverse Effects That May Mimic Natural Diseases or Disorders**
Liver reactions may suggest viral hepatitis.

Natural Diseases or Disorders That May Be Activated by This Drug
Acute intermittent and/or cutaneous porphyria, systemic lupus erythematosus.

CAUTION
1. Anticonvulsant drug therapy must be carefully individualized. Accu-

rate diagnosis and classification of the seizure pattern are essential to the correct selection of the most appropriate drug for seizure control.

2. Emotional stress or physical trauma (including surgery) may require increased anticonvulsant dosage to control seizures.

3. Prolonged-action dosage forms of this drug are not appropriate for the treatment of seizures and should not be used.

Precautions for Use

By Infants and Children: This drug should not be given to the hyperkinetic child. Observe for possible paradoxical stimulation and hyperactivity; this can occur in 10% to 40% of children. Changes associated with puberty characteristically slow the metabolism of this drug and permit its gradual accumulation. Blood levels of this drug in young adolescents should be monitored every 3 months to detect rising concentrations and early toxicity. Adjust dosage as necessary.

By Those over 60 Years of Age: It is advisable to avoid all barbiturates in the elderly. If use of this drug is attempted, start with small doses until tolerance has been determined. Observe for confusion, delirium, agitation and excitement. Do not use this drug concurrently with other drugs for mental disorders. This drug is conducive to the development of hypothermia (see Glossary).

▷ Advisability of Use During Pregnancy

Pregnancy Category: B (tentative). See Pregnancy Code inside back cover.

Animal studies: Conflicting reports of cleft palate and skeletal defects in mouse, rat and rabbit studies.

Human studies: Information from studies of pregnant women indicates no increase in birth defects in 8037 exposures to this drug.

Avoid use of drug during entire pregnancy if possible. If use is clearly needed to control seizures, the mother should receive vitamin K prior to delivery and the infant should receive it at birth.

Advisability of Use if Breast-Feeding

Presence of this drug in breast milk: Yes.

Monitor nursing infant closely and discontinue drug or nursing if adverse effects develop.

Habit-Forming Potential: Psychological and physical dependence can occur with prolonged use of excessive doses—300 to 700 mg/day for 1 to 2 months. Dependence is not likely to occur with usual sedative or anticonvulsant doses.

Effects of Overdosage: Behavior similar to alcoholic intoxication: confusion, slurred speech, physical incoordination, staggering gait, drowsiness, stupor progressing to coma.

Possible Effects of Long-Term Use: Psychological and/or physical dependence; syndrome of chronic intoxication: headache, depression, impaired vision, dizziness, slurred speech, incoordination. Megaloblastic anemia due to folic acid deficiency. Rickets or osteomalacia due to deficiencies of vitamin D and calcium.

Suggested Periodic Examinations While Taking This Drug (at physician's discretion)

Complete blood cell counts, liver function tests.

During long-term use: blood levels of folic acid, vitamin B-12, calcium and phosphorus; skeletal X-ray studies for demineralization of bone.

▷ **While Taking This Drug, Observe the Following**

Foods: No restrictions. Eat liberally of foods rich in folic acid: fortified breakfast cereals, liver, legumes, green leafy vegetables.

Beverages: No restrictions. May be taken with milk or fruit juices.

▷ *Alcohol*: Avoid completely. Alcohol can increase greatly the sedative and depressant actions of this drug on brain functions.

Tobacco Smoking: May enhance the sedative effects of this drug and increase drowsiness.

Marijuana Smoking: Increased drowsiness, unsteadiness; significantly impaired mental and physical performance.

▷ *Other Drugs*

Phenobarbital may *increase* the effects of

- all other drugs with sedative effects, and cause excessive sedation.

Phenobarbital may *decrease* the effects of

- anticoagulants (Coumadin, etc.), and require dosage adjustments.
- certain beta-blockers (Inderal, Lopressor), and reduce their effectiveness.
- cortisonelike drugs.
- doxycycline (Vibramycin), and reduce its effectiveness.
- griseofulvin (Fulvicin, etc.), and reduce its effectiveness.
- oral contraceptives, and reduce their effectiveness in preventing pregnancy.
- quinidine (Quinaglute, etc.), and reduce its effectiveness.
- theophyllines (Aminophyllin, Theo-Dur, etc.), and reduce their antiasthmatic effectiveness.

Phenobarbital *taken concurrently* with

- phenytoin (Dilantin) may alter phenytoin blood levels: a high phenobarbital level will increase the phenytoin level; a low phenobarbital level will decrease the phenytoin level. Periodic determination of blood levels of both drugs is advised.

The following drugs may *increase* the effects of phenobarbital

- valproic acid (Depakene).

▷ *Driving, Hazardous Activities*: This drug may cause drowsiness and may impair mental alertness, judgment, physical coordination and reaction time. Restrict activities as necessary.

Aviation Note: The use of this drug *is a disqualification* for piloting. Consult a designated Aviation Medical Examiner.

Exposure to Sun: Use caution until sensitivity has been determined. This drug may cause photosensitivity.

Exposure to Cold: Observe the elderly for possible hypothermia (see Glossary) while taking this drug.

Discontinuation: If used as an anticonvulsant, this drug must not be discontinued abruptly. Sudden withdrawal can precipitate status epilepticus (repetitive seizures). Gradual reduction in dosage should be made over a period of 3 months. Total drug withdrawal may be attempted after a period of 3 to 5 years without a seizure. However, seizures are likely to recur in 40% of adults and in 20% to 30% of children.

PHENYLBUTAZONE
(fen il BYU ta zohn)

Introduced: 1949

Class: Mild Analgesic, Anti-inflammatory

Prescription: USA: Yes
Canada: Yes

Controlled Drug: USA: No
Canada: No

Available as Generic: Yes

Brand Names: ❧Apo-Phenylbutazone, Azolid, Butazolidin, ❧Intrabutazone, ❧Neo-Zoline, ❧Novobutazone, ❧Phenbuff

---

BENEFITS versus RISKS

Possible Benefits	*Possible Risks*
PROMPT, EFFECTIVE RELIEF OF INFLAMMATION AND PAIN IN MODERATELY SEVERE ARTHRITIS, GOUT, BURSITIS AND SUPERFICIAL PHLEBITIS (FOR SHORT-TERM USE)	BONE MARROW DEPRESSION MAY BE SEVERE DRUG-INDUCED HEPATITIS KIDNEY DAMAGE, IMPAIRED FUNCTION GASTROINTESTINAL ULCER FORMATION AND BLEEDING HYPERTENSION HEART MUSCLE DAMAGE EYE DAMAGE: OPTIC NEURITIS EAR DAMAGE: HEARING LOSS

▷ **Principal Uses**

As a Single Drug Product: This potent anti-inflammatory drug is used primarily for the short-term relief of pain and inflammation associated with moderately severe arthritis, gout, bursitis, tendinitis and superficial phlebitis. Because of its potential for severe toxicity, it is not considered to be an "aspirin substitute." Its use should be limited to those conditions that do not respond to less toxic drugs.

How This Drug Works: Not completely established. It is thought that this drug acts somewhat like aspirin, by suppressing the formation of prostaglandins and related substances that are involved in the production of inflammation.

Available Dosage Forms and Strengths
Capsules — 100 mg
Tablets — 100 mg

▷ **Usual Adult Dosage Range:** For arthritis: Initially, 100 to 200 mg 3 times/day; for maintenance, 100 mg 1 to 4 times/day. For acute gout: Initially, 400 mg as a single dose; then 100 mg/4 hours for 4 days or until the acute attack is relieved; continual use should not exceed 1 week. Alternate course for gout: 200 mg/4 hours for 4 days or until acute attack is relieved; continual use should not exceed 2 weeks. **Note: Actual dosage and administration schedule must be determined by the physician for each patient individually.**

▷ **Dosing Instructions:** Take with or following food to reduce stomach irritation. The tablet may be crushed and the capsule may be opened for administration.

Usual Duration of Use: Continual use on a regular schedule for 2 to 5 days is usually necessary to determine this drug's effectiveness in relieving acute pain in arthritis, gout and related conditions. This drug should be limited to short-term use only. If significant improvement does not occur within 1 week, this drug should be discontinued. The maximal period of continual use should not exceed 10 to 14 days.

▷ **This Drug Should Not Be Taken If**
- you have had an allergic reaction to it previously, or to oxyphenbutazone (Tandearil), a closely related drug.
- you have a history of serious adverse effects from drugs.
- you have a history of a blood cell or bone marrow disorder.
- you have a history of stomach or intestinal ulceration or bleeding.
- you have a history of disease or impaired function of the thyroid, heart, liver or kidneys.
- you have high blood pressure.

▷ **Inform Your Physician Before Taking This Drug If**
- you are allergic to aspirin or aspirin substitutes (anti-inflammatory analgesics).
- you are taking any other drugs at this time, either prescription or over-the-counter drugs.
- you are taking anticoagulants.
- you have glaucoma.

Possible Side-Effects (natural, expected and unavoidable drug actions)
Salt and water retention, reduced urine output.

▷ **Possible Adverse Effects** (unusual, unexpected and infrequent reactions)
If any of the following develop, consult your physician promptly.
Mild Adverse Effects
Allergic Reactions: Skin rashes, hives, itching, drug fever (see Glossary).
Headache, drowsiness, lethargy, nervousness, confusion, tremors.

Indigestion, stomach pain, nausea, vomiting, diarrhea.

Progressive gain in weight and rise in blood pressure; these are indications to discontinue this drug.

Serious Adverse Effects

Allergic Reactions: Severe skin reactions, high fever, swollen and painful joints, salivary gland enlargement, anaphylactic reaction (see Glossary).

Bone marrow depression (see Glossary): fatigue, weakness, fever, sore throat, abnormal bleeding or bruising.

Drug-induced hepatitis, with or without jaundice (see Glossary).

Kidney damage, impaired kidney function, kidney failure.

Stomach and intestinal ulceration and/or bleeding.

Damage to heart muscle (myocarditis) and heart covering (pericarditis).

Eye damage: injuries to optic nerve and retina, impaired vision.

Ear damage: loss of hearing.

Possible Delayed Adverse Effects

The development of leukemia following the use of this drug has been reported. A cause-and-effect relationship (see Glossary) has not been established.

▷ **Adverse Effects That May Mimic Natural Diseases or Disorders**

Liver reactions may suggest viral hepatitis.

Natural Diseases or Disorders That May Be Activated by This Drug

Latent hypertension, peptic ulcer disease, ulcerative colitis.

CAUTION

1. This drug should never be used for mild and trivial conditions. It has high potential for serious and life-threatening adverse effects.
2. Follow your physician's instructions fully regarding periodic examinations while taking this drug. These are essential for the early detection of possible adverse effects.

Precautions for Use

By Infants and Children: Safety and effectiveness for use by those under 15 years of age have not been established.

By Those over 60 Years of Age: Many authorities advise that this drug should not be used by this age group. More than 60% of users over 61 years of age experience adverse effects from this drug. The elderly and the debilitated are clearly more vulnerable to the toxic effects of this drug. Its use is not recommended.

▷ **Advisability of Use During Pregnancy**

Pregnancy Category: D (tentative). See Pregnancy Code inside back cover.

Animal studies: Evidence of embryo toxicity reported.

Human studies: Information from adequate studies of pregnant women is not available. Two cases of birth defects following use of this drug have been reported. A causal relationship has not been established.

One manufacturer of this drug recommends that it not be used during pregnancy.

Advisability of Use if Breast-Feeding
Presence of this drug in breast milk: Yes.
Avoid drug or refrain from nursing.

Habit-Forming Potential: None.

Effects of Overdosage: Headache, dizziness, insomnia, mental and behavioral disturbances, hallucinations, seizures, coma.

Possible Effects of Long-Term Use: Bone marrow depression. Development of thyroid gland enlargement (goiter), with or without altered function.

Suggested Periodic Examinations While Taking This Drug (at physician's discretion)
Complete blood cell counts and urine analysis should be made before the drug is taken and during the course of treatment at intervals of 1 to 2 weeks.
Liver function tests.

▷ **While Taking This Drug, Observe the Following**
Foods: No restrictions. Avoid excessive salt.
Beverages: No restrictions. May be taken with milk.
▷ *Alcohol*: Avoid completely because of its irritant effect on the stomach, increasing the risk of ulceration and bleeding.
Tobacco Smoking: No interactions expected.
▷ *Other Drugs*
Phenylbutazone may *increase* the effects of
- anticoagulants (Coumadin, etc.), and cause bleeding.
- lithium (Lithane, Lithotabs, etc.), and increase the risk of lithium toxicity.
- phenytoin (Dilantin), and cause phenytoin toxicity.
- sulfonylureas (see Drug Class, Section Four), and increase the risk of hypoglycemia.
▷ *Driving, Hazardous Activities*: This drug may cause dizziness, confusion and impaired vision or hearing. Restrict activities as necessary.
Aviation Note: The use of this drug *may be a disqualification* for piloting. Consult a designated Aviation Medical Examiner.
Exposure to Sun: Use caution until sensitivity has been determined. This drug may cause photosensitivity (see Glossary).

PHENYLEPHRINE
(fen il EF rin)

Introduced: 1949

Prescription: USA: No
Canada: No

Available as Generic: USA: Yes
Canada: Yes

Class: Decongestant

Controlled Drug: USA: No
Canada: No

Brand Names: Alconefrin, Clistin-D [CD], Coricidin Nasal Mist, Duo-Medihaler [CD], 4-Way Nasal Spray [CD], Hycomine Compound [CD], ♣Mydfrin, ♣Naldecol [CD], Naldecon [CD], Neo-Synephrine, Nostril, ♣Prefin Liquifilm, Sinarest Nasal Spray, Sinex

---

BENEFITS versus RISKS

Possible Benefits	*Possible Risks*
EFFECTIVE DECONGESTION OF NASAL AND SINUS TISSUES	"REBOUND" CONGESTION WITH EXCESSIVE USE
EFFECTIVE DECONGESTION OF INFLAMED EYES	Mild irritation of ocular or nasal tissues
	Systemic effects (via absorption with excessive use): nervousness, insomnia, hypertension

---

▷ **Principal Uses**

As a Single Drug Product: Used primarily as a decongestant nose drop or spray to relieve swelling and congestion of the nasal membranes due to colds or allergy. It is also used as an eye drop to relieve inflammation and swelling of the conjunctival membranes ("red eyes") due to allergy or chemical irritation.

As a Combination Drug Product [CD]: This drug is available in a variety of combinations. Combined with another decongestant and two antihistamines, the product is widely used to treat infections and allergic conditions of the upper respiratory tract. Combined with isoproterenol as an inhalant for the treatment of acute asthma, this drug improves breathing by reducing the swelling and congestion of bronchial passages.

How This Drug Works: By contracting the walls of arterioles and thus reducing their size, this drug decreases the volume of blood in the tissues, resulting in shrinkage of tissue mass (decongestion). This expands the nasal airway and enlarges the openings into the sinuses and eustachian tubes. The same action on the conjunctival vessels in the eye results in clearing of the capillary congestion (redness) and swelling.

Available Dosage Forms and Strengths
Nasal jelly — 0.5%
Ophthalmic solutions — 0.12%, 2.5%, 10%

Solutions — 0.125%, 0.16%, 0.2%, 0.25%, 0.5%, 1%
Tablets — only in combination with other drugs

▷ **Usual Adult Dosage Range:**   Eye drops: 1 or 2 drops in affected eye every 4 to 6 hours. Nose drops and spray: 2 or 3 drops or sprays into each nostril every 4 hours as needed. For long-term use, consult your physician.

▷ **Dosing Instructions:**   Do not exceed the recommended doses. The nasal spray is more effective than the drops and is less likely to cause systemic absorption. Oral preparations that contain this drug may be taken with or following food to reduce stomach irritation. Prolonged action capsules or tablets should be swallowed whole without alteration.

Usual Duration of Use: Continual use on a regular schedule for 2 to 3 days is usually necessary to determine this drug's effectiveness in relieving eye and nasal congestion. If there is no significant improvement after 1 week of use, consult your physician for further evaluation.

▷ **This Drug Should Not Be Taken If**
- you have had an allergic reaction to it previously.
- for the eye drops: you have untreated narrow-angle glaucoma or an active eye infection.

▷ **Inform Your Physician Before Taking This Drug If**
- you have high blood pressure or heart disease.
- you have diabetes or an overactive thyroid gland (hyperthyroidism).
- you are taking any beta-blocker drug (see Drug Class, Section Four).
- you are taking, or have taken within the past 14 days, any monoamine oxidase (MAO) inhibitor drug (see Drug Class, Section Four).

Possible Side-Effects   (natural, expected and unavoidable drug actions)
Dryness or irritation of the nose, nervousness, insomnia.

▷ **Possible Adverse Effects**   (unusual, unexpected and infrequent reactions)
If any of the following develop, consult your physician promptly.
Mild Adverse Effects
Headache, light-headedness, burning or stinging of the nose, heart palpitation, tremors.
Serious Adverse Effects
None reported.

CAUTION
1. Too frequent use, or extended use, of nose drops or sprays containing this drug may cause a secondary "rebound" congestion resulting in a form of functional dependence (see Glossary).
2. Many over-the-counter drug products for allergies, colds and coughs contain drugs that may interact unfavorably with this drug. Ask your physician or pharmacist for guidance before using such medications.

Precautions for Use
By Infants and Children: Children may be especially susceptible to systemic absorption of this drug. Avoid excessive use. Nasal drops of all strengths

should not be used in infants less than 1 year of age; rebound nasal congestion can impair breathing and be potentially life-threatening.

By Those over 60 Years of Age: Use small doses until your tolerance has been determined. Observe for possible nervousness, insomnia, palpitation or angina.

▷ **Advisability of Use During Pregnancy**

Pregnancy Category: C (tentative). See Pregnancy Code inside back cover.

Animal studies: Significant birth defects due to this drug found in rabbits.

Human studies: Information from studies of pregnant women is conflicting. Limited studies indicate a possible increased risk for birth defects during the first 3 months. Larger studies indicate no increase in defects in 4194 exposures during entire pregnancy.

Avoid completely during the first 3 months. Limit use to small, infrequent doses as needed during the last 6 months.

Advisability of Use if Breast-Feeding

Presence of this drug in breast milk: Unknown.

Monitor nursing infant closely and discontinue drug or nursing if adverse effects develop.

Habit-Forming Potential: Frequent or excessive use may cause functional dependence (see Glossary).

Effects of Overdosage: Headache, restlessness, anxiety, agitation, palpitation, sweating.

Possible Effects of Long-Term Use: Secondary "rebound" congestion and chemical irritation of nasal tissues.

Suggested Periodic Examinations While Taking This Drug   (at physician's discretion)

None required.

▷ **While Taking This Drug, Observe the Following**

Foods: No restrictions.

Beverages: Heavy use of coffee or tea may add to the nervousness or insomnia experienced by sensitive individuals.

▷   *Alcohol*: No interactions expected.

Tobacco Smoking: No interactions expected.

▷   *Other Drugs*

Phenylephrine *taken concurrently* with

 • beta-blocker drugs or monoamine oxidase (MAO) inhibitor drugs may cause dangerous elevations of blood pressure. Observe for headache or palpitation.

▷   *Driving, Hazardous Activities*: No restrictions.

Aviation Note: The use of this drug *may be a disqualification* for piloting. Consult a designated Aviation Medical Examiner.

Exposure to Sun: No restrictions.

PHENYLPROPANOLAMINE
(fen il proh pa NOHL a meen)

Introduced: 1948

Class: Decongestant, Appetite Suppressant

Prescription: USA: No
Canada: No

Controlled Drug: USA: No
Canada: No

Available as Generic: USA: Yes
Canada: No

Brand Names: Acutrim, Allerest [CD], Contac Perma-Seal Capsules [CD], Contac Severe Cold Formula Caplets [CD], Contac 12-Hour Caplets [CD], ♣Corsym [CD], Dimetapp [CD], Dexatrim-15, Hycomine Pediatric Syrup [CD], Hycomine Syrup [CD], Naldecon [CD], Naldecon-CX [CD], Ornade [CD], Ornex [CD], Sine-Off Extra Strength Tablets [CD], Sinubid [CD], ♣Sinutab Capsules [CD], Triaminic Allergy Tablets [CD], Triaminic Cold Syrup [CD], Triaminic Expectorant DH [CD], Triaminicin [CD], Tuss-Ornade Liquid [CD], Tuss-Ornade Spansules [CD]

BENEFITS versus RISKS

Possible Benefits	*Possible Risks*
EFFECTIVE DECONGESTION OF NASAL AND SINUS TISSUES	HYPERTENSIVE CRISIS IN SENSITIVE INDIVIDUALS
Moderate suppression of appetite for short-term aid in weight reduction	Nervous system reactions: anxiety, agitation, dizziness, tremors, hallucinations

---

▷ **Principal Uses**

As a Single Drug Product: This drug is currently used for two purposes: (1) As a nasal decongestant, and (2) as an appetite suppressant for weight reduction and control.

As a Combination Drug Product [CD]: This drug is available in a variety of combinations. Combined with other decongestants and antihistamines, the products are widely used to treat infections and allergic conditions of the upper respiratory tract. Similar formulas are combined with aspirin or acetaminophen for treatment of sinus headache. This drug is also combined with expectorants and cough suppressants, such as codeine and dextromethorphan, in the formulation of cough syrups.

How This Drug Works: By contracting the walls of arterioles and thus reducing their size, this drug decreases the volume of blood in the tissues, resulting in shrinkage of tissue mass (decongestion). This expands the nasal airway and enlarges the openings into the sinuses and eustachian tubes. By altering the chemical control of nerve impulse transmission within the appetite-regulating center of the brain, this drug can temporarily reduce hunger in some individuals.

Available Dosage Forms and Strengths

> Capsules — 37.5 mg
> Capsules, prolonged action — 50 mg, 75 mg
> Lozenges — 25 mg
> Syrup — 12.5 mg per 5 ml teaspoonful
> Tablets — 25 mg, 50 mg
> Tablets, prolonged action — 75 mg

▷ **Usual Adult Dosage Range:** As decongestant: 12.5 to 37.5 mg every 4 to 6 hours as needed. As appetite suppressant: 25 to 50 mg 1 hour before meals, or 50 to 75 mg of the prolonged action form once daily in the morning. The total daily dosage should not exceed 200 mg. **Note: Actual dosage and administration schedule must be determined by the physician for each patient individually.**

▷ **Dosing Instructions:** Do not exceed the recommended doses. This drug may be taken with or following food to reduce stomach irritation. Prolonged action capsules or tablets should be swallowed whole without alteration.

Usual Duration of Use: Continual use on a regular schedule for 2 to 3 days is usually necessary to determine this drug's effectiveness in relieving nasal congestion. If there is no significant improvement after 1 week of use, consult your physician for further evaluation.

▷ **This Drug Should Not Be Taken If**
- you have had an allergic reaction to any dosage form of it previously.

▷ **Inform Your Physician Before Taking This Drug If**
- you have high blood pressure or heart disease.
- you have diabetes or an overactive thyroid gland (hyperthyroidism).
- you are taking any beta-blocker drug (see Drug Class, Section Four).
- you are taking, or have taken within the past 14 days, any monoamine oxidase (MAO) inhibitor drug (see Drug Class, Section Four).
- you plan to have surgery under general anesthesia in the near future.

Possible Side-Effects   (natural, expected and unavoidable drug actions)
Nervousness, insomnia, increase in blood pressure in sensitive individuals.

▷ **Possible Adverse Effects**   (unusual, unexpected and infrequent reactions)
If any of the following develop, consult your physician promptly.
Mild Adverse Effects
Headache, dizziness, heart palpitation, tremors.
Nausea, vomiting.
Serious Adverse Effects
Excessive rise in blood pressure, hypertensive crises.
Anxiety, agitation, hallucinations.
Acute temporary mental derangement (psychotic episodes).

Natural Diseases or Disorders That May Be Activated by This Drug
Latent hypertension, angina pectoris, heart rhythm disorders.

CAUTION
1. Many over-the-counter drug products for allergies, colds and coughs contain drugs that may interact unfavorably with this drug. Ask your physician or pharmacist for guidance before using such medications.
2. This drug is an amphetaminelike substance. It is capable of excessive and sometimes dangerous stimulation in sensitive individuals. If you experience any unusual increase in nervousness, restlessness, insomnia or overstimulation, discontinue this drug and consult your physician.

Precautions for Use
By Infants and Children: Children may be especially susceptible to the stimulant effects of this drug. Use small, infrequent doses and observe closely for adverse effects.
By Those over 60 Years of Age: Use small doses until your tolerance has been determined. Observe for possible nervousness, insomnia, palpitation or angina.

▷ **Advisability of Use During Pregnancy**
Pregnancy Category: D (tentative). See Pregnancy Code inside back cover.
Animal studies: No information available.
Human studies: Information from studies of pregnant women is conflicting. Limited studies indicate a possible increased risk for birth defects during the first 3 months. Larger studies indicate no increase in defects in 2489 exposures during entire pregnancy.
Avoid completely during the first 3 months. Limit use to small, infrequent doses as needed during the last 6 months.

Advisability of Use if Breast-Feeding
Presence of this drug in breast milk: Yes.
Avoid drug or refrain from nursing.

Habit-Forming Potential: None.

Effects of Overdosage: Headache, restlessness, anxiety, agitation, palpitation, sweating, tremors, confusion, delirium, rapid pulse, irregular heart rhythm.

Possible Effects of Long-Term Use: Hypertension in susceptible individuals.

Suggested Periodic Examinations While Taking This Drug (at physician's discretion)
None required.

▷ **While Taking This Drug, Observe the Following**
Foods: No restrictions.
Beverages: Heavy use of coffee or tea may add to the nervousness or insomnia experienced by sensitive individuals.
▷ *Alcohol*: No interactions expected.
Tobacco Smoking: No interactions expected.
▷ *Other Drugs*
Phenylpropanolamine *taken concurrently* with
• beta-blocker drugs or monoamine oxidase (MAO) inhibitor drugs may

cause dangerous elevations of blood pressure. Observe for headache or palpitation.

▷ *Driving, Hazardous Activities*: No restrictions.
Aviation Note: The use of this drug *may be a disqualification* for piloting. Consult a designated Aviation Medical Examiner.
Exposure to Sun: No restrictions.

PHENYLTOLOXAMINE
(fen il toh LOX a meen)

Introduced: 1959

Prescription: USA: Varies
Canada: Varies

Class: Antihistamines

Controlled Drug: USA: Tussionex is C-III*
Canada: Tussionex is <N>

Available as Generic: USA: No
Canada: No

Brand Names: ✿Naldecol [CD], Naldecon [CD], Percogesic [CD], ✿Sinutab Tablets [CD], ✿Sinutab Tablets w/Codeine [CD], Tussionex [CD]

BENEFITS versus RISKS	
Possible Benefits	*Possible Risks*
EFFECTIVE RELIEF OF ALLERGIC RHINITIS AND ALLERGIC TRACHEO-BRONCHITIS	Mild sedation Atropinelike effects

▷ **Principal Uses**
As a Single Drug Product: This drug is not available in a single entity preparation.
As a Combination Drug Product [CD]: This drug is available in combination with another antihistamine and two decongestants for use in treating nasal allergies, headcolds and sinusitis. It is also combined with acetaminophen for the treatment of sinus headache. A combination of this drug and hydrocodone is a widely used cough remedy.

How This Drug Works: Antihistamines reduce the intensity of the allergic response by blocking the action of histamine after it has been released from sensitized tissue cells in the eyes, nose and respiratory passages.

Available Dosage Forms and Strengths
Combination drug products containing this drug are available in the following forms: capsules, pediatric drops, elixirs, syrups, tablets and prolonged action tablets. Read the product label carefully to learn the contents and the strength of each ingredient.

*See Schedules of Controlled Drugs inside back cover.

▷ **Usual Adult Dosage Range:** 7.5 to 30 mg every 4 to 6 hours as needed. The total daily dosage should not exceed 130 mg. **Note: For long-term use, actual dosage and administration schedule must be determined by the physician for each patient individually.**

▷ **Dosing Instructions:** Take with food or milk to prevent stomach irritation. The prolonged-action forms should be swallowed whole (not crushed or chewed).

Usual Duration of Use: Continual use on a regular schedule for 2 to 3 days is usually necessary to determine this drug's effectiveness in relieving the symptoms of allergic rhinitis or bronchitis. Antihistamines should not be taken continually (without interruption) for long-term use. Limit their use to periods that require symptomatic relief.

▷ **This Drug Should Not Be Taken If**
- you have had an allergic reaction to any dosage form of it previously.
- you are currently undergoing allergy skin tests.
- you are subject to acute attacks of asthma.
- you have narrow-angle glaucoma.

▷ **Inform Your Physician Before Taking This Drug If**
- you have had any allergic reactions or unfavorable responses to the previous use of antihistamines.
- you have difficulty emptying the urinary bladder, especially if due to prostate gland enlargement. (See Prostatism in Glossary.)
- you plan to have surgery under general anesthesia in the near future.

Possible Side-Effects (natural, expected and unavoidable drug actions)
Drowsiness; sense of weakness; blurred vision; dryness of the nose, mouth and throat; impaired urination; constipation.

▷ **Possible Adverse Effects** (unusual, unexpected and infrequent reactions)
If any of the following develop, consult your physician promptly.
Mild Adverse Effects
Allergic Reactions: Skin rash, hives.
Headache, dizziness, inability to concentrate, impaired coordination, nervousness, insomnia, tremors.
Reduced tolerance for contact lenses.
Thickening of bronchial secretions in asthma or bronchitis.
Indigestion, nausea, vomiting, diarrhea.
Serious Adverse Effects
Drop in blood pressure, palpitation, seizures.

Natural Diseases or Disorders That May Be Activated by This Drug
Latent glaucoma, prostatism (see Glossary).

CAUTION
1. Discontinue this drug 4 days before diagnostic skin testing procedures in order to prevent false negative test results.
2. Do not use this drug if you have active bronchial asthma, bronchitis or

pneumonia. It can thicken bronchial mucus and make it more difficult to remove (by absorption or coughing).

Precautions for Use

By Infants and Children: This drug should not be used in premature or full-term newborn infants. Doses for children should be small. The young child is especially sensitive to the effects of antihistamines on the brain and nervous system.

By Those over 60 Years of Age: You may be more susceptible to the development of drowsiness, dizziness and unsteadiness, and to impairment of thinking, judgment and memory. This drug can increase the degree of impaired urination associated with prostate gland enlargement (prostatism). The sedative effects of antihistamines in the elderly can cause a syndrome of underactivity that may be misinterpreted as senility or emotional depression.

▷ **Advisability of Use During Pregnancy**

Pregnancy Category: C (tentative). See Pregnancy Code inside back cover.

Animal studies: No information available.

Human studies: Information from adequate studies of pregnant women is not available.

Avoid during the first 3 months. Ask your physician for guidance during the last 6 months.

Advisability of Use if Breast-Feeding

Presence of this drug in breast milk: Probably yes.

Avoid drug or refrain from nursing.

Habit-Forming Potential: None.

Effects of Overdosage: Drowsiness; unsteadiness; faintness; marked dryness of mouth, nose and throat; flushing of face; shortness of breath; hallucinations; convulsions; stupor progressing to coma.

Possible Effects of Long-Term Use: Tardive dyskinesia (see Glossary) has been reported in association with the long-term use of several widely used antihistamines. It is advisable to avoid the prolonged, continual use of antihistamines without interruption.

Suggested Periodic Examinations While Taking This Drug   (at physician's discretion)

None required.

▷ **While Taking This Drug, Observe the Following**

Foods: No restrictions.

Beverages: No restrictions. May be taken with milk.

▷   *Alcohol*: Use with extreme caution until the combined effects have been determined. The combination of antihistamine and alcohol can produce rapid and marked sedation.

Tobacco Smoking: No interactions expected.

▷ *Other Drugs*

Phenyltoloxamine may *increase* the effects of
- all sedatives, sleep-inducing drugs, tranquilizers, analgesics and narcotic drugs, and produce oversedation.

Phenyltoloxamine *taken concurrently* with
- phenytoin (Dantoin, Dilantin) may alter the pattern of epileptic seizures. Dosage adjustments may be necessary.

▷ *Driving, Hazardous Activities*: This drug may impair mental alertness, judgment, coordination and reaction time. Avoid hazardous activities until the full sedative effects have been determined.

Aviation Note: The use of this drug *is a disqualification* for piloting. Consult a designated Aviation Medical Examiner.

Exposure to Sun: Use caution. Some drugs of this class can cause photosensitivity (see Glossary).

✍ PHENYTOIN
(FEN i toh in)

Other Names: Diphenylhydantoin

Introduced: 1938	**Class:** Anticonvulsant, Hydantoins
Prescription: USA: Yes Canada: Yes	**Controlled Drug:** USA: No Canada: No

Available as Generic: USA: Yes
Canada: No

Brand Names: Dilantin, Dilantin w/Phenobarbital [CD], Diphenylan

BENEFITS versus RISKS	
Possible Benefits	*Possible Risks*
EFFECTIVE CONTROL OF TONIC-CLONIC (GRAND MAL), PSYCHOMOTOR (TEMPORAL LOBE), MYOCLONIC AND FOCAL SEIZURES IN 80% OF USERS	VERY NARROW TREATMENT MARGIN POSSIBLE BIRTH DEFECTS Overgrowth of gums Excessive hair growth Rare blood cell disorders: Impaired production of all blood cells Drug-induced hepatitis Drug-induced nephritis

▷ **Principal Uses**

As a Single Drug Product: Used primarily as an antiepileptic drug to control grand mal, psychomotor, myoclonic and focal seizures. Though not officially approved, this drug is also used to initiate treatment of trigeminal

neuralgia; it is sometimes effective in relieving the severe facial pain of
this disorder.

As a Combination Drug Product [CD]: This drug is available in combination
with phenobarbital, another effective anticonvulsant. Some seizure disorders require the combined actions of these two drugs for effective control.

How This Drug Works: Not completely established. It is thought that by promoting the loss of sodium from nerve fibers, this drug lowers and stabilizes their excitability and thereby inhibits the repetitive spread of
electrical impulses along nerve pathways. This action may prevent
seizures altogether, or it may reduce their frequency and severity.

Available Dosage Forms and Strengths
    Capsules (extended) — 30 mg, 100 mg
    Capsules (prompt) — 30 mg, 100 mg
               Injection — 50 mg per ml
        Oral suspension — 30 mg per 5 ml, 125 mg per 5 ml teaspoonful
    Tablets, chewable — 50 mg

▷ **Usual Adult Dosage Range:**   Initially, 100 mg 3 times/day. Dose may be
increased cautiously by 100 mg/week as needed and tolerated. After the
optimal maintenance dose has been determined, the total daily dose may
be taken as a single dose every 24 hours if Dilantin capsules are used. No
other formulation is approved for once-a-day use. The total daily dosage
should not exceed 600 mg. **Note: Actual dosage and administration schedule must be determined by the physician for each patient individually.**

▷ **Dosing Instructions:**   May be taken with or after food to reduce stomach irritation. The capsule may be opened and the tablet may be crushed for
administration.

Usual Duration of Use: Continual use on a regular schedule for 2 to 3 weeks is
usually necessary to determine this drug's effectiveness in reducing the
frequency and severity of seizures. Optimal control will require careful
dosage adjustments over a period of several months. Long-term use
(months to years) requires ongoing supervision and periodic evaluation
by your physician.

▷ **This Drug Should Not Be Taken If**
    • you have had an allergic reaction to this drug or to other hydantoin
      drugs previously.

▷ **Inform Your Physician Before Taking This Drug If**
    • you are taking any other drugs at this time.
    • you have a history of liver disease or impaired liver function.
    • you have low blood pressure, diabetes or any type of heart disease.
    • you plan to have surgery under general anesthesia in the near future.

Possible Side-Effects   (natural, expected and unavoidable drug actions)
    Mild fatigue, sluggishness and drowsiness (in sensitive individuals).
    Pink to red to brown coloration of urine (of no significance).

▷ **Possible Adverse Effects**   (unusual, unexpected and infrequent reactions)
   If any of the following develop, consult your physician promptly.
   Mild Adverse Effects
      Allergic Reactions: Skin rashes (5% to 10%), hives, drug fever (see Glossary).
      Headache, dizziness, nervousness, insomnia, muscle twitching.
      Nausea, vomiting, constipation.
      Overgrowth of gum tissues (most common in children).
      Excessive growth of body hair (most common in young girls).
   Serious Adverse Effects
      Allergic Reactions: Drug-induced hepatitis, with or without jaundice (see Glossary). Drug-induced nephritis, with acute kidney failure. Severe skin reactions. Generalized enlargement of lymph glands (pseudolymphoma).
      Idiosyncratic Reactions: Hemolytic anemia (see Glossary). Acute psychotic episodes (rare).
      Bone marrow depression (see Glossary): fatigue, weakness, fever, sore throat, abnormal bleeding or bruising.
      Mental confusion, unsteadiness, double vision, jerky eye movements, slurred speech.
      Joint pain and swelling.
      Elevated blood sugar, due to inhibition of insulin release.

▷ **Adverse Effects That May Mimic Natural Diseases or Disorders**
   Drug-induced hepatitis may suggest viral hepatitis.
   Skin reactions may resemble lupus erythematosus.

Natural Diseases or Disorders That May Be Activated by This Drug
   Latent diabetes, porphyria, systemic lupus erythematosus.

CAUTION
   1. Some brand name capsules of this drug have a significantly longer duration of action than generic name capsules of the same strength. To assure a correct dosing schedule, it is necessary to distinguish between "prompt" action and "extended" action capsules. Do not substitute one for the other without your physician's knowledge and guidance.
   2. When used for the treatment of epilepsy, *this drug must not be stopped abruptly.*
   3. The wide variation of this drug's action from person to person requires careful individualization of dosage schedules. Periodic measurements of blood levels of this drug can be very helpful in determining appropriate dosage. (See Therapeutic Drug Monitoring in Section One.)
   4. Regularity of drug use is essential for successful management of seizure disorders. Take this drug at the same time each day.
   5. Shake the suspension form of this drug thoroughly before measuring the dose. Use a standard measuring device to assure that the dose is based upon a 5 ml teaspoon.
   6. Side-effects and mild adverse effects are usually most apparent during the first several days of treatment, and often subside with continued use.

7. It may be necessary to take folic acid to prevent anemia while taking this drug. Consult your physician regarding this.
8. It is advisable to carry a card of personal identification with a notation that you are taking this drug.

Precautions for Use

By Infants and Children: Elimination of this drug varies widely with age. Careful monitoring by periodic measurement of blood levels is essential for all ages. Some children will require more than one dose daily for good control. Observe for early indications of drug toxicity: jerky eye movements, unsteadiness in stance and gait, slurred speech, abnormal involuntary movements of the extremities and odd behavior.

By Those over 60 Years of Age: You may be more sensitive to all of the actions of this drug and require smaller doses. Observe closely for any indications of early toxicity: drowsiness, fatigue, confusion, unsteadiness, disturbances of vision, slurred speech, muscle twitching.

▷ Advisability of Use During Pregnancy

Pregnancy Category: D (tentative). See Pregnancy Code inside back cover.

Animal studies: Cleft lip and palate, skeletal and visceral defects in mice; skeletal and visceral defects in rats.

Human studies: Available information is conflicting. Some studies suggest a small but significant increase in the occurrence of birth defects associated with the use of phenytoin during pregnancy. The incidence of birth defects in children of epileptics not taking anticonvulsant drugs is 3.2%; the incidence with the use of anticonvulsant drugs during pregnancy increases to 6.4%. The "fetal hydantoin syndrome" in the newborn infant exposed to phenytoin during pregnancy consists of birth defects of the skull, face and limbs, deficient growth and development, and subnormal intelligence and performance. Other effects on the infant include reduction in blood clotting factors that predispose it to severe bruising and hemorrhage.

Discuss with your physician the advantages and possible disadvantages of using this drug during pregnancy. It is advisable to use the smallest maintenance dose that will control seizures. In addition, you should be given vitamin K during the last month of pregnancy to prevent a deficiency of blood clotting factors in the fetus.

Advisability of Use if Breast-Feeding

Presence of this drug in breast milk: Yes, in trace amounts.

Monitor nursing infant closely and discontinue drug or nursing if adverse effects develop.

Habit-Forming Potential: None.

Effects of Overdosage: Drowsiness, jerky eye movements, hand tremor, unsteadiness, slurred speech, hallucinations, delusions, nausea, vomiting, stupor progressing to coma.

Possible Effects of Long-Term Use: Low blood calcium resulting in rickets or osteomalacia; megaloblastic anemia; peripheral neuropathy (see Glos-

sary); schizophreniclike psychosis. Lymphosarcoma, malignant lymphoma and leukemia have been associated with long-term use; a cause-and-effect relationship (see Glossary) has not been established.

Suggested Periodic Examinations While Taking This Drug (at physician's discretion)

Monitoring of blood phenytoin levels to guide dosage.

Complete blood cell counts, liver function tests.

Measurements of the following blood levels: glucose, calcium, phosphorus, folic acid, vitamin B-12.

Skeletal X-ray studies for demineralization of bone.

▷ **While Taking This Drug, Observe the Following**

Foods: No restrictions.

Nutritional Support: Supplements of folic acid, calcium, vitamin D and vitamin K may be necessary.

Beverages: No restrictions. May be taken with milk.

▷ *Alcohol*: Use extreme caution until the combined effects have been determined. Alcohol (in large quantities or with continual use) may reduce this drug's effectiveness in preventing seizures.

Tobacco Smoking: No interactions expected.

▷ *Other Drugs*

Phenytoin may *decrease* the effects of

- cortisonelike drugs (see Drug Class, Section Four).
- cyclosporine.
- doxycycline (Vibramycin, etc.).
- levodopa (Larodopa, Sinemet).
- methadone (Dolophine).
- mexiletine (Mexitil).
- oral contraceptives.
- quinidine (Quinaglute, etc.).

Phenytoin *taken concurrently* with

- oral anticoagulants (Coumadin, etc.) can either increase or decrease the anticoagulant effect; monitor this combination very closely with serial prothrombin testing.
- primidone (Mysoline) may alter primidone actions and enhance its toxicity.
- theophyllines (Aminophyllin, Theo-Dur, etc.) may cause a decrease in the effectiveness of both drugs.

The following drugs may *increase* the effects of phenytoin

- chloramphenicol (Chloromycetin).
- cimetidine (Tagamet).
- disulfiram (Antabuse).
- isoniazid (INH, Niconyl, etc.).
- phenacemide (Phenurone).
- phenylbutazone (Butazolidin).
- sulfonamides (see Drug Class, Section Four).
- trimethoprim (Proloprim, Trimpex).
- valproic acid (Depakene).

The following drugs may *decrease* the effects of phenytoin
- bleomycin.
- carmustine.
- cisplatin.
- diazoxide.
- folic acid.
- methotrexate.
- rifampin.
- vinblastine.

▷ *Driving, Hazardous Activities*: This drug may impair mental alertness, vision and coordination. Restrict activities as necessary.

Aviation Note: The use of this drug *is a disqualification* for piloting. Consult a designated Aviation Medical Examiner.

Exposure to Sun: Use caution. This drug may cause photosensitivity (see Glossary).

Occurrence of Unrelated Illness: Intercurrent infections may slow the elimination of this drug and increase the risk of toxicity due to higher blood levels.

Discontinuation: **This drug must not be discontinued abruptly**. Sudden withdrawal can precipitate severe and repeated seizures. If this drug is to be discontinued, gradual reduction in dosage should be made over a period of 3 months. Total drug withdrawal may be attempted after a period of 3 to 4 years without a seizure. However, seizures are likely to recur in 40% of adults and in 20% to 30% of children.

PILOCARPINE
(pi loh KAR peen)

Introduced: 1875

Class: Antiglaucoma

Prescription: USA: Yes
Canada: No

Controlled Drug: USA: No
Canada: No

Available as Generic: Yes

Brand Names: Almocarpine, E-Pilo Preparations, Isopto Carpine, ✤Minims, ✤Miocarpine, Ocusert Pilo-20,-40, PE Preparations [CD], Pilocar, ✤Pilopine HS, ✤P.V.Carpine

BENEFITS versus RISKS	
Possible Benefits	*Possible Risks*
EFFECTIVE REDUCTION OF INTERNAL EYE PRESSURE FOR CONTROL OF ACUTE AND CHRONIC GLAUCOMA	Mild side-effects with systemic absorption
	Minor eye discomfort
	Altered vision

▷ **Principal Uses**

As a Single Drug Product: This drug is used exclusively for the management of all types of glaucoma. Selection of the appropriate dosage form and strength must be carefully individualized.

As a Combination Drug Product [CD]: This drug is combined with epinephrine (in eye drop solutions) to utilize the actions of both drugs in lowering internal eye pressure. The opposite effects of these two drugs on the size of the pupil (pilocarpine constricts, epinephrine dilates) provides a balance that prevents excessive constriction or dilation.

How This Drug Works: By directly stimulating constriction of the pupil, this drug enlarges the outflow canal in the anterior chamber of the eye and promotes the drainage of excess fluid (aqueous humor), thus lowering the internal eye pressure.

Available Dosage Forms and Strengths

Eye drop solutions — 0.25%, 0.5%, 1%, 2%, 3%, 4%, 5%, 6%, 8%, 10%

Gel — 4%

Ocuserts — 20 mcg, 40 mcg

▷ **Usual Adult Dosage Range:** For chronic glaucoma: Eye drop solutions—1 drop of a 0.5% to 4% solution 4 times/day. Eye gel—apply 0.5 inch strip of gel into the eye once daily at bedtime. Ocusert—insert one into affected eye and replace every 7 days with a new one. **Note: Actual dosage and administration schedule must be determined by the physician for each patient individually.**

▷ **Dosing Instructions:** To avoid excessive absorption into the body, press finger against inner corner of the eye (to close off the tear duct) during and for 2 minutes following instillation of the eye drop. Place the gel and the Ocusert in the eye at bedtime.

Usual Duration of Use: Continual use on a regular schedule for 1 to 2 weeks is usually necessary to determine this drug's effectiveness in controlling internal eye pressure. Long-term use (months to years) requires supervision and periodic evaluation by your physician.

▷ **This Drug Should Not Be Taken If**
- you have had an allergic reaction to it previously.
- you have active bronchial asthma.

▷ **Inform Your Physician Before Taking This Drug If**
- you have a history of bronchial asthma.
- you have a history acute iritis.

Possible Side-Effects (natural, expected and unavoidable drug actions)
Temporary impairment of vision, usually lasting 2 to 3 hours following instillation of drops.

▷ **Possible Adverse Effects** (unusual, unexpected and infrequent reactions)
If any of the following develop, consult your physician promptly.

Mild Adverse Effects

Allergic Reactions: Itching of the eyes, itching and/or swelling of the eyelids.

Headache, heart palpitation, tremors.

Serious Adverse Effects

Provocation of acute asthma in susceptible individuals.

Precautions for Use

By Those over 60 Years of Age: Maintain personal cleanliness to prevent eye infections. Report promptly any indication of possible infection involving the eyes.

▷ **Advisability of Use During Pregnancy**

Pregnancy Category: C (tentative). See Pregnancy Code inside back cover.

Animal studies: Significant birth defects due to this drug reported in rats.

Human studies: Information from adequate studies of pregnant women is not available.

Limit use to the smallest effective dose. Minimize systemic absorption (see Dosing Instructions).

Advisability of Use if Breast-Feeding

Presence of this drug in breast milk: May be present in small amounts.

Monitor nursing infant closely and discontinue drug or nursing if adverse effects develop.

Habit-Forming Potential: None.

Effects of Overdosage: Flushing of face, increased flow of saliva, sweating. If solution is swallowed: nausea, vomiting, diarrhea, profuse sweating, rapid pulse, difficult breathing, loss of consciousness.

Possible Effects of Long-Term Use: Development of tolerance (see Glossary), temporary loss of effectiveness.

Suggested Periodic Examinations While Taking This Drug   (at physician's discretion)

Measurement of internal eye pressure on a regular basis.

Examination of eyes for development of cataracts.

▷ **While Taking This Drug, Observe the Following**

Foods: No restrictions.

Beverages: No restrictions.

▷ *Alcohol*: Use caution until the combined effect has been determined. If this drug is absorbed, it may prolong the effect of alcohol on the brain.

Tobacco Smoking: No interactions expected.

Marijuana Smoking: Sustained additional decrease in internal eye pressure.

▷ *Other Drugs*

The following drugs may *decrease* the effects of pilocarpine

- atropine and drugs with atropinelike actions (see Drug Class, Section Four).

▷ *Driving, Hazardous Activities*: This drug may impair your ability to focus your vision properly. Restrict activities as necessary.

Aviation Note: The use of this drug *may be a disqualification* for piloting. Consult a designated Aviation Medical Examiner.

Exposure to Sun: No restrictions.

Discontinuation: Do not discontinue the regular use of this drug without consulting your physician. Periodic discontinuation and temporary substitution of another drug may be necessary to preserve its effectiveness in treating glaucoma.

PINDOLOL
(PIN doh lohl)

Introduced: 1972

Class: Antihypertensive, Beta-Adrenergic Blocker

Prescription: USA: Yes
Canada: Yes

Controlled Drug: USA: No
Canada: No

Available as Generic: No

Brand Names: ✦Viskazide [CD], Visken

BENEFITS versus RISKS	
Possible Benefits	*Possible Risks*
EFFECTIVE, WELL-TOLERATED ANTIHYPERTENSIVE in mild to moderate high blood pressure	CONGESTIVE HEART FAILURE in advanced heart disease Worsening of angina in coronary heart disease (abrupt withdrawal) Masking of low blood sugar (hypoglycemia) in drug-treated diabetes Provocation of asthma (with high doses)

▷ **Principal Uses**

As a Single Drug Product: The treatment of mild to moderately severe high blood pressure. May be used alone or concurrently with other antihypertensive drugs, such as diuretics.

As a Combination Drug Product [CD]: This drug is available in combination with hydrochlorothiazide (in Canada). The addition of a thiazide diuretic to this beta-blocker drug enhances its effectiveness as an antihypertensive.

How This Drug Works: By blocking certain actions of the sympathetic nervous system, this drug

- reduces the rate and contraction force of the heart, thus lowering the ejection pressure of the blood leaving the heart.
- reduces the degree of contraction of blood vessel walls, resulting in their relaxation and expansion and consequent lowering of blood pressure.

Available Dosage Forms and Strengths
Tablets — 5 mg, 10 mg

▷ **Usual Adult Dosage Range:**   Initially, 5 mg twice daily (12 hours apart). The dose may be increased gradually by 10 mg/day at intervals of 2 to 3 weeks as needed and tolerated up to 60 mg/day. For maintenance, 5 to 10 mg 2 or 3 times/day. The total daily dose should not exceed 60 mg. **Note: Actual dosage and administration schedule must be determined by the physician for each patient individually.**

▷ **Dosing Instructions:**   May be taken without regard to eating. The tablet may be crushed for administration. Do not discontinue this drug abruptly.

Usual Duration of Use: Continual use on a regular schedule for 2 to 3 weeks is usually necessary to determine this drug's effectiveness in lowering blood pressure. The long-term use of this drug (months to years) will be determined by the course of your blood pressure over time and your response to the overall treatment program (weight reduction, salt restriction, smoking cessation, etc.).

▷ **This Drug Should Not Be Taken If**
- you have had an allergic reaction to it previously.
- you have congestive heart failure.
- you have an abnormally slow heart rate or a serious form of heart block.
- you are taking, or have taken within the past 14 days, any monoamine oxidase (MAO) inhibitor drug (see Drug Class, Section Four).

▷ **Inform Your Physician Before Taking This Drug If**
- you have had an adverse reaction to any "beta-blocker" drug in the past (see Drug Class, Section Four).
- you have a history of serious heart disease, with or without episodes of heart failure.
- you have a history of hay fever (allergic rhinitis), asthma, chronic bronchitis or emphysema.
- you have a history of overactive thyroid function (hyperthyroidism).
- you have a history of low blood sugar (hypoglycemia).
- you have impaired liver or kidney function.
- you have diabetes or myasthenia gravis.
- you are currently taking any form of digitalis, quinidine or reserpine, or any "calcium-blocker" drug (see Drug Class, Section Four).
- you plan to have surgery under general anesthesia in the near future.

Possible Side-Effects   (natural, expected and unavoidable drug actions)
Lethargy and fatigability (15%), cold extremities, slow heart rate, lightheadedness in upright position (see orthostatic hypotension in Glossary).

▷ **Possible Adverse Effects**   (unusual, unexpected and infrequent reactions)
If any of the following develop, consult your physician promptly.
Mild Adverse Effects
Allergic Reactions: Skin rash, itching.
Headache (5%), dizziness (17%), insomnia (19%), abnormal dreams.

Indigestion, nausea (7%), vomiting, constipation, diarrhea.

Joint and muscle discomfort (11%), fluid retention (edema) (11%).

Serious Adverse Effects

Mental depression, anxiety, impotence (rare).

Chest pain, shortness of breath, precipitation of congestive heart failure.

Induction of bronchial asthma (in asthmatic individuals).

CAUTION

1. ***Do not discontinue this drug suddenly*** without the knowledge and guidance of your physician. Carry a notation on your person that you are taking this drug.
2. Consult your physician or pharmacist before using nasal decongestants usually present in over-the-counter cold preparations and nose drops. These can cause sudden increases in blood pressure when taken concurrently with beta-blocker drugs.
3. Report the development of any tendency to emotional depression.

Precautions for Use

By Infants and Children: Safety and effectiveness for use by those under 12 years of age have not been established. However, if this drug is used, observe for the development of low blood sugar (hypoglycemia) during periods of reduced food intake.

By Those over 60 Years of Age: Proceed *cautiously* with all antihypertensive drugs. Unacceptably high blood pressure should be reduced without creating the risks associated with excessively low blood pressure. Start treatment with small doses, and monitor the blood pressure response frequently. Sudden, rapid and excessive reduction of blood pressure can predispose to stroke or heart attack. Observe for dizziness, unsteadiness, tendency to fall, confusion, hallucinations, depression or urinary frequency.

▷ **Advisability of Use During Pregnancy**

Pregnancy Category: B (tentative). See Pregnancy Code inside back cover.

Animal studies: No significant increase in birth defects due to this drug.

Human studies: Information from adequate studies of pregnant women is not available.

Use this drug only if clearly needed. Ask physician for guidance.

Advisability of Use if Breast-Feeding

Presence of this drug in breast milk: Yes.

Avoid drug or refrain from nursing.

Habit-Forming Potential: None.

Effects of Overdosage: Weakness, slow pulse, low blood pressure, fainting, cold and sweaty skin, congestive heart failure, possible coma and convulsions.

Possible Effects of Long-Term Use: Reduced heart reserve and eventual heart failure in susceptible individuals with advanced heart disease.

Suggested Periodic Examinations While Taking This Drug (at physician's discretion)

Measurements of blood pressure, evaluation of heart function.

▷ **While Taking This Drug, Observe the Following**

Foods: No restrictions. Avoid excessive salt intake.

Beverages: No restrictions. May be taken with milk.

▷ *Alcohol*: Use with caution until the combined effect has been determined. Alcohol may exaggerate this drug's ability to lower the blood pressure and may increase its mild sedative effect.

Tobacco Smoking: Nicotine may reduce this drug's effectiveness in treating high blood pressure. In addition, high doses of this drug may potentiate the constriction of the bronchial tubes caused by regular smoking.

▷ *Other Drugs*

Pindolol may *increase* the effects of

- other antihypertensive drugs, and cause excessive lowering of the blood pressure. Dosage adjustments may be necessary.
- reserpine (Ser-Ap-Es, etc.), and cause sedation, depression, slowing of the heart rate and lowering of the blood pressure.
- verapamil (Calan, Isoptin), and cause excessive depression of heart function; monitor this combination closely.

Pindolol *taken concurrently* with

- clonidine (Catapres) requires close monitoring for rebound high blood pressure if clonidine is withdrawn while pindolol is still being taken.
- insulin requires close monitoring to avoid undetected hypoglycemia (see Glossary).

The following drugs may *increase* the effects of pindolol

- cimetidine (Tagamet).
- methimazole (Tapazole).
- oral contraceptives.
- propylthiouracil (Propacil).

The following drugs may *decrease* the effects of pindolol

- barbiturates (phenobarbital, etc.).
- indomethacin (Indocin), and possibly other "aspirin substitutes," may impair pindolol's antihypertensive effect.
- rifampin (Rifadin, Rimactane).

▷ *Driving, Hazardous Activities*: Use caution until the full extent of fatigue, dizziness and blood pressure change have been determined.

Aviation Note: The use of this drug *is a disqualification* for piloting. Consult a designated Aviation Medical Examiner.

Exposure to Sun: No restrictions.

Exposure to Heat: Caution advised. Hot environments can lower the blood pressure and exaggerate the effects of this drug.

Exposure to Cold: Caution advised. Cold environments can enhance the circulatory deficiency in the extremities that may occur with this drug. The elderly should take precautions to prevent hypothermia (see Glossary).

Heavy Exercise or Exertion: It is advisable to avoid exertion that produces

light-headedness, excessive fatigue or muscle cramping. The use of this
drug may intensify the hypertensive response to isometric exercise.

Occurrence of Unrelated Illness: The fever that accompanies systemic infections can lower the blood pressure and require adjustment of dosage.
Illnesses that cause nausea or vomiting may interrupt the regular dosage
schedule. Ask your physician for guidance.

Discontinuation: It is advisable to avoid sudden discontinuation of this drug
in all situations. If possible, gradual reduction of dose over a period of 2
to 3 weeks is recommended. Ask your physician for specific guidance.

PIROXICAM
(peer OX i kam)

Introduced: 1978

Class: Mild Analgesic, Anti-
inflammatory

Prescription: USA: Yes
Canada: Yes

Controlled Drug: USA: No
Canada: No

Available as Generic: No

Brand Names: Feldene

BENEFITS versus RISKS

Possible Benefits	*Possible Risks*
EFFECTIVE RELIEF OF MILD TO MODERATE PAIN AND INFLAMMATION	Gastrointestinal pain, ulceration, bleeding (rare)
	Drug-induced hepatitis (rare)
	Rare kidney damage
	Mild fluid retention
	Reduced white blood cell and platelet counts

▷ **Principal Uses**

As a Single Drug Product: Used primarily to relieve mild to moderately severe
pain and inflammation associated with (1) rheumatoid arthritis, (2)
osteoarthritis and (3) acute and chronic gout.

How This Drug Works: Not completely established. It is thought that this
drug suppresses the formation of prostaglandins (and related compounds), chemicals involved in the production of inflammation and pain.

Available Dosage Forms and Strengths
Capsules — 10 mg, 20 mg

▷ **Usual Adult Dosage Range:** As antiarthritic: 10 mg twice daily, 12 hours
apart; or 20 mg once daily. The total daily dosage should not exceed 40
mg, and then for no more than 5 days. **Note: Actual dosage and adminis-**

tration schedule must be determined by the physician for each patient individually.

▷ **Dosing Instructions:** Take with or following food to prevent stomach irritation. Take with a full glass of water and remain upright (do not lie down) for 30 minutes. The capsule may be opened for administration.

Usual Duration of Use: Continual use on a regular schedule for 2 weeks is usually necessary to determine this drug's effectiveness in relieving the discomfort of arthritis. Long-term use (months to years) requires supervision and periodic evaluation by your physician.

▷ **This Drug Should Not Be Taken If**
- you have had an allergic reaction to it previously.
- you are subject to asthma or nasal polyps caused by aspirin.
- you have active peptic ulcer disease or any form of gastrointestinal bleeding.
- you have a bleeding disorder or a blood cell disorder.
- you have active liver disease.
- you have severe impairment of kidney function.

▷ **Inform Your Physician Before Taking This Drug If**
- you are allergic to aspirin or to other aspirin substitutes.
- you have a history of peptic ulcer disease, regional enteritis or ulcerative colitis.
- you have a history of any type of bleeding disorder.
- you have impaired liver or kidney function.
- you have high blood pressure or a history of heart failure.
- you are taking any of the following: acetaminophen, aspirin or other aspirin substitutes, anticoagulants, oral antidiabetic drugs.
- you plan to have surgery of any type in the near future.

Possible Side-Effects   (natural, expected and unavoidable drug actions)
Fluid retention (weight gain), prolongation of bleeding time.

▷ **Possible Adverse Effects**   (unusual, unexpected and infrequent reactions)
If any of the following develop, consult your physician promptly.
Mild Adverse Effects
Allergic Reactions: Skin rash, itching, spontaneous bruising.
Headache, dizziness, altered or blurred vision, ringing in the ears, drowsiness, fatigue, inability to concentrate.
Indigestion, nausea, vomiting, abdominal pain, diarrhea.
Serious Adverse Effects
Active peptic ulcer, stomach or intestinal bleeding.
Drug-induced liver damage.
Kidney damage with painful urination, bloody urine, reduced urine formation.
Rare bone marrow depression (see Glossary): fatigue, weakness, fever, sore throat, abnormal bleeding or bruising.

Possible Delayed Adverse Effects
Mild anemia due to "silent" blood loss from the stomach (less than that caused by aspirin).

▷ **Adverse Effects That May Mimic Natural Diseases or Disorders**
Liver reaction may suggest viral hepatitis.

Natural Diseases or Disorders That May Be Activated by This Drug
Peptic ulcer disease, ulcerative colitis.

CAUTION
1. Dosage should always be limited to the smallest amount that produces reasonable improvement.
2. This drug may mask early indications of infection. Inform your physician if you think you are developing an infection of any kind.

Precautions for Use
By Infants and Children: Indications and dosage recommendations for use by those under 12 years of age have not been established.
By Those over 60 Years of Age: Small doses are advisable until tolerance is determined. Observe for any indications of liver or kidney toxicity, fluid retention, dizziness, confusion, impaired memory, stomach bleeding or constipation.

▷ **Advisability of Use During Pregnancy**
Pregnancy Category: B (tentative). See Pregnancy Code inside back cover.
Animal studies: No birth defects reported due to this drug.
Human studies: Information from adequate studies of pregnant women is not available.
The manufacturer does not recommend the use of this drug during pregnancy.

Advisability of Use if Breast-Feeding
Presence of this drug in breast milk: Unknown.
Avoid drug or refrain from nursing.

Habit-Forming Potential: None.

Effects of Overdosage: Possible drowsiness, dizziness, ringing in the ears, nausea, vomiting, indigestion.

Possible Effects of Long-Term Use: Development of anemia due to "silent" bleeding from the gastrointestinal tract.

Suggested Periodic Examinations While Taking This Drug (at physician's discretion)
Complete blood cell counts, liver and kidney function tests.
Complete eye examinations if vision is altered in any way.
Hearing examinations if ringing in the ears or hearing loss develops.

▷ **While Taking This Drug, Observe the Following**
Foods: No restrictions.
Beverages: No restrictions. May be taken with milk.

▷ *Alcohol*: Use with caution. The irritant action of alcohol on the stomach lining, added to the irritant action of this drug in sensitive individuals, can increase the risk of stomach ulceration and/or bleeding.

Tobacco Smoking: No interactions expected.

▷ *Other Drugs*

Piroxicam may *increase* the effects of

- acetaminophen (Tylenol, etc.), and increase the risk of kidney damage; avoid prolonged use of this combination.
- anticoagulants (Coumadin, etc.), and increase the risk of bleeding; monitor prothrombin time, adjust dose accordingly.

Piroxicam *taken concurrently* with the following drugs may increase the risk of bleeding; avoid these combinations:

- aspirin.
- dipyridamole (Persantine).
- indomethacin (Indocin).
- sulfinpyrazone (Anturane).
- valproic acid (Depakene).

▷ *Driving, Hazardous Activities*: This drug may cause drowsiness or dizziness. Restrict activities as necessary.

Aviation Note: The use of this drug *may be a disqualification* for piloting. Consult a designated Aviation Medical Examiner.

Exposure to Sun: No restrictions.

POTASSIUM
(poh TAS ee um)

Introduced: 1939

Class: Potassium Preparations

Prescription: USA: Yes
   Canada: No

Controlled Drug: USA: No
   Canada: No

Available as Generic: Yes

Brand Names: ❦Apo-K, Kaochlor, Kaochlor-Eff, Kaon, Kaon-Cl, Kay Ciel, K-Lor, Klorvess, Klotrix, K-Lyte, K-Lyte/Cl, K-Tab, Micro-K, ❦Micro-K Extencaps, ❦Neo-K, SK-Potassium Chloride, Slow-K

BENEFITS versus RISKS

Possible Benefits	*Possible Risks*
EFFECTIVE PREVENTION AND TREATMENT OF POTASSIUM DEFICIENCY (HYPOKALEMIA)	DEVELOPMENT OF EXCESSIVE POTASSIUM (HYPERKALEMIA) Ulceration and perforation of stomach or intestine with use of slow-release or enteric-coated tablets (these forms no longer recommended)

▷ **Principal Uses**

As a Single Drug Product: This drug is used primarily in conjunction with those diuretics that cause excessive loss of potassium from the body. Potassium preparations are usually given to stabilize the blood level within the normal range. Dosage adjustments may be necessary from time to time.

How This Drug Works: By maintaining or replenishing the normal potassium content of cells, this drug preserves or restores such normal cellular functions as the transmission of nerve impulses, the contraction of muscle fibers, the regulation of kidney function and the secretion of stomach juices.

Available Dosage Forms and Strengths

Capsules, prolonged action — 8 mEq, 10 mEq

Elixirs — 10 mEq, 20 mEq, 40 mEq per 15 ml tablespoonful

Liquids — 15 mEq, 20 mEq, 30 mEq, 45 mEq per 15 ml tablespoonful

Powders — 15 mEq per packet, 20 mEq per packet, 25 mEq per packet

Tablets — 2 mEq, 2.5 mEq, 5 mEq

Tablets, chewable — 1 mEq, 2.5 mEq

Tablets, effervescent — 20 mEq, 25 mEq, 50 mEq

Tablets, enteric-coated — 4 mEq

Tablets, wax matrix — 6.7 mEq, 8 mEq, 10 mEq

▷ **Usual Adult Dosage Range:** Depends upon the dosage form prescribed. Follow your physician's prescribed dose exactly. **Note: Actual dosage and administration schedule must be determined by the physician for each patient individually.**

▷ **Dosing Instructions:** Take each dose with food or immediately following a meal to reduce stomach irritation. Regular tablets should be swallowed whole. Soluble tablets and powders should be dissolved completely in 4 ounces of cold water or juice and sipped slowly over a period of 5 to 10 minutes. Liquid forms should be diluted in 4 ounces of water or juice. The prolonged action capsules should be swallowed whole and not opened for administration. Wax matrix and enteric-coated tablets are not recommended because of their potential for causing localized erosion and ulceration of gastrointestinal tissues.

Usual Duration of Use: This must be determined by your physician. Periods of use will depend upon your concurrent use of diuretics, the potassium content of your diet and periodic measurement of your blood potassium level.

▷ **This Drug Should Not Be Taken If**
- you have had an allergic reaction to it previously.
- you have severe impairment of kidney function.

- you are taking any drug that contains amiloride, spironolactone or triamterene.

▷ **Inform Your Physician Before Taking This Drug If**
- you are taking any of the following: a cortisonelike drug, a digitalis preparation, a diuretic (see Drug Classes, Section Four).
- you have Addison's disease (adrenal gland deficiency).
- you have diabetes or any form of heart disease.
- you have a history of kidney disease or impaired kidney function.
- you have a history of familial periodic paralysis.

Possible Side-Effects   (natural, expected and unavoidable drug actions)
A mild laxative effect for some individuals.

▷ **Possible Adverse Effects**   (unusual, unexpected and infrequent reactions)
If any of the following develop, consult your physician promptly.
Mild Adverse Effects
Nausea, vomiting, abdominal discomfort, diarrhea. (These usually occur if potassium is taken undiluted or on an empty stomach.)
Serious Adverse Effects
Potassium accumulation, resulting in abnormally high blood levels. Immediate treatment is mandatory.
Potassium in enteric-coated tablets or slow-release (wax matrix) tablets can cause ulceration of the stomach or intestine with risk of bleeding and/or perforation.

CAUTION
1. Dosage must be carefully individualized. Periodic evaluation of overall condition and blood potassium levels is essential to safe and effective management. Excessively high blood levels of potassium can occur without warning. Do not exceed the prescribed dose.
2. Inform your physician promptly if you are taking a tablet form of this drug and you become aware of any difficulty in swallowing.
3. If you have chronic constipation, it is advisable that you avoid potassium in tablet form.
4. Some salt substitutes contain a large amount of potassium. If you are using a salt substitute, consult your physician regarding its continued use or any necessary adjustment in the dosage of your potassium preparation.

Precautions for Use
By Those over 60 Years of Age: Your potassium balance must be maintained within strict limitations. Serious adverse effects can occur when the potassium level is either above or below the normal range. Adhere to your dosage schedule exactly.

▷ **Advisability of Use During Pregnancy**
Pregnancy Category: A (tentative). See Pregnancy Code inside back cover.
Animal studies: No information available.

Human studies: Information from adequate studies of pregnant women is not available.

Potassium is a normal and essential constituent of body tissues. Potassium preparations can be used safely during pregnancy. Adhere strictly to prescribed dosage schedules.

Advisability of Use if Breast-Feeding

Presence of this drug in breast milk: Yes.

Monitor nursing infant closely and discontinue drug or nursing if adverse effects develop.

Habit-Forming Potential: None.

Effects of Overdosage: Lethargy, weakness and heaviness of legs, numbness and tingling in the extremities, confusion, irregular heart rhythm, drop in blood pressure, seizures, coma, heart arrest.

Possible Effects of Long-Term Use: Reduced absorption of vitamin B-12, resulting in anemia in some individuals.

Suggested Periodic Examinations While Taking This Drug (at physician's discretion)

Measurement of blood potassium levels.

▷ **While Taking This Drug, Observe the Following**

Foods: No restrictions. Consult your physician regarding any special modifications of your diet.

Beverages: No restrictions.

▷ *Alcohol*: No interactions expected.

Tobacco Smoking: No interactions expected.

▷ *Other Drugs*

Potassium *taken concurrently* with

- amiloride, spironolactone or triamterene may cause an excessive rise in blood potassium levels. This can be extremely dangerous; avoid the concurrent use of these diuretics and any form of potassium.
- digitalis preparations requires very careful monitoring of dosage and heart status.

▷ *Driving, Hazardous Activities:* No restrictions.

Aviation Note: The use of this drug *may be a disqualification* for piloting. Consult a designated Aviation Medical Examiner.

Exposure to Sun: No restrictions.

Discontinuation: Do not discontinue this drug suddenly if you are taking digitalis. Ask your physician for guidance if you find it necessary to discontinue potassium medication for any reason.

PRAZEPAM
(PRA ze pam)

Introduced: 1969

Class: Mild Tranquilizer, Benzodiazepines

Prescription: USA: Yes

Controlled Drug: USA: C-IV*

Available as Generic: USA: No

Brand Names: Centrax

BENEFITS versus RISKS

Possible Benefits	*Possible Risks*
RELIEF OF ANXIETY AND NERVOUS TENSION in 70% to 80% of users	Habit-forming potential with prolonged use
Wide margin of safety with therapeutic doses	Minor impairment of mental functions
Very few drug interactions	

▷ **Principal Uses**

   As a Single Drug Product: Used primarily to (1) provide short-term relief of mild to moderate anxiety; (2) relieve the symptoms of acute alcohol withdrawal: agitation, tremors, hallucinations, incipient delirium tremens.

How This Drug Works: It is thought that this drug produces a calming effect by enhancing the action of the nerve transmitter gamma-aminobutyric acid (GABA), which in turn blocks the arousal of higher brain centers.

Available Dosage Forms and Strengths
   Capsules — 5 mg, 10 mg, 20 mg
   Tablets — 10 mg

▷ **Usual Adult Dosage Range:**   20 to 60 mg/24 hours, in 3 or 4 divided doses. The total daily dosage should not exceed 60 mg. **Note: Actual dosage and administration schedule must be determined by the physician for each patient individually.**

▷ **Dosing Instructions:**   May be taken on empty stomach or with food or milk as needed to prevent stomach irritation. The tablet may be crushed and the capsule may be opened for administration. Do not discontinue this drug abruptly if taken for more than 4 weeks.

Usual Duration of Use: Continual use on a regular schedule for 3 to 5 days is usually necessary to determine this drug's effectiveness in relieving moderate anxiety. Limit continual use to 1 to 3 weeks. Avoid uninterrupted and prolonged use.

*See Schedules of Controlled Drugs inside back cover.

▷ **This Drug Should Not Be Taken If**
  • you have had an allergic reaction to any dosage form of it previously.
  • you have acute narrow-angle glaucoma.
  • it is prescribed for a child under 18 years of age.

▷ **Inform Your Physician Before Taking This Drug If**
  • you are allergic to any benzodiazepine drug (see Drug Class, Section Four).
  • you have a history of alcoholism or drug abuse.
  • you are pregnant or planning pregnancy.
  • you have impaired liver or kidney function.
  • you have a history of serious depression or mental disorder.
  • you have any of the following: asthma, emphysema, epilepsy, myasthenia gravis.
  • you are taking any drugs with sedative effects.

Possible Side-Effects (natural, expected and unavoidable drug actions)
  Drowsiness (6%), lethargy (11%), unsteadiness (5%), "hangover" effects on the day following bedtime use.

▷ **Possible Adverse Effects** (unusual, unexpected and infrequent reactions)
  If any of the following develop, consult your physician promptly.
  Mild Adverse Effects
  Allergic Reactions: Skin rashes, hives, itching.
  Dizziness (8%), fainting, weakness (7%), confusion, blurred vision, double vision, slurred speech, sweating, nausea.
  Serious Adverse Effects
  Paradoxical responses of excitement, agitation, anger, rage.

CAUTION
  1. This drug should not be discontinued abruptly if it has been taken continually for more than 4 weeks.
  2. The concurrent use of some over-the-counter drug products that contain antihistamines (allergy and cold preparations, sleep aids) can cause excessive sedation in sensitive individuals.

Precautions for Use
  By Infants and Children: Safety and effectiveness for use by those under 18 years of age have not been established. This drug should not be used in the hyperactive or psychotic child of any age. Observe for excessive sedation and incoordination.
  By Those over 60 Years of Age: It is advisable to use smaller doses at longer intervals to avoid overdosage. Observe for the possible development of lethargy, indifference, fatigue, weakness, unsteadiness, disturbing dreams, nightmares and paradoxical reactions of excitement, agitation, anger, hostility and rage.

▷ **Advisability of Use During Pregnancy**
  Pregnancy Category: C (tentative). See Pregnancy Code inside back cover.
  Animal studies: No information available.
  Human studies: Information from adequate studies of pregnant women is

not available. No birth defects have been reported with the use of this drug. However, available information regarding the use of other drugs of this class (benzodiazepines) is conflicting and inconclusive. Some studies found an increase in serious birth defects associated with the use of 2 benzodiazepines. Other studies have found no significant increase in birth defects.

Frequent use in late pregnancy can cause the "floppy infant" syndrome in the newborn: weakness, lethargy, unresponsiveness, depressed breathing, low body temperature.

Avoid use during entire pregnancy if possible.

Advisability of Use if Breast-Feeding
Presence of this drug in breast milk: Probably yes.
Avoid drug or refrain from nursing.

Habit-Forming Potential: This drug can produce psychological and/or physical dependence (see Glossary) if used in large doses for an extended period of time.

Effects of Overdosage: Marked drowsiness, weakness, feeling of drunkenness, staggering gait, tremor, stupor progressing to deep sleep or coma.

Possible Effects of Long-Term Use: Psychological and/or physical dependence.

Suggested Periodic Examinations While Taking This Drug (at physician's discretion)
Complete blood cell counts during long-term use.

▷ **While Taking This Drug, Observe the Following**
Foods: No restrictions.
Beverages: Avoid excessive intake of caffeine-containing beverages: coffee, tea, cola. May be taken with milk.
▷ *Alcohol*: Use with extreme caution until the combined effect has been determined. Alcohol may increase the depressant effects of this drug on the brain. It is advisable to avoid alcohol completely—throughout the day and night—if it is necessary to drive or to engage in any hazardous activity.
Tobacco Smoking: Heavy smoking may reduce the calming action of this drug.
Marijuana Smoking: Increased sedation and significant impairment of intellectual and physical performance.
▷ *Other Drugs*
The following drugs may *increase* the effects of prazepam
- cimetidine (Tagamet).
- disulfiram (Antabuse).
- oral contraceptives.
▷ *Driving, Hazardous Activities*: This drug can impair mental alertness, judgment, physical coordination and reaction time. Avoid hazardous activities accordingly.

Aviation Note: The use of this drug *is a disqualification* for piloting. Consult a designated Aviation Medical Examiner.

Exposure to Sun: No restrictions.

Exposure to Heat: Use caution until the effect of excessive perspiration is determined. Because of reduced urine volume, this drug may accumulate in the body and produce effects of overdosage.

Exposure to Cold: The elderly should dress warmly and avoid situations and environments conducive to hypothermia (see Glossary).

Discontinuation: Avoid sudden discontinuation if this drug has been taken for over 4 weeks without interruption. Dosage should be tapered gradually to prevent a withdrawal syndrome that could include depression, confusion, hallucinations, tremor, seizures, muscle cramping, sweating and vomiting.

PRAZOSIN
(PRA zoh sin)

Introduced: 1970

Prescription: USA: Yes
Canada: Yes

Available as Generic: No

Class: Antihypertensive

Controlled Drug: USA: No
Canada: No

Brand Names: Minipress, Minizide [CD]

BENEFITS versus RISKS

Possible Benefits	*Possible Risks*
EFFECTIVE "STEP 2 OR 3" ANTIHYPERTENSIVE IN 60% TO 70% OF CASES OF MILD TO SEVERE HYPERTENSION when used adjunctively with other antihypertensive drugs	"First dose" drop in blood pressure with fainting (1%)
EFFECTIVE CONTROL OF HYPERTENSION IN PHEOCHROMOCYTOMA	Induction of paroxysmal tachycardia (rare)
Effective in presence of impaired kidney function	

▷ **Principal Uses**

As a Single Drug Product: Used primarily as a "step 2" or "step 3" antihypertensive drug, in conjunction with other drugs, to treat moderate to severe hypertension.

As a Combination Drug Product [CD]: This drug is available in combination with polythiazide, a diuretic of the thiazide class of drugs that are usually used as "step 1" medications to initiate treatment for hypertension. By utilizing two different methods of drug action, this combination product is more effective and more convenient for long-term use.

How This Drug Works: It is thought that by blocking certain actions of the sympathetic nervous system, this drug causes direct relaxation and expansion of blood vessel walls, thus lowering the pressure of the blood within the vessels.

Available Dosage Forms and Strengths
Capsules — 1 mg, 2 mg, 5 mg

▷ **Usual Adult Dosage Range:** Initiate treatment with a "test dose" of 1 mg to determine the patient's response within the first 2 hours. If tolerated satisfactorily, increase dose cautiously up to 15 mg/24 hours in 2 or 3 divided doses. The total daily dosage should not exceed 20 mg. **Note: Actual dosage and administration schedule must be determined by the physician for each patient individually.**

▷ **Dosing Instructions:** May be taken without regard to eating. The capsule may be opened for administration.

Usual Duration of Use: Continual use on a regular schedule for 4 to 6 weeks is usually necessary to determine this drug's effectiveness in controlling hypertension. Long-term use (months to years) requires supervision and periodic evaluation by your physician.

▷ **This Drug Should Not Be Taken If**
- you have had an allergic reaction to it previously.
- you are experiencing mental depression.
- you have angina (active coronary artery disease) and you are not taking a beta-blocking drug.

▷ **Inform Your Physician Before Taking This Drug If**
- you have experienced orthostatic hypotension (see Glossary) when using other antihypertensive drugs.
- you have a history of mental depression.
- you have impaired circulation to the brain, or a history of stroke.
- you have coronary artery disease.
- you have active liver disease or impaired liver function.
- you plan to have surgery under general anesthesia in the near future.

Possible Side-Effects   (natural, expected and unavoidable drug actions)
Orthostatic hypotension, drowsiness (7%), salt and water retention, dry mouth, nasal congestion, constipation.

▷ **Possible Adverse Effects**   (unusual, unexpected and infrequent reactions)
If any of the following develop, consult your physician promptly.
Mild Adverse Effects
Allergic Reactions: Skin rash, itching.

Headache (7.8%), dizziness (10.3%), fatigue (6.9%), weakness (6.5%), nervousness, sweating, numbness and tingling, blurred vision, reddened eyes, ringing in the ears.

Palpitation (5.3%), rapid heart rate, shortness of breath.

Nausea (4.9%), vomiting, diarrhea, abdominal pain.

Urinary frequency and incontinence.

Serious Adverse Effects

Mental depression, sleep disturbance.

Paroxysmal tachycardia (heart rates of 120 to 160).

Sexual impotence (less than 1%); painful erection of penis.

Natural Diseases or Disorders That May Be Activated by This Drug

Latent coronary artery insufficiency.

CAUTION

1. Observe for the possible "first dose" response of precipitous drop in blood pressue, with or without fainting; this usually occurs within 30 to 90 minutes. Limit initial doses to 1 mg taken at bedtime for the first 3 days; remain supine after taking these trial doses.
2. Impaired kidney function may increase your sensitivity to this drug and require smaller than usual doses.

Precautions for Use

By Infants and Children: Safety and effectiveness for use by those under 12 years of age have not been established.

By Those over 60 Years of Age: Begin treatment with no more than 1 mg/day for the first 3 days. Subsequent increases in dose must be very gradual and carefully supervised by your physician. The occurrence of orthostatic hypotension can cause unexpected falls and injury; sit or lie down promptly if you feel light-headed or dizzy. Report any indications of dizziness or chest pain promptly.

▷ Advisability of Use During Pregnancy

Pregnancy Category: B (tentative). See Pregnancy Code inside back cover.

Animal studies: No birth defects found.

Human studies: Information from adequate studies of pregnant women is not available.

Use this drug only if clearly needed. Ask your physician for guidance.

Advisability of Use if Breast-Feeding

Presence of this drug in breast milk: Yes.

Monitor nursing infant closely and discontinue drug or nursing if adverse effects develop.

Habit-Forming Potential: None.

Effects of Overdosage: Orthostatic hypotension, headache, generalized flushing, rapid heart rate, extreme weakness, irregular heart rhythm, circulatory collapse.

Possible Effects of Long-Term Use: None reported.

Suggested Periodic Examinations While Taking This Drug   (at physician's
   discretion)
   Measurements of blood pressure in lying, sitting and standing positions.
   Measurements of body weight to detect fluid retention.

▷ **While Taking This Drug, Observe the Following**
   Foods: No restrictions. Avoid excessive salt intake.
   Beverages: No restrictions. May be taken with milk.
▷   *Alcohol*: Use with extreme caution until the combined effects have been
      determined. Alcohol can exaggerate the blood-pressure-lowering actions
      of this drug and cause excessive reduction.
   Tobacco Smoking: Nicotine can contribute significantly to this drug's ability
      to intensify coronary insufficiency in susceptible individuals. All forms of
      tobacco should be avoided.
▷   *Other Drugs*
      The following drugs may *increase* the effects of prazosin
      • beta-adrenergic blocking drugs (see Drug Class, Section Four); the sever-
        ity and duration of the "first dose" hypotensive response may be
        increased.
▷   *Driving, Hazardous Activities*: This drug may cause dizziness or drowsiness.
      Restrict activities as necessary.
   Aviation Note: The use of this drug *is a disqualification* for piloting. Consult a
      designated Aviation Medical Examiner.
   Exposure to Sun: No restrictions.
   Exposure to Cold: Use caution until combined effect has been determined.
      Cold environments may increase this drug's ability to cause coronary
      insufficiency (angina) in susceptible individuals.
   Heavy Exercise or Exertion: Excessive exertion can augment this drug's abil-
      ity to induce angina. See Profile of Angina in Section Two.
   Discontinuation: If you are taking this drug as part of your treatment pro-
      gram for congestive heart failure, do not discontinue it abruptly. Ask
      your physician for guidance.

PREDNISOLONE
(pred NIS oh lohn)

Introduced: 1955

Class: Cortisonelike Drugs

Prescription: USA: Yes
   Canada: Yes

Controlled Drug: USA: No
   Canada: No

Available as Generic: USA: Yes
   Canada: Yes

Brand Names: Delta-Cortef, Fernisolone-P, ✦Inflamase, ✦Inflamase Forte,
   ✦Nova-Pred, ✦Novoprednisolone, ✦Pred Forte, ✦Pred Mild, Sterane

```
┌─────────────────────────────────────────────────────────────────┐
│                    BENEFITS versus RISKS                          │
│                                                                   │
│      Possible Benefits                  Possible Risks            │
│   EFFECTIVE RELIEF OF           Short-term use (up to 10 days) is  │
│     SYMPTOMS IN A WIDE            usually well tolerated. Long-term│
│     VARIETY OF INFLAMMATORY       use (exceeding 2 weeks) is       │
│     AND ALLERGIC DISORDERS        associated with many possible    │
│   EFFECTIVE IMMUNO-               adverse effects:                 │
│     SUPPRESSION in selected     ALTERED MOOD AND                   │
│     benign and malignant disorders  PERSONALITY                   │
│   Prevention of rejection in organ  CATARACTS, GLAUCOMA            │
│     transplantation             HYPERTENSION                       │
│                                 OSTEOPOROSIS                       │
│                                 ASEPTIC BONE NECROSIS              │
│                                 INCREASED SUSCEPTIBILITY TO        │
│                                   INFECTIONS                       │
│                                 (See Possible Adverse Effects and  │
│                                   Possible Effects of Long-Term    │
│                                   Use below)                       │
└─────────────────────────────────────────────────────────────────┘
```

▷ **Principal Uses**

As a Single Drug Product: This potent drug of the cortisone class is used in the treatment of a wide variety of allergic and inflammatory conditions. It is used most commonly in the management of serious skin disorders, asthma, regional enteritis, ulcerative colitis and all types of major rheumatic disorders including bursitis, tendinitis and most forms of arthritis.

How This Drug Works: Not fully established. It is thought that this drug's anti-inflammatory effect is due to its ability to inhibit the normal defensive functions of certain white blood cells. Its immunosuppressant effect is attributed to a reduced production of lymphocytes and antibodies.

Available Dosage Forms and Strengths
Tablets — 1 mg, 5 mg

▷ **Usual Adult Dosage Range:**   5 to 60 mg daily as a single dose or in divided doses. The total daily dosage should not exceed 250 mg. **Note: Actual dosage and administration schedule must be determined by the physician for each patient individually.**

▷ **Dosing Instructions:**   Take with or following food to prevent stomach irritation, preferably in the morning. The tablet may be crushed for administration.

Usual Duration of Use: For acute disorders: 4 to 10 days. For chronic disorders: according to individual requirements. The duration of use should not exceed the time necessary to obtain adequate symptomatic relief in acute self-limiting conditions; or the time required to stabilize a chronic condition and permit gradual withdrawal. Because of its intermediate duration of action, this drug is appropriate for alternate day administration.

▷ **This Drug Should Not Be Taken If**
- you have had an allergic reaction to any dosage form of it previously.
- you have active peptic ulcer disease.
- you have an active infection of the eye caused by the herpes simplex virus.
- you have active tuberculosis.

▷ **Inform Your Physician Before Taking This Drug If**
- you have had an unfavorable reaction to any cortisonelike drug in the past.
- you have a history of peptic ulcer disease, thrombophlebitis or tuberculosis.
- you have any of the following: diabetes, glaucoma, high blood pressure, deficient thyroid function or myasthenia gravis.
- you plan to have surgery of any kind in the near future.

Possible Side-Effects   (natural, expected and unavoidable drug actions)

Increased appetite, weight gain, retention of salt and water, excretion of potassium, increased susceptibility to infection.

▷ **Possible Adverse Effects**   (unusual, unexpected and infrequent reactions)
If any of the following develop, consult your physician promptly.

Mild Adverse Effects

Allergic Reactions: Skin rash.

Headache, dizziness, insomnia.

Acid indigestion, abdominal distention.

Muscle cramping and weakness.

Irregular or altered menstruation.

Acne, excessive growth of facial hair.

Serious Adverse Effects

Mental and emotional disturbances of serious magnitude.

Reactivation of latent tuberculosis.

Development of peptic ulcer.

Increased blood pressure.

Development of inflammation of the pancreas.

Thrombophlebitis (inflammation of a vein with the formation of blood clot)—pain or tenderness in thigh or leg, with or without swelling of the foot, ankle or leg.

Pulmonary embolism (movement of a blood clot to the lung)—sudden shortness of breath, pain in the chest, coughing, bloody sputum.

▷ **Adverse Effects That May Mimic Natural Diseases or Disorders**

Pattern of symptoms and signs resembling Cushing's syndrome.

Natural Diseases or Disorders That May Be Activated by This Drug

Latent diabetes, glaucoma, peptic ulcer disease, tuberculosis.

CAUTION

1. It is advisable to carry a card of personal identification with a notation that you are taking this drug, if your course of treatment is to exceed 1 week.

2. Do not discontinue this drug abruptly if you are using it for long-term treatment.
3. If vaccination against measles, rabies, smallpox or yellow fever is required, discontinue this drug 72 hours before vaccination and do not resume it for at least 14 days after vaccination.

Precautions for Use

By Infants and Children: Avoid prolonged use if possible. During long-term use, observe for suppression of normal growth and the possibility of increased intracranial pressure. Following long-term use, the child may be at risk for adrenal gland deficiency during stress for as long as 18 months after cessation of this drug.

By Those over 60 Years of Age: Cortisonelike drugs should be used very sparingly after 60 and only when the disorder under treatment is unresponsive to adequate trials of unrelated drugs. Avoid prolonged use of this drug. Continual use (even in small doses) can increase the severity of diabetes, enhance fluid retention, raise blood pressure, weaken resistance to infection, induce stomach ulcer and accelerate the development of cataract and osteoporosis.

▷ **Advisability of Use During Pregnancy**

Pregnancy Category: C (tentative). See Pregnancy Code inside back cover.
Animal studies: Birth defects reported in mice, rats and rabbits.
Human studies: Information from adequate studies of pregnant women is not available.
Avoid completely during the first 3 months. Limit use during the last 6 months as much as possible. If used, examine infant for possible deficiency of adrenal gland function.

Advisability of Use if Breast-Feeding

Presence of this drug in breast milk: Yes.
Avoid drug or refrain from nursing.

Habit-Forming Potential: Use of this drug to suppress symptoms over an extended period of time may produce a state of functional dependence (see Glossary). In the treatment of conditions like asthma and rheumatoid arthritis, it is advisable to keep the dose as small as possible and to attempt drug withdrawal after periods of reasonable improvement. Such procedures may reduce the degree of "steroid rebound"—the return of symptoms as the drug is withdrawn.

Effects of Overdosage: Fatigue, muscle weakness, stomach irritation, acid indigestion, excessive sweating, facial flushing, fluid retention, swelling of extremities, increased blood pressure.

Possible Effects of Long-Term Use: Increased blood sugar (possible diabetes), increased fat deposits on the trunk of the body ("buffalo hump"), rounding of the face ("moon face"), thinning and fragility of skin, loss of texture and strength of bones (osteoporosis, aseptic necrosis), cataracts, glaucoma, retarded growth and development in children.

Suggested Periodic Examinations While Taking This Drug   (at physician's discretion)

Measurements of blood pressure, blood sugar and potassium levels.

Complete eye examinations at regular intervals.

Chest X-ray if history of tuberculosis.

Determination of the rate of development of the growing child to detect retardation of normal growth.

▷ **While Taking This Drug, Observe the Following**

Foods: No interactions expected. Ask physician regarding need to restrict salt intake or to eat potassium-rich foods. During long-term use of this drug, it is advisable to eat a high-protein diet.

Nutritional Support: During long-term use, take a vitamin D supplement. During wound repair, take a zinc supplement.

Beverages: No restrictions. Drink all forms of milk liberally.

▷ *Alcohol*: No interactions expected. Use caution if you are prone to peptic ulcer disease.

Tobacco Smoking: Nicotine increases the blood levels of naturally produced cortisone and related hormones. Heavy smoking may add to the expected actions of this drug and requires close observation for excessive effects.

Marijuana Smoking: May cause additional impairment of immunity.

▷ *Other Drugs*

Prednisolone may *decrease* the effects of

• isoniazid (INH, Niconyl, etc.).

• salicylates (aspirin, sodium salicylate, etc.).

Prednisolone *taken concurrently* with

• oral anticoagulants may either increase or decrease their effectiveness; consult physician regarding the need for prothrombin time testing and dosage adjustment.

The following drugs may *decrease* the effects of prednisolone

• antacids may reduce its absorption.

• barbiturates (Amytal, Butisol, phenobarbital, etc.).

• phenytoin (Dilantin, etc.).

• rifampin (Rifadin, Rimactane, etc.).

▷ *Driving, Hazardous Activities*: Usually no restrictions. Be alert to the rare occurrence of dizziness.

Aviation Note: The use of this drug *may be a disqualification* for piloting. Consult a designated Aviation Medical Examiner.

Exposure to Sun: No restrictions.

Occurrence of Unrelated Illness: This drug may decrease natural resistance to infection. Inform your physician if you develop an infection of any kind. It may also reduce your body's ability to respond to the stress of acute illness, injury or surgery. Keep your physician fully informed of any significant changes in your state of health.

Discontinuation: If you have been taking this drug for an extended period of time, do not discontinue it abruptly. Ask physician for guidance regarding gradual withdrawal. For a period of 2 years after discontinuing this drug, it is essential in the event of illness, injury or surgery that you inform attending medical personnel that you have used this drug in the past. The period of impaired response to stress following the use of cortisonelike drugs may last for 1 to 2 years.

PREDNISONE
(PRED ni sohn)

Introduced: 1955

Prescription: USA: Yes
   Canada: Yes

Available as Generic: USA: Yes
   Canada: Yes

Class: Cortisonelike Drugs

Controlled Drug: USA: No
   Canada: No

Brand Names: ♣Apo-Prednisone, Deltasone, Meticorten, ♣Novoprednisone, Orasone, SK-Prednisone, ♣Winpred

---

BENEFITS versus RISKS

Possible Benefits	*Possible Risks*
EFFECTIVE RELIEF OF SYMPTOMS IN A WIDE VARIETY OF INFLAMMATORY AND ALLERGIC DISORDERS EFFECTIVE IMMUNO-SUPPRESSION in selected benign and malignant disorders Prevention of rejection in organ transplantation	Short-term use (up to 10 days) is usually well tolerated. Long-term use (exceeding 2 weeks) is associated with many possible adverse effects: ALTERED MOOD AND PERSONALITY CATARACTS, GLAUCOMA HYPERTENSION OSTEOPOROSIS ASEPTIC BONE NECROSIS INCREASED SUSCEPTIBILITY TO INFECTIONS (See Possible Adverse Effects and Possible Effects of Long-Term Use below)

▷ **Principal Uses**

   As a Single Drug Product: This potent drug of the cortisone class is used in the treatment of a wide variety of allergic and inflammatory conditions. It is used most commonly in the management of serious skin disorders, asthma, regional enteritis, ulcerative colitis and all types of major rheumatic disorders including bursitis, tendinitis and most forms of arthritis.

How This Drug Works: Not fully established. It is thought that this drug's anti-inflammatory effect is due to its ability to inhibit the normal defensive functions of certain white blood cells. Its immunosuppressant effect is attributed to a reduced production of lymphocytes and antibodies.

Available Dosage Forms and Strengths
Oral solution — 5 mg per 5 ml teaspoonful
    Syrup — 5 mg per 5 ml teaspoonful (alcohol 5%)
    Tablets — 1 mg, 2.5 mg, 5 mg, 10 mg, 20 mg, 25 mg, 50 mg

▷ **Usual Adult Dosage Range:**   5 to 60 mg daily as a single dose or in divided doses. The total daily dosage should not exceed 250 mg. **Note: Actual dosage and administration schedule must be determined by the physician for each patient individually.**

▷ **Dosing Instructions:**   Take with or following food to prevent stomach irritation, preferably in the morning. The tablet may be crushed for administration.

Usual Duration of Use: For acute disorders: 4 to 10 days. For chronic disorders: according to individual requirements. The duration of use should not exceed the time necessary to obtain adequate symptomatic relief in acute self-limiting conditions; or the time required to stabilize a chronic condition and permit gradual withdrawal. Because of its intermediate duration of action, this drug is appropriate for alternate day administration.

▷ **This Drug Should Not Be Taken If**
- you have had an allergic reaction to any dosage form of it previously.
- you have active peptic ulcer disease.
- you have an active infection of the eye caused by the herpes simplex virus.
- you have active tuberculosis.

▷ **Inform Your Physician Before Taking This Drug If**
- you have had an unfavorable reaction to any cortisonelike drug in the past.
- you have a history of peptic ulcer disease, thrombophlebitis or tuberculosis.
- you have any of the following: diabetes, glaucoma, high blood pressure, deficient thyroid function or myasthenia gravis.
- you plan to have surgery of any kind in the near future.

Possible Side-Effects   (natural, expected and unavoidable drug actions)
Increased appetite, weight gain, retention of salt and water, excretion of potassium, increased susceptibility to infection.

▷ **Possible Adverse Effects**   (unusual, unexpected and infrequent reactions)
If any of the following develop, consult your physician promptly.
Mild Adverse Effects
Allergic Reactions: Skin rash.
Headache, dizziness, insomnia.
Acid indigestion, abdominal distention.
Muscle cramping and weakness.

Irregular or altered menstruation.

Acne, excessive growth of facial hair.

Serious Adverse Effects

Mental and emotional disturbances of serious magnitude.

Reactivation of latent tuberculosis.

Development of peptic ulcer.

Increased blood pressure.

Development of inflammation of the pancreas.

Thrombophlebitis (inflammation of a vein with the formation of blood clot)—pain or tenderness in thigh or leg, with or without swelling of the foot, ankle or leg.

Pulmonary embolism (movement of a blood clot to the lung)—sudden shortness of breath, pain in the chest, coughing, bloody sputum.

▷ **Adverse Effects That May Mimic Natural Diseases or Disorders**

Pattern of symptoms and signs resembling Cushing's syndrome.

Natural Diseases or Disorders That May Be Activated by This Drug

Latent diabetes, glaucoma, peptic ulcer disease, tuberculosis.

CAUTION

1. It is advisable to carry a card of personal identification with a notation that you are taking this drug, if your course of treatment is to exceed 1 week.
2. Do not discontinue this drug abruptly if you are using it for long-term treatment.
3. If vaccination against measles, rabies, smallpox or yellow fever is required, discontinue this drug 72 hours before vaccination and do not resume it for at least 14 days after vaccination.

Precautions for Use

By Infants and Children: Avoid prolonged use if possible. During long-term use, observe for suppression of normal growth and the possibility of increased intracranial pressure. Following long-term use, the child may be at risk for adrenal gland deficiency during stress for as long as 18 months after cessation of this drug.

By Those over 60 Years of Age: Cortisonelike drugs should be used very sparingly after 60 and only when the disorder under treatment is unresponsive to adequate trials of unrelated drugs. Avoid prolonged use of this drug. Continual use (even in small doses) can increase the severity of diabetes, enhance fluid retention, raise blood pressure, weaken resistance to infection, induce stomach ulcer and accelerate the development of cataract and osteoporosis.

▷ **Advisability of Use During Pregnancy**

Pregnancy Category: C (tentative). See Pregnancy Code inside back cover.

Animal studies: Birth defects reported in mice, rats and rabbits.

Human studies: Information from adequate studies of pregnant women is not available.

Avoid completely during the first 3 months. Limit use during the last 6 months as much as possible. If used, examine infant for possible deficiency of adrenal gland function.

Advisability of Use if Breast-Feeding
Presence of this drug in breast milk: Yes.
Avoid drug or refrain from nursing.

Habit-Forming Potential: Use of this drug to suppress symptoms over an extended period of time may produce a state of functional dependence (see Glossary). In the treatment of conditions like asthma and rheumatoid arthritis, it is advisable to keep the dose as small as possible and to attempt drug withdrawal after periods of reasonable improvement. Such procedures may reduce the degree of "steroid rebound"—the return of symptoms as the drug is withdrawn.

Effects of Overdosage: Fatigue, muscle weakness, stomach irritation, acid indigestion, excessive sweating, facial flushing, fluid retention, swelling of extremities, increased blood pressure.

Possible Effects of Long-Term Use: Increased blood sugar (possible diabetes), increased fat deposits on the trunk of the body ("buffalo hump"), rounding of the face ("moon face"), thinning and fragility of skin, loss of texture and strength of bones (osteoporosis, aseptic necrosis), cataracts, glaucoma, retarded growth and development in children.

Suggested Periodic Examinations While Taking This Drug (at physician's discretion)
Measurements of blood pressure, blood sugar and potassium levels.
Complete eye examinations at regular intervals.
Chest X-ray if history of tuberculosis.
Determination of the rate of development of the growing child to detect retardation of normal growth.

▷ **While Taking This Drug, Observe the Following**
Foods: No interactions expected. Ask physician regarding need to restrict salt intake or to eat potassium-rich foods. During long-term use of this drug, it is advisable to eat a high-protein diet.
Nutritional Support: During long-term use, take a vitamin D supplement. During wound repair, take a zinc supplement.
Beverages: No restrictions. Drink all forms of milk liberally.
▷ *Alcohol*: No interactions expected. Use caution if you are prone to peptic ulcer disease.
Tobacco Smoking: Nicotine increases the blood levels of naturally produced cortisone and related hormones. Heavy smoking may add to the expected actions of this drug and requires close observation for excessive effects.
Marijuana Smoking: May cause additional impairment of immunity.
▷ *Other Drugs*
Prednisone may *decrease* the effects of
• isoniazid (INH, Niconyl, etc.).
• salicylates (aspirin, sodium salicylate, etc.).

Prednisone *taken concurrently* with
- oral anticoagulants may either increase or decrease their effectiveness; consult physician regarding the need for prothrombin time testing and dosage adjustment.

The following drugs may *decrease* the effects of prednisone
- antacids may reduce its absorption.
- barbiturates (Amytal, Butisol, phenobarbital, etc.).
- phenytoin (Dilantin, etc.).
- rifampin (Rifadin, Rimactane, etc.).

▷ *Driving, Hazardous Activities*: Usually no restrictions. Be alert to the rare occurrence of dizziness.

Aviation Note: The use of this drug *may be a disqualification* for piloting. Consult a designated Aviation Medical Examiner.

Exposure to Sun: No restrictions.

Occurrence of Unrelated Illness: This drug may decrease natural resistance to infection. Inform your physician if you develop an infection of any kind. It may also reduce your body's ability to respond to the stress of acute illness, injury or surgery. Keep your physician fully informed of any significant changes in your state of health.

Discontinuation: If you have been taking this drug for an extended period of time, do not discontinue it abruptly. Ask physician for guidance regarding gradual withdrawal. For a period of 2 years after discontinuing this drug, it is essential in the event of illness, injury or surgery that you inform attending medical personnel that you have used this drug in the past. The period of impaired response to stress following the use of cortisonelike drugs may last for 1 to 2 years.

PRIMIDONE
(PRI mi dohn)

Introduced: 1953

Class: Anticonvulsant

Prescription: USA: Yes
Canada: Yes

Controlled Drug: USA: No
Canada: No

Available as Generic: USA: Yes
Canada: No

Brand Names: ✤Apo-Primidone, Mysoline, ✤Sertan

BENEFITS versus RISKS	
Possible Benefits	*Possible Risks*
EFFECTIVE CONTROL OF TONIC-CLONIC (GRAND MAL) AND ALL TYPES OF PARTIAL SEIZURES	Allergic skin reactions Rare blood cell disorders: megaloblastic anemia, deficient white blood cells and platelets

▷ **Principal Uses**

As a Single Drug Product: This drug is used exclusively to control generalized grand mal seizures and all types of partial seizures. It can be used to supplement the anticonvulsant action of phenytoin.

How This Drug Works: Not completely established. This drug reduces and stabilizes the excitability of nerve fibers and inhibits the repetitious spread of electrical impulses along nerve pathways. This action may prevent seizures altogether, or it may reduce their frequency and severity. (Part of this drug's action is attributable to phenobarbital, one of its conversion products in the body.)

Available Dosage Forms and Strengths
Oral suspensions — 250 mg per 5 ml teaspoonful
Tablets — 50 mg, 250 mg

▷ **Usual Adult Dosage Range:**   Initially, 250 mg/24 hours as a single dose at bedtime for 1 week; 2nd week, 250 mg/12 hours; 3rd week, 250 mg 3 times/day, 6 to 8 hours apart; 4th week, 250 mg 4 times/day, 4 to 6 hours apart. The total daily dosage should not exceed 2000 mg. **Note: Actual dosage and administration schedule must be determined by the physician for each patient individually.**

▷ **Dosing Instructions:**   May be taken with or following food to reduce stomach irritation. The tablet may be crushed for administration. Shake the suspension well before measuring the dose.

Usual Duration of Use: Continual use on a regular schedule for 2 to 4 weeks is usually necessary to determine this drug's effectiveness in reducing the frequency and severity of seizures. Long-term use (months to years) requires supervision and periodic evaluation by your physician.

▷ **This Drug Should Not Be Taken If**
- you have had an allergic reaction to it previously.
- you are allergic to phenobarbital.
- you have a history of porphyria.

▷ **Inform Your Physician Before Taking This Drug If**
- you have had an allergic or idiosyncratic reaction to any barbiturate drug in the past.
- you have a family history of intermittent porphyria.
- you have impaired liver, kidney or thyroid gland function.
- you have asthma, emphysema or myasthenia gravis.
- you are pregnant or planning pregnancy.
- you plan to have surgery under general anesthesia in the near future.

Possible Side-Effects   (natural, expected and unavoidable drug actions)
Drowsiness, impaired concentration, mental and physical sluggishness.

▷ **Possible Adverse Effects**   (unusual, unexpected and infrequent reactions)
If any of the following develop, consult your physician promptly.

Mild Adverse Effects
Allergic Reactions: Skin rashes, hives, localized swellings.
"Hangover" effect, dizziness, unsteadiness, impaired vision, double vision, fatigue, emotional disturbances.
Low blood pressure, faintness.
Nausea, vomiting, thirst, increased urine volume.

Serious Adverse Effects
Allergic Reactions: Swelling of lymph glands.
Idiosyncratic Reactions: Paradoxical anxiety, agitation, restlessness, rage.
Visual hallucinations, sexual impotence.
Blood cell disorders: megaloblastic anemia due to folic acid depletion; deficient production of white blood cells and blood platelets.

▷ **Adverse Effects That May Mimic Natural Diseases or Disorders**
Allergic swelling of lymph glands may suggest a naturally occurring lymphoma.

Natural Diseases or Disorders That May Be Activated by This Drug
Acute intermittent and/or cutaneous porphyria (see Glossary).
Systemic lupus erythematosus.

CAUTION
1. This drug must not be stopped abruptly.
2. The wide variation of this drug's action from person to person requires careful individualization of dosage schedules.
3. Regularity of drug use is essential for the successful management of seizure disorders. Take your medication at the same time each day.
4. Side-effects and mild adverse effects are usually most apparent during the first several weeks of treatment and often subside with continued use.
5. It may be necessary to take folic acid to prevent anemia while taking this drug. Consult your physician.
6. It is advisable to carry a card of personal identification with a notation that you are taking this drug.

Precautions for Use
By Infants and Children: This drug should be used with caution in the hyperkinetic (overactive) child. Observe for possible paradoxical hyperactivity. Changes associated with puberty characteristically slow the metabolism of phenobarbital and permit its gradual accumulation. Measurements of blood levels in young adolescents can detect rising concentrations of this drug that could lead to toxicity. (See Therapeutic Drug Monitoring in Section One.)
By Those over 60 Years of Age: It is advisable to avoid all barbiturates in the elderly. If use of this drug is attempted, start with small doses until tolerance has been determined. Observe for confusion, delirium, agitation or paradoxical excitement. This drug may be conducive to hypothermia (see Glossary).

▷ **Advisability of Use During Pregnancy**

Pregnancy Category: D (tentative). See Pregnancy Code inside back cover.

Animal studies: Birth defects due to this drug reported in mice.

Human studies: Information from adequate studies of pregnant women is not available. However, recent reports suggest a possible association between the use of this drug during the first 3 months of pregnancy and the development of birth defects in the fetus. Discuss with your physician the advantages and possible disadvantages of using this drug during pregnancy. If it is used, determine the smallest maintenance dose that will prevent seizures.

The newborn infants of mothers who take this drug during pregnancy may develop abnormal bleeding or bruising due to the deficiency of certain blood clotting factors in the blood. Consult your physician regarding the need to take vitamin K during the last month of pregnancy.

Advisability of Use if Breast-Feeding

Presence of this drug in breast milk: Yes.

Monitor nursing infant closely and discontinue drug or nursing if adverse effects develop.

Habit-Forming Potential: None.

Effects of Overdosage: Drowsiness, jerky eye movements, blurred vision, staggering gait, incoordination, slurred speech, stupor progressing to coma.

Possible Effects of Long-Term Use: Enlargement of lymph glands; enlargement of thyroid gland. Megaloblastic anemia due to folic acid deficiency. Reduced blood levels of calcium and phosphorus, leading to rickets in children and loss of bone texture (osteomalacia) in adults.

Suggested Periodic Examinations While Taking This Drug   (at physician's discretion)

Complete blood cell counts. Measurements of blood levels of calcium and phosphorus. Evaluation of lymph and thyroid glands. Skeletal X-ray examinations for bone demineralization during long-term use.

▷ **While Taking This Drug, Observe the Following**

Foods: No restrictions.

Nutritional Support: Consult your physician regarding the need for supplements of calcium, vitamin D, folic acid and vitamin K.

Beverages: No restrictions. May be taken with milk or fruit juice.

▷ *Alcohol*: Avoid completely. Alcohol can increase greatly the sedative and depressant effects of this drug on brain function.

Tobacco Smoking: May enhance the sedative effects of this drug and increase drowsiness.

▷ *Other Drugs*

Note: 15% of primidone is converted to phenobarbital in the body. See the Drug Profile of Phenobarbital for possible interactions with other drugs.

▷ *Driving, Hazardous Activities*: This drug may cause drowsiness and dizziness; it can also impair mental alertness, vision and physical coordination. Restrict activities as necessary.

Aviation Note: The use of this drug *is a disqualification* for piloting. Consult a designated Aviation Medical Examiner.

Exposure to Sun: No restrictions.

Occurrence of Unrelated Illness: Notify your physician of any illness or injury that prevents the use of this drug according to your regular dosage schedule.

Discontinuation: Do not discontinue this drug without your physician's knowledge and approval. Sudden withdrawal of any anticonvulsant drug can cause severe and repeated seizures.

PROBENECID
(proh BEN e sid)

Introduced: 1951

Class: Antigout

Prescription: USA: Yes
Canada: No

Controlled Drug: USA: No
Canada: No

Available as Generic: USA: Yes
Canada: No

Brand Names: Benemid, ✦Benuryl, ColBenemid [CD], Probalan, ✦Pro-Biosan 500 Kit [CD], SK-Probenecid

---

BENEFITS versus RISKS

Possible Benefits	*Possible Risks*
EFFECTIVE LONG-TERM PREVENTION OF ACUTE ATTACKS OF GOUT	Formation of uric acid kidney stones
Useful adjunct to penicillin therapy (to achieve high blood and tissue levels of penicillin)	Bone marrow depression (aplastic anemia) (rare)
	Drug-induced liver and kidney damage (both rare)

▷ **Principal Uses**

As a Single Drug Product: Used primarily in the long-term management of gout to prevent acute attacks. While effective for prevention, it has no beneficial effects in relieving the joint inflammation and pain of the acute episode. In fact, it may aggravate and prolong the symptoms of acute gout.

As a Combination Drug Product [CD]: This drug is available in combination with colchicine, a drug often used for the treatment of acute gout. Each drug has a different mechanism of action; when used in combination they provide both relief of the acute manifestations of gout and some measure of protection from recurrence of acute attacks.

How This Drug Works: By acting on the tubular systems of the kidney to increase the amount of uric acid excreted in the urine, this drug reduces the levels of uric acid in the blood and body tissues. By acting on the tubular systems of the kidney to decrease the amount of penicillin excreted in the urine, this drug prolongs the presence of penicillin in the blood and helps achieve higher concentrations in body tissues.

Available Dosage Forms and Strengths
Tablets — 500 mg

▷ **Usual Adult Dosage Range:**   Antigout: Initially, 250 mg twice/day for 1 week; then 500 mg twice/day. Adjunct to penicillin therapy: 500 mg 4 times/day. **Note: Actual dosage and administration schedule must be determined by the physician for each patient individually.**

▷ **Dosing Instructions:**   Take with or following food to reduce stomach irritation. Drink 2.5 to 3 quarts of liquids daily. The tablet may be crushed for administration.

Usual Duration of Use: Continual use on a regular schedule for several months is usually necessary to determine this drug's effectiveness in preventing acute attacks of gout. Long-term use (months to years) requires supervision and periodic evaluation by your physician.

▷ **This Drug Should Not Be Taken If**
- you have had an allergic reaction to it previously.
- you have active liver disease.
- you have an active blood cell or bone marrow disorder.
- you are experiencing an attack of acute gout at the present time.

▷ **Inform Your Physician Before Taking This Drug If**
- you have a history of kidney disease or kidney stones.
- you have a history of liver disease or impaired liver function.
- you have a history of peptic ulcer disease.
- you have a history of a blood cell or bone marrow disorder.
- you are taking any drug product that contains aspirin or aspirinlike drugs.

Possible Side-Effects   (natural, expected and unavoidable drug actions)
Development of kidney stones (composed of uric acid); this is preventable. Consult your physician regarding the use of sodium bicarbonate (or other urine alkalizer) to prevent stone formation.

▷ **Possible Adverse Effects**   (unusual, unexpected and infrequent reactions)
If any of the following develop, consult your physician promptly.
Mild Adverse Effects
Allergic Reactions: Skin rash, itching, drug fever (see Glossary).

Headache, dizziness, flushing of face.

Reduced appetite, sore gums, nausea, vomiting.

Serious Adverse Effects

Allergic Reactions: Anaphylactic reaction (see Glossary).

Idiosyncratic Reactions: Hemolytic anemia (see Glossary).

Bone marrow depression (see Glossary): fatigue, weakness, fever, sore throat, abnormal bleeding or bruising.

Drug-induced liver damage with jaundice (see Glossary).

Drug-induced kidney damage: marked fluid retention, reduced urine formation.

▷ **Adverse Effects That May Mimic Natural Diseases or Disorders**

Liver reactions may suggest viral hepatitis.

Kidney reactions may suggest nephrosis.

CAUTION
1. This drug should not be started until 2 to 3 weeks after an acute attack of gout has subsided.
2. This drug may increase the frequency of acute attacks of gout during the first few months of treatment. Concurrent use of colchicine is advised to prevent acute attacks. See the Profile of Gout in Section Two.
3. Aspirin (and aspirin-containing drug products) can reduce the effectiveness of this drug. Use acetaminophen or a nonaspirin analgesic for pain relief as needed.

Precautions for Use

By Infants and Children: Safety and effectiveness for use by those under 2 years of age have not been established.

By Those over 60 Years of Age: The natural decline in kidney function that occurs after 60 may require adjustment of your dosage. You may be more susceptible to the serious adverse effects of this drug. Report any unusual symptoms promptly for evaluation.

▷ **Advisability of Use During Pregnancy**

Pregnancy Category: C (tentative). See Pregnancy Code inside back cover.

Animal studies: No information available.

Human studies: Information from adequate studies of pregnant women is not available.

This drug has been used during pregnancy with no reports of birth defects or adverse effects on the fetus. Ask your physician for guidance.

Advisability of Use if Breast-Feeding

Presence of this drug in breast milk: Unknown.

Avoid drug or refrain from nursing.

Habit-Forming Potential: None.

Effects of Overdosage: Stomach irritation, nausea, vomiting, nervous agitation, delirium, seizures, coma.

Possible Effects of Long-Term Use: Formation of kidney stones. Kidney damage in sensitive individuals.

Suggested Periodic Examinations While Taking This Drug (at physician's discretion)
Complete blood cell counts, measurements of blood uric acid, liver and kidney function tests.

▷ **While Taking This Drug, Observe the Following**
Foods: Follow physician's advice regarding the need for a low-purine diet.
Beverages: A large intake of coffee, tea or cola beverages may reduce the effectiveness of treatment.

▷ *Alcohol*: No interactions expected. However, large amounts of alcohol can raise the blood uric acid level and reduce the effectiveness of treatment.
Tobacco Smoking: No interactions expected.

▷ *Other Drugs*
Probenecid may *increase* the effects of
• clofibrate (Atromid S).
• dyphylline (Neothylline).
• methotrexate (Mexate), and increase its toxicity.
• thiopental (Pentothal), and prolong its anesthetic effect.
Probenecid *taken concurrently* with
• penicillins may cause a threefold to fivefold increase in penicillin blood levels, greatly increasing the effectiveness of each penicillin dose.
The following drugs may *decrease* the effects of probenecid
• aspirin and other salicylates may reduce its effectiveness in promoting the excretion of uric acid.

▷ *Driving, Hazardous Activities*: This drug may cause dizziness. Restrict activities as necessary.
Aviation Note: The use of this drug *may be a disqualification* for piloting. Consult a designated Aviation Medical Examiner.
Exposure to Sun: No restrictions.
Discontinuation: Do not discontinue this drug without consulting your physician.

PROCAINAMIDE
(proh kayn A mide)

Introduced: 1950

Class: Antiarrhythmic

Prescription: USA: Yes
Canada: Yes

Controlled Drug: USA: No
Canada: No

Available as Generic: USA: Yes
Canada: No

Brand Names: Procan SR, Pronestyl, Pronestyl-SR

```
┌─────────────────────────────────────────────────────────────┐
│                    BENEFITS versus RISKS                       │
│                                                                 │
│     Possible Benefits              Possible Risks              │
│  EFFECTIVE TREATMENT OF      NARROW TREATMENT RANGE           │
│    SELECTED HEART RHYTHM     INDUCTION OF SYSTEMIC            │
│    DISORDERS                   LUPUS ERYTHEMATOSUS            │
│                                SYNDROME in 20% of long-term   │
│                                users                          │
│                              Provocation of abnormal heart    │
│                                rhythms                        │
│                              Blood cell disorders: insufficient│
│                                white blood cells and platelets │
└─────────────────────────────────────────────────────────────┘
```

▷ **Principal Uses**

As a Single Drug Product: This drug is classified as a Type 1 antiarrhythmic agent, similar to disopyramide and quinidine in its actions. It is used primarily to abolish and prevent the recurrence of premature beats arising in the atria (upper chambers) and the ventricles (lower chambers) of the heart. It is also useful in the treatment and prevention of atrial fibrillation, atrial flutter and abnormally rapid heart rates (tachycardia) that originate in the atria or the ventricles.

How This Drug Works: By slowing the activity of the pacemaker and delaying the transmission of electrical impulses through the conduction system and muscle of the heart, this drug assists in restoring normal heart rate and rhythm.

Available Dosage Forms and Strengths

Capsules — 250 mg, 375 mg, 500 mg
Injections — 100 mg per ml, 500 mg per ml
Tablets — 250 mg, 375 mg, 500 mg
Tablets, prolonged action — 250 mg, 500 mg, 750 mg, 1000 mg

▷ **Usual Adult Dosage Range:** Dose varies according to indication for use. Premature atrial or ventricular contractions: 250 to 500 mg/3 hours. Paroxysmal atrial tachycardia: initially, 1250 mg, followed in 1 hour by 750 mg; then 500 to 1000 mg/2 hours as needed and tolerated. Atrial fibrillation and flutter: the heart should be digitalized first; then initiate procainamide with 1250 mg, followed in 1 hour by 750 mg; follow with 500 to 1000 mg/2 hours as needed and tolerated. For maintenance: 500 to 1000 mg/4 to 6 hours. The total daily dosage should not exceed 6000 mg. **Note: Actual dosage and administration schedule must be determined by the physician for each patient individually.**

▷ **Dosing Instructions:** Preferably taken on an empty stomach, 1 hour before or 2 hours after eating. However, it may be taken with or following food to reduce stomach irritation. The regular capsules may be opened and the regular tablets may be crushed for administration; however, the prolonged-action tablets should be swallowed whole without alteration.

Usual Duration of Use: Continual use on a regular schedule for 24 to 48 hours is usually necessary to determine this drug's effectiveness in correcting or preventing responsive rhythm disorders. Long-term use requires supervision and periodic evaluation by your physician.

▷ **This Drug Should Not Be Taken If**
  • you have had an allergic reaction to it previously.
  • you have second-degree or third-degree heart block (determined by electrocardiogram).

▷ **Inform Your Physician Before Taking This Drug If**
  • you are allergic to procaine (Novocain) or to other local anesthetics of the "-caine" drug class, such as those commonly used for glaucoma testing and for dental procedures.
  • you have had any unfavorable reactions to other antiarrhythmic drugs in the past.
  • you have a history of heart disease of any kind, especially "heart block."
  • you have a history of low blood pressure.
  • you have a history of lupus erythematosus.
  • you have a history of abnormally low blood platelet counts from any cause.
  • you have impaired liver or kidney function.
  • you have myasthenia gravis.
  • you have an enlarged prostate gland.
  • you are taking any form of digitalis or any diuretic drug that can cause excessive loss of body potassium (ask physician).
  • you plan to have surgery under general anesthesia in the near future.

Possible Side-Effects   (natural, expected and unavoidable drug actions)
Drop in blood pressure in susceptible individuals.

▷ **Possible Adverse Effects**   (unusual, unexpected and infrequent reactions)
  If any of the following develop, consult your physician promptly.
  Mild Adverse Effects
  Allergic Reactions: Skin rash, hives, itching, drug fever (see Glossary).
  Weakness, light-headedness.
  Loss of appetite, bitter taste, indigestion, nausea, vomiting, diarrhea.
  Serious Adverse Effects
  Allergic Reactions: Systemic lupus erythematosuslike syndrome: fever, skin eruptions, joint and muscle pains, pleurisy. (This is reported to occur in at least 20% of users.)
  Idiosyncratic Reactions: Mental depression, hallucinations, psychotic behavior, hemolytic anemia (see Glossary).
  Severe drop in blood pressure, fainting.
  Asthmalike breathing difficulties.
  Induction of new heart rhythm disturbances.
  Inability to empty urinary bladder, prostatism (see Glossary).
  Blood cell disorders: abnormally low white blood cell count, causing fever,

sore throat, infections; abnormally low blood platelet count, causing abnormal bleeding or bruising.

▷ **Adverse Effects That May Mimic Natural Diseases or Disorders**
Rare liver reaction may suggest viral hepatitis.

Natural Diseases or Disorders That May Be Activated by This Drug
Systemic lupus erythematosus, myasthenia gravis.

CAUTION
1. Thorough evaluation of your heart function (including electrocardiograms) is necessary prior to using this drug.
2. Periodic evaluation of your heart function is necessary to determine your response to this drug. Some individuals may experience worsening of their heart rhythm disorder and/or deterioration of heart function. Close monitoring of heart rate, rhythm and overall performance is essential.
3. Dosage must be adjusted carefully for each individual. Do not change your dosage without the knowledge and supervision of your physician.
4. Do not take any other antiarrhythmic drug while taking this drug unless directed to do so by your physician.

Precautions for Use
By Infants and Children: Blood cell counts should be monitored for loss of white blood cells.
By Those over 60 Years of Age: Reduced kidney function may require reduction in dosage. Observe carefully for light-headedness, dizziness, unsteadiness and tendency to fall.

▷ **Advisability of Use During Pregnancy**
Pregnancy Category: C (tentative). See Pregnancy Code inside back cover.
Animal studies: No information available.
Human studies: Information from adequate studies of pregnant women is not available.
Use this drug only if clearly needed.

Advisability of Use if Breast-Feeding
Presence of this drug in breast milk: Unknown.
Avoid drug or refrain from nursing.

Habit-Forming Potential: None.

Effects of Overdosage: Loss of appetite, nausea, vomiting, weakness, faintness, irregular heart rhythm, stupor, circulatory collapse, heart arrest.

Possible Effects of Long-Term Use: Lupus erythematosuslike syndrome (see above).

Suggested Periodic Examinations While Taking This Drug (at physician's discretion)
Complete blood cell counts.

Blood tests for the development of lupus erythematosus (LE) cells and antinuclear antibodies.

Electrocardiograms to monitor the full effect of this drug on the mechanisms that influence heart rate and rhythm.

▷ **While Taking This Drug, Observe the Following**

Foods: No restrictions.

Beverages: Avoid excessive intake of coffee, tea and cola beverages. Avoid iced drinks. May be taken with milk.

▷ *Alcohol*: Use caution until the combined effects have been determined. Alcohol can increase the blood-pressure-lowering effects of this drug.

Tobacco Smoking: Nicotine can cause irritability of the heart and reduce the effectiveness of this drug. Follow physician's advice regarding smoking.

▷ *Other Drugs*

Procainamide may *increase* the effects of

• antihypertensive drugs, and cause excessive lowering of blood pressure.

The following drugs may *increase* the effects of procainamide

• amiodarone.

• cimetidine (Tagamet).

▷ *Driving, Hazardous Activities*: This drug may cause dizziness or weakness. Restrict activities as necessary.

Aviation Note: The use of this drug *may be a disqualification* for piloting. Consult a designated Aviation Medical Examiner.

Exposure to Sun: No restrictions.

Exposure to Heat: Use caution. Hot environments are conducive to lower blood pressure.

Occurrence of Unrelated Illness: Disorders that cause vomiting, diarrhea or dehydration can affect this drug's action adversely. Report such developments promptly.

Discontinuation: This drug should not be discontinued abruptly following long-term use. Ask your physician for guidance regarding gradual dose reduction.

PROCHLORPERAZINE
(proh klor PER a zeen)

Introduced: 1956

Class: Strong Tranquilizer, Antiemetic, Phenothiazines

Prescription: USA: Yes
Canada: Yes

Controlled Drug: USA: No
Canada: No

Available as Generic: USA: Yes
Canada: No

Brand Names: Compazine, ♣Stemetil

BENEFITS versus RISKS

Possible Benefits	*Possible Risks*
EFFECTIVE CONTROL OF ACUTE MENTAL DISORDERS in the majority of patients: beneficial effects on thinking, mood and behavior	SERIOUS TOXIC EFFECTS ON BRAIN with long-term use
	Liver damage with jaundice (infrequent)
EFFECTIVE CONTROL OF NAUSEA AND VOMITING	Rare blood cell disorders: abnormally low white cell and platelet counts
Relief of anxiety and nervous tension	

▷ **Principal Uses**

As a Single Drug Product: This member of the phenothiazine class is used primarily to relieve severe nausea and vomiting. Although it has sedative and antipsychotic effects characteristic of this class, it is used less often as a major tranquilizer.

How This Drug Works: Not completely established. Present theory is that by inhibiting the action of dopamine, this drug acts to correct an imbalance of nerve impulse transmissions that is thought to be responsible for certain mental disorders. By blocking the action of dopamine in the chemoreceptor trigger zone of the brain, this drug prevents excessive stimulation of the vomiting center.

Available Dosage Forms and Strengths

Capsules, prolonged action — 10 mg, 15 mg, 30 mg
Injection — 5 mg per ml
Suppositories — 2.5 mg, 5 mg, 25 mg
Syrup — 5 mg per 5 ml teaspoonful
Tablets — 5 mg, 10 mg, 25 mg

▷ **Usual Adult Dosage Range:**   Initially, 5 mg/6 to 8 hours. If needed and tolerated, dose may be increased by 5 mg at intervals of 3 to 4 days. Usual range is 35 to 60 mg/24 hours. The total daily dosage should not exceed 150 mg. **Note: Actual dosage and administration schedule must be determined by the physician for each patient individually.**

▷ **Dosing Instructions:**   May be taken with or following food to reduce stomach irritation. The tablets may be crushed for administration. Prolonged-action capsules should be swallowed whole without alteration.

Duration of Use: Continual use on a regular schedule for 12 to 24 hours is usually necessary to determine this drug's effectiveness in controlling nausea and vomiting. If used for severe anxiety-tension states or acute psychotic behavior, a trial of several weeks is usually necessary to determine effectiveness. If not significantly beneficial within 6 weeks, it should be discontinued.

▷ **This Drug Should Not Be Taken If**
  • you have had an allergic reaction to it previously.
  • you have active liver disease.
  • you have cancer of the breast.
  • you have a current blood cell or bone marrow disorder.

▷ **Inform Your Physician Before Taking This Drug If**
  • you are allergic or abnormally sensitive to any phenothiazine drug (see Drug Class, Section Four).
  • you have impaired liver or kidney function.
  • you have any type of seizure disorder.
  • you have diabetes, glaucoma or heart disease.
  • you have a history of lupus erythematosus.
  • you are taking any drug with sedative effects.
  • you plan to have surgery under general or spinal anesthesia in the near future.

Possible Side-Effects   (natural, expected and unavoidable drug actions)
  Drowsiness (usually during the first 2 weeks), orthostatic hypotension (see Glossary), blurred vision, dry mouth, nasal congestion, constipation, impaired urination.
  Pink or purple coloration of urine, of no significance.

▷ **Possible Adverse Effects**   (unusual, unexpected and infrequent reactions)
  If any of the following develop, consult your physician promptly.
  Mild Adverse Effects
  Allergic Reactions: Skin rash, hives, low-grade fever.
  Lowering of body temperature, especially in the elderly. (See Hypothermia in Glossary.)
  Increased appetite and weight gain.
  Breast fullness, tenderness, milk production, menstrual irregularity.
  Dizziness, weakness, agitation, insomnia, impaired day and night vision.
  Chronic constipation, fecal impaction.
  Serious Adverse Effects
  Allergic Reactions: Hepatitis with jaundice (see Glossary), usually between second and fourth week; high fever; asthma; anaphylactic reaction (see Glossary).
  Idiosyncratic Reactions: Toxic dermatitis.
  Depression, disorientation, seizures.
  Disturbances of heart rhythm, rapid heart rate.
  Bone marrow depression (see Glossary): fever, sore throat, abnormal bleeding or bruising.
  Parkinson-like disorders (see Glossary); muscle spasms of face, jaw, neck, back, extremities; extreme restlessness; slowed movements, muscle rigidity, tremors; tardive dyskinesias (see Glossary).

▷ **Adverse Effects That May Mimic Natural Diseases or Disorders**
  Nervous system reactions may suggest Parkinson's disease.

Liver reactions may suggest viral hepatitis.
Reactions resembling systemic lupus erythematosus can occur.

Natural Diseases or Disorders That May Be Activated by This Drug
Latent epilepsy, glaucoma, diabetes mellitus, prostatism (see Glossary).

CAUTION
1. Many over-the-counter medications (see OTC Drugs in Glossary) for allergies, colds and coughs contain drugs that can interact unfavorably with this drug. Ask your physician or pharmacist for guidance before using any such medications.
2. Antacids that contain aluminum and/or magnesium can prevent the absorption of this drug and reduce its effectiveness.
3. Obtain prompt evaluation of any change or disturbance of vision.

Precautions for Use
By Infants and Children: Do not use this drug in infants under 2 years of age, or in children of any age with symptoms suggestive of Reye syndrome (see Glossary). Children with acute illnesses ("flulike" infections, measles, chicken pox, etc.) are very susceptible to adverse effects when this drug is given to control nausea and vomiting.

By Those over 60 Years of Age: Small doses are advisable until individual response has been determined. You may be more susceptible to the development of drowsiness, lethargy, constipation, lowering of body temperature (hypothermia) and orthostatic hypotension (see Glossary). This drug can enhance existing prostatism (see Glossary). You may also be more susceptible to the development of Parkinson-like reactions and/or tardive dyskinesia (see discussion of these terms in Glossary). These reactions must be recognized early since they may become unresponsive to treatment and irreversible.

▷ **Advisability of Use During Pregnancy**
Pregnancy Category: C (tentative). See Pregnancy Code inside back cover.
Animal studies: Cleft palate reported in mouse and rat studies.
Human studies: No increase in birth defects reported in 2023 exposures. Information from adequate studies of pregnant women is not available.
Limit use to small and infrequent doses. Avoid drug during the last month because of possible effects on the newborn infant.

Advisability of Use if Breast-Feeding
Presence of this drug in breast milk: Yes, in small amounts.
Monitor nursing infant closely and discontinue drug or nursing if adverse effects develop.

Habit-Forming Potential: None.

Effects of Overdosage: Marked drowsiness, weakness, tremor, agitation, unsteadiness, deep sleep, coma, convulsions.

Possible Effects of Long-Term Use: Tardive dyskinesias. Eye changes: opacities in cornea or lens, retinal pigmentation.

Suggested Periodic Examinations While Taking This Drug   (at physician's discretion)

Complete blood cell counts, especially between the fourth and tenth weeks of treatment.

Liver function tests, electrocardiograms.

Complete eye examinations—eye structures and vision.

Careful inspection of the tongue for early evidence of fine, involuntary, wavelike movements that could indicate the beginning of tardive dyskinesia.

▷ **While Taking This Drug, Observe the Following**

Foods: No restrictions.

Nutritional Support: A riboflavin (vitamin B-2) supplement should be taken with long-term use.

Beverages: No restrictions. May be taken with milk.

▷   *Alcohol:* Avoid completely. Alcohol can increase the sedative action of phenothiazines and accentuate their depressant effects on brain function and blood pressure. Phenothiazines can increase the intoxicating effects of alcohol.

Tobacco Smoking: Possible reduction of drowsiness from drug.

Marijuana Smoking: Moderate increase in drowsiness; accentuation of orthostatic hypotension; increased risk of precipitating latent psychoses, confusing the interpretation of mental status and drug responses.

▷   *Other Drugs*

Prochlorperazine may *increase* the effects of

- all sedative drugs, especially meperidine (Demerol), and cause excessive sedation.
- all atropinelike drugs, and cause nervous system toxicity.

Prochlorperazine may *decrease* the effects of

- guanethidine (Ismelin, Esimil), and reduce its effectiveness in lowering blood pressure.

Prochlorperazine *taken concurrently* with

- propranolol (Inderal) may cause increased effects of both drugs; monitor drug effects closely and adjust dosages as necessary.

The following drugs may *decrease* the effects of prochlorperazine

- antacids containing aluminum and/or magnesium.
- benztropine (Cogentin).
- trihexyphenidyl (Artane).

▷   *Driving, Hazardous Activities:* This drug can impair mental alertness, judgment and physical coordination. Avoid hazardous activities.

Aviation Note: The use of this drug *is a disqualification* for piloting. Consult a designated Aviation Medical Examiner.

Exposure to Sun: Use caution until sensitivity has been determined. Some phenothiazines can cause photosensitivity (see Glossary).

Exposure to Heat: Use caution and avoid excessive heat as much as possible. This drug may impair the regulation of body temperature and increase the risk of heat stroke.

Exposure to Cold: Use caution and dress warmly. This drug can increase the risk of hypothermia in the elderly.

Discontinuation: After a period of long-term use, do not discontinue this drug suddenly. Gradual withdrawal over 2 to 3 weeks under physician supervision is recommended.

PROMETHAZINE
(proh METH a zeen)

Introduced: 1945

Class: Antiemetic, Antihistamines, Phenothiazines

Prescription: USA: Yes
Canada: No

Controlled Drug: USA: No
Canada: No

Available as Generic: USA: Yes
Canada: No

Brand Names: ✚Histanil, Ganphen, K-Phen, Pentazine, Phenergan, ✚PMS Promethazine, Prorex, Provigan, Remsed, Zipan-25/50

BENEFITS versus RISKS	
Possible Benefits	*Possible Risks*
EFFECTIVE SYMPTOMATIC RELIEF OF ALLERGIC RHINITIS AND DERMATOSIS	EXCESSIVE SEDATION in sensitive individuals
Moderately effective prevention and treatment of motion sickness, nausea and vomiting	Atropinelike effects Rare blood cell disorders: abnormally low white cell and platelet counts
Effective as mild sedative and hypnotic	

▷ **Principal Uses**

As a Single Drug Product: This versatile drug shares the characteristics of two major drug classes, the antihistamines and the phenothiazines. It is used to provide symptomatic relief in allergic disorders (hay fever, hives, etc.), to control nausea and vomiting and to produce mild sedation.

As a Combination Drug Product [CD]: This drug is often combined with analgesics such as aspirin or codeine to enhance their pain-relieving action by producing mild sedation. It is also used in cough mixtures for its drying (antihistaminic) effect.

How This Drug Works: Not completely established. This drug reduces the intensity of the allergic response by blocking the action of histamine after it has been released from sensitized tissue cells. It reduces the sensitivity of the nerve endings in the labyrinth (inner ear) and blocks the transmission of excessive nerve impulses to the vomiting center in the brain. The way this drug produces sedation and light sleep is not known.

Available Dosage Forms and Strengths
Injections — 25 mg per ml, 50 mg per ml
Suppositories — 12.5 mg, 25 mg
Syrups — 6.25 mg per 5 ml teaspoonful, 25 mg per 5 ml
teaspoonful (alcohol 1.5%)
Tablets — 12.5 mg, 25 mg, 50 mg

▷ **Usual Adult Dosage Range:** 12.5 to 25 mg/4 to 6 hours as needed. The total daily dosage should not exceed 150 mg. **Note: Actual dosage and administration schedule must be determined by the physician for each patient individually.**

▷ **Dosing Instructions:** Preferably taken with or following food to reduce stomach irritation. The tablets may be crushed for administration.

Usual Duration of Use: Continual use on a regular schedule for 3 to 5 days is usually necessary to determine this drug's effectiveness in relieving allergic symptoms or controlling vomiting. If not effective within 5 days, it should be discontinued.

▷ **This Drug Should Not Be Taken If**
- you have had an allergic reaction to it previously.
- you have a blood cell or bone marrow disorder.
- you have narrow-angle glaucoma (not adequately treated).

▷ **Inform Your Physician Before Taking This Drug If**
- you are allergic or overly sensitive to any phenothiazine drug (see Drug Class, Section Four).
- you are taking any drugs with sedative effects.
- you have a seizure disorder or bronchial asthma.
- you have impaired liver function.
- you have a history of peptic ulcer disease.
- you have an enlarged prostate gland or prostatism (see Glossary).

Possible Side-Effects (natural, expected and unavoidable drug actions)
Drowsiness (25% of users), lethargy, impaired concentration, dry mouth, constipation, impaired urination, reduced tolerance for contact lenses.

▷ **Possible Adverse Effects** (unusual, unexpected and infrequent reactions)
If any of the following develop, consult your physician promptly.
Mild Adverse Effects
Allergic Reactions: Skin rash, hives.
Headache, dizziness, unsteadiness, confusion, nervousness, excitation, irritability, tremor, insomnia, numbness and tingling, blurred vision, double vision, ringing in ears.
Loss of appetite, stomach irritation, nausea, vomiting, diarrhea.
Rapid heart rate, palpitation, low blood pressure.
Chest tightness, asthmatic wheezing, thickening of bronchial secretions.
Serious Adverse Effects
Allergic Reactions: Drug-induced hepatitis with jaundice (see Glossary).
Idiosyncratic Reactions: Euphoria, hysteria.

Nervous system reactions: Muscle spasms of the face, neck, back and extremities: rolling of the eyes, twisting of the neck, arching of the back, spasms of the hands and feet.

Blood cell disorders: abnormally low white blood cell and blood platelet counts, causing fever, sore throat, infections, abnormal bleeding or bruising (all very rare).

▷ **Adverse Effects That May Mimic Natural Diseases or Disorders**
Drug-induced hepatitis may suggest viral hepatitis.

Natural Diseases or Disorders That May Be Activated by This Drug
Latent epilepsy, glaucoma, prostatism (see Glossary).

CAUTION
1. This drug should not be used alone to treat symptoms of lower respiratory tract disease, including asthma.
2. Avoid this drug for at least 5 days before skin testing for possible allergens.

Precautions for Use
By Infants and Children: This drug should not be used in premature or full-term newborn infants. The young child is especially sensitive to the nervous system effects of antihistamines and phenothiazines. Children with acute illnesses ("flulike" infections, measles, chicken pox, etc.) are very susceptible to muscular spasms of the face, neck, back or extremities when this drug is used to control nausea and vomiting. Avoid this drug completely during such infections; there is evidence to suggest that it may contribute to the development of Reye syndrome (see Glossary).
By Those over 60 Years of Age: You may be more susceptible to the development of drowsiness, dizziness and lethargy and to impaired thinking, judgment and memory. The sedative effect of this drug can cause a hypoactive syndrome that may be misinterpreted as senility or emotional depression. This drug can increase the symptoms of prostatism (see Glossary).

▷ **Advisability of Use During Pregnancy**
Pregnancy Category: B (tentative). See Pregnancy Code inside back cover.
Animal studies: No birth defects reported in rats.
Human studies: No significant increase in birth defects reported in 746 exposures to this drug.
Avoid use of this drug during the last 3 months; it can reduce certain blood clotting factors in the fetus and cause bleeding in the newborn infant.

Advisability of Use if Breast-Feeding
Presence of this drug in breast milk: Yes.
Avoid drug or refrain from nursing.

Habit-Forming Potential: None.

Effects of Overdosage: Marked drowsiness, weakness, unsteadiness, agitation, delirium, deep sleep, coma, seizures.

Possible Effects of Long-Term Use: The development of tolerance and loss of effectiveness.

Suggested Periodic Examinations While Taking This Drug (at physician's
　　discretion)
　　Complete blood cell counts.

▷ **While Taking This Drug, Observe the Following**
　　Foods: No restrictions.
　　Beverages: No restrictions. May be taken with milk.
▷　*Alcohol*: Use extreme caution until the combined effects have been deter-
　　　　mined. The combination of alcohol and antihistamines can cause rapid
　　　　and marked sedation.
　　Tobacco Smoking: No interactions expected.
▷　*Other Drugs*
　　Promethazine may *increase* the effects of
　　　• all sedative drugs, and cause excessive sedation.
　　　• atropine and atropinelike drugs (see Drug Class, Section Four).
▷　*Driving, Hazardous Activities*: This drug may cause dizziness or drowsiness.
　　　Restrict activities as necessary.
　　Aviation Note: The use of this drug *is a disqualification* for piloting. Consult a
　　　designated Aviation Medical Examiner.
　　Exposure to Sun: Use caution until sensitivity has been determined. This drug
　　　may cause photosensitivity (see Glossary).

PROPOXYPHENE
(proh POX i feen)

Introduced: 1955

Class: Analgesic, Narcotic

Prescription: USA: Yes
　Canada: Yes

Controlled Drug: USA: C-IV*
　Canada: <N>

Available as Generic: Yes

Brand Names: Darvocet-N 50/100 [CD], Darvon, Darvon-N, Darvon w/ASA
[CD], Darvon Compound [CD], Darvon Compound-65 [CD], Darvon-N
w/ASA [CD], ✤Darvon-N Compound [CD], Dolene, Dolene AP-65 [CD],
Dolene Compound-65 [CD], ✤Novopropoxyn, ✤Novopropoxyn Com-
pound [CD], ✤642, SK-65, SK-65 APAP [CD], SK-65 Compound [CD],
Wygesic [CD]

BENEFITS versus RISKS

Possible Benefits	*Possible Risks*
EFFECTIVE RELIEF OF MILD TO MODERATE PAIN	POTENTIAL FOR HABIT FORMATION (DEPENDENCE) Sedative effects Drug-induced hepatitis (very rare)

---

*See Schedules of Controlled Drugs inside back cover.

▷ **Principal Uses**

As a Single Drug Product: This drug is used exclusively as an analgesic to relieve mild to moderate pain.

As a Combination Drug Product [CD]: It is available in combinations with acetaminophen and with aspirin. These milder pain relievers are added to enhance the analgesic effect and to reduce fever when present. Some combinations also contain caffeine to counteract the sedative effects of the analgesics.

How This Drug Works: Acting primarily as a depressant of certain brain functions, this drug suppresses the perception of pain and calms the emotional response to pain.

Available Dosage Forms and Strengths

Capsules — 32 mg, 65 mg

Oral suspension — 50 mg per 5 ml teaspoonful

Tablets — 100 mg

▷ **Usual Adult Dosage Range:**   For propoxyphene: 65 mg/4 hours as needed. The total daily dosage should not exceed 390 mg. For propoxyphene napsylate (Darvon-N): 100 mg/4 hours as needed. The total daily dose should not exceed 600 mg. **Note: Actual dosage and administration schedule must be determined by the physician for each patient individually.**

▷ **Dosing Instructions:**   May be taken with or following food to reduce stomach irritation or nausea. The tablet may be crushed and the capsule may be opened for administration.

Usual Duration of Use: As required to control pain. Continual use should not exceed 5 to 7 days without interruption and reassessment of need.

▷ **This Drug Should Not Be Taken If**
- you have had an allergic reaction to any dosage form of it previously.
- you are having an acute attack of asthma.

▷ **Inform Your Physician Before Taking This Drug If**
- you have had an unfavorable reaction to any narcotic drug in the past.
- you have a history of drug abuse or alcoholism.
- you have chronic lung disease with impaired breathing.
- you have impaired liver or kidney function.
- you are taking any other drugs that have a sedative effect.

Possible Side-Effects   (natural, expected and unavoidable drug actions)

Drowsiness, light-headedness, constipation.

▷ **Possible Adverse Effects**   (unusual, unexpected and infrequent reactions)

If any of the following develop, consult your physician promptly.

Mild Adverse Effects

Allergic Reactions: Skin rash, itching.

Headache, dizziness, weakness, confusion, blurred vision.

Nausea, vomiting, abdominal discomfort.

Serious Adverse Effects
   Allergic Reactions: Hepatitis with jaundice (see Glossary).
   Paradoxical excitement, agitation, insomnia.

Precautions for Use
   By Infants and Children: Safety and effectiveness for use by those under 12
   years of age have not been established.
   By Those over 60 Years of Age: Use small doses initially and increase dosage
   as needed and tolerated. Limit use to short-term treatment only. There
   may be increased susceptibility to the development of drowsiness, dizziness, unsteadiness, falling and constipation (possibly leading to fecal
   impaction).

▷ **Advisability of Use During Pregnancy**
   Pregnancy Category: C (tentative). See Pregnancy Code inside back cover.
   Animal studies: No birth defects due to this drug were found.
   Human studies: Information from studies of pregnant women indicates no
   significant increase in birth defects in 2914 exposures to this drug.
   Use this drug only if clearly needed and in small, infrequent doses.

Advisability of Use if Breast-Feeding
   Presence of this drug in breast milk: Yes, in small amounts.
   Monitor nursing infant closely and discontinue drug or nursing if adverse
   effects develop.

Habit-Forming Potential: Psychological and/or physical dependence can
   develop with use of large doses for an extended period of time.

Effects of Overdosage: Drowsiness, restlessness, agitation, nausea, vomiting,
   dry mouth, vertigo, weakness, lethargy, stupor, coma, seizures.

Possible Effects of Long-Term Use: Psychological and physical dependence,
   chronic constipation.

Suggested Periodic Examinations While Taking This Drug   (at physician's
   discretion)
   None.

▷ **While Taking This Drug, Observe the Following**
   Foods: No restrictions.
   Beverages: No restrictions. May be taken with milk.
▷   *Alcohol*: Use extreme caution until the combined effects have been deter-
   mined. Propoxyphene can intensify the intoxicating effects of alcohol,
   and alcohol can intensify the depressant effects of propoxyphene on
   brain function.
   Tobacco Smoking: Heavy smoking may reduce the effectiveness of this drug.
   Marijuana Smoking: Increase in drowsiness and pain relief; impairment of
   mental and physical performance.
▷   *Other Drugs*
      Propoxyphene may *increase* the effects of
      • other drugs with sedative effects.

- oral anticoagulants (Coumadin, etc.), and increase the risk of bleeding.
- carbamazepine (Tegretol), and increase its toxicity.
- doxepin (Sinequan), and increase its toxicity.

▷ *Driving, Hazardous Activities*: This drug can impair mental alertness, judgment, reaction time and physical coordination. Avoid hazardous activities accordingly.

Aviation Note: The use of this drug *is a disqualification* for piloting. Consult a designated Aviation Medical Examiner.

Exposure to Sun: No restrictions.

Discontinuation: It is advisable to limit this drug to short-term use. If it is necessary to use it for extended periods of time, discontinuation should be gradual to minimize possible effects of withdrawal.

PROPRANOLOL
(proh PRAN oh lohl)

Introduced: 1966

Class: Antianginal, Antiarrhythmic, Antihypertensive, Migraine Preventive, Beta-Adrenergic Blocker

Prescription: USA: Yes
Canada: Yes

Controlled Drug: USA: No
Canada: No

Available as Generic: Yes

Brand Names: ✿Apo-Propranolol, ✿Detensol, Inderal, Inderal-LA, Inderide [CD], Inderide LA [CD], ✿Novopranol, ✿PMS Propranolol

---

BENEFITS versus RISKS

Possible Benefits	*Possible Risks*
EFFECTIVE, WELL-TOLERATED AS: ANTIANGINAL DRUG in effort-induced angina; ANTIARRHYTHMIC DRUG in certain heart rhythm disorders; ANTIHYPERTENSIVE DRUG in mild to moderate hypertension EFFECTIVE PREVENTION OF MIGRAINE HEADACHES Effective adjunct in the prevention of recurrent heart attack (myocardial infarction) Effective adjunct in the management of pheochromocytoma	CONGESTIVE HEART FAILURE in advanced heart disease Worsening of angina in coronary heart disease (if drug is abruptly withdrawn) Masking of low blood sugar (hypoglycemia) in drug-treated diabetes Provocation of asthma Rare blood cell disorders: low white cell and platelet counts

---

▷ **Principal Uses**

As a Single Drug Product: This first "beta-blocker" drug is used primarily to treat several serious cardiovascular disorders: classical effort-induced angina, certain types of heart rhythm disturbance and high blood pressure. It is also beneficial in preventing the recurrence of heart attacks (myocardial infarction). In addition, it is used to reduce the frequency and severity of migraine headaches. Other uses (not "officially approved" at this time) include the control of physical manifestations of anxiety and nervous tension (as in stage fright), the control of familial tremors and the control of symptoms associated with markedly overactive thyroid gland function (thyrotoxicosis).

As a Combination Drug Product [CD]: This drug is available in combination with hydrochlorothiazide for the treatment of hypertension. This combination product includes two "step 1" drugs with different mechanisms of action; it is intended to provide greater effectiveness and convenience for long-term use.

How This Drug Works: By blocking certain actions of the sympathetic nervous system, this drug
- reduces the rate and contraction force of the heart, thus lowering the ejection pressure of the blood leaving the heart and reducing the oxygen requirement for heart function.
- reduces the degree of contraction of blood vessel walls, resulting in their relaxation and expansion and consequent lowering of blood pressure.
- prolongs the conduction time of nerve impulses through the heart, of benefit in the management of certain heart rhythm disorders.

Available Dosage Forms and Strengths

Capsules, prolonged action — 80 mg, 120 mg, 160 mg

Injection — 1 mg per ml

Tablets — 10 mg, 20 mg, 40 mg, 60 mg, 80 mg, 90 mg

▷ **Usual Adult Dosage Range:**   Varies with indication.

Antianginal: Initially, 10 to 20 mg 3 or 4 times/day; increase dose gradually every 3 to 7 days as needed and tolerated. The total daily dosage should not exceed 320 mg.

Antiarrhythmic: 10 to 30 mg 3 or 4 times/day as needed and tolerated.

Antihypertensive: Initially, 40 mg twice/day; increase dose gradually as needed and tolerated. The total daily dosage should not exceed 640 mg.

Migraine headache prevention: Initially, 20 mg 4 times/day; increase dose gradually as needed and tolerated. The total daily dosage should not exceed 240 mg.

Note: Actual dosage and administration schedule must be determined by the physician for each patient individually.

▷ **Dosing Instructions:**   Preferably taken 1 hour before eating to maximize absorption. The tablet may be crushed for administration. The prolonged action capsules should be swallowed whole without alteration. Do not discontinue this drug abruptly.

Usual Duration of Use: Continual use on a regular schedule for 10 to 14 days is usually necessary to determine this drug's effectiveness in preventing angina, controlling heart rhythm disorders and lowering blood pressure. Maximal effectiveness may require continual use for 6 to 8 weeks. The long-term use of this drug (months to years) will be determined by the course of your symptoms over time and your response to the overall treatment program (weight reduction, salt restriction, smoking cessation, etc.).

▷ **This Drug Should Not Be Taken If**
- you have had an allergic reaction to it previously.
- you have Prinzmetal's variant angina (coronary artery spasm).
- you have congestive heart failure.
- you have an abnormally slow heart rate or a serious form of heart block.
- you are taking, or have taken within the past 14 days, any monoamine oxidase (MAO) inhibitor drug (see Drug Class, Section Four).

▷ **Inform Your Physician Before Taking This Drug If**
- you have had an adverse reaction to any "beta-blocker" drug in the past (see Drug Class, Section Four).
- you have a history of serious heart disease, with or without episodes of heart failure.
- you have a history of hay fever (allergic rhinitis), asthma, chronic bronchitis or emphysema.
- you have a history of overactive thyroid function (hyperthyroidism).
- you have a history of low blood sugar (hypoglycemia).
- you have impaired liver or kidney function.
- you have diabetes or myasthenia gravis.
- you are currently taking any form of digitalis, quinidine or reserpine, or any "calcium-blocker" drug (see Drug Class, Section Four).
- you plan to have surgery under general anesthesia in the near future.

Possible Side-Effects (natural, expected and unavoidable drug actions)
Lethargy and fatigability, cold extremities, slow heart rate, light-headedness in upright position (see orthostatic hypotension in Glossary).

▷ **Possible Adverse Effects** (unusual, unexpected and infrequent reactions)
If any of the following develop, consult your physician promptly.
Mild Adverse Effects
Allergic Reactions: Skin rash, temporary loss of hair, drug fever (see Glossary).
Headache, dizziness, insomnia, vivid dreams.
Indigestion, nausea, vomiting, diarrhea.
Serious Adverse Effects
Idiosyncratic Reactions: Acute behavioral disturbances: disorientation, confusion, hallucinations, amnesia.
Mental depression, anxiety, impotence (rare).
Chest pain, shortness of breath, precipitation of congestive heart failure.
Induction of bronchial asthma (in asthmatic individuals).

Rare blood cell disorders: abnormally low white blood cell count, causing fever and sore throat; abnormally low blood platelet count, causing abnormal bleeding or bruising.

▷ **Adverse Effects That May Mimic Natural Diseases or Disorders**
Reduced blood flow to extremities may resemble Raynaud's phenomenon (see Glossary).

Natural Diseases or Disorders That May Be Activated by This Drug
Prinzmetal's variant angina, Raynaud's disease, intermittent claudication, myasthenia gravis (questionable).

CAUTION
1. *Do not discontinue this drug suddenly* without the knowledge and guidance of your physician. Carry a notation on your person that you are taking this drug.
2. Consult your physician or pharmacist before using nasal decongestants usually present in over-the-counter cold preparations and nose drops. These can cause sudden increases in blood pressure when taken concurrently with beta-blocker drugs.
3. Report the development of any tendency to emotional depression.

Precautions for Use
By Infants and Children: Safety and effectiveness for use by those under 12 years of age have not been established. However, if this drug is used, observe for the development of low blood sugar (hypoglycemia) during periods of reduced food intake.
By Those over 60 Years of Age: Proceed *cautiously* with all antihypertensive drugs. Unacceptably high blood pressure should be reduced without creating the risks associated with excessively low blood pressure. Start treatment with small doses, and monitor the blood pressure response frequently. Sudden, rapid and excessive reduction of blood pressure can predispose to stroke or heart attack. Observe for dizziness, unsteadiness, tendency to fall, confusion, hallucinations, depression or urinary frequency.

▷ **Advisability of Use During Pregnancy**
Pregnancy Category: C (tentative). See Pregnancy Code inside back cover.
Animal studies: No significant increase in birth defects due to this drug. Some toxic effects on embryo reported.
Human studies: Information from adequate studies of pregnant women is not available.
Avoid use of drug during the first 3 months if possible. Use this drug only if clearly needed. Ask your physician for guidance.

Advisability of Use if Breast-Feeding
Presence of this drug in breast milk: Yes.
Monitor nursing infant closely and discontinue drug or nursing if adverse effects develop.

Habit-Forming Potential: None.

Effects of Overdosage: Weakness, slow pulse, low blood pressure, fainting, cold and sweaty skin, congestive heart failure, possible coma and convulsions.

Possible Effects of Long-Term Use: Reduced heart reserve and eventual heart failure in susceptible individuals with advanced heart disease.

Suggested Periodic Examinations While Taking This Drug   (at physician's discretion)
Complete blood cell counts.
Measurements of blood pressure, evaluation of heart function.

▷ **While Taking This Drug, Observe the Following**
Foods: No restrictions. Avoid excessive salt intake.
Beverages: No restrictions. May be taken with milk.
▷ *Alcohol*: Use with caution until the combined effect has been determined. Alcohol may exaggerate this drug's ability to lower the blood pressure and may increase its mild sedative effect.
Tobacco Smoking: Nicotine may reduce this drug's effectiveness in treating angina, heart rhythm disorders and high blood pressure. Smoking increases the rate of elimination of this drug and decreases its blood levels, especially in younger individuals. In addition, high doses of this drug may potentiate the constriction of the bronchial tubes caused by regular smoking.
▷ *Other Drugs*
Propranolol may *increase* the effects of
- other antihypertensive drugs, and cause excessive lowering of blood pressure. Dosage adjustments may be necessary.
- lidocaine (Xylocaine, etc.).
- reserpine (Ser-Ap-Es, etc.), and cause sedation, depression, slowing of the heart rate and lowering of the blood pressure.
- verapamil (Calan, Isoptin), and cause excessive depression of heart function; monitor this combination closely.
Propranolol may *decrease* the effects of
- theophyllines (Aminophyllin, Theo-Dur, etc.), and reduce their anti-asthmatic effectiveness.
Propranolol *taken concurrently* with
- clonidine (Catapres) requires close monitoring for rebound high blood pressure if clonidine is withdrawn while propranolol is still being taken.
- epinephrine (Adrenalin, etc.) may cause marked rise in blood pressure and slowing of the heart rate.
- insulin requires close monitoring to avoid undetected hypoglycemia (see Glossary).
The following drugs may *increase* the effects of propranolol
- chlorpromazine (Thorazine, etc.).
- cimetidine (Tagamet).
- methimazole (Tapazole).
- propylthiouracil (Propacil).

The following drugs may *decrease* the effects of propranolol

- barbiturates (phenobarbital, etc.).
- indomethacin (Indocin), and possibly other "aspirin substitutes," may impair propranolol's antihypertensive effect.
- rifampin (Rifadin, Rimactane).

▷ *Driving, Hazardous Activities*: Use caution until the full extent of drowsiness, lethargy and blood pressure change have been determined.

Aviation Note: The use of this drug *may be a disqualification* for piloting. Consult a designated Aviation Medical Examiner.

Exposure to Sun: No restrictions.

Exposure to Heat: Caution advised. Hot environments can lower blood pressure and exaggerate the effects of this drug.

Exposure to Cold: Caution advised. Cold environments can enhance the circulatory deficiency in the extremities that may occur with this drug. The elderly should take precautions to prevent hypothermia (see Glossary).

Heavy Exercise or Exertion: It is advisable to avoid exertion that produces light-headedness, excessive fatigue or muscle cramping. The use of this drug may intensify the hypertensive response to isometric exercise.

Occurrence of Unrelated Illness: The fever that accompanies systemic infections can lower blood pressure and require adjustment of dosage. Illnesses that cause nausea or vomiting may interrupt the regular dosage schedule. Ask your physician for guidance.

Discontinuation: It is advisable to avoid sudden discontinuation of this drug in all situations; this is especially true in the presence of coronary artery disease. If possible, gradual reduction of dose over a period of 2 to 3 weeks is recommended. Ask your physician for specific guidance.

PSEUDOEPHEDRINE
(soo doh e FED rin)

Other Names: Isoephedrine

Introduced: 1957

Class: Decongestant

Prescription: USA: No
Canada: No

Controlled Drug: USA: No
Canada: No

Available as Generic: USA: Yes
Canada: No

Brand Names: Actifed [CD], ✦Actifed-A [CD], Actifed w/Codeine [CD], ✦Actifed DM [CD], Afrinol Repetabs, Cenafed, Deconamine [CD], Dimacol [CD], Dimacol Liquid [CD], Disophrol [CD], Drixoral Syrup [CD], Drixoral Tablets [CD], ✦Eltor AF [CD], ✦Eltor-120, Fedahist [CD], Fedahist Expectorant [CD], Fedrazil [CD], Isoclor [CD], Neo-Synephrinol, Novafed, Novafed A Capsules [CD], Novafed A Liquid [CD], Novafed Liquid, Phenergan-D [CD], Sudafed, Sudafed Cough Syrup [CD], Sudafed Plus [CD], Sudafed S.A., Tussend [CD], Tussend Expectorant [CD]

BENEFITS versus RISKS

Possible Benefits	*Possible Risks*
EFFECTIVE DECONGESTION OF NASAL AND SINUS TISSUES	Nervousness
	Palpitation
	Insomnia

▷ **Principal Uses**

As a Single Drug Product: Used exclusively as a decongestant in the treatment of allergic and infectious conditions of the nose, sinuses and eustachian tubes, such as allergic rhinitis (hay fever), headcolds, sinusitis and the "ear blockage" that occurs with air travel.

As a Combination Drug Product [CD]: This drug is frequently combined with antihistamines to enhance the drying effect on tissues of the upper respiratory tract. It is also present in cough mixtures to provide decongestion in conditions of the lower respiratory tract, such as tracheobronchitis.

How This Drug Works: By contracting the walls of arterioles and thus reducing their size, this drug decreases the volume of blood in the tissues, resulting in shrinkage of tissue mass (decongestion). This expands the nasal airway and enlarges the openings into the sinuses and eustachian tubes.

Available Dosage Forms and Strengths

Capsules, prolonged action — 120 mg

Liquid — 15 mg per 5 ml teaspoonful, 30 mg per 5 ml teaspoonful

Tablets — 30 mg, 60 mg

Tablets, prolonged action — 120 mg

▷ **Usual Adult Dosage Range:** 30 to 60 mg/4 to 6 hours as needed. Prolonged action forms: 120 mg/8 to 12 hours. The total daily dosage should not exceed 240 mg. **Note: For prolonged use, the actual dosage and administration schedule should be determined by the physician for each patient individually.**

▷ **Dosing Instructions:** Do not exceed the recommended doses. This drug may be taken with or following food to reduce stomach irritation. Prolonged action capsules or tablets should be swallowed whole without alteration.

Usual Duration of Use: Continual use on a regular schedule for 2 to 3 days is usually necessary to determine this drug's effectiveness in relieving nasal and sinus congestion. If there is no significant improvement after 1 week of use, consult your physician for further evaluation.

▷ **This Drug Should Not Be Taken If**
- you have had an allergic reaction to any dosage form of it previously.

▷ **Inform Your Physician Before Taking This Drug If**
- you are overly sensitive to other decongestants or to stimulants of the sympathetic nervous system.
- you have high blood pressure or heart disease.
- you have diabetes or an overactive thyroid gland (hyperthyroidism).
- you have an enlarged prostate gland (prostatism, see Glossary).
- you are taking any form of digitalis (digitoxin, digoxin).
- you are taking any beta-blocker drug (see Drug Class, Section Four).
- you are taking, or have taken within the past 14 days, any monoamine oxidase (MAO) inhibitor drug (see Drug Class, Section Four).

Possible Side-Effects   (natural, expected and unavoidable drug actions)
Nervousness, insomnia.

▷ **Possible Adverse Effects**   (unusual, unexpected and infrequent reactions)
If any of the following develop, consult your physician promptly.
Mild Adverse Effects
Headache, dizziness, light-headedness, heart palpitation, tremors.
Nausea, vomiting, difficult urination.
Serious Adverse Effects
None reported.

CAUTION
1. Many over-the-counter drug products for allergies, colds and coughs contain drugs that may interact unfavorably with this drug. Ask your physician or pharmacist for guidance before using such medications.
2. Avoid this drug within 6 hours of bedtime to reduce the possibility of insomnia.

Precautions for Use
By Infants and Children: The prolonged action dosage forms should not be given to children under 6 years of age.
By Those over 60 Years of Age: Use small doses until your tolerance has been determined. Observe for possible nervousness, insomnia, palpitation or angina. Prostatism may be increased.

▷ **Advisability of Use During Pregnancy**
Pregnancy Category: C (tentative). See Pregnancy Code inside back cover.
Animal studies: No significant birth defects due to this drug found.
Human studies: Information from studies of pregnant women is inconclusive. Limited studies indicate a possible increased risk for birth defects during the first 3 months with use of drugs of this class.
Avoid completely during the first 3 months. Limit use to small, infrequent doses as needed during the last 6 months.

Advisability of Use if Breast-Feeding
Presence of this drug in breast milk: Yes.
Avoid drug or refrain from nursing.

Habit-Forming Potential: None.

Effects of Overdosage: Headache, restlessness, anxiety, agitation, palpitation, sweating, nausea, vomiting, tremors, delirium, hallucinations, seizures.

Possible Effects of Long-Term Use: None reported.

Suggested Periodic Examinations While Taking This Drug   (at physician's discretion)
None required.

▷ **While Taking This Drug, Observe the Following**
Foods: No restrictions.
Beverages: Heavy use of coffee or tea may add to the nervousness or insomnia experienced by sensitive individuals.
▷ *Alcohol*: No interactions expected.
Tobacco Smoking: No interactions expected.
▷ *Other Drugs*
Pseudoephedrine may *decrease* the effects of
- guanethidine (Esimil, Ismelin), and reduce its antihypertensive effectiveness.

Pseudoephedrine *taken concurrently* with
- beta-blocker drugs or monoamine oxidase (MAO) inhibitor drugs may cause dangerous elevations of blood pressure. Observe for headache or palpitation.

The following drugs may *increase* the effects of pseudoephedrine
- sodium bicarbonate (soda mint, etc.).
▷ *Driving, Hazardous Activities*: This drug may cause dizziness. Restrict activities as necessary.
Aviation Note: The use of this drug *may be a disqualification* for piloting. Consult a designated Aviation Medical Examiner.
Exposure to Sun: No restrictions.

QUINIDINE
(KWIN i deen)

Introduced: 1918

Prescription: USA: Yes
Canada: No

Available as Generic: Yes

Class: Antiarrhythmic

Controlled Drug: USA: No
Canada: No

Brand Names: ✤Apo-Quinidine, ✤Biquin Durules, Cardioquin, Cin-Quin, Duraquin, ✤Novoquinidine, Quinaglute Dura-Tabs, ✤Quinate, Quinidex Extentabs, ✤Quinobarb [CD]*, Quinora

*Quinobarb contains phenylethylbarbiturate, a sedative of the barbiturate class.

BENEFITS versus RISKS

Possible Benefits	*Possible Risks*
EFFECTIVE TREATMENT OF SELECTED HEART RHYTHM DISORDERS	NARROW TREATMENT RANGE FREQUENT ADVERSE EFFECTS (30% of users) NUMEROUS ALLERGIC AND IDIOSYNCRATIC REACTIONS Dose-related toxicity Provocation of abnormal heart rhythms Abnormally low blood platelet count (rare)

▷ **Principal Uses**

As a Single Drug Product: Used primarily to control the following types of abnormal heart rhythm: atrial fibrillation and flutter, paroxysmal atrial tachycardia, paroxysmal ventricular tachycardia, premature atrial and ventricular contractions.

As a Combination Drug Product [CD]: This drug is available (in Canada) in combination with a barbiturate, a mild sedative that is added to allay the anxiety and nervous tension that often accompany heart rhythm disorders.

How This Drug Works: By slowing the activity of the pacemaker and delaying the transmission of electrical impulses through the conduction system and muscle of the heart, this drug assists in restoring normal heart rate and rhythm.

Available Dosage Forms and Strengths

Capsules — 300 mg, 1200 mg
Injections — 180 mg per ml, 200 mg per ml
Tablets — 200 mg, 275 mg, 300 mg, 1100 mg
Tablets, prolonged action — 300 mg, 324 mg, 330 mg

▷ **Usual Adult Dosage Range:**   Test dose: 200 mg, then observe for 2 hours for evidence of idiosyncrasy.

Dose varies with indication:

Premature atrial or ventricular contractions: 200 to 300 mg 3 or 4 times/day.

Paroxysmal atrial tachycardia: 400 to 600 mg/2 to 3 hours until paroxysm is terminated.

Atrial flutter: digitalize first; then individualize dosage schedule as appropriate.

Atrial fibrillation: digitalize first; then try 200 mg/2 to 3 hours for 5 to 8 doses; increase dose daily until normal rhythm is restored or toxic effects develop.

Maintenance schedule: 200 to 300 mg 3 or 4 times/day.

The total daily dosage should not exceed 4000 mg.

Note: Actual dosage and administration schedule must be determined by the physician for each patient individually.

▷ **Dosing Instructions:**   Preferably taken on an empty stomach to achieve high blood levels rapidly. However, it may be taken with or following food to reduce stomach irritation. The regular tablets may be crushed and the capsules opened for administration. The prolonged action forms should be swallowed whole without alteration.

Usual Duration of Use: Continual use on a regular schedule for 2 to 4 days is usually necessary to determine this drug's effectiveness in correcting or preventing responsive abnormal rhythms. Long-term use (months to years) requires supervision and periodic evaluation by your physician.

▷ **This Drug Should Not Be Taken If**
- you have had an allergic or idiosyncratic reaction to any dosage form of it previously.
- you currently have an acute infection of any kind.

▷ **Inform Your Physician Before Taking This Drug If**
- you have coronary artery disease or myasthenia gravis.
- you have a history of hyperthyroidism.
- you have had a deficiency of blood platelets in the past from any cause.
- you are now taking, or have taken recently, any digitalis preparation (digitoxin, digoxin, etc.).
- you plan to have surgery under general anesthesia in the near future.

Possible Side-Effects   (natural, expected and unavoidable drug actions)
Drop in blood pressure, may be marked in sensitive individuals.

▷ **Possible Adverse Effects**   (unusual, unexpected and infrequent reactions)
If any of the following develop, consult your physician promptly.
Mild Adverse Effects
Allergic Reactions: Skin rash, hives, itching, drug fever (rare).
Dose-related toxicity (cinchonism): blurred vision, ringing in the ears, loss of hearing, dizziness.
Nausea, vomiting, diarrhea (20% to 30% of users).
Serious Adverse Effects
Allergic Reactions: Severe skin reactions, hemolytic anemia (see Glossary), joint and muscle pains, anaphylactic reaction (see Glossary), reduced blood platelet count, drug-induced hepatitis (see Glossary).
Idiosyncratic Reactions: Skin rash, rapid heart rate, acute delirium and combative behavior, difficult breathing.
Heart conduction abnormalities.
Optic neuritis, impaired vision.
Abnormally low white blood cell count: fever, sore throat, infections.

▷ **Adverse Effects That May Mimic Natural Diseases or Disorders**
Drug-induced hepatitis may suggest viral hepatitis.

Natural Diseases or Disorders That May Be Activated by This Drug
Systemic lupus erythematosus, myasthenia gravis, psoriasis (in sensitive individuals).

CAUTION
1. The effects of this drug are very unpredictable because of the wide variation in response from person to person. Dosage adjustments must be based upon individual reaction. Notify your physician of any events that you suspect may be drug related.
2. It is advisable to carry a card of personal identification that includes a notation that you are taking this drug.

Precautions for Use
By Infants and Children: A test for drug idiosyncrasy should be made before starting treatment with this drug. If there is no beneficial response after 3 days of adequate dosage, this drug should be discontinued.
By Those over 60 Years of Age: Small doses are mandatory until your individual response has been determined. Observe for the development of lightheadedness, dizziness, weakness or sense of impending faint. Use caution to prevent falls.

▷ **Advisability of Use During Pregnancy**
Pregnancy Category: C (tentative). See Pregnancy Code inside back cover.
Animal studies: No information available.
Human studies: Information from adequate studies of pregnant women is not available. No birth defects have been reported following use of this drug during pregnancy.
Use this drug only if clearly needed.

Advisability of Use if Breast-Feeding
Presence of this drug in breast milk: Yes.
Avoid drug or refrain from nursing.

Habit-Forming Potential: None.

Effects of Overdosage: Nausea, vomiting, ringing in the ears, headache, jerky eye movements, double vision, altered color vision, confusion, delirium, hot skin, seizures, coma.

Possible Effects of Long-Term Use: None reported.

Suggested Periodic Examinations While Taking This Drug   (at physician's discretion)
Complete blood cell counts, electrocardiograms.

▷ **While Taking This Drug, Observe the Following**
Foods: No restrictions.
Beverages: No restrictions. May be taken with milk.
▷   *Alcohol*: Use caution until the combined effects have been determined. Alcohol may enhance the blood-pressure-lowering effects of this drug.
Tobacco Smoking: Nicotine can increase irritability of the heart and aggravate rhythm disorders. Avoid all forms of tobacco.

▷   *Other Drugs*
Quinidine may *increase* the effects of
- anticoagulants (Coumadin, etc.), and increase the risk of bleeding.
- digitoxin and digoxin (Lanoxin), and cause digitalis toxicity.

The following drugs may *increase* the effects of quinidine
- amiodarone.
- cimetidine (Tagamet).

The following drugs may *decrease* the effects of quinidine
- barbiturates (phenobarbital, etc.).
- phenytoin (Dilantin).
- rifampin (Rifadin, Rimactane).

▷   *Driving, Hazardous Activities*: This drug may cause dizziness and alter vision. Restrict activities as necessary.

Aviation Note: The use of this drug *may be a disqualification* for piloting. Consult a designated Aviation Medical Examiner.

Exposure to Sun: No restrictions.

RANITIDINE
(ra NI te deen)

Introduced: 1981

Prescription: USA: Yes
Canada: Yes

Available as Generic: No

Brand Names: Zantac

Class: Antiulcer, H-2 Receptor Blocker

Controlled Drug: USA: No
Canada: No

BENEFITS versus RISKS

Possible Benefits	*Possible Risks*
EFFECTIVE TREATMENT OF PEPTIC ULCER DISEASE: Relief of symptoms Acceleration of healing Prevention of recurrence CONTROL OF HYPERSECRETORY STOMACH DISORDERS Beneficial in treatment of reflux esophagitis	Drug-induced hepatitis (rare) Confusion (in severely ill elderly patients) Rare blood cell disorders

---

▷ **Principal Uses**
As a Single Drug Product: Used primarily in the treatment of peptic ulcer disease, both benign stomach (gastric) ulcer and duodenal ulcer. It is used specifically to hasten the healing of ulcer and to prevent recurrence.

Also used to control the excessive production of stomach acid in the Zollinger-Ellison syndrome. Though its effectiveness has not been fully established, this drug is also widely used in the management of esophagitis (as with hiatal hernia) and upper gastrointestinal bleeding.

How This Drug Works: By blocking the action of histamine, this drug effectively inhibits the secretion of stomach acid and thus creates a more favorable environment for the healing of peptic ulcers.

Available Dosage Forms and Strengths
    Injection — 25 mg per ml
    Tablets — 150 mg, 300 mg

▷ **Usual Adult Dosage Range:**   For active peptic ulcer and hypersecretory states: 150 mg 2 times daily, 12 hours apart. For prevention of recurrent ulcer: 150 mg at bedtime. **Note: Actual dosage and administration schedule must be determined by the physician for each patient individually.**

▷ **Dosing Instructions:**   To obtain the longest period of stomach acid reduction, this drug should be taken with or immediately following meals. The tablet may be crushed for administration.

Usual Duration of Use: Continual use on a regular schedule for 4 to 6 weeks is usually necessary to determine this drug's effectiveness in healing active peptic ulcer. Long-term use (months to years) for prevention of ulcer recurrence requires individual consideration by your physician.

▷ **This Drug Should Not Be Taken If**
- you have had an allergic reaction to any dosage form of it previously.

▷ **Inform Your Physician Before Taking This Drug If**
- you are allergic to cimetidine (Tagamet).
- you have impaired liver or kidney function.
- you are taking an oral anticoagulant.

Possible Side-Effects   (natural, expected and unavoidable drug actions)
    None reported.

▷ **Possible Adverse Effects**   (unusual, unexpected and infrequent reactions)
    If any of the following develop, consult your physician promptly.
    Mild Adverse Effects
    Allergic Reactions: Skin rash.
    Headache, malaise, dizziness.
    Nausea, constipation, diarrhea.
    Serious Adverse Effects
    Idiosyncratic Reactions: Confusion in the elderly and debilitated.
    Drug-induced hepatitis (see Glossary).
    Bone marrow depression (see Glossary)—weakness, fever, sore throat, abnormal bleeding or bruising.

▷ **Adverse Effects That May Mimic Natural Diseases or Disorders**
    Liver reactions may suggest viral hepatitis.

CAUTION
1. Do not discontinue this drug abruptly. (Ulcer activation and perforation have occurred following abrupt cessation of cimetidine, a closely related drug.)
2. After discontinuation of this drug, inform your physician promptly if you experience a return of symptoms indicative of ulcer reactivation.

Precautions for Use
By Infants and Children: Safety and effectiveness for use by those under 12 years of age have not been established.
By Those over 60 Years of Age: Observe for the development of nervous agitation or confusion. This drug may contribute to the formation of stomach phytobezoars (masses of undigested vegetable fibers). Individuals with poor chewing ability (missing teeth) and those who have had partial gastrectomy or vagotomy (stomach surgery) are most susceptible. Observe for loss of appetite, stomach fullness, nausea and vomiting.

▷ **Advisability of Use During Pregnancy**
Pregnancy Category: B (tentative). See Pregnancy Code inside back cover.
Animal studies: No birth defects reported.
Human studies: Information from adequate studies of pregnant women is not available.
Use this drug only if clearly needed. Ask physician for guidance.

Advisability of Use if Breast-Feeding
Presence of this drug in breast milk: Yes.
Avoid drug or refrain from nursing.

Habit-Forming Potential: None.

Effects of Overdosage: Confusion, delirium, slurred speech, flushing, sweating, drowsiness, muscle twitching, seizures, coma.

Possible Effects of Long-Term Use: None reported.

Suggested Periodic Examinations While Taking This Drug (at physician's discretion)
Complete blood cell counts, liver function tests.

▷ **While Taking This Drug, Observe the Following**
Foods: Protein-rich foods produce maximal stomach acid secretion. Follow the diet prescribed to derive optimal benefit from this drug.
Beverages: No restrictions. May be taken with milk.
▷ *Alcohol*: No interactions with drug. However, alcoholic beverages increase stomach acidity and can reduce the effectiveness of this drug.
▷ *Other Drugs*
Ranitidine may *increase* the effects of
• oral anticoagulants, and increase the risk of bleeding.
▷ *Driving, Hazardous Activities*: This drug may cause dizziness. Restrict activities as necessary.
Aviation Note: The use of this drug *may be a disqualification* for piloting. Consult a designated Aviation Medical Examiner.

Exposure to Sun: No restrictions.

Discontinuation: Do not discontinue this drug suddenly if taken for peptic ulcer disease. Consult physician for withdrawal instructions. This drug does not provide an extended protective effect. Be alert to the possibility of ulcer recurrence anytime after discontinuation.

RESERPINE
(re SER peen)

Other Names: Deserpidine, Rauwolfia

Introduced: 1953   **Class:**   Antihypertensive

Prescription: USA: Yes   **Controlled Drug:**   USA: No
  Canada: Yes   Canada: No

Available as Generic: Yes

Brand Names: Demi-Regroton [CD], ✤Novoreserpine, Rauzide [CD], Regroton [CD], ✤Reserfia, Sandril, Ser-Ap-Es [CD], Serpalan, Serpasil, Serpate

---

BENEFITS versus RISKS

Possible Benefits	*Possible Risks*
Moderately effective "step 2" antihypertensive in mild to moderate hypertension when used concurrently with a diuretic	INDUCTION OF MENTAL DEPRESSION (can be severe and prolonged)
	ACTIVATION OF PEPTIC ULCER, GASTROINTESTINAL BLEEDING
	Frequent nasal congestion and diarrhea
	Reduced libido, sexual impotence
	Mental disturbances

▷ **Principal Uses**

As a Single Drug Product: Used primarily as a "step 2" antihypertensive drug in the treatment of mild to moderate hypertension. Originally introduced as a tranquilizer for the treatment of schizophrenia, it is seldom used for this purpose currently.

As a Combination Drug Product [CD]: This drug is available in combination with most of the thiazide diuretics, the conventional "step 1" antihypertensive medication. One popular product combines reserpine, hydrochlorothiazide and hydralazine, a "step 2 or 3" antihypertensive. These combinations are more effective for treating moderate to severe hypertension.

How This Drug Works: By depleting the nerve impulse transmitter norepinephrine from nerve terminals, this drug reduces the ability of the sympathetic nervous system to maintain the degree of blood vessel constriction that is responsible for high blood pressure. The reduced availability of norepinephrine results in relaxation of blood vessel walls and lowering of blood pressure.

Available Dosage Forms and Strengths
Capsules, prolonged action — 0.5 mg
Tablets — 0.1 mg, 0.25 mg, 1 mg

▷ **Usual Adult Dosage Range:** As antihypertensive: Initially, 0.1 to 0.5 mg/24 hours for 1 to 2 weeks. Adjust dose as needed and tolerated. The usual maintenance dose is 0.1 to 0.25 mg/24 hours. The total daily dosage should not exceed 1.0 mg/24 hours. **Note: Actual dosage and administration schedule must be determined by the physician for each patient individually.**

▷ **Dosing Instructions:** Take with or following food to reduce stomach irritation. The tablet may be crushed for administration. The prolonged action capsule should be swallowed whole without alteration.

Usual Duration of Use: Continual use on a regular schedule for 3 to 6 weeks is usually necessary to determine this drug's full effectiveness in controlling hypertension. Long-term use (months to years) requires supervision and periodic evaluation by your physician.

▷ **This Drug Should Not Be Taken If**
  - you have had an allergic reaction to any form of reserpine previously.
  - you are mentally depressed, or you have had a depression in the past.
  - you have an active peptic ulcer, or a history of peptic ulcer disease.
  - you have active regional enteritis, ulcerative colitis or a history of ulcerative bowel disease.

▷ **Inform Your Physician Before Taking This Drug If**
  - you have a seizure disorder.
  - you are subject to migraine headaches.
  - you have any form of heart disease.
  - you have gallbladder disease.
  - you are taking any of the following drugs: anticoagulants, a digitalis preparation, quinidine, levodopa, antidepressants, sedatives or a monoamine oxidase (MAO) inhibitor (see Drug Classes, Section Four).
  - you plan to have surgery under general anesthesia in the near future.

Possible Side-Effects (natural, expected and unavoidable drug actions)
Drowsiness and lethargy (especially during the first few weeks), reddening of the eyes, nasal stuffiness (frequent), dry mouth, increased hunger contractions, acid indigestion, intestinal cramping, diarrhea, water retention.

▷ **Possible Adverse Effects** (unusual, unexpected and infrequent reactions)
If any of the following develop, consult your physician promptly.

Mild Adverse Effects
Allergic Reactions: Skin rashes, itching.
Headache, dizziness, nosebleeds.
Nausea, vomiting, persistent diarrhea.
Altered menstrual pattern.

Serious Adverse Effects
Allergic Reactions: Reduction of blood platelet count, with or without spontaneous bruising.
Idiosyncratic Reactions: Paradoxical nervousness, agitation, confusion, nightmares, hallucinations.
Bronchospasm, asthmatic wheezing.
Mental depression, reduced libido, sexual impotence.
Peptic ulcer activation, with or without bleeding.
Breast enlargement and tenderness, milk production.

▷ **Adverse Effects That May Mimic Natural Diseases or Disorders**
Parkinson-like muscle rigidity and lethargic behavior may suggest true Parkinson's disease.

Natural Diseases or Disorders That May Be Activated by This Drug
Migraine headaches, mental depression, peptic ulcer disease, systemic lupus erythematosus.

CAUTION
1. Discontinue this drug at the first indication of despondency, loss of appetite, early morning awakening (insomnia), or impaired sex drive or performance.
2. Avoid concurrent use of drugs with strong sedative effects, antidepressants, levodopa and monoamine oxidase (MAO) inhibitors.
3. If surgery is planned, consult your surgeon and/or anesthesiologist regarding the need to discontinue this drug prior to surgery.

Precautions for Use
By Infants and Children: Continual use for a minimum of 7 to 14 days is necessary to determine this drug's effectiveness as an antihypertensive. Observe carefully for excessive drowsiness, emotional instability or gastrointestinal disturbances.
By Those over 60 Years of Age: Start treatment with small doses and proceed cautiously. Unacceptably high blood pressure should be reduced without creating the risks associated with excessively low blood pressure. Sudden, rapid and excessive reduction of blood pressure can predispose to stroke or heart attack. This age group is more susceptible to the development of impaired thinking, depression (6%), confusion, nightmares and orthostatic hypotension (see Glossary).

▷ **Advisability of Use During Pregnancy**
Pregnancy Category: D (tentative). See Pregnancy Code inside back cover.
Animal studies: Significant eye defects reported in rats.
Human studies: Information from adequate studies of pregnant women is not available. Significant birth defects have been reported with the use

of this drug during the first 3 months. Use of this drug during the last
month of pregnancy can cause lethargy, nasal congestion, breathing difficulties and poor feeding in the newborn infant.
Avoid this drug during the first 3 months and the last month. Use it otherwise only if clearly needed.

Advisability of Use if Breast-Feeding
Presence of this drug in breast milk: Yes.
Avoid drug or refrain from nursing.

Habit-Forming Potential: None.

Effects of Overdosage: Marked drowsiness, flushed skin, incoordination,
tremors, slow and weak pulse, slow and shallow breathing, diarrhea, stupor progressing to coma.

Possible Effects of Long-Term Use: None reported.

Suggested Periodic Examinations While Taking This Drug (at physician's
discretion)
Complete blood cell counts.
Assessment of emotional status for unrecognized depression.

▷ **While Taking This Drug, Observe the Following**
Foods: No restrictions. Avoid excessive salt intake.
Beverages: No restrictions. May be taken with milk.
▷ *Alcohol*: Use with extreme caution until the combined effects have been
determined. This drug can increase the intoxicating effects of alcohol.
Both of these drugs depress brain function.
Tobacco Smoking: No interactions expected.
Marijuana Smoking: Significant increase in drowsiness; possible accentuation of hypotension; possible preciptation of depression.
▷ *Other Drugs*
Reserpine may *decrease* the effects of
• levodopa (Dopar, Sinemet), and reduce its effectiveness in treating Parkinson's disease.
Reserpine *taken concurrently* with
• anticonvulsants may lower the convulsive threshold in susceptible individuals and alter seizure patterns.
• digitalis preparations may cause rhythm disorders in susceptible individuals.
• monoamine oxidase (MAO) inhibitors may cause excessive stimulation
of the nervous system (theoretical).
• quinidine may cause rhythm disorders in susceptible individuals.
• warfarin (Coumadin, etc.) may cause decreased anticoagulant effect with
short-term use and increased anticoagulant effect with long-term use.
▷ *Driving, Hazardous Activities*: This drug may impair mental alertness, judgment, physical coordination and reaction time. Restrict activities as necessary.

Aviation Note: The use of this drug *is a disqualification* for piloting. Consult a designated Aviation Medical Examiner.

Exposure to Sun: No restrictions.

Exposure to Cold: Use caution. Monitor the elderly for excessive hypotension and other changes conducive to hypothermia (see Glossary).

RIFAMPIN
(RIF am pin)

Other Names: Rifampicin

Introduced: 1967   **Class:**   Antibiotic, Rifamycins

Prescription: USA: Yes   **Controlled Drug:**   USA: No
    Canada: Yes   Canada: No

Available as Generic: No

Brand Names: Rifadin, Rifamate [CD], Rimactane, ♣Rofact

BENEFITS versus RISKS

Possible Benefits	*Possible Risks*
EFFECTIVE TREATMENT OF TUBERCULOSIS in combination with other drugs	DRUG-INDUCED HEPATITIS
	DRUG-INDUCED NEPHRITIS
	Flulike syndrome
EFFECTIVE PREVENTION OF MENINGITIS by the elimination of meningococcus from the throat of carriers	Rare blood cell disorder: abnormally low blood platelet count

---

▷ **Principal Uses**

As a Single Drug Product: This antibiotic drug is used primarily to treat active tuberculosis. It is usually given concurrently with other antitubercular drugs to enhance its effectiveness. It is also used to eliminate the meningitis germ (meningococcus) from the throats of healthy carriers so it cannot be spread to others. It is not effective in the treatment of active meningitis.

As a Combination Drug Product [CD]: This drug is available in combination with isoniazid, another antitubercular drug that delays the development of drug-resistant strains of the tuberculosis germ.

How This Drug Works: This drug prevents the growth and multiplication of susceptible tuberculosis organisms by blocking specific enzyme systems that are involved in the formation of essential proteins.

Available Dosage Forms and Strengths
Capsules — 150 mg, 300 mg

▷ **Usual Adult Dosage Range:**   For tuberculosis: 600 mg once/day. For meningococcus carriers: 600 mg once/day for 4 days. The total daily dosage should not exceed 600 mg. **Note: Actual dosage and administration schedule must be determined by the physician for each patient individually.**

▷ **Dosing Instructions:** Preferably taken with 8 ounces of water on an empty stomach (1 hour before or 2 hours after eating). However, it may be taken with food if necessary to reduce stomach irritation. The capsule may be opened and the contents mixed with applesauce or jelly for administration.

Usual Duration of Use: Continual use on a regular schedule for several months is usually necessary to determine this drug's effectiveness in promoting recovery from tuberculosis. Long-term use (possibly 1 to 2 years) requires ongoing supervision and periodic evaluation by your physician.

▷ **This Drug Should Not Be Taken If**
- you have had an allergic reaction to it previously.
- you have active liver disease.

▷ **Inform Your Physician Before Taking This Drug If**
- you are pregnant.
- you have a history of liver disease or impaired liver function.
- you consume alcohol daily.
- you are taking an oral contraceptive. (An alternate method of contraception is advised.)
- you are taking an anticoagulant.

Possible Side-Effects   (natural, expected and unavoidable drug actions)
Red, orange or brown discoloration of tears, sweat, saliva, sputum, urine or stool. Yellow discoloration of the skin (not jaundice). Note: In the absence of symptoms indicating illness, any discoloration is a harmless drug effect and does not indicate toxicity.
Possible fungal superinfections (see Glossary).

▷ **Possible Adverse Effects**   (unusual, unexpected and infrequent reactions)
If any of the following develop, consult your physician promptly.
Mild Adverse Effects
Allergic Reactions: Skin rash, hives, itching, drug fever (see Glossary).
Headache, drowsiness, dizziness, blurred vision, impaired hearing, vague numbness and tingling.
Loss of appetite, heartburn, nausea, vomiting, abdominal cramps, diarrhea.
Mild menstrual irregularity.
Serious Adverse Effects
Flulike syndrome: fever, chills, headache, dizziness, musculoskeletal pain, difficult breathing.
Drug-induced liver damage, with or without jaundice.
Drug-induced kidney damage: impaired urine production, bloody or cloudy urine.
Excessively low blood platelet count: abnormal bleeding or bruising.

▷ **Adverse Effects That May Mimic Natural Diseases or Disorders**
Liver reactions may suggest viral hepatitis.
Kidney reactions may suggest an infectious nephritis.

CAUTION
1. This drug may permanently discolor soft contact lenses.
2. This drug may reduce the effectiveness of oral contraceptives; unplanned pregnancy could occur; an alternate method of contraception is advised.
3. When this drug is used alone in the treatment of tuberculosis, bacterial strains that are resistant to this drug can develop rapidly. This drug should only be used in conjunction with other antitubercular drugs.
4. To ensure the best possible response to treatment, take the full course of medication prescribed; this may be for several months or years.

Precautions for Use
By Infants and Children: Monitor closely for possible liver toxicity or deficiency of blood platelets.
By Those over 60 Years of Age: Natural changes in body composition and function make you more susceptible to the adverse effects of this drug. Report promptly any indications of possible drug toxicity.

▷ **Advisability of Use During Pregnancy**
Pregnancy Category: C (tentative). See Pregnancy Code inside back cover.
Animal studies: Cleft palate and spinal defects reported in rodent studies.
Human studies: Information from adequate studies of pregnant women is not available.
If possible, avoid use of drug during the first 3 months.

Advisability of Use if Breast-Feeding
Presence of this drug in breast milk: Yes.
Avoid drug or refrain from nursing.

Habit-Forming Potential: None.

Effects of Overdosage: Nausea, vomiting, drowsiness, unconsciousness, severe liver damage, jaundice.

Possible Effects of Long-Term Use: Superinfections, fungal overgrowth of mouth or tongue.

Suggested Periodic Examinations While Taking This Drug (at physician's discretion)
Complete blood cell counts, liver and kidney function tests.
Hearing acuity tests if hearing loss is suspected.

▷ **While Taking This Drug, Observe the Following**
Foods: No restrictions.
Beverages: No restrictions.
▷ *Alcohol*: It is best to avoid alcohol completely to reduce the risk of potential liver toxicity.
Tobacco Smoking: No interactions expected.

▷ *Other Drugs*
Rifampin may *decrease* the effects of
- anticoagulants (Coumadin, etc.), and reduce their effectiveness.
- beta-blockers: metoprolol, propranolol.
- cortisonelike drugs (see Drug Class, Section Four).
- cyclosporine.
- digitoxin.
- methadone (Dolophine).
- mexiletine (Mexitil).
- oral contraceptives.
- phenytoin (Dilantin).
- progestins.
- quinidine.
- sulfonylureas: chlorpropamide, tolbutamide.
- theophyllines (Aminophyllin, Theo-Dur, etc.).

The following drugs may *decrease* the effects of rifampin
- aminosalicylic acid (PAS), and reduce its antitubercular effectiveness.

▷ *Driving, Hazardous Activities*: This drug may cause dizziness, drowsiness, impaired vision and impaired hearing. Restrict activities as necessary.

Aviation Note: The use of this drug *may be a disqualification* for piloting. Consult a designated Aviation Medical Examiner.

Exposure to Sun: No restrictions.

Discontinuation: It is advisable not to interrupt or discontinue this drug without consulting your physician. Intermittent administration can increase the possibility of developing allergic reactions.

SODIUM BICARBONATE
(SOH dee um bi KAR boh nayt)

Other Names: Antacid

Introduced: 1886   **Class:** Antacids

Prescription: USA: No   **Controlled Drug:** USA: No
            Canada: No   Canada: No

Available as Generic: Yes

Brand Names: Alka-Seltzer Effervescent Antacid, Bell-Ans, Bisodol Powder [CD], Bromo-Seltzer [CD], Soda Mint

BENEFITS versus RISKS	
Possible Benefits	*Possible Risks*
EFFECTIVE, FAST-ACTING ANTACID FOR SHORT-TERM USE	Belching, bloating Fluid retention with excessive use

▷ **Principal Uses**

As a Single Drug Product: Used primarily as an antacid for symptomatic relief of heartburn, sour stomach and acid indigestion. Because it is readily absorbed, it is not appropriate for long-term use as an antacid in the treatment of peptic ulcer disease.

How This Drug Works: By chemically neutralizing some of the acid content of the stomach, this drug temporarily relieves the symptoms of excessive acidity. It does not affect the production of stomach acid.

Available Dosage Forms and Strengths

Powders — 120 grams, 240 grams, 300 grams
Tablets — 325 mg, 520 mg, 650 mg

▷ **Usual Adult Dosage Range:**   325 to 2000 mg 1 to 4 times/day. The total daily dosage should not exceed 16,000 mg (16 grams) for those under 60 years of age, and 8000 mg (8 grams) for those 60 years of age and older.

▷ **Dosing Instructions:**   Take 1 to 3 hours after meals and at bedtime for maximal effectiveness. When possible, do not take this drug within 1 to 2 hours of other medications.

Usual Duration of Use: This drug is for short-term use only. Do not take it continually for more than 2 weeks without consulting your physician. If symptoms of hyperacidity persist, appropriate examinations should be made to determine the cause.

▷ **Inform Your Physician Before Taking This Drug If**

- you have hypertension.
- you have a history of congestive heart failure.
- you have cirrhosis of the liver.
- you have impaired kidney function.

Possible Side-Effects   (natural, expected and unavoidable drug actions)
Bloating, belching, fluid retention with excessive use.

▷ **Advisability of Use During Pregnancy**

Pregnancy Category: C (tentative). See Pregnancy Code inside back cover.
Animal studies: No information available.
Human studies: Information from adequate studies of pregnant women is not available.
Occasional doses of this drug to treat acid indigestion are considered safe. However, this drug should not be used if you have a history of toxemia during a previous pregnancy or any degree of hypertension with a current pregnancy. Use antacids that do not contain sodium. Ask your physician for guidance.

Advisability of Use if Breast-Feeding

Presence of this drug in breast milk: No.
No adverse effects on infant expected.

▷ **While Taking This Drug, Observe the Following**
▷ *Other Drugs*
   Sodium bicarbonate may *increase* the effects of
   • ephedrine.
   • pseudoephedrine.
   Sodium bicarbonate may *decrease* the effects of
   • aspirin, when used in large doses (for arthritis).
   • chlorpropamide (Diabinese).
   • iron preparations.
   • lithium.
   • tetracyclines.
   Note: When possible, do not take any other drugs within 1 to 2 hours of
   taking any antacid.

SPIRONOLACTONE
(speer on oh LAK tohn)

Introduced: 1959

Prescription: USA: Yes
   Canada: Yes

Available as Generic: USA: Yes
   Canada: No

Class: Diuretic

Controlled Drug: USA: No
   Canada: No

Brand Names: Aldactone, Aldactazide [CD], ♣Novospiroton, ♣Sincomen

BENEFITS versus RISKS	
Possible Benefits	*Possible Risks*
EFFECTIVE PREVENTION OF POTASSIUM LOSS when used adjunctively with other diuretics	ABNORMALLY HIGH BLOOD POTASSIUM LEVEL with excessive use
EFFECTIVE DIURETIC IN REFRACTORY CASES OF FLUID RETENTION when used adjunctively with other diuretics	Enlargement of male breast tissue Masculinization effects in women: excessive hair growth, deepening of the voice

▷ **Principal Uses**
   As a Single Drug Product: This mild diuretic is used as part of the treatment
      program for the management of congestive heart failure and disorders
      of the liver and kidney that are accompanied by excessive fluid retention
      (edema). It is also used in conjunction with other measures to treat high
      blood pressure. It is used primarily in situations where it is advisable to
      prevent loss of potassium from the body.
   As a Combination Drug Product [CD]: This drug is available in combination
      with hydrochlorothiazide, a different kind of diuretic that promotes the

loss of potassium from the body. Spironolactone is used in this combination to counteract the potassium-wasting effect of the thiazide diuretic.

How This Drug Works: Not completely established. It is thought that by inhibiting the action of aldosterone (an adrenal gland hormone), this drug prevents the reabsorption of sodium and the excretion of potassium by the kidney. Thus the drug promotes the excretion of sodium (and water with it) and the retention of potassium.

Available Dosage Forms and Strengths
Tablets — 25 mg, 50 mg, 100 mg

▷ **Usual Adult Dosage Range:** Initially, 25 to 100 mg/day for 5 days. The dose is then adjusted according to individual response. The usual maintenance dose is 50 to 200 mg/day, divided into 2 to 4 doses. The total daily dosage should not exceed 400 mg. **Note: Actual dosage and administration schedule must be determined by the physician for each patient individually.**

▷ **Dosing Instructions:** May be taken with or following meals to promote absorption of the drug and to reduce stomach irritation. The tablet may be crushed for administration. Intermittent or alternate day use is recommended to minimize the possibility of sodium and potassium imbalance.

Usual Duration of Use: Continual use on a regular schedule for 5 to 10 days is usually necessary to determine this drug's effectiveness in clearing edema, and for 2 to 3 weeks to determine its effect on hypertension. Long-term use (months to years) requires supervision and periodic evaluation by your physician.

▷ **This Drug Should Not Be Taken If**
- you have had an allergic reaction to it previously.
- you have severely impaired liver or kidney function.

▷ **Inform Your Physician Before Taking This Drug If**
- you have a history of liver or kidney disease.
- you have diabetes.
- you are taking any of the following: an anticoagulant, antihypertensives, a digitalis preparation, another diuretic, lithium or a potassium preparation.
- you plan to have surgery under general anesthesia in the near future.

Possible Side-Effects   (natural, expected and unavoidable drug actions)
Abnormally high blood potassium levels (42%), abnormally low blood sodium levels (12%), dehydration (17%).

▷ **Possible Adverse Effects**   (unusual, unexpected and infrequent reactions)
If any of the following develop, consult your physician promptly.
Mild Adverse Effects
Allergic Reactions: Skin rash, hives, itching, drug fever (see Glossary).
Headache, dizziness, unsteadiness, weakness, drowsiness, lethargy, confusion.
Dry mouth, nausea, vomiting, diarrhea.

Serious Adverse Effects
Allergic Reactions: Abnormally low blood platelet count (rare).
Symptomatic potassium excess: confusion, numbness and tingling in lips and extremities, fatigue, weakness, shortness of breath, slow heart rate, low blood pressure.
Breast enlargement, decreased libido, sexual impotence in men.
Painful breast enlargement, menstrual irregularity, post-menopausal bleeding, masculine hair pattern, deepening of the voice in women.
Stomach ulceration with bleeding (rare).

CAUTION
1. Do not take potassium supplements or increase your intake of potassium-rich foods while taking this drug.
2. Do not discontinue this drug abruptly unless abnormally high blood levels of potassium develop.
3. Ordinary doses of aspirin (600 mg) may reverse the diuretic effect of this drug. Observe response to this drug combination.
4. Avoid the excessive use of salt substitutes that contain potassium; these are a potential cause of potassium excess.

Precautions for Use
By Infants and Children: Limit the continual use of this drug in children to 1 month. Observe closely for indications of potassium accumulation.
By Those over 60 Years of Age: The natural decline in kidney function may predispose to potassium retention in the body. Limit continual use of this drug to periods of 2 to 3 weeks. Observe for indications of potassium excess: slow heart rate, irregular heart rhythms, low blood pressure, confusion, drowsiness. The excessive use of diuretics can cause harmful loss of body water (dehydration), increased viscosity of the blood and an increased tendency of the blood to clot, predisposing to stroke, heart attack or thrombophlebitis.

▷ **Advisability of Use During Pregnancy**
Pregnancy Category: D (tentative). See Pregnancy Code inside back cover.
Animal studies: This drug causes feminization of male rat fetuses.
Human studies: Information from adequate studies of pregnant women is not available.
This drug should not be used during pregnancy unless a very serious complication of pregnancy occurs for which this drug is significantly beneficial.

Advisability of Use if Breast-Feeding
Presence of this drug in breast milk: A metabolic byproduct (canrenone) is present.
Avoid drug or refrain from nursing.

Habit-Forming Potential: None.

Effects of Overdosage: Thirst, drowsiness, fatigue, weakness, nausea, vomiting, confusion, irregular heart rhythm, low blood pressure.

Possible Effects of Long-Term Use: Potassium accumulation to abnormally high blood levels. Male breast enlargement.

Suggested Periodic Examinations While Taking This Drug   (at physician's discretion)
Measurements of blood sodium, potassium and chloride levels.
Kidney function tests.

▷ **While Taking This Drug, Observe the Following**
Foods: No restrictions. Avoid excessive restriction of salt.
Beverages: No restrictions. May be taken with milk.
▷   *Alcohol*: Use with caution until the combined effects have been determined. Alcohol may enhance the drowsiness and the blood-pressure-lowering effect of this drug.
Tobacco Smoking: No interactions expected.
▷   *Other Drugs*
Spironolactone may *increase* the effects of
• digoxin (Lanoxin).
Spironolactone may *decrease* the effects of
• anticoagulants (Coumadin, etc.).
Spironolactone *taken concurrently* with
• captopril (Capoten) may cause excessively high blood potassium levels.
• digitoxin (Crystodigin) may cause either increased or decreased digitoxin effects (unpredictable).
• lithium may cause accumulation of lithium to toxic levels.
• potassium preparations may cause excessively high blood potassium levels.
The following drugs may *decrease* the effects of spironolactone
• aspirin may reduce its diuretic effectiveness.
▷   *Driving, Hazardous Activities*: This drug may cause dizziness and drowsiness. Restrict activities as necessary.
Aviation Note: The use of this drug *may be a disqualification* for piloting. Consult a designated Aviation Medical Examiner.
Exposure to Sun: No restrictions.
Discontinuation: With high dosage or prolonged use, it is advisable to withdraw this drug gradually. Ask your physician for guidance.

SUCRALFATE
(soo KRAL fayt)

Introduced: 1978	**Class:** Antiulcer
Prescription: USA: Yes Canada: Yes	**Controlled Drug:** USA: No Canada: No
Available as Generic: No	
Brand Names: Carafate, ♣Sulcrate	

```
BENEFITS versus RISKS

    Possible Benefits                    Possible Risks
EFFECTIVE TREATMENT IN          Constipation
   PEPTIC ULCER DISEASE         Skin rash, hives, itching
No serious adverse effects
No significant drug interactions
```

▷ **Principal Uses**

As a Single Drug Product: Used exclusively in the management of peptic ulcer disease to promote healing of both stomach (gastric) and duodenal ulcer. It is effective when used alone, but may be used in conjunction with antacids when these are needed for pain relief.

How This Drug Works: Not completely established. It is thought that this drug promotes ulcer healing by several mechanisms: (1) the formation of a protective coating over the ulcer site to prevent further erosion by stomach acid; (2) the inhibition of the digestive action of pepsin; (3) the protection of injured tissue at the ulcer margins; (4) the stimulation of active healing (tissue repair).

Available Dosage Forms and Strengths

Tablets — 0.5 gram, 1 gram

▷ **Usual Adult Dosage Range:** 1 gram 4 times/day. **Note: Actual dosage and administration schedule must be determined by the physician for each patient individually.**

▷ **Dosing Instructions:** Take with water on an empty stomach 1 hour before each meal and at bedtime. Swallow the tablets whole; do not alter or chew. Take the full course prescribed.

Usual Duration of Use: Continual use on a regular schedule for 6 to 8 weeks is usually necessary to determine this drug's effectiveness in promoting the healing of peptic ulcers. Use beyond 8 weeks must be determined by your physician.

▷ **This Drug Should Not Be Taken If**

• you have had an allergic reaction to it previously.

▷ **Inform Your Physician Before Taking This Drug If**

• you have chronic constipation.
• you are taking any other drugs at this time.

Possible Side-Effects   (natural, expected and unavoidable drug actions)

Constipation (2.2%).

▷ **Possible Adverse Effects**   (unusual, unexpected and infrequent reactions)

If any of the following develop, consult your physician promptly.

Mild Adverse Effects

Allergic Reactions: Skin rash, hives, itching.

Dizziness, light-headedness, drowsiness.

Dry mouth, indigestion, nausea, cramping, diarrhea.

Serious Adverse Effects

None reported.

CAUTION

1. If antacids are needed to relieve ulcer pain, do not take them within 1/2 hour before or 1 hour after the dose of sucralfate.
2. This drug may impair the absorption of other drugs if they are taken close together. It is advisable to avoid taking any other drugs within 2 hours of taking sucralfate. This applies especially to cimetidine (Tagamet), phenytoin (Dilantin) and tetracyclines.

▷ **Advisability of Use During Pregnancy**

Pregnancy Category: B (tentative). See Pregnancy Code inside back cover.

Animal studies: No birth defects due to this drug reported in mouse, rat and rabbit studies.

Human studies: Information from adequate studies of pregnant women is not available.

Because only very small amounts of this drug are absorbed, it is probably safe for use at any time during pregnancy. However, it should be used only if clearly needed. Ask your physician for guidance.

Advisability of Use if Breast-Feeding

Presence of this drug in breast milk: Unknown.

Monitor nursing infant closely and discontinue drug or nursing if adverse effects develop.

Habit-Forming Potential: None.

Effects of Overdosage: Nausea, stomach cramping, possible diarrhea.

Possible Effects of Long-Term Use: Deficiencies of vitamins A, D, E and K due to impaired absorption from the intestine.

Suggested Periodic Examinations While Taking This Drug   (at physician's discretion)

None required.

▷ **While Taking This Drug, Observe the Following**

Foods: No restrictions. Follow diet prescribed by your physician.

Beverages: No restrictions. This drug is preferably taken with water.

▷   *Alcohol*: No interactions with drug expected. However, alcohol is best avoided because of its irritant effect on the stomach.

Tobacco Smoking: No interactions expected. However, nicotine can delay ulcer healing and reduce the effectiveness of this drug. Avoid all forms of tobacco.

▷   *Other Drugs*

Sucralfate may *decrease* the effects of
- warfarin (Coumadin, etc.), and reduce its effectiveness as an anticoagulant.

▷ *Driving, Hazardous Activities*: This drug may cause dizziness or drowsiness. Restrict activities as necessary.

Aviation Note: The use of this drug *may be a disqualification* for piloting. Consult a designated Aviation Medical Examiner.

Exposure to Sun: No restrictions.

SULFAMETHOXAZOLE
(sul fa meth OX a zohl)

Introduced: 1961   **Class:** Anti-infective, Sulfonamides

Prescription: USA: Yes   **Controlled Drug:** USA: No
Canada: Yes   Canada: No

Available as Generic: Yes

Brand Names: ✤Apo-Sulfamethoxazole, ✤Apo-Sulfatrim [CD], ✤Apo-Sulfatrim DS [CD], Azo Gantanol [CD], Bactrim [CD], Bactrim DS [CD], Gantanol, ✤Novotrimel [CD], ✤Novotrimel DS [CD], ✤Protrin [CD], ✤Protrin DF [CD], ✤Roubac [CD], Septra [CD], Septra DS [CD], ✤Uro Gantanol [CD]

BENEFITS versus RISKS

Possible Benefits	*Possible Risks*
EFFECTIVE ANTIMICROBIAL ACTION against susceptible bacteria and protozoa	Allergic reactions: mild to severe skin reactions, anaphylaxis, myocarditis Rare blood cell disorders: aplastic anemia, hemolytic anemia, abnormally low white cell and platelet counts Drug-induced liver damage Drug-induced kidney damage

---

▷ **Principal Uses**

As a Single Drug Product: This member of the sulfonamide class is used to treat a variety of bacterial and protozoal infections. It is most commonly used to treat certain infections of the urinary tract.

As a Combination Drug Product [CD]: This drug is available in combination with phenazopyridine, an analgesic drug that relieves the discomfort associated with acute infections of the urinary bladder and urethra. This combination provides early symptomatic relief while the underlying infection is being eradicated. This drug is also available in combination with another antibacterial drug—trimethoprim. This combination is quite effective in the treatment of certain types of middle ear infection, bronchitis, pneumonia and certain infections of the intestinal tract and the urinary tract.

How This Drug Works: This drug prevents the growth and multiplication of susceptible bacteria by interfering with their formation of folic acid, an essential nutrient.

Available Dosage Forms and Strengths
Oral suspension — 500 mg per 5 ml teaspoonful
Tablets — 500 mg, 1 gram

▷ **Usual Adult Dosage Range:** Initially, 2 grams; then 1 gram every 8 to 12 hours, depending upon the severity of the infection. The total daily dosage should not exceed 3 grams. **Note: Actual dosage and administration schedule must be determined by the physician for each patient individually.**

▷ **Dosing Instructions:** Preferably taken on an empty stomach, 1 hour before or 2 hours after eating. However, it may be taken with or following food to reduce stomach irritation. The tablet may be crushed for administration.

Usual Duration of Use: Continual use on a regular schedule for 4 to 7 days is usually necessary to determine this drug's effectiveness in controlling responsive infections. Treatment should be continued until the patient is free of symptoms for 48 hours. Limit treatment to no more than 14 days if possible.

▷ **This Drug Should Not Be Taken If**
  • you are allergic to *any* sulfonamide drug (see Drug Class, Section Four).
  • you are in the last month of pregnancy.
  • you are breast-feeding.

▷ **Inform Your Physician Before Taking This Drug If**
  • you are allergic to any sulfonamide derivative: acetazolamide, thiazide diuretics, sulfonylurea antidiabetic drugs (see Drug Classes, Section Four).
  • you are allergic by nature: history of hay fever, asthma, hives, eczema.
  • you have impaired liver or kidney function.
  • you have a personal or family history of porphyria.
  • you have had a drug-induced blood cell or bone marrow disorder in the past.
  • you are currently taking any oral anticoagulant, antidiabetic drug or phenytoin.
  • you plan to have surgery under pentothal anesthesia while taking this drug.

Possible Side-Effects   (natural, expected and unavoidable drug actions)
Brownish coloration of the urine, of no significance.
Superinfections, bacterial or fungal (see Glossary).

▷ **Possible Adverse Effects**   (unusual, unexpected and infrequent reactions)
  If any of the following develop, consult your physician promptly.
  Mild Adverse Effects
  Allergic Reactions: Skin rashes, hives, itching, localized swellings, reddened eyes.

Headache, dizziness, unsteadiness, ringing in the ears.

Loss of appetite, irritation of the mouth and tongue, nausea, vomiting, abdominal pain, diarrhea.

Serious Adverse Effects

Allergic Reactions: Drug fever (see Glossary), swollen glands, painful joints, anaphylaxis (see Glossary). Allergic reaction in the heart muscle (myocarditis), allergic pneumonitis, allergic hepatitis. Severe skin reactions.

Idiosyncratic Reactions: Hemolytic anemia (see Glossary).

Bone marrow depression (see Glossary): fatigue, weakness, fever, sore throat, abnormal bleeding or bruising.

Pancreatitis; kidney damage: bloody or cloudy urine, reduced urine volume.

Psychotic reactions, hallucinations, seizures, hearing loss, peripheral neuropathy (see Glossary).

▷ **Adverse Effects That May Mimic Natural Diseases or Disorders**

Liver reactions may suggest viral hepatitis.

Lung reactions may suggest an infectious pneumonia.

Natural Diseases or Disorders That May Be Activated by This Drug

Goiter, acute intermittent porphyria, polyarteritis nodosa, systemic lupus erythematosus (questionable).

CAUTION

1. A large intake of water (up to 2 quarts daily) is necessary to ensure an adequate volume of urine.
2. Shake liquid dosage forms thoroughly before measuring each dose.

Precautions for Use

By Infants and Children: This drug should not be used in infants under 2 months of age.

By Those over 60 Years of Age: Small doses taken at longer intervals often achieve adequate blood and tissue drug levels. Observe for the development of reduced urine volume, fever, sore throat, abnormal bleeding or bruising or skin irritation with itching, particularly in the anal or genital regions.

▷ **Advisability of Use During Pregnancy**

Pregnancy Category: C (tentative). See Pregnancy Code inside back cover.

Animal studies: Cleft palate and skeletal birth defects reported in mice and rats.

Human studies: No increase in birth defects reported in 4584 exposures to various sulfonamides during pregnancy.

Avoid use of drug during the last month of pregnancy because of possible adverse effects on the newborn infant.

Advisability of Use if Breast-Feeding

Presence of this drug in breast milk: Yes.

Avoid drug or refrain from nursing.

Habit-Forming Potential: None.

Effects of Overdosage: Headache, dizziness, nausea, vomiting, abdominal cramping, toxic fever, coma, jaundice, kidney failure.

Possible Effects of Long-Term Use: Superinfections, bacterial or fungal. Development of goiter, with or without hypothyroidism. Excessive loss of vitamin C via urine.

Suggested Periodic Examinations While Taking This Drug (at physician's discretion)
Complete blood cell counts, weekly for the first 8 weeks.
Urine analysis weekly.
Liver and kidney function tests.

▷ **While Taking This Drug, Observe the Following**
Foods: No restrictions.
Beverages: No restrictions. May be taken with milk.
▷   *Alcohol*: Use caution until the combined effect has been determined. Sulfonamide drugs can increase the intoxicating effects of alcohol.
Tobacco Smoking: No interactions expected.
▷   *Other Drugs*
Sulfamethoxazole may *increase* the effects of
  • anticoagulants (Coumadin, etc.), and increase the risk of bleeding.
  • sulfonylureas (see Drug Class, Section Four), and increase the risk of hypoglycemia.
Sulfamethoxazole may *decrease* the effects of
  • cyclosporine, and reduce its immunosuppressive effect.
  • penicillins.
▷   *Driving, Hazardous Activities*: This drug may cause dizziness. Restrict activities as necessary.
Aviation Note: The use of this drug *may be a disqualification* for piloting. Consult a designated Aviation Medical Examiner.
Exposure to Sun: Use caution until sensitivity has been determined. Some sulfonamide drugs can cause photosensitivity (see Glossary).

SULFASALAZINE
(sul fa SAL a zeen)

Introduced: 1949

Class: Bowel Anti-inflammatory, Sulfonamides

Prescription: USA: Yes
Canada: Yes

Controlled Drug: USA: No
Canada: No

Available as Generic: USA: Yes
Canada: No

Brand Names: Azaline, Azulfidine, Azulfidine EN-tabs, ✤PMS Sulfasalazine,

♣PMS Sulfasalazine E.C., ♣Salazopyrin, ♣SAS-Enema, ♣SAS Enteric-500, SAS-500

BENEFITS versus RISKS	
Possible Benefits	*Possible Risks*
EFFECTIVE SUPPRESSION OF INFLAMMATORY BOWEL DISEASE SYMPTOMATIC RELIEF IN TREATMENT OF REGIONAL ENTERITIS AND ULCERATIVE COLITIS	Allergic reactions: mild to severe skin reactions Rare blood cell disorders: aplastic anemia, hemolytic anemia, abnormally low white cell and platelet counts Drug-induced liver damage Drug-induced kidney damage

▷ **Principal Uses**

As a Single Drug Product: This member of the sulfonamide class is used exclusively to treat inflammatory disease of the lower intestinal tract: regional enteritis (Crohn's disease) and ulcerative colitis. It is usually taken by mouth, but may also be used in retention enemas.

How This Drug Works: Not completely established. Possible methods of this drug's action include
- an anti-inflammatory action that suppresses the formation of prostaglandins (and related compounds), tissue substances that induce inflammation, tissue destruction and diarrhea.
- an anti-infective action that may prevent the growth and multiplication of certain infective agents in the intestine and colon. (This method of action is questionable.)

Available Dosage Forms and Strengths

Oral suspension — 250 mg per 5 ml teaspoonful

Tablets — 500 mg

Tablets, enteric coated — 500 mg

▷ **Usual Adult Dosage Range:** Initially, 1 to 2 grams every 6 to 8 hours until symptoms are adequately controlled. For maintenance, 500 mg/6 hours. The total daily dosage should not exceed 12 grams. **Note: Actual dosage and administration schedule must be determined by the physician for each patient individually.**

▷ **Dosing Instructions:** Preferably taken with 8 ounces of water on an empty stomach, 1 hour before or 2 hours after eating. However, it may be taken with or following food to reduce stomach irritation. Intervals between doses (day and night) should be no longer than 8 hours. The regular tablet may be crushed for administration; the enteric-coated tablet should be swallowed whole without alteration.

Usual Duration of Use: Continual use on a regular schedule for 1 to 3 weeks is usually necessary to determine this drug's effectiveness in controlling the symptoms of regional enteritis or ulcerative colitis. Long-term use (months to years) requires supervision and periodic evaluation by your physician.

▷ **This Drug Should Not Be Taken If**
- you are allergic to *any* sulfonamide drug (see Drug Class, Section Four), or to aspirin (or other salicylates).
- you are in the last month of pregnancy.
- you are breast-feeding.

▷ **Inform Your Physician Before Taking This Drug If**
- you are allergic to any sulfonamide derivative: acetazolamide, thiazide diuretics, sulfonylurea antidiabetic drugs (see Drug Classes, Section Four).
- you are allergic by nature: history of hay fever, asthma, hives, eczema.
- you have impaired liver or kidney function.
- you have a personal or family history of porphyria.
- you have had a drug-induced blood cell or bone marrow disorder in the past.
- you are currently taking any oral anticoagulant, antidiabetic drug or phenytoin.
- you plan to have surgery under pentothal anesthesia while taking this drug.

Possible Side-Effects   (natural, expected and unavoidable drug actions)
Brownish coloration of the urine, of no significance.
Superinfections, bacterial or fungal (see Glossary).

▷ **Possible Adverse Effects**   (unusual, unexpected and infrequent reactions)
If any of the following develop, consult your physician promptly.
Mild Adverse Effects
Allergic Reactions: Skin rashes, hives, itching.
Headache, dizziness.
Loss of appetite, irritation of the mouth and tongue, nausea, vomiting, abdominal pain, diarrhea.
Serious Adverse Effects
Allergic Reactions: Drug fever (see Glossary), swollen glands, painful joints, anaphylaxis (see Glossary). Allergic pneumonitis, allergic hepatitis. Severe skin reactions.
Idiosyncratic Reactions: Hemolytic anemia (see Glossary).
Bone marrow depression (see Glossary): fatigue, weakness, fever, sore throat, abnormal bleeding or bruising.
Pancreatitis; kidney damage: bloody or cloudy urine, reduced urine volume.
Peripheral neuropathy (see Glossary).
Reduced production of sperm, reversible infertility.

▷ **Adverse Effects That May Mimic Natural Diseases or Disorders**
Liver reactions may suggest viral hepatitis.
Lung reactions may suggest an infectious pneumonia.

Natural Diseases or Disorders That May Be Activated by This Drug
Goiter, acute intermittent porphyria.

CAUTION
1. A large intake of water (up to 2 quarts daily) is necessary to ensure an adequate volume of urine.
2. Shake liquid dosage forms thoroughly before measuring each dose.

Precautions for Use
By Infants and Children: Safety and effectiveness for use by those under 2 years of age have not been established.
By Those over 60 Years of Age: Observe for the development of reduced urine volume, fever, sore throat, abnormal bleeding or bruising or skin irritation with itching, particularly in the anal or genital regions.

▷ **Advisability of Use During Pregnancy**
Pregnancy Category: C (tentative). See Pregnancy Code inside back cover.
Animal studies: Cleft palate and skeletal birth defects due to sulfonamides reported in mice and rats.
Human studies: No increase in birth defects reported in 4584 exposures to various sulfonamides during pregnancy.
Avoid use of drug during the last month of pregnancy because of possible adverse effects on the newborn infant.

Advisability of Use if Breast-Feeding
Presence of this drug in breast milk: Yes.
Avoid drug or refrain from nursing.

Habit-Forming Potential: None.

Effects of Overdosage: Headache, dizziness, nausea, vomiting, abdominal cramping, toxic fever, coma, jaundice, kidney failure.

Possible Effects of Long-Term Use: Development of goiter, with or without hypothyroidism. An orange-yellow discoloration of the skin has been reported. This is not jaundice.

Suggested Periodic Examinations While Taking This Drug   (at physician's discretion)
Complete blood cell counts, weekly for the first 8 weeks.
Urine analysis weekly.
Liver and kidney function tests.

▷ **While Taking This Drug, Observe the Following**
Foods: No restrictions. Follow prescribed diet.
Beverages: No restrictions. May be taken with milk.
▷ *Alcohol*: Use caution until the combined effect has been determined. Sulfonamide drugs can increase the intoxicating effects of alcohol.
Tobacco Smoking: No interactions expected.
▷ *Other Drugs*
Sulfasalazine may *increase* the effects of
• anticoagulants (Coumadin, etc.), and increase the risk of bleeding.

- sulfonylureas (see Drug Class, Section Four), and increase the risk of hypoglycemia.

Sulfasalazine may *decrease* the effects of

- digoxin (Lanoxin).

▷ *Driving, Hazardous Activities*: This drug may cause dizziness. Restrict activities as necessary.

Aviation Note: The use of this drug *may be a disqualification* for piloting. Consult a designated Aviation Medical Examiner.

Exposure to Sun: Use caution until sensitivity has been determined. Some sulfonamide drugs can cause photosensitivity (see Glossary).

SULFISOXAZOLE
(sul fi SOX a zohl)

Introduced: 1949

Prescription: USA: Yes
Canada: Yes

Available as Generic: Yes

Class: Anti-infective, Sulfonamides

Controlled Drug: USA: No
Canada: No

Brand Names: ❦Apo-Sulfisoxazole, Azo Gantrisin [CD], Gantrisin, Lipo Gantrisin, ❦Novosoxazole, SK-Soxazole

BENEFITS versus RISKS	
Possible Benefits	*Possible Risks*
EFFECTIVE ANTIMICROBIAL ACTION against susceptible bacteria and protozoa	Allergic reactions: mild to severe skin reactions, anaphylaxis
	Rare blood cell disorders: aplastic anemia, hemolytic anemia, abnormally low white cell and platelet counts
	Drug-induced liver damage
	Drug-induced kidney damage

▷ **Principal Uses**

As a Single Drug Product: This member of the sulfonamide class is used to treat a variety of bacterial and protozoal infections. It is most commonly used to treat certain infections of the urinary tract.

As a Combination Drug Product [CD]: This drug is available in combination with phenazopyridine, an analgesic drug that relieves the discomfort associated with acute infections of the urinary bladder and urethra. This combination provides early symptomatic relief while the underlying infection is being eradicated.

How This Drug Works: This drug prevents the growth and multiplication of susceptible bacteria by interfering with their formation of folic acid, an essential nutrient.

Available Dosage Forms and Strengths
Emulsion, prolonged action — 1 gram per 5 ml teaspoonful
Injection — 400 mg per ml
Ointment, ophthalmic — 4%
Suspension, pediatric — 500 mg per 5 ml teaspoonful
Syrup — 500 mg per 5 ml teaspoonful
Tablets — 500 mg

▷ **Usual Adult Dosage Range:**   Initially, 2 to 4 grams; then 750 to 1500 mg (1.5 grams) every 4 hours, or 1 to 2 grams every 6 hours, depending upon the severity of the infection. The total daily dosage should not exceed 12 grams. **Note: Actual dosage and administration schedule must be determined by the physician for each patient individually.**

▷ **Dosing Instructions:**   Preferably taken with 8 ounces of water on an empty stomach, 1 hour before or 2 hours after eating. However, it may be taken with or following food to reduce stomach irritation. The tablet may be crushed for administration.

Usual Duration of Use: Continual use on a regular schedule for 7 to 10 days is usually necessary to determine this drug's effectiveness in controlling responsive infections. Treatment should be continued until the patient is free of symptoms for 48 hours. Limit treatment to no more than 14 days if possible.

▷ **This Drug Should Not Be Taken If**
- you are allergic to *any* sulfonamide drug (see Drug Class, Section Four).
- you are in the last month of pregnancy.
- you are breast-feeding.

▷ **Inform Your Physician Before Taking This Drug If**
- you are allergic to any sulfonamide derivative: acetazolamide, thiazide diuretics, sulfonylurea antidiabetic drugs (see Drug Classes, Section Four).
- you are allergic by nature: history of hay fever, asthma, hives, eczema.
- you have impaired liver or kidney function.
- you have a personal or family history of porphyria.
- you have had a drug-induced blood cell or bone marrow disorder in the past.
- you are currently taking any oral anticoagulant, antidiabetic drug or phenytoin.
- you plan to have surgery under pentothal anesthesia while taking this drug.

Possible Side-Effects   (natural, expected and unavoidable drug actions)
Brownish coloration of the urine, of no significance.
Superinfections, bacterial or fungal (see Glossary).

▷ **Possible Adverse Effects**   (unusual, unexpected and infrequent reactions)
If any of the following develop, consult your physician promptly.

Mild Adverse Effects
Allergic Reactions: Skin rashes, hives, itching, localized swellings, reddened eyes.
Headache, dizziness, unsteadiness, ringing in the ears.
Loss of appetite, irritation of the mouth and tongue, nausea, vomiting, abdominal pain, diarrhea.

Serious Adverse Effects
Allergic Reactions: Drug fever (see Glossary), swollen glands, painful joints, anaphylaxis (see Glossary). Allergic hepatitis. Severe skin reactions.
Idiosyncratic Reactions: Hemolytic anemia (see Glossary).
Bone marrow depression (see Glossary): fatigue, weakness, fever, sore throat, abnormal bleeding or bruising.
Kidney damage: bloody or cloudy urine, reduced urine volume.
Peripheral neuropathy (see Glossary).

▷ **Adverse Effects That May Mimic Natural Diseases or Disorders**
Liver reactions may suggest viral hepatitis.

Natural Diseases or Disorders That May Be Activated by This Drug
Goiter, acute intermittent porphyria.

CAUTION
1. A large intake of water (up to 2 quarts daily) is necessary to ensure an adequate volume of urine.
2. Shake liquid dosage forms thoroughly before measuring each dose.

Precautions for Use
By Infants and Children: This drug should not be used in infants under 2 months of age.
By Those over 60 Years of Age: Small doses taken at longer intervals often achieve adequate blood and tissue drug levels. Observe for the development of reduced urine volume, fever, sore throat, abnormal bleeding or bruising or skin irritation with itching, particularly in the anal or genital regions.

▷ **Advisability of Use During Pregnancy**
Pregnancy Category: C (tentative). See Pregnancy Code inside back cover.
Animal studies: Cleft palate and skeletal birth defects due to sulfonamides reported in mice and rats.
Human studies: No increase in birth defects reported in 4287 exposures to this drug during pregnancy.
Avoid use of drug during the last month of pregnancy because of possible adverse effects on the newborn infant.

Advisability of Use if Breast-Feeding
Presence of this drug in breast milk: Yes.
Avoid drug or refrain from nursing.

Habit-Forming Potential: None.

Effects of Overdosage: Headache, dizziness, nausea, vomiting, abdominal cramping, toxic fever, coma, jaundice, kidney failure.

Possible Effects of Long-Term Use: Superinfections, bacterial or fungal. Development of goiter, with or without hypothyroidism. Excessive loss of vitamin C via urine.

Suggested Periodic Examinations While Taking This Drug   (at physician's discretion)
Complete blood cell counts, weekly for the first 8 weeks.
Urine analysis weekly.
Liver and kidney function tests.

▷ **While Taking This Drug, Observe the Following**
Foods: No restrictions.
Beverages: No restrictions. May be taken with milk.
▷ *Alcohol*: Use caution until the combined effect has been determined. Sulfonamide drugs can increase the intoxicating effects of alcohol.
Tobacco Smoking: No interactions expected.
▷ *Other Drugs*
Sulfisoxazole may *increase* the effects of
• anticoagulants (Coumadin, etc.), and increase the risk of bleeding.
• sulfonylureas (see Drug Class, Section Four), and increase the risk of hypoglycemia.
Sulfisoxazole may *decrease* the effects of
• penicillins.
▷ *Driving, Hazardous Activities*: This drug may cause dizziness. Restrict activities as necessary.
Aviation Note: The use of this drug *may be a disqualification* for piloting. Consult a designated Aviation Medical Examiner.
Exposure to Sun: Use caution until sensitivity has been determined. Some sulfonamide drugs can cause photosensitivity (see Glossary).

SULINDAC
(sul IN dak)

Introduced: 1976

Class: Mild Analgesic, Anti-inflammatory

Prescription: USA: Yes
    Canada: Yes

Controlled Drug: USA: No
    Canada: No

Available as Generic: No

Brand Names: Clinoril

```
┌─────────────────────────────────────────────────────────────────┐
│                     BENEFITS versus RISKS                         │
│                                                                   │
│      Possible Benefits              Possible Risks                │
│   EFFECTIVE RELIEF OF MILD TO    Gastrointestinal pain, ulceration,│
│      MODERATE PAIN AND              bleeding (rare)               │
│      INFLAMMATION                Rare liver damage               │
│                                  Rare kidney damage              │
│                                  Rare bone marrow depression     │
│                                     (aplastic anemia)            │
└─────────────────────────────────────────────────────────────────┘
```

▷ **Principal Uses**

As a Single Drug Product: Used primarily to relieve mild to moderately severe pain associated with (1) rheumatoid arthritis and osteoarthritis; (2) acute and chronic gout; and (3) bursitis, tendinitis and related disorders.

How This Drug Works: Not completely established. It is thought that this drug reduces the tissue concentrations of prostaglandins (and related compounds), substances involved in the production of inflammation and pain.

Available Dosage Forms and Strengths

Tablets — 150 mg, 200 mg

▷ **Usual Adult Dosage Range:** 150 to 200 mg twice/day, 12 hours apart. The total daily dosage should not exceed 400 mg. **Note: Actual dosage and administration schedule must be determined by the physician for each patient individually.**

▷ **Dosing Instructions:** Preferably taken on an empty stomach, 1 hour before or 2 hours after eating. However, it may be taken with or after food if necessary to reduce stomach irritation. Take with a full glass of water and remain upright (do not lie down) for 30 minutes. The tablet may be crushed for administration.

Usual Duration of Use: Continual use on a regular schedule for 2 to 3 weeks is usually necessary to determine this drug's effectiveness in relieving the discomfort of arthritis. Acute gout usually responds within 7 days. Shoulder bursitis or tendinitis usually responds within 7 to 14 days. Long-term use (months to years) requires supervision and periodic evaluation by your physician.

▷ **This Drug Should Not Be Taken If**
- you have had an allergic reaction to it previously.
- you are subject to asthma or nasal polyps caused by aspirin.
- you have active peptic ulcer disease or any form of gastrointestinal bleeding.
- you have a bleeding disorder or a blood cell disorder.
- you have severe impairment of liver or kidney function.

▷ **Inform Your Physician Before Taking This Drug If**
- you are allergic to aspirin or to other aspirin substitutes.

- you have a history of peptic ulcer disease or any type of bleeding disorder.
- you have impaired liver or kidney function.
- you have high blood pressure or a history of heart failure.
- you are taking any of the following: acetaminophen, aspirin or other aspirin substitutes, anticoagulants, oral antidiabetic drugs.

Possible Side-Effects   (natural, expected and unavoidable drug actions)
Fluid retention (edema). Drowsiness in sensitive individuals.

▷ **Possible Adverse Effects**   (unusual, unexpected and infrequent reactions)
If any of the following develop, consult your physician promptly.
Mild Adverse Effects
Allergic Reactions: Skin rash, hives, itching.
Headache, dizziness, mild numbness and tingling, blurred vision, ringing in the ears.
Mouth sores, indigestion, nausea, vomiting, constipation, diarrhea.
Serious Adverse Effects
Allergic Reactions: Anaphylactic reaction (see Glossary), severe skin reactions.
Idiosyncratic Reactions: Drug-induced pneumonitis with fever.
Active peptic ulcer, with or without bleeding.
Liver damage with jaundice (see Glossary).
Kidney damage with painful urination, bloody urine, reduced urine formation.
Rare bone marrow depression (see Glossary): fatigue, weakness, fever, sore throat, abnormal bleeding or bruising.

Possible Delayed Adverse Effects
Mild anemia due to "silent" blood loss from the stomach (less than that caused by aspirin).

▷ **Adverse Effects That May Mimic Natural Diseases or Disorders**
Liver reaction may suggest viral hepatitis.

Natural Diseases or Disorders That May Be Activated by This Drug
Peptic ulcer disease, ulcerative colitis.

CAUTION
1. Dosage should always be limited to the smallest amount that produces reasonable improvement.
2. This drug may mask early indications of infection. Inform your physician if you think you are developing an infection of any kind.

Precautions for Use
By Infants and Children: Safety and effectiveness for use by those under 12 years of age have not been established.
By Those over 60 Years of Age: Small doses are advisable until tolerance is determined. Observe for any indications of liver or kidney toxicity, fluid retention, dizziness, confusion, impaired memory, stomach bleeding or constipation.

▷ **Advisability of Use During Pregnancy**
    Pregnancy Category: C (tentative). See Pregnancy Code inside back cover.
        Animal studies: A low incidence of birth defects has been reported but not confirmed.
        Human studies: Information from adequate studies of pregnant women is not available.
        The manufacturer does not recommend the use of this drug during pregnancy.

Advisability of Use if Breast-Feeding
    Presence of this drug in breast milk: Unknown.
    Avoid drug or refrain from nursing.

Habit-Forming Potential: None.

Effects of Overdosage: Stomach irritation, nausea, vomiting, diarrhea.

Possible Effects of Long-Term Use: Fluid retention.

Suggested Periodic Examinations While Taking This Drug   (at physician's discretion)
    Complete blood cell counts, liver and kidney function tests, complete eye examinations if vision is altered in any way.

▷ **While Taking This Drug, Observe the Following**
    Foods: No restrictions.
    Beverages: No restrictions. May be taken with milk.
▷   *Alcohol*: Use with caution. The irritant action of alcohol on the stomach lining, added to the irritant action of this drug in sensitive individuals, can increase the risk of stomach ulceration and/or bleeding.
    Tobacco Smoking: No interactions expected.
▷   *Other Drugs*
    Sulindac may *increase* the effects of
    • acetaminophen (Tylenol, etc.), and increase the risk of kidney damage; avoid prolonged use of this combination.
    • anticoagulants (Coumadin, etc.), and increase the risk of bleeding; monitor prothrombin time, adjust dose accordingly.
    Sulindac *taken concurrently* with the following drugs may increase the risk of bleeding; avoid these combinations:
    • aspirin.
    • dipyridamole (Persantine).
    • indomethacin (Indocin).
    • sulfinpyrazone (Anturane).
    • valproic acid (Depakene).
▷   *Driving, Hazardous Activities*: This drug may cause drowsiness or dizziness. Restrict activities as necessary.
    Aviation Note: The use of this drug *may be a disqualification* for piloting. Consult a designated Aviation Medical Examiner.
    Exposure to Sun: No restrictions.

SUPROFEN
(soo PROH fen)

Other Names: Sutoprofen

Introduced: 1985   **Class:** Mild Analgesic

Prescription: USA: Yes   **Controlled Drug:** USA: No

Available as Generic: No

Brand Names: Suprol

BENEFITS versus RISKS

Possible Benefits	*Possible Risks*
EFFECTIVE RELIEF OF MILD TO MODERATE PAIN	Gastrointestinal pain, ulceration, bleeding (rare) Rare kidney damage Blood cell disorder: abnormally low blood platelet count

---

▷ **Principal Uses**

As a Single Drug Product: Used primarily to relieve mild to moderately severe pain associated with (1) dental, obstetric or orthopedic surgery; (2) muscular sprains and strains; and (3) menstrual cramping.

How This Drug Works: Not completely established. It is thought that this drug reduces the tissue concentrations of prostaglandins (and related compounds), substances involved in the production of inflammation and pain.

Available Dosage Forms and Strengths

Capsules — 200 mg

▷ **Usual Adult Dosage Range:** 200 mg every 4 to 6 hours as needed. The total daily dosage should not exceed 800 mg. **Note: Actual dosage and administration schedule must be determined by the physician for each patient individually.**

▷ **Dosing Instructions:** Preferably taken on an empty stomach, 1 hour before or 2 hours after eating. However, it may be taken with or following food if necessary to reduce stomach irritation. Take with a full glass of water and remain upright (do not lie down) for 30 minutes. The capsule may be opened for administration.

Usual Duration of Use: Continual use on a regular schedule for 24 to 48 hours is usually necessary to determine this drug's effectiveness in relieving postoperative pain and the pain of sprains, strains and menstrual cramping. Limit continual use to 1 to 2 weeks.

▷ **This Drug Should Not Be Taken If**
- you have had an allergic reaction to it previously.
- you are subject to asthma or nasal polyps caused by aspirin.

- you have active peptic ulcer disease or any form of gastrointestinal bleeding.
- you have a bleeding disorder or a blood cell disorder.
- you have severe impairment of liver or kidney function.

▷ **Inform Your Physician Before Taking This Drug If**
- you are allergic to aspirin or to other aspirin substitutes.
- you are pregnant.
- you have a history of peptic ulcer disease or any type of bleeding disorder.
- you have impaired liver or kidney function.
- you have high blood pressure or a history of heart failure.
- you are taking any of the following: acetaminophen, aspirin or other aspirin substitutes, anticoagulants, oral antidiabetic drugs.

Possible Side-Effects   (natural, expected and unavoidable drug actions)
Fluid retention (edema). Drowsiness in sensitive individuals.

▷ **Possible Adverse Effects**   (unusual, unexpected and infrequent reactions)
If any of the following develop, consult your physician promptly.
Mild Adverse Effects
Allergic Reactions: Skin rash, hives, itching.
Headache, dizziness, mild numbness and tingling, blurred vision, ringing in the ears, nasal congestion, nosebleeds.
Unusual weakness, heart palpitation.
Mouth sores, indigestion (13%), nausea (15%), vomiting, constipation, diarrhea (10%).
Serious Adverse Effects
Allergic Reactions: Asthmatic breathing; anaphylactic reaction (see Glossary).
Idiosyncratic Reactions: Sudden pain in side or flank following the first or second dose, with transient impairment of kidney function.
Active peptic ulcer, with or without bleeding.
Kidney damage with painful urination, bloody urine, reduced urine formation.
Insufficient blood platelets: abnormal bleeding or bruising.

Possible Delayed Adverse Effects
Mild anemia due to "silent" blood loss from the stomach (less than that caused by aspirin).

Natural Diseases or Disorders That May Be Activated by This Drug
Peptic ulcer disease.

Precautions for Use
By Infants and Children: Safety and effectiveness for use by those under 12 years of age have not been established.
By Those over 60 Years of Age: Small doses are advisable until tolerance is determined. Observe for any indications of kidney toxicity, fluid reten-

tion, dizziness, confusion, impaired memory, stomach bleeding or constipation.

▷ **Advisability of Use During Pregnancy**
Pregnancy Category: B (tentative). See Pregnancy Code inside back cover.
Animal studies: No birth defects due to this drug found in rats or rabbits.
Human studies: Information from adequate studies of pregnant women is not available.
Avoid this drug during the last month. Use it otherwise only if clearly needed. Ask your physician for guidance.

Advisability of Use if Breast-Feeding
Presence of this drug in breast milk: Yes.
Avoid drug or refrain from nursing.

Habit-Forming Potential: None.

Effects of Overdosage: Stomach irritation, nausea, vomiting, diarrhea.

Possible Effects of Long-Term Use: Fluid retention.

Suggested Periodic Examinations While Taking This Drug   (at physician's discretion)
Complete blood cell counts, kidney function tests, complete eye examinations if vision is altered in any way.

▷ **While Taking This Drug, Observe the Following**
Foods: No restrictions.
Beverages: No restrictions. May be taken with milk.
▷ *Alcohol*: Use with caution. The irritant action of alcohol on the stomach lining, added to the irritant action of this drug in sensitive individuals, can increase the risk of stomach ulceration and/or bleeding.
Tobacco Smoking: No interactions expected.
▷ *Other Drugs*
Suprofen may *increase* the effects of
• acetaminophen (Tylenol, etc.), and increase the risk of kidney damage; avoid prolonged use of this combination.
• anticoagulants (Coumadin, etc.), and increase the risk of bleeding; monitor prothrombin time, adjust dose accordingly.
Suprofen *taken concurrently* with the following drugs may increase the risk of bleeding; avoid these combinations:
• aspirin.
• dipyridamole (Persantine).
• indomethacin (Indocin).
• sulfinpyrazone (Anturane).
• valproic acid (Depakene).
▷ *Driving, Hazardous Activities*: This drug may cause drowsiness or dizziness. Restrict activities as necessary.
Aviation Note: The use of this drug *may be a disqualification* for piloting. Consult a designated Aviation Medical Examiner.
Exposure to Sun: No restrictions.

TAMOXIFEN
(ta MOX i fen)

Introduced: 1973

Prescription: USA: Yes
Canada: Yes

Available as Generic: No

Brand Names: Nolvadex, ♣Nolvadex-D

Class: Antiestrogen, Anticancer

Controlled Drug: USA: No
Canada: No

BENEFITS versus RISKS

Possible Benefits	*Possible Risks*
EFFECTIVE ADJUNCTIVE TREATMENT IN ADVANCED BREAST CANCER in 30% to 40% of cases	Severe increase in tumor or bone pain, transient Thromophlebitis, pulmonary embolism Abnormally high blood calcium levels Eye changes: corneal opacities, retinal injury

---

▷ **Principal Uses**

As a Single Drug Product: Used primarily as an alternative to estrogens and androgens (male sex hormones) to treat advanced breast cancer in postmenopausal women. It is also used to stimulate ovulation in premenopausal women with infertility.

How This Drug Works: Not completely established. It is thought that by blocking the uptake of estradiol (estrogen), this drug removes or reduces a stimulus to breast cancer cells.

Available Dosage Forms and Strengths
Tablets — 10 mg, 20 mg (in Canada)

▷ **Usual Adult Dosage Range:** 10 to 20 mg twice/day, morning and evening. **Note: Actual dosage and administration schedule must be determined by the physician for each patient individually.**

▷ **Dosing Instructions:** May be taken either on an empty stomach or with food. The tablet may be crushed for administration.

Usual Duration of Use: Continual use on a regular schedule for 4 to 10 weeks is usually necessary to determine this drug's effectiveness in controlling the growth and spread of advanced breast cancer. In the presence of bone involvement, treatment for several months may be required to evaluate effectiveness. Long-term use (months to years) requires supervision and periodic evaluation by your physician.

▷ **This Drug Should Not Be Taken If**
- you have had a serious allergic or adverse reaction to it previously.

- you have active phlebitis.
- you have a significant deficiency of white blood cells or blood platelets.

▷ **Inform Your Physician Before Taking This Drug If**
- you have a history of thrombophlebitis or pulmonary embolism.
- you have a history of abnormally high blood calcium levels.
- you have a history of any type of blood cell or bone marrow disorder.
- you have cataracts or other visual impairment.
- you have impaired liver function.
- you plan to have surgery in the near future.

Possible Side-Effects   (natural, expected and unavoidable drug actions)
Hot flashes, fluid retention, weight gain.

▷ **Possible Adverse Effects**   (unusual, unexpected and infrequent reactions)
If any of the following develop, consult your physician promptly.
Mild Adverse Effects
Allergic Reactions: Skin rash.
Headache, dizziness, drowsiness, depression, fatigue, confusion.
Nausea, vomiting, itching in genital area, loss of hair.
Postmenopausal: vaginal bleeding.
Premenopausal: alteration of menstrual pattern.
Serious Adverse Effects
Initial "flare" of severe pain in tumor or involved bone.
Development of thrombophlebitis, risk of pulmonary embolism.
Eye changes: corneal opacities, retinal injury.
Development of abnormally high blood calcium levels.
Transient decreases in white blood cells and blood platelets.

CAUTION
1. If this drug is used prior to your menopause, it may induce ovulation and predispose to pregnancy. Since this drug should not be used during pregnancy, some method of contraception (other than oral contraceptives) is advised.
2. Do not take any form of estrogen while taking this drug; estrogens can inhibit tamoxifen's effectiveness.

▷ **Advisability of Use During Pregnancy**
Pregnancy Category: X (tentative). See Pregnancy Code inside back cover.
Animal studies: No birth defects due to this drug reported.
Human studies: Information from adequate studies of pregnant women is not available.
This drug can have estrogenic effects. It should not be used during pregnancy.

Advisability of Use if Breast-Feeding
Presence of this drug in breast milk: Unknown.
Avoid drug or refrain from nursing.

Habit-Forming Potential: None.

Effects of Overdosage: No information available.

Possible Effects of Long-Term Use: Development of abnormally high blood calcium levels.

Suggested Periodic Examinations While Taking This Drug   (at physician's discretion)
Complete blood cell counts, measurements of blood calcium levels.
Complete eye examinations if impaired vision occurs.

▷ **While Taking This Drug, Observe the Following**
Foods: No restrictions.
Beverages: No restrictions. May be taken with milk.
▷ *Alcohol*: No interactions expected.
Tobacco Smoking: No interactions expected.
▷ *Other Drugs*
The following drugs may *decrease* the effects of tamoxifen
• estrogens.
• oral contraceptives (those that contain estrogens).
▷ *Driving, Hazardous Activities*: This drug may cause dizziness or drowsiness. Restrict activities as necessary.
Aviation Note: The use of this drug *may be a disqualification* for piloting. Consult a designated Aviation Medical Examiner.
Exposure to Sun: No restrictions.

TEMAZEPAM
(tem AZ e pam)

Introduced: 1978

Prescription: USA: Yes
Canada: Yes

Available as Generic: USA: No
Canada: No

Brand Names: Restoril

Class: Hypnotic, Benzodiazepines

Controlled Drug: USA: C-IV*
Canada: No

BENEFITS versus RISKS

Possible Benefits	*Possible Risks*
EFFECTIVE HYPNOTIC after 4 weeks of continual use	Habit-forming potential with long-term use
Wide margin of safety with therapeutic doses	Minor impairment of mental functions ("hangover" effect)

▷ **Principal Uses**
As a Single Drug Product: This member of the benzodiazepine class of "minor tranquilizers" is used exclusively as a bedtime sedative to induce sleep.

*See Schedules of Controlled Drugs inside back cover.

How This Drug Works: It is thought that this drug produces a calming effect by enhancing the action of the nerve transmitter gamma-aminobutyric acid (GABA), which in turn blocks the arousal of higher brain centers and helps to induce sleep.

Available Dosage Forms and Strengths
Capsules — 15 mg, 30 mg

▷ **Usual Adult Dosage Range:**   15 to 30 mg at bedtime. Total daily dosage should not exceed 90 mg. **Note: Actual dosage and administration schedule must be determined by the physician for each patient individually.**

▷ **Dosing Instructions:**   Preferably taken on an empty stomach to hasten absorption and induce sleep rapidly. The capsule may be opened for administration. Do not discontinue this drug abruptly if taken for more than 4 weeks.

Usual Duration of Use: Periods of 3 to 5 nights intermittently, repeated as needed with appropriate dosage adjustment. Avoid uninterrupted and prolonged use. The duration of use should not exceed 2 weeks without reappraisal of continued need.

▷ **This Drug Should Not Be Taken If**
  • you have had an allergic reaction to it previously.
  • you have acute narrow-angle glaucoma, inadequately treated.

▷ **Inform Your Physician Before Taking This Drug If**
  • you are allergic to any benzodiazepine drug (see Drug Class, Section Four).
  • you have a history of alcoholism or drug abuse.
  • you are pregnant or planning pregnancy.
  • you have impaired liver or kidney function.
  • you have a history of serious depression or mental disorder.
  • you are taking other drugs with sedative effects.
  • you have any of the following: asthma, emphysema, epilepsy, myasthenia gravis.

Possible Side-Effects   (natural, expected and unavoidable drug actions)
"Hangover" effects on arising: drowsiness, lethargy and unsteadiness.

Possible Adverse Effects   (unusual, unexpected and infrequent reactions)
If any of the following develop, consult your physician promptly.
Mild Adverse Effects
Allergic Reactions: Skin rash, hives.
Dizziness, fainting, slurred speech, nausea, indigestion.
Serious Adverse Effects
Idiosyncratic Reactions: Nervousness, talkativeness, irritability, apprehension, euphoria, excitement, hallucinations.

CAUTION
  1.   This drug should not be discontinued abruptly if it has been taken continually for more than 4 weeks.

2. The concurrent use of some over-the-counter drug products that contain antihistamines (allergy and cold preparations, sleep aids) can cause excessive sedation in sensitive individuals.
3. Regular nightly use of any hypnotic drug should be avoided.
4. If you experience a "hangover" effect, avoid hazardous activities (driving, etc.) and the use of alcohol.

Precautions for Use
By Infants and Children: Safety and effectiveness for use by those under 18 years of age have not been established.

By Those over 60 Years of Age: It is advisable to use smaller doses (15 mg) at first to determine your response. Observe for the possible development of lethargy, indifference, fatigue, weakness, unsteadiness, disturbing dreams, nightmares and paradoxical reactions of excitement, agitation, anger, hostility and rage.

▷ **Advisability of Use During Pregnancy**
Pregnancy Category: X (tentative). See Pregnancy Code inside back cover.
Animal studies: Rib defects reported in rats; skull and rib defects reported in rabbits.
Human studies: Information from adequate studies of pregnant women is not available.
Avoid use during entire pregnancy.

Advisability of Use if Breast-Feeding
Presence of this drug in breast milk: Probably yes.
Avoid drug or refrain from nursing.

Habit-Forming Potential: This drug can produce psychological and/or physical dependence (see Glossary) if used in large doses for an extended period of time. Avoid continual use.

Effects of Overdosage: Marked drowsiness, weakness, feeling of drunkenness, staggering gait, tremor, stupor progressing to deep sleep or coma.

Possible Effects of Long-Term Use: Psychological and/or physical dependence.

Periodic Examinations While Taking This Drug (at physician's discretion)
Complete blood cell counts during long-term use.

▷ **While Taking This Drug, Observe the Following**
Foods: No restrictions.
Beverages: Avoid excessive intake of caffeine-containing beverages (coffee, tea, cola) within 4 hours of taking this drug. May be taken with milk.
▷ *Alcohol*: Use with extreme caution until the combined effect has been determined. Alcohol may increase the absorption of this drug and add to its depressant effects on the brain. It is advisable to avoid alcohol completely—throughout the day and night—if it is necessary to drive or to engage in any hazardous activity.

Tobacco Smoking: Heavy smoking may reduce the hypnotic action of this drug.

Marijuana Smoking: Increased sedation and significant impairment of intellectual and physical performance.

▷ *Other Drugs*

Temazepam may *increase* the effects of
- digoxin (Lanoxin), and cause digoxin toxicity.
- phenytoin (Dilantin), and cause phenytoin toxicity.

Temazepam may *decrease* the effects of
- levodopa (Sinemet, etc.), and reduce its effectiveness in treating Parkinson's disease.

The following drugs may *increase* the effects of temazepam
- cimetidine (Tagamet).
- disulfiram (Antabuse).
- isoniazid (INH, Rifamate, etc.).
- oral contraceptives.
- valproic acid (Depakene).

The following drugs may *decrease* the effects of temazepam
- rifampin (Rimactane, etc.).
- theophylline (aminophylline, Theo-Dur, etc.).

▷ *Driving, Hazardous Activities*: This drug can impair mental alertness, judgment, physical coordination and reaction time. Avoid hazardous activities accordingly.

Aviation Note: The use of this drug *is a disqualification* for piloting. Consult a designated Aviation Medical Examiner.

Exposure to Sun: No restrictions.

Exposure to Heat: Use caution until the effect of excessive perspiration is determined. Because of reduced urine volume, this drug may accumulate in the body and produce effects of overdosage.

Discontinuation: Avoid sudden discontinuation if this drug has been taken for over 4 weeks without interruption. Dosage should be tapered gradually to prevent a withdrawal syndrome that could include depression, confusion, hallucinations, tremor, seizures, muscle cramping, sweating and vomiting.

TERBUTALINE
(ter BYU ta leen)

Introduced: 1974

Class: Antiasthmatic, Bronchodilator

Prescription: USA: Yes
Canada: Yes

Controlled Drug: USA: No
Canada: No

Available as Generic: No

Brand Names: Brethaire, Brethine, Bricanyl, ✤Bricanyl Spacer

BENEFITS versus RISKS

Possible Benefits	*Possible Risks*
VERY EFFECTIVE RELIEF OF BRONCHOSPASM	Increased blood pressure
	Fine hand tremor
	Irregular heart rhythm (with excessive use)

▷ **Principal Uses**

As a Single Drug Product: To relieve acute bronchial asthma and to reduce the frequency and severity of chronic, recurrent asthmatic attacks; also used to relieve reversible bronchospasm associated with chronic bronchitis and emphysema.

How This Drug Works: By stimulating certain sympathetic nerve terminals, this drug acts to dilate those bronchial tubes that are in sustained constriction, thereby increasing the size of the airway and improving the ability to breathe.

Available Dosage Forms and Strengths
Aerosol — 0.2 mg/actuation, 0.25 mg/actuation (Canada)
Injection — 1 mg per ml
Tablets — 2.5 mg, 5 mg

▷ **Usual Adult Dosage Range:**   Aerosol: 0.4 mg taken in 2 separate inhalations 1 minute apart; repeat every 4 to 6 hours as needed. Tablets: 2.5 to 5 mg taken 3 times/day, 6 hours apart. The total daily dosage should not exceed 15 mg. **Note: Actual dosage and administration schedule must be determined by the physician for each patient individually.**

▷ **Dosing Instructions:**   May be taken on empty stomach or with food or milk. Tablets may be crushed for administration. For aerosol, follow the written instructions carefully. Do not overuse.

Usual Duration of Use: According to individual requirements. Do not use beyond the time necessary to terminate episodes of asthma.

▷ **This Drug Should Not Be Taken If**
- you have had an allergic reaction to any dosage form of it previously.
- you currently have an irregular heart rhythm.
- you are taking, or have taken within the past 2 weeks, any monoamine oxidase (MAO) inhibitor drug (see Drug Class, Section Four).

▷ **Inform Your Physician Before Taking This Drug If**
- you are overly sensitive to other drugs that stimulate the sympathetic nervous system.
- you are currently using epinephrine (Adrenalin, Primatene Mist, etc.) to relieve asthmatic breathing.

- you have a seizure disorder.
- you have any type of heart or circulatory disorder, especially high blood pressure or coronary heart disease.
- you have diabetes or an overactive thyroid gland (hyperthyroidism).
- you are taking any form of digitalis or any stimulant drug.

Possible Side-Effects   (natural, expected and unavoidable drug actions)
Aerosol: dryness or irritation of mouth or throat, altered taste. Tablet: nervousness, tremor, palpitation.

▷ **Possible Adverse Effects**   (unusual, unexpected and infrequent reactions)
If any of the following develop, consult your physician promptly.
Mild Adverse Effects
Headache, dizziness, drowsiness, restlessness, insomnia.
Rapid, pounding heartbeat; increased sweating; muscle cramps in arms and legs.
Nausea, heartburn, vomiting.
Serious Adverse Effects
Rapid or irregular heart rhythm, intensification of angina, increased blood pressure.

Natural Diseases or Disorders That May Be Activated By This Drug
Latent coronary artery disease, diabetes or high blood pressure.

CAUTION
1. Concurrent use of this drug by aerosol inhalation with beclomethasone aerosol (Beclovent, Vanceril) may increase the risk of toxicity due to fluorocarbon propellants. It is advisable to use this aerosol 20 to 30 minutes *before* beclomethasone aerosol. This will reduce the risk of toxicity and will enhance the penetration of beclomethasone.
2. *Avoid excessive use of aerosol inhalation.* The excessive or prolonged use of this drug by inhalation can reduce its effectiveness and cause serious heart rhythm disturbances, including cardiac arrest.
3. Do not use this drug concurrently with epinephrine. These two drugs may be used alternately if an interval of 4 hours is allowed between doses.
4. If you do not respond to your usually effective dose, ask your physician for guidance. Do not increase the size or frequency of the dose without your physician's approval.

Precautions for Use
By Infants and Children: Safety and effectiveness for use by those under 12 years of age have not been established.
By Those over 60 Years of Age: Avoid excessive and continual use. If acute asthma is not relieved promptly, other drugs will have to be tried. Observe for the development of nervousness, palpitations, irregular

heart rhythm and muscle tremors. Use with extreme caution if you have hardening of the arteries, heart disease or high blood pressure.

▷ **Advisability of Use During Pregnancy**
Pregnancy Category: B (tentative). See Pregnancy Code inside back cover.
Animal studies: No significant birth defects reported in mouse and rat studies.
Human studies: Information from adequate studies of pregnant women is not available.
Use only if clearly needed. Ask your physician for guidance.

Advisability of Use if Breast-Feeding
Presence of this drug in breast milk: Yes.
Monitor nursing infant closely and discontinue drug or nursing if adverse effects develop.

Habit-Forming Potential: None.

Effects of Overdosage: Nervousness, palpitation, rapid heart rate, sweating, headache, tremor, vomiting, chest pain.

Possible Effects of Long-Term Use: Loss of effectiveness. See *CAUTION* category above.

Suggested Periodic Examinations While Taking This Drug   (at physician's discretion)
Blood pressure measurements, evaluation of heart status.

▷ **While Taking This Drug, Observe the Following**
Foods: No restrictions.
Beverages: Avoid excessive use of caffeine-containing beverages: coffee, tea, cola, chocolate.
▷ *Alcohol*: No interactions expected.
Tobacco Smoking: No interactions expected.
▷ *Other Drugs*
Terbutaline *taken concurrently* with
• monoamine oxidase (MAO) inhibitor drugs may cause excessive increase in blood pressure and undesirable heart stimulation (see Drug Class, Section Four).
The following drugs may *decrease* the effects of terbutaline
• beta-blocker drugs may impair its effectiveness (see Drug Class, Section Four).
▷ *Driving, Hazardous Activities*: Usually no restrictions. Use caution if excessive nervousness or dizziness occurs.
Aviation Note: The use of this drug *is a disqualification* for piloting. Consult a designated Aviation Medical Examiner.
Exposure to Sun: No restrictions.
Heavy Exercise or Exertion: Use caution. Excessive exercise can induce asthma in sensitive individuals.

TERFENADINE
(ter FEN a deen)

Introduced: 1977

Prescription: USA: Yes
   Canada: No

Available as Generic: No

Brand Names: Seldane

Class: Antihistamines

Controlled Drug: USA: No
   Canada: No

BENEFITS versus RISKS

Possible Benefits	*Possible Risks*
EFFECTIVE RELIEF OF ALLERGIC RHINITIS AND ALLERGIC SKIN DISORDERS	Infrequent headache Mild fatigue Minor digestive disturbances Slight atropinelike effects

---

▷ **Principal Uses**

As a Single Drug Product: Used primarily to provide symptomatic relief in allergic and related disorders: seasonal and perennial allergic rhinitis (hay fever), allergic conjunctivitis and vasomotor rhinitis; also in hives and localized swellings (angioedema) of allergic origin.

How This Drug Works: Antihistamines reduce the intensity of the allergic response by blocking the action of histamine after it has been released from sensitized tissue cells in the eyes, nose and skin.

Available Dosage Forms and Strengths

Suspension — 30 mg per 5 ml teaspoonful (Canada)
   Tablets — 60 mg

▷ **Usual Adult Dosage Range:** 60 mg every 8 to 12 hrs as needed. The total daily dosage should not exceed 360 mg. **Note: Actual dosage and administration schedule must be determined by the physician for each patient individually.**

▷ **Dosing Instructions:** May be taken with food or milk to prevent stomach irritation. The tablet may be crushed for administration.

Usual Duration of Use: Continual use on a regular schedule for 2 to 3 days is usually necessary to determine this drug's effectiveness in relieving the symptoms of allergic rhinitis and dermatosis. It may be necessary to take this drug throughout the entire pollen season, depending upon individual sensitivity. However, antihistamines should not be taken continually (without interruption) for long-term use. Limit their use to periods that require symptomatic relief.

▷ **This Drug Should Not Be Taken If**

- you have had an allergic reaction to any dosage form of it previously.
- you are currently undergoing allergy skin tests.

▷ **Inform Your Physician Before Taking This Drug If**
- you have had any allergic reactions or unfavorable responses to the previous use of antihistamines.

Possible Side-Effects   (natural, expected and unavoidable drug actions)
Dry nose, mouth or throat.

▷ **Possible Adverse Effects**   (unusual, unexpected and infrequent reactions)
If any of the following develop, consult your physician promptly.
Mild Adverse Effects
Allergic Reactions: Skin rash, itching.
Headache, nervousness, fatigue.
Increased appetite, indigestion, nausea, vomiting.
Serious Adverse Effects
None reported.

CAUTION
1. Discontinue this drug 4 days before diagnostic skin testing procedures in order to prevent false negative test results.
2. Do not use this drug if you have active bronchial asthma, bronchitis or pneumonia. It may thicken bronchial mucus and make it more difficult to remove (by absorption or coughing).

Precautions for Use
By Infants and Children: Safety and effectiveness for use by those under 12 years of age have not been established.
By Those over 60 Years of Age: You may be more susceptible to the development of headache and fatigue. Use smaller doses at longer intervals if necessary.

▷ **Advisability of Use During Pregnancy**
Pregnancy Category: C (tentative). See Pregnancy Code inside back cover.
Animal studies: No birth defects due to this drug reported.
Human studies: Information from adequate studies of pregnant women is not available.
Use this drug only if clearly needed. Ask your physician for guidance.

Advisability of Use if Breast-Feeding
Presence of this drug in breast milk: Unknown.
Avoid drug or refrain from nursing.

Habit-Forming Potential: None.

Effects of Overdosage: No information available. No serious or threatening effects expected.

Possible Effects of Long-Term Use: None reported.

Suggested Periodic Examinations While Taking This Drug   (at physician's discretion)
None required.

▷ **While Taking This Drug, Observe the Following**
Foods: No restrictions.

Beverages: No restrictions. May be taken with milk.
▷ *Alcohol*: No interactions expected.
Tobacco Smoking: No interactions expected.
▷ *Other Drugs*: No significant interactions reported to date.
Hazardous Activities: No restrictions.
Aviation Note: The use of this drug *is probably not a disqualification* for piloting. Consult a designated Aviation Medical Examiner.
Exposure to Sun: No restrictions.

TETRACYCLINE
(te trah SI kleen)

Introduced: 1953

Class: Antibiotic, Tetracyclines

Prescription: USA: Yes
Canada: Yes

Controlled Drug: USA: No
Canada: No

Available as Generic: Yes

Brand Names: Achromycin, Achromycin V, ✤Apo-Tetra, Cyclopar, ✤Medicycline, Mysteclin-F [CD], ✤Neo-Tetrine, Nor-Tet, ✤Novotetra, Panmycin, Retet, Robitet, SK-Tetracycline, Sumycin, Tetra-C, Tetracyn, Tetralan, Tetram, ✤Tetrex, Tropicycline

---

BENEFITS versus RISKS

Possible Benefits	*Possible Risks*
EFFECTIVE TREATMENT OF INFECTIONS due to susceptible bacteria and protozoa	ALLERGIC REACTIONS, mild to severe: ANAPHYLAXIS, DRUG-INDUCED HEPATITIS (rare) Drug-induced colitis Superinfections (bacterial or fungal) Rare blood cell disorders: hemolytic anemia, abnormally low white cell and platelet counts

---

▷ **Principal Uses**

As a Single Drug Product: This member of the tetracycline drug class is used primarily to (1) treat a broad range of infections caused by susceptible bacteria and protozoa (short-term use); and (2) treat severe, resistant pustular acne (long-term use).

As a Combination Drug Product [CD]: This drug is available in combination with amphotericin B, an antifungal antibiotic that is provided to reduce the risk of developing an overgrowth of yeast organisms (superinfection) of the gastrointestinal tract.

How This Drug Works: This drug prevents the growth and multiplication of susceptible bacteria by interfering with their formation of essential proteins.

Available Dosage Forms and Strengths

> Capsules — 100 mg, 250 mg, 500 mg
> Ointment — 3%
> Ointment, ophthalmic — 10 mg per gram
> Solution, topical — 2.2 mg per ml
> Suspension, ophthalmic — 10 mg per ml
> Suspension, oral — 125 mg per 5 ml teaspoonful
> Tablets — 250 mg, 500 mg

▷ **Usual Adult Dosage Range:** 250 to 500 mg/6 hours, or 500 to 1000 mg/12 hours. The total daily dosage should not exceed 4000 mg (4 grams). **Note: Actual dosage and administration schedule must be determined by the physician for each patient individually.**

▷ **Dosing Instructions:** Preferably taken on an empty stomach, 1 hour before or 2 hours after eating. However, to reduce stomach irritation it may be taken with crackers that contain insignificant amounts of iron, calcium, magnesium or zinc. Avoid all dairy products for 2 hours before and after taking this drug. Take at the same time each day, with a full glass of water. Take the full course prescribed. The tablet may be crushed and the capsule may be opened for administration.

Usual Duration of Use: The time required to control the infection and be free of fever and symptoms for 48 hours. This varies with the nature of the infection.

▷ **This Drug Should Not Be Taken If**
- you are allergic to any tetracycline drug (see Drug Class, Section Four).
- you are pregnant or breast-feeding.

▷ **Inform Your Physician Before Taking This Drug If**
- it is prescribed for a child under 8 years of age.
- you have a history of liver or kidney disease.
- you have systemic lupus erythematosus.
- you are taking any penicillin drug.
- you are taking any anticoagulant drug.
- you plan to have surgery under general anesthesia in the near future.

Possible Side-Effects (natural, expected and unavoidable drug actions)
Superinfections (see Glossary), often due to yeast organisms. These can occur in the mouth, intestinal tract, rectum and/or vagina, resulting in rectal and vaginal itching.

▷ **Possible Adverse Effects** (unusual, unexpected and infrequent reactions)
If any of the following develop, consult your physician promptly.
Mild Adverse Effects
Allergic Reactions: Skin rash, hives, itching of hands and feet, swelling of face or extremities.
Loss of appetite, stomach irritation, nausea, vomiting, diarrhea.
Irritation of mouth or tongue, "black tongue," sore throat, abdominal cramping or pain.

Serious Adverse Effects

Allergic Reactions: Anaphylactic reaction (see Glossary), asthma, fever, swollen joints and lymph glands.

Drug-induced hepatitis with jaundice.

Permanent discoloration and/or malformation of teeth when taken under 8 years of age, including unborn child and infant.

Impaired vision, increased intracranial pressure.

Drug-induced colitis.

Rare blood cell disorders: hemolytic anemia (see Glossary); abnormally low white blood cell count, causing fever, sore throat and infections; abnormally low blood platelet count, causing abnormal bleeding or bruising.

▷ **Adverse Effects That May Mimic Natural Diseases or Disorders**

Drug-induced hepatitis may suggest viral hepatitis.

Natural Diseases or Disorders That May Be Activated by This Drug

Systemic lupus erythematosus.

CAUTION

1. Antacids, dairy products and preparations containing aluminum, bismuth, calcium, iron, magnesium or zinc can prevent adequate absorption of this drug and reduce its effectiveness significantly.
2. Troublesome and persistent diarrhea can develop in sensitive individuals. If diarrhea persists for more than 24 hours, discontinue this drug and consult your physician.
3. If surgery under general anesthesia is required while taking this drug, the choice of anesthetic agent must be considered carefully to prevent serious kidney damage.

Precautions for Use

By Infants and Children: If possible, tetracyclines should not be given to children under 8 years of age because of the risk of permanent discoloration and deformity of the teeth. Rarely, young infants may develop increased intracranial pressure within the first 4 days of receiving this drug. Tetracyclines may inhibit normal bone growth and development.

By Those over 60 Years of Age: Dosage must be carefully individualized and based upon determinations of kidney function. Natural skin changes may predispose to severe and prolonged itching reactions in the genital and anal regions.

▷ **Advisability of Use During Pregnancy**

Pregnancy Category: D (tentative). See Pregnancy Code inside back cover.

Animal studies: Tetracycline causes limb defects in rats, rabbits and chickens.

Human studies: Information from studies of pregnant women indicates that this drug can cause impaired development and discoloration of teeth and other developmental defects.

It is advisable to avoid this drug completely during entire pregnancy.

Advisability of Use if Breast-Feeding
Presence of this drug in breast milk: Yes.
Avoid drug or refrain from nursing.

Habit-Forming Potential: None.

Effects of Overdosage: Stomach burning, nausea, vomiting, diarrhea.

Possible Effects of Long-Term Use: Superinfections; rarely, impairment of bone marrow, liver or kidney function.

Suggested Periodic Examinations While Taking This Drug (at physician's discretion)
Complete blood cell counts, liver and kidney function tests.
During extended use, sputum and stool examinations may detect early superinfection due to yeast organisms.

▷ **While Taking This Drug, Observe the Following**
Foods: Avoid cheeses, yogurt, ice cream, iron-fortified cereals and supplements and meats for 2 hours before and after taking this drug. Calcium and iron can combine with this drug and reduce its absorption significantly.
Beverages: Avoid all forms of milk for 2 hours before and after taking this drug.

▷ *Alcohol*: No interactions expected. However, it is best avoided if you have active liver disease.
Tobacco Smoking: No interactions expected.

▷ *Other Drugs*
Tetracyclines may *increase* the effects of
- oral anticoagulants, and make it necessary to reduce their dosage.
- digoxin (Lanoxin), and cause digitalis toxicity.
- lithium (Eskalith, Lithane, etc.), and increase the risk of lithium toxicity.

Tetracyclines may *decrease* the effects of
- oral contraceptives, and impair their effectiveness in preventing pregnancy.
- penicillins, and impair their effectiveness in treating infections.

Tetracyclines *taken concurrently* with
- methoxyflurane anesthesia may impair kidney function.

The following drugs may *decrease* the effects of tetracyclines
- antacids (aluminum and magnesium preparations, sodium bicarbonate, etc.) may reduce drug absorption.
- iron and mineral preparations may reduce drug absorption.

▷ *Driving, Hazardous Activities*: Usually no restrictions. However, this drug may cause nausea or diarrhea. Restrict activities as necessary.
Aviation Note: The use of this drug *may be a disqualification* for piloting. Consult a designated Aviation Medical Examiner.
Exposure to Sun: Use caution until sensitivity has been determined. Some tetracyclines can cause photosensitivity (see Glossary).

THEOPHYLLINE
(thee OFF i lin)

Other Names: Aminophylline, Oxtriphylline

Introduced: 1929

Class: Antiasthmatic, Bronchodilator, Xanthines

Prescription: USA: Yes
Canada: No

Controlled Drug: USA: No
Canada: No

Available as Generic: Yes

Brand Names: Accurbron, Amesec [CD], Brondecon [CD], Bronkaid Tablets [CD], Bronkodyl, Bronkolixir [CD], Bronkotabs [CD], Choledyl, Constant-T, Elixicon, Elixophyllin, LaBID, Lodrane, Mudrane GG Elixir & Tablets [CD], ♣PMS Theophylline, ♣Pulmophylline, Quadrinal [CD], Quibron [CD], Quibron-T Dividose, Respbid, Slo-bid, Slo-Phyllin, Slo-Phyllin GG [CD], Slo-Phyllin Gyrocaps, Somophyllin-CRT, Somophyllin-DF, Somophyllin-T, ♣Somophyllin-12, Sustaire, ♣Tedral Preparations [CD], Theobid Duracaps, Theo-Dur, Theolair, ♣Theolixir, Theophyl-SR, Theo-24, Theovent

---

BENEFITS versus RISKS

Possible Benefits	*Possible Risks*
EFFECTIVE RELIEF OF ACUTE BRONCHIAL ASTHMA	NARROW TREATMENT RANGE
MODERATELY EFFECTIVE CONTROL OF CHRONIC, RECURRENT BRONCHIAL ASTHMA	FREQUENT STOMACH DISTRESS
	Gastrointestinal bleeding
	Central nervous system toxicity, seizures
Moderately effective symptomatic relief in chronic bronchitis and emphysema	Heart rhythm disturbances

---

▷ **Principal Uses**

As a Single Drug Product: Used primarily to relieve the shortness of breath and wheezing characteristic of acute bronchial asthma, and to prevent the recurrence of asthmatic episodes. It is also useful in relieving the asthmaticlike symptoms that are associated with some types of chronic bronchitis and emphysema.

As a Combination Drug Product [CD]: This drug is available in combination with several other drugs that are beneficial in the overall management of bronchial asthma and related conditions. Ephedrine is added to enhance the bronchodilator effects; guaifenesin is added to provide an expectorant effect that thins the mucus secretions in the bronchial tubes; mild sedatives such as phenobarbital are added to allay the anxiety that often accompanies acute attacks of asthma.

How This Drug Works: By inhibiting the enzyme phosphodiesterase, this drug produces an increase in the tissue chemical cyclic AMP. This causes relaxation of the muscles in the bronchial tubes and blood vessels of the lung, resulting in relief of bronchospasm, expanded lung capacity and improved lung circulation.

Available Dosage Forms and Strengths

Capsules —	100 mg, 200 mg, 250 mg
Capsules, prolonged action —	50 mg, 65 mg, 75 mg, 100 mg, 125 mg, 130 mg, 200 mg, 250 mg, 260 mg, 300 mg
Elixir —	80 mg per 15 ml tablespoonful, 150 mg per 15 ml tablespoonful
Liquid —	80 mg per 15 ml tablespoonful, 160 mg per 15 ml tablespoonful
Suspension —	300 mg per 15 ml tablespoonful
Syrup —	80 mg per 15 ml tablespoonful, 150 mg per 15 ml tablespoonful
Tablets —	100 mg, 125 mg, 200 mg, 250 mg, 300 mg
Tablets, prolonged action —	100 mg, 200 mg, 250 mg, 300 mg, 400 mg, 500 mg

▷ **Usual Adult Dosage Range:**   Because of its potential toxicity, this drug is given according to body weight. For acute asthma: Initially, 6 mg/kg as the first dose; then 3 mg/kg every 6 hours for 12 hours; then 3 mg/kg every 8 hours as needed. For maintenance: 16 mg/kg/24 hours, or 400 mg/24 hours, whichever is less, taken in 3 or 4 divided doses at intervals of 6 to 8 hours. The total daily dosage should not exceed 900 mg. **Note: Actual dosage and administration schedule must be determined by the physician for each patient individually.**

▷ **Dosing Instructions:**   May be taken with or following food to reduce stomach irritation. The regular capsules may be opened and the regular tablets may be crushed for administration. The prolonged action dosage forms should be swallowed whole and not altered.

Usual Duration of Use: Continual use on a regular schedule for 48 to 72 hours is usually necessary to determine this drug's effectiveness in controlling the breathing impairment associated with bronchial asthma and chronic lung disease. Long-term use (months to years) requires supervision and periodic evaluation by your physician.

▷ **This Drug Should Not Be Taken If**
- you have had an allergic reaction to it previously.
- you have active peptic ulcer disease.

▷ **Inform Your Physician Before Taking This Drug If**
- you have had an unfavorable reaction to any xanthine drug previously (see Drug Class, Section Four).
- you have a history of peptic ulcer disease.
- you have impaired liver or kidney function.
- you have hypertension, heart disease or any type of heart rhythm disorder.

Possible Side-Effects   (natural, expected and unavoidable drug actions)
Nervousness, insomnia, rapid heart rate, increased urine volume.

▷ **Possible Adverse Effects**   (unusual, unexpected and infrequent reactions)
If any of the following develop, consult your physician promptly.
Mild Adverse Effects
Allergic Reactions: Skin rash, hives.
Headache, dizziness, irritability, tremor, fatigue, weakness.
Loss of appetite, nausea, vomiting, abdominal pain, diarrhea, excessive
thirst.
Flushing of face.
Serious Adverse Effects
Idiosyncratic Reactions: Marked anxiety, confusion, behavioral distur-
bances.
Central nervous system toxicity: muscle twitching, seizures.
Heart rhythm abnormalities, rapid breathing, low blood pressure.
Gastrointestinal bleeding.

Natural Diseases or Disorders That May Be Activated by This Drug
Latent peptic ulcer disease.

CAUTION
1. This drug should not be taken concurrently with other antiasthmatic
   drugs unless you are directed to do so by your physician. Serious overdosage could result.
2. It has been reported that influenza vaccine may delay the elimination
   of this drug and cause accumulation to toxic levels.

Precautions for Use
By Infants and Children: Observe for indications of toxicity: irritability, agitation, tremors, lethargy, fever, vomiting, rapid heart rate and breathing,
seizures.
By Those over 60 Years of Age: Start treatment with small doses until your
tolerance has been determined. You may be more susceptible to the
development of stomach irritation, nausea, vomiting or diarrhea. When
used concurrently with coffee (caffeine) or with nasal decongestants, this
drug may cause excessive stimulation and a hyperactivity syndrome.

▷ **Advisability of Use During Pregnancy**
Pregnancy Category: C (tentative). See Pregnancy Code inside back cover.
Animal studies: Significant birth defects due to this drug reported in mice.
Human studies: Information from adequate studies of pregnant women is
not available. No increase in birth defects reported in 394 exposures to
this drug.
Avoid this drug during the first 3 months. Use it otherwise only if clearly
needed. Ask your physician for guidance.

Advisability of Use if Breast-Feeding
Presence of this drug in breast milk: Yes.
Avoid drug or refrain from nursing.

Habit-Forming Potential: None.

Effects of Overdosage: Nausea, vomiting, restlessness, irritability, confusion, delirium, seizures, high fever, weak pulse, coma.

Possible Effects of Long-Term Use: Gastrointestinal irritation.

Suggested Periodic Examinations While Taking This Drug   (at physician's discretion)
Measurement of blood theophylline levels, especially with high dosage or long-term use. (See Therapeutic Drug Monitoring in Section One.)

▷ **While Taking This Drug, Observe the Following**
Foods: No restrictions.
Beverages: Avoid excessive use of caffeine-containing beverages: coffee, tea, cola; this combination could cause nervousness and insomnia.
▷ *Alcohol:* No interactions expected. May have additive effect on stomach irritation.
Tobacco Smoking: May hasten the elimination of this drug and reduce its effectiveness. Higher doses may be necessary to maintain a therapeutic blood level.
▷ *Other Drugs*
Theophylline may *decrease* the effects of
• lithium (Lithane, Lithobid, etc.), and reduce its effectiveness.
Theophylline *taken concurrently* with
• halothane (anesthesia) may cause heart rhythm abnormalities.
• phenytoin (Dilantin) may cause decreased effects of both drugs.
The following drugs may *increase* the effects of theophylline
• cimetidine (Tagamet) may cause theophylline toxicity.
• erythromycin (E-Mycin, Erythrocin, etc.) may cause theophylline toxicity.
• oral contraceptives.
• troleandomycin (TAO).
The following drugs may *decrease* the effects of theophylline
• barbiturates (phenobarbital, etc.).
• beta-blocker drugs (see Drug Class, Section Four).
• rifampin (Rifadin, Rimactane, etc.).
▷ *Driving, Hazardous Activities:* This drug may cause dizziness. Restrict activities as necessary.
Aviation Note: The use of this drug *may be a disqualification* for piloting. Consult a designated Aviation Medical Examiner.
Exposure to Sun: No restrictions.
Occurrence of Unrelated Illness: Acute viral respiratory infections can delay the elimination of this drug significantly. Observe closely for indications of toxicity and the need to reduce dosage or lengthen the dosage interval.
Discontinuation: Avoid prolonged and unnecessary use of this drug. When you have achieved an asthma-free state, withdraw this drug gradually over several days.

THIORIDAZINE
(thi oh RID a zeen)

Introduced: 1959

Class: Strong Tranquilizer, Phenothiazines

Prescription: USA: Yes
Canada: Yes

Controlled Drug: USA: No
Canada: No

Available as Generic: USA: Yes
Canada: Yes

Brand Names: ✿Apo-Thioridazine, Mellaril, Mellaril-S, ✿Novoridazine, ✿PMS Thioridazine

---

BENEFITS versus RISKS

Possible Benefits	*Possible Risks*
EFFECTIVE CONTROL OF ACUTE MENTAL DISORDERS in the majority of patients: beneficial effects on thinking, mood and behavior	SERIOUS TOXIC EFFECTS ON BRAIN with long-term use
Relief of anxiety, agitation and tension	Liver damage with jaundice (infrequent)
Possibly effective in the management of the hyperactivity syndrome in children	Rare blood cell disorders: abnormally low white blood cell count

---

▷ **Principal Uses**

As a Single Drug Product: This antipsychotic drug is used primarily in the management of the following conditions: moderate to marked depression with significant anxiety and nervous tension; agitation, anxiety, depression and exaggerated fears in the elderly; severe behavioral problems in children characterized by hyperexcitability, combativeness, short attention span and rapid swings in mood.

How This Drug Works: Not completely established. Present theory is that by inhibiting the action of dopamine in certain brain centers, this drug acts to correct an imbalance of nerve impulse transmissions that is thought to be responsible for certain mental disorders.

Available Dosage Forms and Strengths
Concentrate — 30 mg per ml, 100 mg per ml
Suspension — 25 mg per 5 ml teaspoonful, 100 mg per 5 ml teaspoonful
Tablets — 10 mg, 15 mg, 25 mg, 50 mg, 100 mg, 150 mg, 200 mg

▷ **Usual Adult Dosage Range:** Initially, 25 to 100 mg 3 times/day. Dose may be increased by 25 to 50 mg at 3 to 4 day intervals as needed and tolerated. Usual dosage range is 200 to 800 mg daily, divided into 2 to 4 doses. The total daily dosage should not exceed 800 mg. **Note: Actual dosage and** administration schedule must be determined by the physician for each patient individually.

▷ **Dosing Instructions:**   May be taken with or following meals to reduce stomach irritation. The tablets may be crushed for administration.

Usual Duration of Use: Continual use on a regular schedule for 3 to 4 weeks is usually necessary to determine this drug's effectiveness in controlling psychotic disorders. If not significantly beneficial within 6 weeks, it should be discontinued. Long-term use (months to years) requires periodic evaluation of response, appropriate dosage adjustment and consideration of continued need.

▷ **This Drug Should Not Be Taken If**
- you are allergic to any of the drugs bearing the brand names listed above.
- you have active liver disease.
- you have cancer of the breast.
- you have a current blood cell or bone marrow disorder.

▷ **Inform Your Physician Before Taking This Drug If**
- you are allergic or abnormally sensitive to any phenothiazine drug (see Drug Class, Section Four).
- you have impaired liver or kidney function.
- you have any type of seizure disorder.
- you have diabetes, glaucoma or heart disease.
- you have a history of lupus erythematosus.
- you are taking any drug with sedative effects.
- you plan to have surgery under general or spinal anesthesia in the near future.

Possible Side-Effects   (natural, expected and unavoidable drug actions)
Drowsiness (usually during the first 2 weeks), orthostatic hypotension (see Glossary), blurred vision, dry mouth, nasal congestion, constipation, impaired urination.
Pink or purple coloration of urine, of no significance.

▷ **Possible Adverse Effects**   (unusual, unexpected and infrequent reactions)
If any of the following develop, consult your physician promptly.
Mild Adverse Effects
Allergic Reactions: Skin rash, hives, low-grade fever.
Lowering of body temperature, especially in the elderly. (See Hypothermia in Glossary.)
Increased appetite and weight gain.
Breast fullness, tenderness, milk production, menstrual irregularity.
Weakness, agitation, insomnia, impaired day and night vision.
Chronic constipation, fecal impaction.
Serious Adverse Effects
Allergic Reactions: Hepatitis with jaundice (see Glossary), severe skin reactions.
Depression, disorientation, seizures, loss of peripheral vision.

Rapid heart rate, heart rhythm disorders.

Enlargement of male breast tissue, sexual impotence, inhibition of ejaculation (common), reduced libido in women.

Blood cell disorders: reduced white blood cell count (more common in the elderly).

Nervous system reactions: Parkinson-like disorders (see Glossary), severe restlessness, muscle spasms involving the face and neck, tardive dyskinesia (see Glossary).

▷ **Adverse Effects That May Mimic Natural Diseases or Disorders**

Nervous system reactions may suggest true Parkinson's disease.

Liver reactions may suggest viral hepatitis.

Reactions resembling systemic lupus erythematosus can occur.

Natural Diseases or Disorders That May Be Activated by This Drug

Latent epilepsy, glaucoma, diabetes mellitus, prostatism (see Glossary).

CAUTION
1. Many over-the-counter medications (see OTC Drugs in Glossary) for allergies, colds and coughs contain drugs that can interact unfavorably with this drug. Ask your physician or pharmacist for guidance before using any such medications.
2. Antacids that contain aluminum and/or magnesium can prevent the absorption of this drug and reduce its effectiveness.
3. Obtain prompt evaluation of any change or disturbance of vision.

Precautions for Use
By Infants and Children: Use of this drug is not recommended in children under 2 years of age. Do not use this drug in the presence of symptoms suggestive of Reye syndrome (see Glossary). Children with acute infectious diseases ("flulike" infections, chicken pox, measles, etc.) are more prone to develop muscular spasms of the face, back and extremities when this drug is given for any reason.

By Those over 60 Years of Age: Small doses are advisable until individual response has been determined. You may be more susceptible to the development of drowsiness, lethargy, constipation, lowering of body temperature (hypothermia) and orthostatic hypotension (see Glossary). This drug can enhance existing prostatism (see Glossary). You may also be more susceptible to the development of parkinsonlike reactions and/or tardive dyskinesia (see discussion of these terms in Glossary). These reactions must be recognized early since they may become unresponsive to treatment and irreversible.

▷ **Advisability of Use During Pregnancy**
Pregnancy Category: C (tentative). See Pregnancy Code inside back cover.

Animal studies: The results of rodent studies are conflicting.

Human studies: No increase in birth defects reported in 23 exposures. Information from adequate studies of pregnant women is not available.

Avoid drug during the first 3 months. Use it otherwise only if clearly needed. Ask your physician for guidance.

Advisability of Use if Breast-Feeding
Presence of this drug in breast milk: Yes, in minute amounts.
Monitor nursing infant closely and discontinue drug or nursing if adverse effects develop.

Habit-Forming Potential: None.

Effects of Overdosage: Marked drowsiness, weakness, tremor, agitation, unsteadiness, deep sleep, coma, convulsions.

Possible Effects of Long-Term Use: Opacities in the cornea or lens of the eye, pigmentation of the retina. Tardive dyskinesia (see Glossary).

Suggested Periodic Examinations While Taking This Drug (at physician's discretion)
Complete blood cell counts, especially between the fourth and tenth weeks of treatment.
Liver function tests, electrocardiograms.
Complete eye examinations—eye structures and vision.
Careful inspection of the tongue for early evidence of fine, involuntary, wavelike movements that could indicate the beginning of tardive dyskinesia.

▷ **While Taking This Drug, Observe the Following**
Foods: No restrictions.
Nutritional Support: A riboflavin (vitamin B-2) supplement should be taken with long-term use.
Beverages: No restrictions. May be taken with milk.
▷ *Alcohol*: Avoid completely. Alcohol can increase the sedative action of phenothiazines and accentuate their depressant effects on brain function and blood pressure. Phenothiazines can increase the intoxicating effects of alcohol.
Tobacco Smoking: Possible reduction of drowsiness from drug.
Marijuana Smoking: Moderate increase in drowsiness; accentuation of orthostatic hypotension; increased risk of precipitating latent psychoses, confusing the interpretation of mental status and drug responses.
▷ *Other Drugs*
Thioridazine may ***increase*** the effects of
• all sedative drugs, especially meperidine (Demerol), and cause excessive sedation.
• all atropinelike drugs, and cause nervous system toxicity.
Thioridazine may ***decrease*** the effects of
• guanethidine (Ismelin, Esimil), and reduce its effectiveness in lowering blood pressure.
Thioridazine ***taken concurrently*** with
• lithium (Lithobid, Lithotabs) may impair the effectiveness of lithium and cause nervous system toxicity.
The following drugs may ***decrease*** the effects of thioridazine
• antacids containing aluminum and/or magnesium.

- barbiturates (see Drug Class, Section Four).
- benztropine (Cogentin).
- disulfiram (Antabuse).
- trihexyphenidyl (Artane).

▷ *Driving, Hazardous Activities*: This drug can impair mental alertness, judgment and physical coordination. Avoid hazardous activities.

Aviation Note: The use of this drug *is a disqualification* for piloting. Consult a designated Aviation Medical Examiner.

Exposure to Sun: Use caution until sensitivity has been determined. Some phenothiazines can cause photosensitivity (see Glossary).

Exposure to Heat: Use caution and avoid excessive heat as much as possible. This drug may impair the regulation of body temperature and increase the risk of heat stroke.

Exposure to Cold: Use caution and dress warmly. This drug can increase the risk of hypothermia in the elderly.

Discontinuation: After a period of long-term use, do not discontinue this drug suddenly. Gradual withdrawal over 2 to 3 weeks under physician supervision is recommended. Do not discontinue this drug without your physician's knowledge and approval.

THIOTHIXENE
(thi oh THIX een)

Introduced: 1967

Prescription: USA: Yes
Canada: Yes

Available as Generic: USA: No
Canada: No

Brand Names: Navane

Class: Strong Tranquilizer,
Thioxanthenes

Controlled Drug: USA: No
Canada: No

BENEFITS versus RISKS

Possible Benefits	*Possible Risks*
EFFECTIVE CONTROL OF ACUTE MENTAL DISORDERS in the majority of patients: beneficial effects on thinking, mood and behavior	SERIOUS TOXIC EFFECTS ON BRAIN with long-term use Liver damage with jaundice (rare) Rare blood cell disorders: abnormally low white blood cell count

---

▷ **Principal Uses**

As a Single Drug Product: This antipsychotic drug is used to ameliorate the psychotic thinking and behavior associated with acute psychoses of unknown nature, episodes of mania and paranoia, and acute schizophrenia.

How This Drug Works: Not completely established. Present theory is that, by inhibiting the action of dopamine, this drug acts to correct an imbalance of nerve impulse transmissions that is thought to be responsible for certain mental disorders.

Available Dosage Forms and Strengths

    Capsules — 1 mg, 2 mg, 5 mg, 10 mg, 20 mg
Concentrate — 5 mg per ml
Injections — 2 mg per ml, 5 mg per ml

▷ **Usual Adult Dosage Range**   Initially, 2 to 5 mg 2 or 3 times daily. Dose may be increased by 2 mg at 3 to 4 day intervals as needed and tolerated. Usual dosage range is 20 to 30 mg daily. The total daily dosage should not exceed 60 mg. **Note: Actual dosage and administration schedule must be determined by the physician for each patient individually.**

▷ **Dosing Instructions:**   May be taken with or following meals to reduce stomach irritation. The capsules may be opened for administration. The liquid concentrate must be diluted just before administration by adding it to 8 ounces of water, milk, fruit juice or carbonated beverage.

Usual Duration of Use: Continual use on a regular schedule for several weeks is usually necessary to determine this drug's effectiveness in controlling psychotic disorders. If not significantly beneficial within 6 weeks, it should be discontinued. Long-term use (months to years) requires periodic evaluation of response, appropriate dosage adjustment and consideration of continued need.

▷ **This Drug Should Not Be Taken If**
- you have had an allergic reaction to it previously.
- you have active liver disease.
- you have cancer of the breast.
- you have a current blood cell or bone marrow disorder.

▷ **Inform Your Physician Before Taking This Drug If**
- you are allergic or abnormally sensitive to other thioxanthene drugs or any phenothiazine drug (see Drug Classes, Section Four).
- you have impaired liver or kidney function.
- you have any type of seizure disorder.
- you have diabetes, glaucoma or heart disease.
- you have a history of lupus erythematosus.
- you are taking any drug with sedative effects.
- you drink alcohol daily.
- you plan to have surgery under general or spinal anesthesia in the near future.

Possible Side-Effects   (natural, expected and unavoidable drug actions)

    Mild drowsiness (usually during the first 2 weeks), orthostatic hypotension (see Glossary), blurred vision, dry mouth, nasal congestion, constipation, impaired urination.

▷ **Possible Adverse Effects**   (unusual, unexpected and infrequent reactions)
If any of the following develop, consult your physician promptly.
Mild Adverse Effects
  Allergic Reactions: Skin rash, hives, itching.
  Lowering of body temperature, especially in the elderly. (See Hypothermia in Glossary.)
  Fluid retention, weight gain.
  Breast fullness, tenderness, milk production, menstrual irregularity.
  Dizziness, weakness, agitation, insomnia, impaired vision.
  Nausea, vomiting.
Serious Adverse Effects
  Allergic Reactions: Rare hepatitis with jaundice (see Glossary), anaphylactic reaction (see Glossary).
  Idiosyncratic Reactions: Paradoxical worsening of psychotic symptoms. Development of the neuroleptic malignant syndrome: high fever, high (or low) blood pressure, severe muscle rigidity, impaired breathing, rapid heart rate, seizures.
  Depression, disorientation, seizures, deposits in cornea and lens.
  Rapid heart rate, heart rhythm disorders.
  Blood cell disorders: reduced white blood cell count.
  Nervous system reactions: Parkinson-like disorders (see Glossary), severe restlessness, muscle spasms involving the face and neck, tardive dyskinesia (see Glossary).

▷ **Adverse Effects That May Mimic Natural Diseases or Disorders**
  Nervous system reactions may suggest true Parkinson's disease or Reye syndrome (see Glossary).
  Liver reactions may suggest viral hepatitis.

Natural Diseases or Disorders That May Be Activated by This Drug
  Latent epilepsy, glaucoma, prostatism (see Glossary).

CAUTION
  1. Many over-the-counter medications (see OTC Drugs in Glossary) for allergies, colds and coughs contain drugs that can interact unfavorably with this drug. Ask your physician or pharmacist for guidance before using any such medications.
  2. Antacids that contain aluminum and/or magnesium may prevent the absorption of this drug and reduce its effectiveness.
  3. Obtain prompt evaluation of any change or disturbance of vision.

Precautions for Use
  By Infants and Children: Use of this drug is not recommended in children under 12 years of age. Do not use this drug in the presence of symptoms suggestive of Reye syndrome (see Glossary). Children with acute infectious diseases ("flulike" infections, chicken pox, measles, etc.) are more

prone to develop muscular spasms of the face, back and extremities when this drug is given.

By Those over 60 Years of Age: Small doses are advisable until individual response has been determined. You may be more susceptible to the development of drowsiness, lethargy, constipation, lowering of body temperature (hypothermia) and orthostatic hypotension (see Glossary). This drug can enhance existing prostatism (see Glossary). You may also be more susceptible to the development of Parkinson-like reactions and/or tardive dyskinesia (see discussion of these terms in Glossary). These reactions must be recognized early since they may become unresponsive to treatment and irreversible.

▷ **Advisability of Use During Pregnancy**
Pregnancy Category: B (tentative). See Pregnancy Code inside back cover.
Animal studies: No birth defects reported in rats, rabbits or monkeys.
Human studies: Information from adequate studies of pregnant women is not available.
Avoid drug during the first 3 months if possible. Avoid during the last month because of possible effects on the newborn infant.

Advisability of Use if Breast-Feeding
Presence of this drug in breast milk: Unknown.
Avoid drug or refrain from nursing.

Habit-Forming Potential: None.

Effects of Overdosage: Marked drowsiness, weakness, tremor, agitation, unsteadiness, deep sleep, coma, convulsions.

Possible Effects of Long-Term Use: Opacities in the cornea or lens of the eye, pigmentation of the retina. Tardive dyskinesia (see Glossary).

Suggested Periodic Examinations While Taking This Drug   (at physician's discretion)
Complete blood cell counts, especially between the fourth and tenth weeks of treatment.
Liver function tests, electrocardiograms.
Complete eye examinations—eye structures and vision.
Careful inspection of the tongue for early evidence of fine, involuntary, wavelike movements that could indicate the beginning of tardive dyskinesia.

▷ **While Taking This Drug, Observe the Following**
Foods: No restrictions.
Beverages: No restrictions. May be taken with milk.
▷   *Alcohol*: Avoid completely. Alcohol can increase the sedative action of thiothixene and accentuate its depressant effects on brain function and blood pressure. Thiothixene can increase the intoxicating effects of alcohol.
Tobacco Smoking: No interactions expected.

Marijuana Smoking: Moderate increase in drowsiness; accentuation of orthostatic hypotension; increased risk of precipitating latent psychoses, confusing the interpretation of mental status and drug responses.

▷ *Other Drugs*
Thiothixene may *increase* the effects of
- all sedative drugs, especially barbiturates and narcotic analgesics, and
cause excessive sedation.
- all atropinelike drugs, and cause nervous system toxicity.

Thiothixene may *decrease* the effects of
- guanethidine (Ismelin, Esimil), and reduce its effectiveness in lowering
blood pressure.

The following drugs may *decrease* the effects of thiothixene
- antacids containing aluminum and/or magnesium.
- barbiturates (see Drug Class, Section Four).
- benztropine (Cogentin).
- trihexyphenidyl (Artane).

▷ *Driving, Hazardous Activities*: This drug can impair mental alertness, judgment and physical coordination. Avoid hazardous activities.

Aviation Note: The use of this drug *is a disqualification* for piloting. Consult a
designated Aviation Medical Examiner.

Exposure to Sun: Use caution until sensitivity has been determined. This drug
can cause photosensitivity (see Glossary).

Exposure to Heat: Use caution and avoid excessive heat as much as possible.
This drug may impair the regulation of body temperature and increase
the risk of heat stroke.

Exposure to Cold: Use caution and dress warmly. This drug can increase the
risk of hypothermia in the elderly.

Discontinuation: After a period of long-term use, do not discontinue this drug
suddenly. Gradual withdrawal over 2 to 3 weeks under physician supervision is recommended. Do not discontinue this drug without your physician's knowledge and approval. The relapse rate of schizophrenia after
discontinuation is 50% to 60%.

THYROID
(THI royd)

Introduced: 1896

Class: Thyroid Hormones

Prescription: USA: Yes
Canada: Yes

Controlled Drug: USA: No
Canada: No

Available as Generic: Yes

Brand Names: Armour Thyroid, Proloid, S-P-T, Thyrar, Thyroid Strong, Thyroid USP Enseals

---

BENEFITS versus RISKS

Possible Benefits
EFFECTIVE REPLACEMENT
THERAPY IN STATES OF
THYROID HORMONE
DEFICIENCY
(HYPOTHYROIDISM)
EFFECTIVE TREATMENT OF
SIMPLE GOITER AND
CHRONIC THYROIDITIS
EFFECTIVE TREATMENT OF
THYROID GLAND CANCER

Possible Risks
Intensification of angina in presence
of coronary artery disease

▷ **Principal Uses**

As a Single Drug Product: This natural form of thyroid hormones (derived from animal thyroid glands) is used primarily to correct a deficiency of these hormones (hypothyroidism). In the absence of true thyroid deficiency, the use of this drug to treat nonspecific fatigue, obesity, infertility or slow growth is inappropriate and possibly harmful.

How This Drug Works: Not completely established. By altering the processes of cellular chemistry that store energy in an inactive (reserve) form, this drug makes more energy available for biochemical activity and increases the rate of cellular metabolism of all tissues throughout the body.

Available Dosage Forms and Strengths

Capsules — 65 mg, 130 mg, 195 mg, 325 mg
Tablets — 16 mg, 32 mg, 65 mg, 98 mg, 100 mg, 130 mg, 195 mg, 200 mg, 260 mg, 325 mg
Tablets, enteric coated — 32 mg, 65 mg, 130 mg
Tablets, sugar coated — 32 mg, 65 mg, 130 mg, 195 mg

▷ **Usual Adult Dosage Range:** Initially, 60 mg/day; increase dose by 60 mg at intervals of 1 month as needed and tolerated. The usual maintenance dose is 60 to 180 mg/day. **Note: Actual dosage and administration schedule must be determined by the physician for each patient individually.**

▷ **Dosing Instructions:** Preferably taken in the morning on an empty stomach to ensure maximal absorption and uniform results. The capsules may be opened and the uncoated tablets may be crushed for administration.

Usual Duration of Use: Continual use on a regular schedule for 4 to 6 weeks is usually necessary to determine this drug's effectiveness in correcting the symptoms of thyroid deficiency. Long-term use (months to years, possibly for life) requires supervision and periodic evaluation by your physician.

▷ **This Drug Should Not Be Taken If**
  • you have had an allergic reaction to it previously.

- you are recovering from a recent heart attack; ask your physician for guidance.
- you are using it to lose weight and your thyroid function is normal (no deficiency).

▷ **Inform Your Physician Before Taking This Drug If**
- you have high blood pressure, any form of heart disease or diabetes.
- you have a history of Addison's disease or adrenal gland deficiency.
- you are taking any antiasthmatic medications.
- you are taking an anticoagulant.

Possible Side-Effects   (natural, expected and unavoidable drug actions)
None if dosage is adjusted correctly.

▷ **Possible Adverse Effects**   (unusual, unexpected and infrequent reactions)
If any of the following develop, consult your physician promptly.
Mild Adverse Effects
Allergic Reactions: Skin rash, hives.
Headache in sensitive individuals, even with proper dosage adjustment.
Changes in menstrual pattern during dosage adjustments.
Serious Adverse Effects
Increased frequency or intensity of angina in the presence of coronary artery disease.

Natural Diseases or Disorders That May Be Activated by This Drug
Latent coronary artery disease.

CAUTION
1. The need for and response to thyroid hormone treatment varies greatly from person to person. Careful supervision of individual response is necessary to determine correct dosage. Do not change your dosage schedule without consulting your physician.
2. Thyroid hormonal content of drug products may vary significantly among commercial brands. To ensure consistent results from your medication, it is advisable to continue using the same brand throughout your treatment program.

Precautions for Use
By Infants and Children: This drug is not appropriate for treating hypothyroidism in infants and young children. The drug of choice for this purpose is thyroxine. (See the Drug Profile of Thyroxine that follows.)
By Those over 60 Years of Age: This drug must be used cautiously by this age group. Usually the requirements for thyroid hormone replacement are about 25% lower than in younger adults. Observe closely for any indications that suggest possible overdosage.

▷ **Advisability of Use During Pregnancy**
Pregnancy Category: A (tentative). See Pregnancy Code inside back cover.
Animal studies: No information available.
Human studies: Thyroid hormones do not reach the fetus (cross the pla-

centa) in significant amounts. Clinical experience has shown that appropriate use of thyroid hormones causes no adverse effects on the fetus. Use this drug only if clearly needed and with carefully adjusted dosage.

Advisability of Use if Breast-Feeding
Presence of this drug in breast milk: Yes.
Breast-feeding is considered safe with correctly adjusted dosage.

Habit-Forming Potential: None.

Effects of Overdosage: Headache, sense of increased body heat, nervousness, increased sweating, hand tremors, insomnia, rapid and irregular heart action, diarrhea, muscle cramping, weight loss.

Possible Effects of Long-Term Use: None with correct dosage.

Suggested Periodic Examinations While Taking This Drug   (at physician's discretion)
Measurement of thyroid hormone levels in blood.

▷ **While Taking This Drug, Observe the Following**
Foods: No restrictions.
Beverages: No restrictions.
▷   *Alcohol*: No interactions expected.
Tobacco Smoking: No interactions expected.
▷   *Other Drugs*
Thyroid may *increase* the effects of
- warfarin (Coumadin), and increase the risk of bleeding; reduction in the dosage of anticoagulant is usually necessary.

Thyroid may *decrease* the effects of
- digoxin (Lanoxin), when correcting hypothyroidism; a larger dose of digoxin may be needed.

Thyroid *taken concurrently* with
- all antidiabetic drugs (insulin and sulfonylureas) may require an increase in the dosage of the antidiabetic agent to obtain proper control of blood sugar levels. After correct doses of both drugs have been determined, a reduction in the dose of thyroid may require a simultaneous reduction in the dose of the antidiabetic drug to prevent hypoglycemia.
- tricyclic antidepressants (see Drug Class, Section Four) may cause an increase in the activity of both drugs; monitor for indications of overdosage of each drug.

The following drugs may *decrease* the effects of thyroid
- cholestyramine (Cuemid, Questran) may reduce its absorption; intake of the two drugs should be separated by 5 hours.
▷   *Driving, Hazardous Activities*: No restrictions.
Aviation Note: The use of this drug is probably not a disqualification for piloting. Consult a designated Aviation Medical Examiner.
Exposure to Sun: No restrictions.
Exposure to Heat: This drug may decrease individual tolerance to warm environments, increasing discomfort due to heat. Consult your physician if

you develop symptoms of overdosage during the warm months of the year.

Heavy Exercise or Exertion: Use caution if you have angina (coronary artery disease). This drug may increase the frequency or severity of angina during physical activity.

Discontinuation: This drug must be taken continually on a regular schedule to correct thyroid deficiency. Do not discontinue it without consulting your physician.

THYROXINE
(thi ROX een)

Other Names: Levothyroxine, L-thyroxine, T-4

Introduced: 1953

Class: Thyroid Hormones

Prescription: USA: Yes
Canada: Yes

Controlled Drug: USA: No
Canada: No

Available as Generic: USA: Yes
Canada: No

Brand Names: ✦Eltroxin, Euthroid [CD], Levothroid, Synthroid, Thyrolar [CD]

BENEFITS versus RISKS	
Possible Benefits	*Possible Risks*
EFFECTIVE REPLACEMENT THERAPY IN STATES OF THYROID HORMONE DEFICIENCY (HYPOTHYROIDISM) EFFECTIVE TREATMENT OF SIMPLE GOITER AND CHRONIC THYROIDITIS EFFECTIVE TREATMENT OF THYROID GLAND CANCER	Intensification of angina in presence of coronary artery disease Drug-induced hyperthyroidism (with excessive dosage)

▷ **Principal Uses**

As a Single Drug Product: This synthetic thyroid hormone is used primarily to correct thyroid deficiency (hypothyroidism). In addition, it is used to suppress thyroid function in the treatment of simple goiter and the management of Hashimoto's thyroiditis. It is also of value as adjunctive therapy in the management of thyroid gland cancer.

As a Combination Drug Product [CD]: This thyroid hormone is available in combination with the other principal thyroid hormone, liothyronine, in a preparation that resembles the natural hormone material produced by the thyroid gland.

How This Drug Works: Not completely established. By altering the processes of cellular chemistry that store energy in an inactive (reserve) form, this drug makes more energy available for biochemical activity and increases the rate of cellular metabolism of all tissues throughout the body.

Available Dosage Forms and Strengths
Injections — 100 mcg per ml, 200 mcg per vial
Tablets — 0.025 mg, 0.05 mg, 0.075 mg, 0.1 mg, 0.125 mg, 0.15 mg, 0.175 mg, 0.2 mg, 0.3 mg

▷ **Usual Adult Dosage Range:**   Initially, 0.05 to 0.10 mg/day. The dose may be increased at intervals of 2 to 3 weeks as needed and tolerated. The usual maintenance dose is 0.025 to 0.3 mg/day. The total daily dosage should not exceed 0.4 mg. **Note: Actual dosage and administration schedule must be determined by the physician for each patient individually.**

▷ **Dosing Instructions:**   Preferably taken in the morning on an empty stomach to ensure maximal absorption and uniform results. The tablets may be crushed for administration.

Usual Duration of Use: Continual use on a regular schedule for 4 to 6 weeks is usually necessary to determine this drug's effectiveness in correcting the symptoms of thyroid deficiency. Long-term use (months to years, possibly for life) requires supervision and periodic evaluation by your physician.

▷ **This Drug Should Not Be Taken If**
- you have had an allergic reaction to it previously.
- you are recovering from a recent heart attack; ask your physician for guidance.
- you are using it to lose weight and your thyroid function is normal (no deficiency).

▷ **Inform Your Physician Before Taking This Drug If**
- you have high blood pressure, any form of heart disease or diabetes.
- you have a history of Addison's disease or adrenal gland deficiency.
- you are taking any antiasthmatic medications.
- you are taking an anticoagulant.

Possible Side-Effects   (natural, expected and unavoidable drug actions)
None if dosage is adjusted correctly.

▷ **Possible Adverse Effects**   (unusual, unexpected and infrequent reactions)
If any of the following develop, consult your physician promptly.
Mild Adverse Effects
Allergic Reactions: Skin rash, hives.
Headache in sensitive individuals, even with proper dosage adjustment.
Changes in menstrual pattern during dosage adjustments.
Serious Adverse Effects
Increased frequency or intensity of angina in the presence of coronary artery disease.

Note: Other adverse effects are manifestations of excessive dosage. See Effects of Overdosage category.

Natural Diseases or Disorders That May Be Activated by This Drug
Latent coronary artery insufficiency (angina), diabetes.

CAUTION
1. The need for and response to thyroid hormone treatment varies greatly from person to person. Careful supervision of individual response is necessary to determine correct dosage. Do not change your dosage schedule without consulting your physician.
2. In the absence of verified thyroid deficiency, this drug should not be used to treat nonspecific fatigue, obesity, infertility or slow growth. Such use is inappropriate and could be harmful.

Precautions for Use
By Infants and Children: To facilitate normal growth and development, the thyroid-deficient child often requires higher dosage than the adult. A transient loss of hair may occur during the early months of treatment.
By Those over 60 Years of Age: This drug must be used cautiously by this age group. Usually the requirements for thyroid hormone replacement are about 25% lower than in younger adults. Observe closely for any indications that suggest possible overdosage.

▷ **Advisability of Use During Pregnancy**
Pregnancy Category: A (tentative). See Pregnancy Code inside back cover.
Animal studies: Cataract formation reported in rat studies. Other defects reported in rabbit and guinea pig studies.
Human studies: Thyroid hormones do not reach the fetus (cross the placenta) in significant amounts. Clinical experience has shown that appropriate use of thyroid hormones causes no adverse effects on the fetus.
Use this drug only if clearly needed and with carefully adjusted dosage.

Advisability of Use if Breast-Feeding
Presence of this drug in breast milk: Yes, in minimal amounts.
Breast-feeding is considered safe with correctly adjusted dosage.

Habit-Forming Potential: None.

Effects of Overdosage: Headache, sense of increased body heat, nervousness, increased sweating, hand tremors, insomnia, rapid and irregular heart action, diarrhea, muscle cramping, weight loss.

Possible Effects of Long-Term Use: None with correct dosage.

Suggested Periodic Examinations While Taking This Drug   (at physician's discretion)
Measurement of thyroid hormone levels in blood.

▷ **While Taking This Drug, Observe the Following**
Foods: No restrictions.
Beverages: No restrictions.
▷   *Alcohol*: No interactions expected.
Tobacco Smoking: No interactions expected.

▷   *Other Drugs*

Thyroxine may *increase* the effects of
- warfarin (Coumadin), and increase the risk of bleeding; reduction in the dosage of anticoagulant is usually necessary.

Thyroxine may *decrease* the effects of
- digoxin (Lanoxin), when correcting hypothyroidism; a larger dose of digoxin may be needed.

Thyroxine *taken concurrently* with
- all antidiabetic drugs (insulin and sulfonylureas) may require an increase in the dosage of the antidiabetic agent to obtain proper control of blood sugar levels. After correct doses of both drugs have been determined, a reduction in the dose of thyroid may require a simultaneous reduction in the dose of the antidiabetic drug to prevent hypoglycemia.
- tricyclic antidepressants (see Drug Class, Section Four) may cause an increase in the activity of both drugs; monitor for indications of overdosage of each drug.

The following drugs may *decrease* the effects of thyroxine
- cholestyramine (Cuemid, Questran) may reduce its absorption; intake of the two drugs should be separated by 5 hours.

▷   *Driving, Hazardous Activities*: No restrictions.

Aviation Note: The use of this drug is probably not a disqualification for piloting. Consult a designated Aviation Medical Examiner.

Exposure to Sun: No restrictions.

Exposure to Heat: This drug may decrease individual tolerance to warm environments, increasing discomfort due to heat. Consult your physician if you develop symptoms of overdosage during the warm months of the year.

Heavy Exercise or Exertion: Use caution if you have angina (coronary artery disease). This drug may increase the frequency or severity of angina during physical activity.

Discontinuation: This drug must be taken continually on a regular schedule to correct thyroid deficiency. Do not discontinue it without consulting your physician.

TIMOLOL
(TI moh lohl)

Introduced: 1972

Class: Antianginal, Antiglaucoma, Antihypertensive, Migraine Preventive, Beta-Adrenergic Blocker

Prescription: USA: Yes
Canada: Yes

Controlled Drug: USA: No
Canada: No

Available as Generic: USA: No
Canada: Yes

Brand Names: Blocadren, Timolide [CD], Timoptic

BENEFITS versus RISKS

Possible Benefits	*Possible Risks*
EFFECTIVE, WELL-TOLERATED AS: ANTIANGINAL DRUG in effort-induced angina; ANTIGLAUCOMA DRUG in open-angle glaucoma; ANTIHYPERTENSIVE DRUG in mild to moderate hypertension EFFECTIVE PREVENTION OF MIGRAINE HEADACHES Effective adjunct in the prevention of recurrent heart attack (myocardial infarction)	CONGESTIVE HEART FAILURE in advanced heart disease Worsening of angina in coronary heart disease (if drug is abruptly withdrawn) Masking of low blood sugar (hypoglycemia) in drug-treated diabetes Provocation of asthma

---

▷ **Principal Uses**

As a Single Drug Product: This member of the "beta-blocker" drug class is used primarily to treat (1) classical effort-induced angina, certain types of heart rhythm disturbance and high blood pressure; (2) increased internal eye pressure and chronic open-angle glaucoma. It is also beneficial in preventing the recurrence of heart attacks (myocardial infarction). In addition, it is used to reduce the frequency and severity of migraine headaches.

As a Combination Drug Product [CD]: This drug is available in combination with hydrochlorothiazide for the treatment of hypertension. This combination product includes two "step 1" drugs with different mechanisms of action; it is intended to provide greater effectiveness and convenience for long-term use.

How This Drug Works: By blocking certain actions of the sympathetic nervous system, this drug

- reduces the rate and contraction force of the heart, thus lowering the ejection pressure of the blood leaving the heart and reducing the oxygen requirement for heart function.
- reduces the degree of contraction of blood vessel walls, resulting in their relaxation and expansion and consequent lowering of blood pressure.
- prolongs the conduction time of nerve impulses through the heart, of benefit in the management of certain heart rhythm disorders.
- slows the formation of fluid (aqueous humor) in the anterior chamber of the eye and improves its drainage from the eye, thus lowering the internal eye pressure.

Available Dosage Forms and Strengths

Eye solutions — 0.25%, 0.5%

    Tablets — 5 mg, 10 mg, 20 mg

▷ **Usual Adult Dosage Range:**   Varies with indication.

Antianginal and antihypertensive: Initially, 10 mg 2 times/day; increase dose gradually every 7 days as needed and tolerated. Usual maintenance dose is 10 to 20 mg twice/day. The total daily dosage should not exceed 60 mg.

Migraine headache prevention: Initially, 10 mg 2 times/day; increase dose as needed to 10 mg in the morning and 20 mg at night.

Recurrent heart attack prevention: 10 mg twice/day.

Antiglaucoma: 1 drop in affected eye every 12 to 24 hours.

Note: Actual dosage and administration schedule must be determined by the physician for each patient individually.

▷ **Dosing Instructions:**   Preferably taken 1 hour before eating to maximize absorption. The tablet may be crushed for administration. Do not discontinue this drug abruptly.

Usual Duration of Use: Continual use on a regular schedule for 10 to 14 days is usually necessary to determine this drug's effectiveness in preventing angina, controlling heart rhythm disorders and lowering blood pressure. Maximal effectiveness may require continual use for 6 to 8 weeks. The long-term use of this drug (months to years) will be determined by the course of your symptoms over time and your response to the overall treatment program (weight reduction, salt restriction, smoking cessation, etc.).

▷ **This Drug Should Not Be Taken If**
- you have had an allergic reaction to it previously.
- you have Prinzmetal's variant angina (coronary artery spasm).
- you have congestive heart failure.
- you have an abnormally slow heart rate or a serious form of heart block.
- you are taking, or have taken within the past 14 days, any monoamine oxidase (MAO) inhibitor drug (see Drug Class, Section Four).

▷ **Inform Your Physician Before Taking This Drug If**
- you have had an adverse reaction to any "beta-blocker" drug in the past (see Drug Class, Section Four).
- you have a history of serious heart disease, with or without episodes of heart failure.
- you have a history of hay fever (allergic rhinitis), asthma, chronic bronchitis or emphysema.
- you have a history of overactive thyroid function (hyperthyroidism).
- you have a history of low blood sugar (hypoglycemia).
- you have impaired liver or kidney function.
- you have diabetes or myasthenia gravis.
- you are currently taking any form of digitalis, quinidine or reserpine, or any "calcium-blocker" drug (see Drug Class, Section Four).
- you plan to have surgery under general anesthesia in the near future.

Possible Side-Effects   (natural, expected and unavoidable drug actions)
Lethargy and fatigability, cold extremities, slow heart rate, light-headedness in upright position (see Orthostatic Hypotension in Glossary).

▷ **Possible Adverse Effects**   (unusual, unexpected and infrequent reactions)
If any of the following develop, consult your physician promptly.

Mild Adverse Effects
　Allergic Reactions: Skin rash, itching.
　Headache, dizziness, visual disturbances, vivid dreams.
　Indigestion, nausea, vomiting, diarrhea.
　Numbness and tingling in extremities.
Serious Adverse Effects
　Allergic Reactions: Laryngospasm, severe dermatitis.
　Idiosyncratic Reactions: Acute behavioral disturbances: depression, hallu-
　　cinations.
　Chest pain, shortness of breath, precipitation of congestive heart failure.
　Induction of bronchial asthma (in asthmatic individuals).
　Reduced libido, sexual impotence.
　Masking of warning signs of impending low blood sugar (hypoglycemia) in
　　drug-treated diabetes.

▷ **Adverse Effects That May Mimic Natural Diseases or Disorders**
　Reduced blood flow to extremities may resemble Raynaud's phenomenon
　(see Glossary).

Natural Diseases or Disorders That May Be Activated by This Drug
　Prinzmetal's variant angina, Raynaud's disease, intermittent claudication,
　myasthenia gravis (questionable).

CAUTION
　1. ***Do not discontinue this drug suddenly*** without the knowledge and
　　 guidance of your physician. Carry a notation on your person that you
　　 are taking this drug.
　2. Consult your physician or pharmacist before using nasal decongestants
　　 usually present in over-the-counter cold preparations and nose drops.
　　 These can cause sudden increases in blood pressure when taken con-
　　 currently with beta-blocker drugs.
　3. Report the development of any tendency to emotional depression (rare
　　 with this drug).

Precautions for Use
　By Infants and Children: Safety and effectiveness for use by those under 12
　　 years of age have not been established. However, if this drug is used,
　　 observe for the development of low blood sugar (hypoglycemia) during
　　 periods of reduced food intake.
　By Those over 60 Years of Age: Proceed *cautiously* with all antihypertensive
　　 drugs. Unacceptably high blood pressure should be reduced without creat-
　　 ing the risks associated with excessively low blood pressure. Start treatment
　　 with small doses, and monitor the blood pressure response frequently. Sud-
　　 den, rapid and excessive reduction of blood pressure can predispose to
　　 stroke or heart attack. Observe for dizziness, unsteadiness, tendency to fall,
　　 confusion, hallucinations, depression or urinary frequency.

▷ **Advisability of Use During Pregnancy**
　Pregnancy Category: C (tentative). See Pregnancy Code inside back cover.
　Animal studies: No significant increase in birth defects due to this drug.

Human studies: Information from adequate studies of pregnant women is not available.

Avoid use of drug during the first 3 months if possible. Use this drug only if clearly needed. Ask your physician for guidance.

Advisability of Use if Breast-Feeding
Presence of this drug in breast milk: Probably yes.

Monitor nursing infant closely and discontinue drug or nursing if adverse effects develop.

Habit-Forming Potential: None.

Effects of Overdosage: Weakness, slow pulse, low blood pressure, fainting, cold and sweaty skin, congestive heart failure, possible coma and convulsions.

Possible Effects of Long-Term Use: Reduced heart reserve and eventual heart failure in susceptible individuals with advanced heart disease.

Suggested Periodic Examinations While Taking This Drug   (at physician's discretion)

Complete blood cell counts (because of adverse effects of other drugs of this class).

Measurements of blood pressure, evaluation of heart function.

▷ **While Taking This Drug, Observe the Following**

Foods: No restrictions. Avoid excessive salt intake.

Beverages: No restrictions. May be taken with milk.

▷   *Alcohol*: Use with caution until the combined effect has been determined. Alcohol may exaggerate this drug's ability to lower the blood pressure and may increase its mild sedative effect.

Tobacco Smoking: Nicotine may reduce this drug's effectiveness in treating angina, heart rhythm disorders and high blood pressure. In addition, high doses of this drug may potentiate the constriction of the bronchial tubes caused by regular smoking.

▷   *Other Drugs*

Timolol may *increase* the effects of

- other antihypertensive drugs, and cause excessive lowering of blood pressure. Dosage adjustments may be necessary.
- lidocaine (Xylocaine, etc.).
- reserpine (Ser-Ap-Es, etc.), and cause sedation, depression, slowing of the heart rate and lowering of the blood pressure.
- verapamil (Calan, Isoptin), and cause excessive depression of heart function; monitor this combination closely.

Timolol may *decrease* the effects of

- theophyllines (Aminophyllin, Theo-Dur, etc.), and reduce their anti-asthmatic effectiveness.

Timolol *taken concurrently* with

- clonidine (Catapres) requires close monitoring for rebound high blood pressure if clonidine is withdrawn while timolol is still being taken.

- epinephrine (Adrenalin, etc.) may cause marked rise in blood pressure and slowing of the heart rate.
- insulin requires close monitoring to avoid undetected hypoglycemia (see Glossary).

The following drugs may *increase* the effects of timolol

- chlorpromazine (Thorazine, etc.).
- cimetidine (Tagamet).
- methimazole (Tapazole).
- propylthiouracil (Propacil).

The following drugs may *decrease* the effects of timolol

- barbiturates (phenobarbital, etc.).
- indomethacin (Indocin), and possibly other "aspirin substitutes," may impair timolol's antihypertensive effect.
- rifampin (Rifadin, Rimactane).

▷ *Driving, Hazardous Activities*: Use caution until the full extent of dizziness, lethargy and blood pressure change have been determined.

Aviation Note: The use of this drug *may be a disqualification* for piloting. Consult a designated Aviation Medical Examiner.

Exposure to Sun: No restrictions.

Exposure to Heat: Caution advised. Hot environments can lower blood pressure and exaggerate the effects of this drug.

Exposure to Cold: Caution advised. Cold environments can enhance the circulatory deficiency in the extremities that may occur with this drug. The elderly should take precautions to prevent hypothermia (see Glossary).

Heavy Exercise or Exertion: It is advisable to avoid exertion that produces light-headedness, excessive fatigue or muscle cramping. The use of this drug may intensify the hypertensive response to isometric exercise.

Occurrence of Unrelated Illness: The fever that accompanies systemic infections can lower blood pressure and require adjustment of dosage. Illnesses that cause nausea or vomiting may interrupt the regular dosage schedule. Ask your physician for guidance.

Discontinuation: It is advisable to avoid sudden discontinuation of this drug in all situations; this is especially true in the presence of coronary artery disease. If possible, gradual reduction of dose over a period of 2 to 3 weeks is recommended. Ask your physician for specific guidance.

TOCAINIDE
(toh KAY nide)

Introduced: 1976

Class: Antiarrhythmic

Prescription: USA: Yes
Canada: Yes

Controlled Drug: USA: No
Canada: No

Available as Generic: USA: No
Canada: No

Brand Names: Tonocard

```
┌─────────────────────────────────────────────────────────────────┐
│                      BENEFITS versus RISKS                        │
│                                                                   │
│      Possible Benefits               Possible Risks               │
│   EFFECTIVE TREATMENT OF        DRUG-INDUCED HEART                 │
│     SELECTED HEART RHYTHM          RHYTHM DISORDERS (10.9%)        │
│     DISORDERS (Ventricular)     CONGESTIVE HEART FAILURE           │
│                                    (4%)                            │
│                                 Rare blood cell disorders:        │
│                                    aplastic anemia, abnormally low │
│                                    white blood cell and platelet  │
│                                    counts                         │
│                                 Drug-induced lung damage          │
└─────────────────────────────────────────────────────────────────┘
```

▷ **Principal Uses**

As a Single Drug Product: This drug is classified as a Type 1 antiarrhythmic agent, similar to procainamide and quinidine in its actions. It is used primarily to correct and prevent the recurrence of (1) abnormally rapid heart rates (tachycardia) that arise in the ventricles (lower heart chambers); and (2) premature beats arising in the ventricles.

How This Drug Works: By slowing the transmission of electrical impulses throughout the conduction system of the heart, this drug assists in restoring normal heart rate and rhythm.

Available Dosage Forms and Strengths

Tablets — 400 mg, 600 mg

▷ **Usual Adult Dosage Range:** Do not take a loading dose. Initiate treatment with 400 mg/8 hours. If needed and tolerated, the dose may be increased gradually to 600 mg/8 hours. The total daily dosage should not exceed 2400 mg. **Note: Actual dosage and administration schedule must be determined by the physician for each patient individually.**

▷ **Dosing Instructions:** May be taken without regard to meals, but may be taken with or following food if desired to reduce stomach irritation. Take at same time each day to obtain uniform results. The tablet may be crushed for administration.

Usual Duration of Use: Continual use on a regular schedule for 1 to 2 weeks is usually necessary to determine this drug's effectiveness in correcting or preventing responsive rhythm disorders. Long-term use requires supervision and periodic evaluation by your physician.

▷ **This Drug Should Not Be Taken If**
- you have had an allergic reaction to it previously.
- you are allergic to local anesthetics of the Novocain type.
- you have second-degree or third-degree heart block (with no pacemaker).

▷ **Inform Your Physician Before Taking This Drug If**
- you have had any unfavorable reactions to other antiarrhythmic drugs in the past.

- you have a history of heart disease of any kind, especially "heart block."
- you have impaired liver or kidney function.
- you are taking any form of digitalis, a potassium supplement or any diuretic drug that can cause excessive loss of body potassium (ask physician).

Possible Side-Effects   (natural, expected and unavoidable drug actions)
Flushing, increased sweating, light-headedness.
The onset of tremors indicates that the dose is reaching the maximum that can be tolerated.

▷ **Possible Adverse Effects**   (unusual, unexpected and infrequent reactions)
If any of the following develop, consult your physician promptly.
Mild Adverse Effects
Allergic Reactions: Skin rash (8%), hives, itching.
Headache (4%), dizziness (15%), visual disturbance (1.5%), fatigue (0.8%), tremor (8%), numbness (9%).
Loss of appetite, indigestion, nausea (14%), vomiting (4%), diarrhea (4%).
Serious Adverse Effects
Idiosyncratic Reactions: Confusion, disorientation, hallucinations (2.7%).
Drug-induced heart rhythm disorders (10%), congestive heart failure (4%), shortness of breath, palpitations, chest pain.
Drug-induced lung damage: pneumonitis and fibrosis, causing cough and breathing difficulty. (Usually occurs after 3 to 18 weeks of drug use.)
Bone marrow depression (see Glossary): fatigue, weakness, fever, sore throat, abnormal bleeding or bruising. (Usually occurs after 2 to 12 weeks of drug use.)

▷ **Adverse Effects That May Mimic Natural Diseases or Disorders**
Lung reactions may suggest an infectious bronchitis or pneumonia.

CAUTION
1. Thorough evaluation of your heart function (including electrocardiograms) is necessary prior to using this drug.
2. Periodic evaluation of your heart function is necessary to determine your response to this drug. Some individuals may experience worsening of their heart rhythm disorder and/or deterioration of heart function. Close monitoring of heart rate, rhythm and overall performance is essential.
3. Dosage must be adjusted carefully for each individual. Do not change your dosage without the knowledge and supervision of your physician.
4. Do not take any other antiarrhythmic drug while taking this drug unless directed to do so by your physician.

Precautions for Use
By Infants and Children: Safety and effectiveness for use by those under 12 years of age have not been established. Initial use of this drug requires hospitalization and supervision by a qualified cardiologist.
By Those over 60 Years of Age: Reduced kidney function may require reduc-

tion in dosage. Observe carefully for light-headedness, dizziness, unsteadiness and tendency to fall.

▷ **Advisability of Use During Pregnancy**
  Pregnancy Category: C (tentative). See Pregnancy Code inside back cover.
  Animal studies: No birth defects reported in rat or rabbit studies; however, an increase in fetal resorptions, stillbirths and abortions was reported.
  Human studies: Information from adequate studies of pregnant women is not available.
  Avoid this drug during first 3 months. Use this drug only if clearly needed. Ask your physician for guidance.

Advisability of Use if Breast-Feeding
  Presence of this drug in breast milk: Unknown.
  Avoid drug or refrain from nursing.

Habit-Forming Potential: None.

Effects of Overdosage: Impaired urination, constipation, marked drop in blood pressure, abnormal heart rhythms, slow heart rate, congestive heart failure, seizures.

Possible Effects of Long-Term Use: None reported.

Suggested Periodic Examinations While Taking This Drug   (at physician's discretion)
  Electrocardiograms, complete blood cell counts, measurements of potassium blood levels.

▷ **While Taking This Drug, Observe the Following**
  Foods: No restrictions. Ask physician regarding need for salt restriction and advisability of eating potassium-rich foods.
  Beverages: No restrictions. May be taken with milk.
▷ *Alcohol*: Use caution until the combined effects have been determined. Alcohol can increase the blood-pressure-lowering effects of this drug.
  Tobacco Smoking: Nicotine can cause irritability of the heart and reduce the effectiveness of this drug. Follow physician's advice regarding smoking.
▷ *Other Drugs*
  Tocainide may *increase* the effects of
  • antihypertensive drugs, and cause excessive lowering of blood pressure.
  • beta-blocker drugs (see Drug Class, Section Four).
  The following drugs may *decrease* the effects of tocainide
  • diuretics that promote potassium loss.
▷ *Driving, Hazardous Activities*: This drug may cause dizziness or blurred vision. Restrict activities as necessary.
  Aviation Note: The use of this drug *may be a disqualification* for piloting. Consult a designated Aviation Medical Examiner.
  Exposure to Sun: No restrictions.
  Occurrence of Unrelated Illness: Disorders that cause vomiting, diarrhea or

dehydration can affect this drug's action adversely. Report such developments promptly.

Discontinuation: This drug should not be discontinued abruptly following long-term use. Ask your physician for guidance regarding gradual dose reduction.

TOLAZAMIDE
(tohl AZ a mide)

Introduced: 1966

Prescription: USA: Yes

Available as Generic: Yes

Brand Names: Tolinase

Class: Antidiabetic, Sulfonylureas

Controlled Drug: USA: No

BENEFITS versus RISKS

Possible Benefits	*Possible Risks*
Assistance in regulating blood sugar in noninsulin-dependent diabetes (adjunctive to appropriate diet and weight control)	HYPOGLYCEMIA, severe and prolonged
	Drug-induced liver damage
	Rare bone marrow depression (see Glossary)
	Hemolytic anemia (see Glossary)

▷ **Principal Uses**

As a Single Drug Product: To assist in the control of mild to moderately severe type II diabetes mellitus (adult, maturity-onset) that does not require insulin, but that cannot be adequately controlled by diet alone.

How This Drug Works: It is thought that this drug (1) stimulates the release of insulin (by a pancreas that is capable of responding to stimulation), and (2) enhances the utilization of insulin by appropriate tissues.

Available Dosage Forms and Strengths

Tablets — 100 mg, 250 mg, 500 mg

▷ **Usual Adult Dosage Range:** Initially, 100 to 250 mg daily with breakfast. At 7 day intervals, the dose may be increased by increments of 100 to 250 mg daily as needed and tolerated. The total daily dosage should not exceed 1000 mg (1 gram). A "loading" or priming dose is not necessary and should not be given. **Note: Actual dosage and administration schedule must be determined by the physician for each patient individually.**

Dosing Instructions: If the daily maintenance dose is found to be more than 500 mg, the total dose should be divided into 2 equal doses: the first taken with the morning meal, the second with the evening meal. The tablet may be crushed for administration.

Usual Duration of Use: Continual use on a regular schedule for several weeks is usually necessary to determine this drug's effectiveness in controlling diabetes. Failure to respond to maximal doses within 1 month constitutes a primary failure. Up to 10% of those who respond initially may develop secondary failure of the drug later. The duration of effective use can only be determined by periodic measurement of the blood sugar.

▷ **This Drug Should Not Be Taken If**
- you have had an allergic reaction to it previously.
- you have severe impairment of liver or kidney function.
- you are pregnant.

▷ **Inform Your Physician Before Taking This Drug If**
- you are allergic to other sulfonylurea drugs or to "sulfa" drugs. (See Drug Classes, Section Four).
- your diabetes has been unstable or "brittle" in the past.
- you do not know how to recognize or treat hypoglycemia (see Glossary).
- you have a history of congestive heart failure, peptic ulcer disease, cirrhosis of the liver, hypothyroidism or porphyria.

Possible Side-Effects (natural, expected and unavoidable drug actions)
If drug dosage is excessive or food intake is delayed or inadequate, abnormally low blood sugar (hypoglycemia) will occur as a predictable drug effect.

▷ **Possible Adverse Effects** (unusual, unexpected and infrequent reactions)
If any of the following develop, consult your physician promptly.
Mild Adverse Effects
Allergic Reactions: Skin rash, hives, itching, drug fever.
Headache, ringing in the ears.
Indigestion, heartburn, nausea, vomiting, diarrhea.
Serious Adverse Effects
Allergic Reactions: Hepatitis with jaundice (see Glossary).
Idiosyncratic Reactions: Hemolytic anemia (see Glossary); disulfiramlike reaction with concurrent use of alcohol (see Glossary), infrequent with this drug.
Bone marrow depression (see Glossary): fatigue, weakness, fever, sore throat, abnormal bleeding or bruising.

▷ **Adverse Effects That May Mimic Natural Diseases or Disorders**
Liver reactions may suggest viral hepatitis.

CAUTION
1. This drug must be regarded as only one part of the total program for the management of your diabetes. It is not a substitute for a properly prescribed diet and regular exercise.
2. Over a period of time (usually several months), this drug may lose its effectiveness in controlling blood sugar levels. Periodic follow-up examinations are necessary to monitor all aspects of response to drug treatment.

Precautions for Use

By Infants and Children: This drug is not effective in type I (juvenile, growth-onset) insulin-dependent diabetes.

By Those over 60 Years of Age: This drug should be used with caution in this age group. Start treatment with 100 mg/day; increase dosage cautiously and monitor closely to prevent hypoglycemic reactions. Repeated episodes of hypoglycemia in the elderly can cause brain damage.

▷ **Advisability of Use During Pregnancy**

Pregnancy Category: C (tentative). See Pregnancy Code inside back cover.

Animal studies: No birth defects due to this drug reported in rats.

Human studies: Information from adequate studies of pregnant women is not available.

Because uncontrolled blood sugar levels during pregnancy are associated with a higher incidence of birth defects, many experts recommend that insulin (instead of an oral agent) be used as necessary to control diabetes during the entire pregnancy.

Use during pregnancy is not recommended by the manufacturer.

Advisability of Use if Breast-Feeding

Presence of this drug in breast milk: Probably yes.

Avoid drug or refrain from nursing.

Habit-Forming Potential: None.

Effects of Overdosage: Symptoms of mild to severe hypoglycemia: headache, light-headedness, faintness, nervousness, confusion, tremor, sweating, heart palpitation, weakness, hunger, nausea, vomiting, stupor progressing to coma.

Possible Effects of Long-Term Use: Reduced function of the thyroid gland (hypothyroidism). Reports of increased frequency and severity of heart and blood vessel diseases associated with long-term use of this class of drugs are highly controversial and inconclusive. A direct cause-and-effect relationship (see Glossary) is tenuous. Ask your physician for guidance.

Suggested Periodic Examinations While Taking This Drug   (at physician's discretion)

Complete blood cell counts, liver function tests, thyroid function tests, periodic evaluation of heart and circulatory system.

▷ **While Taking This Drug, Observe the Following**

Foods: Follow the diabetic diet prescribed by your physician.

Beverages: As directed in the diabetic diet. May be taken with milk.

▷ *Alcohol*: Use with extreme caution until the combined effect has been determined. Alcohol can exaggerate this drug's hypoglycemic effect. This drug infrequently causes a marked intolerance of alcohol resulting in a disulfiramlike reaction (see Glossary): facial flushing, sweating, palpitation.

Tobacco Smoking: No interactions expected.

▷   *Other Drugs*
The following drugs may *increase* the effects of tolazamide
- aspirin, and other salicylates.
- cimetidine (Tagamet).
- clofibrate (Atromid S).
- fenfluramine (Pondimin).
- monoamine oxidase (MAO) inhibitor drugs (see Drug Class, Section Four).
- phenylbutazone (Butazolidin).
- ranitidine (Zantac).

The following drugs may *decrease* the effects of tolazamide
- beta-blocker drugs (see Drug Class, Section Four).
- bumetanide (Bumex).
- diazoxide (Proglycem).
- ethacrynic acid (Edecrin).
- furosemide (Lasix).
- phenytoin (Dilantin).
- thiazide diuretics (see Drug Class, Section Four).

▷   *Driving, Hazardous Activities*: Regulate your dosage schedule, eating schedule and physical activities very carefully to prevent hypoglycemia. Be able to recognize the early symptoms of hypoglycemia so you can avoid hazardous activities and take corrective measures.

Aviation Note: Diabetes *is a disqualification* for piloting. Consult a designated Aviation Medical Examiner.

Exposure to Sun: Use caution until sensitivity has been determined. Some drugs of this class can cause photosensitivity (see Glossary).

Occurrence of Unrelated Illness: Acute infections, illnesses causing vomiting or diarrhea, serious injuries and surgical procedures can interfere with diabetic control and may require the use of insulin. If any of these conditions occur, consult your physician promptly.

Discontinuation: Because of the possibility of secondary failure, it is advisable to evaluate the continued benefit of this drug every 6 months.

TOLBUTAMIDE
(tohl BYU ta mide)

Introduced: 1956

Class: Antidiabetic, Sulfonylureas

Prescription: USA: Yes
  Canada: Yes

Controlled Drug: USA: No
  Canada: No

Available as Generic: Yes

Brand Names: ✿Apo-Tolbutamide, ✿Mobenol, ✿Novobutamide, Orinase, SK-Tolbutamide

---

BENEFITS versus RISKS

Possible Benefits	*Possible Risks*
Assistance in regulating blood sugar in noninsulin-dependent diabetes (adjunctive to appropriate diet and weight control)	HYPOGLYCEMIA, severe and prolonged Drug-induced liver damage Rare bone marrow depression (See Glossary) Hemolytic anemia (See Glossary)

▷ **Principal Uses**

   As a Single Drug Product: To assist in the control of mild to moderately severe type II diabetes mellitus (adult, maturity-onset) that does not require insulin, but that cannot be adequately controlled by diet alone.

How This Drug Works: It is thought that this drug (1) stimulates the release of insulin (by a pancreas that is capable of responding to stimulation), and (2) enhances the utilization of insulin by appropriate tissues.

Available Dosage Forms and Strengths
   Tablets — 250 mg, 500 mg

▷ **Usual Adult Dosage Range:**   Initially, 500 mg twice a day. The dose may be increased or decreased every 48 to 72 hours until the minimal amount required for satisfactory control is determined. The usual range is 500 to 2000 mg/24 hours. The total daily dosage should not exceed 3000 mg (3 grams). A "loading" or priming dose is not necessary and should not be given. **Note: Actual dosage and administration schedule must be determined by the physician for each patient individually.**

Dosing Instructions: May be taken with food (morning and evening meals) to reduce stomach irritation. The tablet may be crushed for administration.

Usual Duration of Use: Continual use on a regular schedule for several weeks is usually necessary to determine this drug's effectiveness in controlling diabetes. Failure to respond to maximal doses within 1 month constitutes a primary failure. Up to 15% of those who respond initially may develop secondary failure of the drug within the first year. The duration of effective use can only be determined by periodic measurement of the blood sugar.

▷ **This Drug Should Not Be Taken If**
   • you have had an allergic reaction to it previously.
   • you have severe impairment of liver or kidney function.
   • you are pregnant.

▷ **Inform Your Physician Before Taking This Drug If**
   • you are allergic to other sulfonylurea drugs or to "sulfa" drugs. (See Drug Classes, Section Four).
   • your diabetes has been unstable or "brittle" in the past.
   • you do not know how to recognize or treat hypoglycemia (see Glossary).

- you have a history of congestive heart failure, peptic ulcer disease, cirrhosis of the liver, hypothyroidism or porphyria.

Possible Side-Effects   (natural, expected and unavoidable drug actions)

If drug dosage is excessive or food intake is delayed or inadequate, abnormally low blood sugar (hypoglycemia) will occur as a predictable drug effect.

▷ **Possible Adverse Effects**   (unusual, unexpected and infrequent reactions)

If any of the following develop, consult your physician promptly.

Mild Adverse Effects

Allergic Reactions: Skin rash, hives, itching, drug fever.

Headache, ringing in the ears, weakness.

Indigestion, heartburn, nausea, vomiting.

Serious Adverse Effects

Allergic Reactions: Hepatitis with jaundice (see Glossary).

Idiosyncratic Reactions: Hemolytic anemia (see Glossary); disulfiramlike reaction with concurrent use of alcohol (see Glossary), infrequent with this drug.

Bone marrow depression (see Glossary): fatigue, weakness, fever, sore throat, abnormal bleeding or bruising.

▷ **Adverse Effects That May Mimic Natural Diseases or Disorders**

Liver reactions may suggest viral hepatitis.

Natural Diseases or Disorders That May Be Activated by This Drug

Acute intermittent porphyria (see Glossary).

CAUTION

1. This drug must be regarded as only one part of the total program for the management of your diabetes. It is not a substitute for a properly prescribed diet and regular exercise.
2. Over a period of time (usually several months), this drug may lose its effectiveness in controlling blood sugar levels. Periodic follow-up examinations are necessary to monitor all aspects of response to drug treatment.

Precautions for Use

By Infants and Children: This drug is not effective in type I (juvenile, growth-onset) insulin-dependent diabetes.

By Those over 60 Years of Age: This drug should be used with caution in this age group. Start treatment with 500 mg/day; increase dosage cautiously and monitor closely to prevent hypoglycemic reactions. Repeated episodes of hypoglycemia in the elderly can cause brain damage.

▷ **Advisability of Use During Pregnancy**

Pregnancy Category: C (tentative). See Pregnancy Code inside back cover.

Animal studies: Ocular and bone birth defects reported in rat studies.

Human studies: Information from adequate studies of pregnant women is not available.

Because uncontrolled blood sugar levels during pregnancy are associated with a higher incidence of birth defects, many experts recommend that insulin (instead of an oral agent) be used as necessary to control diabetes during the entire pregnancy.

Use during pregnancy is not recommended by the manufacturer.

Advisability of Use if Breast-Feeding
Presence of this drug in breast milk: Yes.
Avoid drug or refrain from nursing.

Habit-Forming Potential: None.

Effects of Overdosage: Symptoms of mild to severe hypoglycemia: headache, light-headedness, faintness, nervousness, confusion, tremor, sweating, heart palpitation, weakness, hunger, nausea, vomiting, stupor progressing to coma.

Possible Effects of Long-Term Use: Reduced function of the thyroid gland (hypothyroidism). Reports of increased frequency and severity of heart and blood vessel diseases associated with long-term use of this class of drugs are highly controversial and inconclusive. A direct cause-and-effect relationship (see Glossary) is tenuous. Ask your physician for guidance.

Suggested Periodic Examinations While Taking This Drug   (at physician's discretion)
Complete blood cell counts, liver function tests, thyroid function tests, periodic evaluation of heart and circulatory system.

▷ **While Taking This Drug, Observe the Following**
Foods: Follow the diabetic diet prescribed by your physician.
Beverages: As directed in the diabetic diet. May be taken with milk.
▷ *Alcohol*: Use with extreme caution until the combined effect has been determined. Alcohol can exaggerate this drug's hypoglycemic effect. This drug infrequently causes a marked intolerance of alcohol resulting in a disulfiramlike reaction (see Glossary): facial flushing, sweating, palpitation.
Tobacco Smoking: No interactions expected.
▷ *Other Drugs*
The following drugs may *increase* the effects of tolbutamide
- aspirin, and other salicylates.
- chloramphenicol (Chloromycetin).
- cimetidine (Tagamet).
- clofibrate (Atromid S).
- fenfluramine (Pondimin).
- monoamine oxidase (MAO) inhibitor drugs (see Drug Class, Section Four).
- phenylbutazone (Butazolidin).
- ranitidine (Zantac).
- sulfonamide drugs (see Drug Class, Section Four).
The following drugs may *decrease* the effects of tolbutamide
- beta-blocker drugs (see Drug Class, Section Four).
- bumetanide (Bumex).

- diazoxide (Proglycem).
- ethacrynic acid (Edecrin).
- furosemide (Lasix).
- phenytoin (Dilantin).
- rifampin (Rifadin, Rimactane).
- thiazide diuretics (see Drug Class, Section Four).

▷ *Driving, Hazardous Activities*: Regulate your dosage schedule, eating schedule and physical activities very carefully to prevent hypoglycemia. Be able to recognize the early symptoms of hypoglycemia so you can avoid hazardous activities and take corrective measures.

Aviation Note: Diabetes *is a disqualification* for piloting. Consult a designated Aviation Medical Examiner.

Exposure to Sun: Use caution until sensitivity has been determined. Some drugs of this class can cause photosensitivity (see Glossary).

Occurrence of Unrelated Illness: Acute infections, illnesses causing vomiting or diarrhea, serious injuries and surgical procedures can interfere with diabetic control and may require the use of insulin. If any of these conditions occur, consult your physician promptly.

Discontinuation: Because of the possibility of secondary failure, it is advisable to evaluate the continued benefit of this drug every 6 months.

TOLMETIN
(TOHL met in)

Introduced: 1976

Class: Mild Analgesic, Anti-inflammatory

Prescription: USA: Yes
Canada: Yes

Controlled Drug: USA: No
Canada: No

Available as Generic: No

Brand Names: Tolectin, Tolectin DS

BENEFITS versus RISKS	
Possible Benefits	*Possible Risks*
EFFECTIVE RELIEF OF MILD TO MODERATE PAIN AND INFLAMMATION	Gastrointestinal pain, ulceration, bleeding (rare)
	Rare liver damage
	Rare kidney damage
	Rare blood cell disorders: hemolytic anemia, abnormally low white blood cell and platelet counts

▷ **Principal Uses**

As a Single Drug Product: Used primarily to relieve mild to moderately severe pain and inflammation associated with (1) acute and chronic rheumatoid arthritis; (2) osteoarthritis; and (3) juvenile rheumatoid arthritis.

How This Drug Works: Not completely established. It is thought that this drug reduces the tissue concentrations of prostaglandins (and related compounds), substances involved in the production of inflammation and pain.

Available Dosage Forms and Strengths
Capsules — 400 mg
Tablets — 200 mg

▷ **Usual Adult Dosage Range:**   Initially, 400 mg 3 times/day. For maintenance: adjust dosage from 600 mg to 1600 mg daily as needed, taken in 3 or 4 divided doses. The total daily dosage should not exceed 2000 mg (2.0 grams) for rheumatoid arthritis, or 1600 mg (1.6 grams) for osteoarthritis. **Note: Actual dosage and administration schedule must be determined by the physician for each patient individually.**

▷ **Dosing Instructions:**   Preferably taken on an empty stomach, 1 hour before or 2 hours after eating. However, it may be taken with or after food if necessary to reduce stomach irritation. Take with a full glass of water and remain upright (do not lie down) for 30 minutes. Schedule dosing to include one in the morning and one at bedtime. The capsule may be opened and the tablet may be crushed for administration.

Usual Duration of Use: Continual use on a regular schedule for 1 to 2 weeks is usually necessary to determine this drug's effectiveness in relieving the discomfort of arthritis. Long-term use (months to years) requires supervision and periodic evaluation by your physician.

▷ **This Drug Should Not Be Taken If**
- you have had an allergic reaction to it previously.
- you are subject to asthma or nasal polyps caused by aspirin.
- you have active peptic ulcer disease or any form of gastrointestinal bleeding.
- you have a bleeding disorder or a blood cell disorder.
- you have severe impairment of liver or kidney function.

▷ **Inform Your Physician Before Taking This Drug If**
- you are allergic to aspirin or to other aspirin substitutes.
- you have a history of peptic ulcer disease or any type of bleeding disorder.
- you have impaired liver or kidney function.
- you have high blood pressure or a history of heart failure.
- you are taking any of the following: acetaminophen, aspirin or other aspirin substitutes, anticoagulants, oral antidiabetic drugs.

Possible Side-Effects   (natural, expected and unavoidable drug actions)
Fluid retention (edema). Drowsiness in sensitive individuals.

▷ **Possible Adverse Effects**   (unusual, unexpected and infrequent reactions)
If any of the following develop, consult your physician promptly.

Mild Adverse Effects
Allergic Reactions: Skin rash, hives, itching.
Headache, dizziness, blurred vision, ringing in the ears.
Mouth sores, indigestion, nausea, vomiting, constipation, diarrhea.
Serious Adverse Effects
Allergic Reactions: Anaphylactic reaction (see Glossary), severe skin reactions.
Active peptic ulcer, with or without bleeding.
Liver damage with jaundice (see Glossary).
Kidney damage with painful urination, bloody urine, reduced urine formation.
Abnormally low white blood cell count: fever, sore throat.
Abnormally low blood platelet count: abnormal bleeding or bruising.

Possible Delayed Adverse Effects
Mild anemia due to "silent" blood loss from the stomach (less than that caused by aspirin).

▷ Adverse Effects That May Mimic Natural Diseases or Disorders
Liver reaction may suggest viral hepatitis.

Natural Diseases or Disorders That May Be Activated by This Drug
Peptic ulcer disease, ulcerative colitis.

CAUTION
1. Dosage should always be limited to the smallest amount that produces reasonable improvement.
2. This drug may mask early indications of infection. Inform your physician if you think you are developing an infection of any kind.

Precautions for Use
By Infants and Children: Safety and effectiveness for use by those under 2 years of age have not been established.
By Those over 60 Years of Age: Small doses are advisable until tolerance is determined. Observe for any indications of liver or kidney toxicity, fluid retention, dizziness, confusion, impaired memory, stomach bleeding or constipation.

▷ Advisability of Use During Pregnancy
Pregnancy Category: B (tentative). See Pregnancy Code inside back cover.
Animal studies: No birth defects due to this drug reported.
Human studies: Information from adequate studies of pregnant women is not available.
The manufacturer does not recommend the use of this drug during pregnancy.

Advisability of Use if Breast-Feeding
Presence of this drug in breast milk: Unknown.
Avoid drug or refrain from nursing.

Habit-Forming Potential: None.

Effects of Overdosage: Stomach irritation, nausea, vomiting, diarrhea.

Possible Effects of Long-Term Use: Fluid retention.

Suggested Periodic Examinations While Taking This Drug   (at physician's
discretion)
Complete blood cell counts, liver and kidney function tests, complete eye
examinations if vision is altered in any way.

▷ **While Taking This Drug, Observe the Following**
Foods: No restrictions.
Beverages: No restrictions. May be taken with milk.
▷ *Alcohol*: Use with caution. The irritant action of alcohol on the stomach lin-
ing, added to the irritant action of this drug in sensitive individuals, can
increase the risk of stomach ulceration and/or bleeding.
Tobacco Smoking: No interactions expected.
▷ *Other Drugs*
Tolmetin may *increase* the effects of
  • acetaminophen (Tylenol, etc.), and increase the risk of kidney damage;
    avoid prolonged use of this combination.
  • anticoagulants (Coumadin, etc.), and increase the risk of bleeding; moni-
    tor prothrombin time, adjust dose accordingly.
Tolmetin *taken concurrently* with the following drugs may increase the risk
of bleeding; avoid these combinations:
  • aspirin.
  • dipyridamole (Persantine).
  • indomethacin (Indocin).
  • sulfinpyrazone (Anturane).
  • valproic acid (Depakene).
▷ *Driving, Hazardous Activities*: This drug may cause drowsiness or dizziness.
Restrict activities as necessary.
Aviation Note: The use of this drug *may be a disqualification* for piloting.
Consult a designated Aviation Medical Examiner.
Exposure to Sun: No restrictions.

TRAZODONE
(TRAZ oh dohn)

Introduced: 1967

Prescription: USA: Yes
Canada: Yes

Available as Generic: No

Brand Names: Desyrel

Class: Antidepressants

Controlled Drug: USA: No
Canada: No

```
┌─────────────────────────────────────────────────────────────┐
│                    BENEFITS versus RISKS                     │
│                                                              │
│      Possible Benefits                 Possible Risks        │
│  EFFECTIVE TREATMENT IN ALL    Adverse behavioral effects:   │
│     TYPES OF DEPRESSIVE            confusion, disorientation, │
│     ILLNESS, with or without       delusions, hallucinations (all │
│     anxiety                        infrequent)               │
│                                 Potential for inducing heart rhythm │
│                                    disorders (in individuals with │
│                                    heart disease)            │
└─────────────────────────────────────────────────────────────┘
```

▷ **Principal Uses**

As a Single Drug Product: Used to provide symptomatic relief in all types of depression, with or without anxiety or agitation. The primary intent is to initiate restoration of normal mood with a minimum of adverse drug effects.

How This Drug Works: Not completely established. It is thought that this drug increases the availability of the nerve impulse transmitter serotonin within certain brain centers and thereby relieves the symptoms of emotional depression.

Available Dosage Forms and Strengths
Tablets — 50 mg, 100 mg

▷ **Usual Adult Dosage Range:** Initially, 50 mg 3 times/day. The dose may be increased by 50 mg daily at intervals of 3 or 4 days as needed and tolerated. The total daily dosage should not exceed 400 mg. **Note: Actual dosage and administration schedule must be determined by the physician for each patient individually.**

▷ **Dosing Instructions:** Best taken with food to improve absorption. The tablet may be crushed for administration. If excessive drowsiness or dizziness occurs, it is advisable to take a larger portion of the total daily dose at bedtime and to divide the remaining amount into 2 or 3 smaller doses to be taken during the day.

Usual Duration of Use: Continual use on a regular schedule for 2 to 4 weeks is usually necessary to determine this drug's effectiveness in relieving the symptoms of depression. Long-term use (weeks to months) requires supervision and periodic evaluation by your physician.

▷ **This Drug Should Not Be Taken If**
- you have had an allergic reaction to it previously.
- you are recovering from a recent heart attack (myocardial infarction).
- you are taking, or have taken within the past 14 days, any monoamine oxidase (MAO) inhibitor drug (see Drug Class, Section Four).

▷ **Inform Your Physician Before Taking This Drug If**
- you have a history of any of the following: alcoholism, epilepsy, heart disease (especially heart rhythm disorders).
- you have impaired liver or kidney function.

- you are taking any antihypertensive drugs.
- you plan to have surgery under general anesthesia in the near future.

Possible Side-Effects   (natural, expected and unavoidable drug actions)
Drowsiness, light-headedness, blurred vision, dry mouth, constipation.

▷ **Possible Adverse Effects**   (unusual, unexpected and infrequent reactions)
  If any of the following develop, consult your physician promptly.
  Mild Adverse Effects
  Allergic Reactions: Skin rash.
  Headache, dizziness, fatigue, impaired concentration, nervousness, tremors.
  Rapid heart rate, palpitations.
  Peculiar taste, stomach discomfort, nausea, vomiting, diarrhea.
  Altered libido, altered menstrual pattern, muscular aches and pains.
  Serious Adverse Effects
  Behavioral effects: Confusion, anger, hostility, disorientation, impaired memory, delusions, hallucinations, nightmares.
  Irregular heart rhythms, low blood pressure, fainting.
  Inappropriate, prolonged and painful erections of the penis (priapism).

CAUTION
  1. If you experience a significant degree of mouth dryness while using this drug, consult your dentist regarding the risk of gum erosion or tooth decay. Ask for his guidance in ways to keep the mouth comfortably moist.
  2. It is advisable to withhold this drug if electroconvulsive therapy (ECT) is to be used.

Precautions for Use
  By Infants and Children: Safety and effectiveness for use by those under 18 years of age have not been established.
  By Those over 60 Years of Age: During the first two weeks of treatment, observe for the development of restlessness, agitation, excitement, forgetfulness, confusion or disorientation. Be aware of possible unsteadiness and incoordination that may predispose to falling. This drug may enhance prostatism (see Glossary).

▷ **Advisability of Use During Pregnancy**
  Pregnancy Category: C (tentative). See Pregnancy Code inside back cover.
  Animal studies: Fetal deaths and birth defects reported.
  Human studies: Information from adequate studies of pregnant women is not available.
  Avoid this drug completely during the first 3 months. Use otherwise only if clearly needed. Ask your physician for guidance.

Advisability of Use if Breast-Feeding
  Presence of this drug in breast milk: Probably yes.
  Avoid drug or refrain from nursing.

Habit-Forming Potential: None.

Effects of Overdosage: Marked drowsiness, weakness, confusion, tremors, low blood pressure, rapid heart rate, stupor, coma, possible seizures.

Possible Effects of Long-Term Use: None reported.

Suggested Periodic Examinations While Taking This Drug   (at physician's discretion)
   Complete blood cell counts. (This drug may cause slight reductions in white blood cell counts. This should be monitored closely if infection, sore throat or fever develops.)
   Serial blood pressure readings and electrocardiograms.

▷ **While Taking This Drug, Observe the Following**
   Foods: No restrictions.
   Beverages: No restrictions. May be taken with milk.
▷ *Alcohol*: Avoid completely. This drug can increase markedly the intoxicating effects of alcohol and accentuate its depressant action on brain functions.
   Tobacco Smoking: No interactions expected.
▷ *Other Drugs*
   Trazodone may *increase* the effects of
   • antihypertensive drugs, and cause excessive lowering of blood pressure; dosage adjustments may be necessary.
   • drugs with sedative effects, and cause excessive sedation.
   • phenytoin (Dilantin), by raising its blood level; observe for phenytoin toxicity.
▷ *Driving, Hazardous Activities*: This drug may cause dizziness or drowsiness. Restrict activities as necessary.
   Aviation Note: The use of this drug *is a disqualification* for piloting. Consult a designated Aviation Medical Examiner.
   Exposure to Sun: No restrictions.
   Discontinuation: It is advisable to discontinue this drug gradually. Ask your physician for guidance in dosage reduction over an appropriate period of time.

TRIAMTERENE
(tri AM ter een)

Introduced: 1964   **Class:**   Diuretic

Prescription: USA: Yes   **Controlled Drug:**   USA: No
   Canada: Yes   Canada: No

Available as Generic: No

Brand Names: ✤Apo-Triazide [CD], Dyazide [CD], Dyrenium

```
┌─────────────────────────────────────────────────────────────────┐
│                    BENEFITS versus RISKS                          │
│                                                                   │
│     Possible Benefits                   Possible Risks            │
│   EFFECTIVE PREVENTION OF           ABNORMALLY HIGH BLOOD          │
│     POTASSIUM LOSS when used          POTASSIUM LEVEL with         │
│     adjunctively with other diuretics excessive use               │
│   EFFECTIVE DIURETIC IN             Rare blood cell disorders:     │
│     REFRACTORY CASES OF               megaloblastic anemia,        │
│     FLUID RETENTION when used         abnormally low white blood cell │
│     adjunctively with other diuretics and platelet counts         │
└─────────────────────────────────────────────────────────────────┘
```

▷ **Principal Uses**

As a Single Drug Product: This mild diuretic is used as part of the treatment program for the management of congestive heart failure and disorders of the liver and kidney that are accompanied by excessive fluid retention (edema). It is also used in conjunction with other measures to treat high blood pressure. It is used primarily in situations where it is advisable to prevent loss of potassium from the body.

As a Combination Drug Product [CD]: This drug is available in combination with hydrochlorothiazide, a different kind of diuretic that promotes the loss of potassium from the body. Triamterene is used in this combination to counteract the potassium-wasting effect of the thiazide diuretic.

How This Drug Works: Not completely established. It is thought that by inhibiting the enzyme system that initiates the sodium-potassium exchange process, this drug prevents the reabsorption of sodium and the excretion of potassium by the kidney. Thus the drug promotes the excretion of sodium (and water with it) and the retention of potassium.

Available Dosage Forms and Strengths

Capsules — 50 mg, 100 mg

▷ **Usual Adult Dosage Range:** Initially, 100 mg twice daily. The dose is then adjusted according to individual response. The usual maintenance dose is 100 to 200 mg/day, divided into 2 doses. The total daily dosage should not exceed 300 mg. **Note: Actual dosage and administration schedule must be determined by the physician for each patient individually.**

▷ **Dosing Instructions:** May be taken with or following meals to promote absorption of the drug and to reduce stomach irritation. The capsule may be opened for administration. Intermittent or alternate-day use is recommended to minimize the possibility of sodium and potassium imbalance.

Usual Duration of Use: Continual use on a regular schedule for 3 to 5 days is usually necessary to determine this drug's effectiveness in clearing edema, and for 2 to 3 weeks to determine its effect on hypertension. Long-term use (months to years) requires supervision and periodic evaluation by your physician.

▷ **This Drug Should Not Be Taken If**
- you have had an allergic reaction to it previously.
- you have severely impaired liver or kidney function.

▷ **Inform Your Physician Before Taking This Drug If**
- you have a history of liver or kidney disease.
- you have diabetes or gout.
- you are taking any of the following: antihypertensives, a digitalis preparation, another diuretic, lithium or a potassium preparation.
- you plan to have surgery under general anesthesia in the near future.

Possible Side-Effects   (natural, expected and unavoidable drug actions)
With excessive use: abnormally high blood potassium levels, abnormally low blood sodium levels, dehydration.
Blue coloration of the urine (of no significance).

▷ **Possible Adverse Effects**   (unusual, unexpected and infrequent reactions)
If any of the following develop, consult your physician promptly.
Mild Adverse Effects
Allergic Reactions: Skin rash, itching.
Headache, dizziness, unsteadiness, weakness, drowsiness, lethargy.
Dry mouth, nausea, vomiting, diarrhea.
Serious Adverse Effects
Allergic Reactions: Anaphylactic reaction (see Glossary).
Symptomatic potassium excess: confusion, numbness and tingling in lips and extremities, fatigue, weakness, shortness of breath, slow heart rate, low blood pressure.
Rare blood cell disorders: megaloblastic anemia, causing weakness and fatigue; abnormally low white blood cell count, causing infection, fever or sore throat; abnormally low blood platelet count, causing abnormal bleeding or bruising.

CAUTION
1. Do not take potassium supplements or increase your intake of potassium-rich foods while taking this drug.
2. Do not discontinue this drug abruptly unless abnormally high blood levels of potassium develop.
3. Avoid the liberal use of salt substitutes that contain potassium; these are a potential cause of potassium excess.

Precautions for Use
By Infants and Children: This drug is not recommended for use in children.
By Those over 60 Years of Age: The natural decline in kidney function may predispose to potassium retention in the body. Limit continual use of this drug to periods of 2 to 3 weeks. Observe for indications of potassium excess: slow heart rate, irregular heart rhythms, low blood pressure, confusion, drowsiness. The excessive use of diuretics can cause harmful loss of body water (dehydration), increased viscosity of the blood and an increased tendency of the blood to clot, predisposing to stroke, heart attack or thrombophlebitis.

▷ **Advisability of Use During Pregnancy**
  Pregnancy Category: D (tentative). See Pregnancy Code inside back cover.
    Animal studies: No birth defects due to this drug reported.
    Human studies: Information from adequate studies of pregnant women is
    not available.
    This drug should not be used during pregnancy unless a very serious com-
    plication of pregnancy occurs for which this drug is significantly benefi-
    cial.

Advisability of Use if Breast-Feeding
  Presence of this drug in breast milk: Yes.
  Avoid drug or refrain from nursing.

Habit-Forming Potential: None.

Effects of Overdosage: Thirst, drowsiness, fatigue, weakness, nausea, vomiting, confusion, irregular heart rhythm, low blood pressure.

Possible Effects of Long-Term Use: Potassium accumulation to abnormally
  high blood levels.

Suggested Periodic Examinations While Taking This Drug (at physician's
  discretion)
  Complete blood cell counts.
  Measurements of blood sodium, potassium and chloride levels.
  Kidney function tests.

▷ **While Taking This Drug, Observe the Following**
  Foods: No restrictions. Avoid excessive restriction of salt.
  Beverages: No restrictions. May be taken with milk.
▷ *Alcohol*: Use with caution until the combined effects have been determined.
    Alcohol may enhance the drowsiness and the blood-pressure-lowering
    effect of this drug.
  Tobacco Smoking: No interactions expected.
▷ *Other Drugs*
    Triamterene may *increase* the effects of
    • amantadine (Symmetrel).
    • digoxin (Lanoxin).
    Triamterene *taken concurrently* with
    • captopril (Capoten) may cause excessively high blood potassium levels.
    • indomethacin (Indocin) may increase the risk of kidney damage.
    • lithium may cause accumulation of lithium to toxic levels.
    • potassium preparations may cause excessively high blood potassium
    levels.
▷ *Driving, Hazardous Activities*: This drug may cause dizziness and drowsiness.
    Restrict activities as necessary.
  Aviation Note: The use of this drug *may be a disqualification* for piloting.
    Consult a designated Aviation Medical Examiner.
  Exposure to Sun: Use caution until your sensitivity has been determined. This
    drug may cause photosensitivity (see Glossary).

Discontinuation: With high dosage or prolonged use, it is advisable to withdraw this drug gradually. Sudden discontinuation may cause rebound potassium excretion and resultant potassium deficiency. Ask your physician for guidance.

TRIAZOLAM
(tri AY zoh lam)

Introduced: 1974

Prescription: USA: Yes
Canada: Yes

Available as Generic: USA: No
Canada: No

Brand Names: Halcion

Class: Hypnotic, Benzodiazepines

Controlled Drug: USA: C-IV*
Canada: No

BENEFITS versus RISKS	
Possible Benefits	*Possible Risks*
EFFECTIVE HYPNOTIC with short duration of action	Habit-forming potential with long-term use
Wide margin of safety with therapeutic doses	Minor impairment of mental functions ("hangover" effect)

▷ **Principal Uses**
As a Single Drug Product: This member of the benzodiazepine class of "minor tranquilizers" is used exclusively as a bedtime sedative to induce sleep. It is useful in the short-term management of insomnia characterized by difficulty in falling asleep, frequent awakenings during the night and early morning awakening.

How This Drug Works: It is thought that this drug produces a calming effect by enhancing the action of the nerve transmitter gamma-aminobutyric acid (GABA), which in turn blocks the arousal of higher brain centers and helps to induce sleep.

Available Dosage Forms and Strengths
Tablets — 0.125 mg, 0.25 mg, 0.5 mg

▷ **Usual Adult Dosage Range:** 0.125 to 0.5 mg at bedtime. The total daily dosage should not exceed 0.5 mg. **Note: Actual dosage and administration schedule must be determined by the physician for each patient individually.**

▷ **Dosing Instructions:** Preferably taken on an empty stomach to hasten absorption and induce sleep rapidly. The tablet may be crushed for

*See Schedules of Controlled Drugs inside back cover.

administration. Do not discontinue this drug abruptly if taken for more than 4 weeks.

Usual Duration of Use: Periods of 3 to 5 nights intermittently, repeated as needed with appropriate dosage adjustment. Avoid uninterrupted and prolonged use. The duration of use should not exceed 2 weeks without reappraisal of continued need.

▷ **This Drug Should Not Be Taken If**
 • you have had an allergic reaction to it previously.

▷ **Inform Your Physician Before Taking This Drug If**
 • you are allergic to any benzodiazepine drug (see Drug Class, Section Four).
 • you have a history of alcoholism or drug abuse.
 • you are pregnant or planning pregnancy.
 • you have impaired liver or kidney function.
 • you have a history of serious depression or mental disorder.
 • you are taking other drugs with sedative effects.
 • you have any of the following: asthma, emphysema, epilepsy, myasthenia gravis.

Possible Side-Effects (natural, expected and unavoidable drug actions)
 "Hangover" effects on arising: drowsiness (14%), lethargy and unsteadiness (4.6%).

Possible Adverse Effects (unusual, unexpected and infrequent reactions)
 If any of the following develop, consult your physician promptly.
 Mild Adverse Effects
 Allergic Reactions: Skin rash, itching.
 Headache, dizziness, fatigue, blurred vision.
 Nausea, indigestion, constipation, diarrhea.
 Serious Adverse Effects
 Idiosyncratic Reactions: Nervousness, talkativeness, irritability, apprehension, euphoria, excitement, hallucinations.
 Confusion, mental depression.

CAUTION
 1. This drug should not be discontinued abruptly if it has been taken continually for more than 4 weeks.
 2. The concurrent use of some over-the-counter drug products that contain antihistamines (allergy and cold preparations, sleep aids) can cause excessive sedation in sensitive individuals.
 3. Regular nightly use of any hypnotic drug should be avoided.
 4. If you experience a "hangover" effect, avoid hazardous activities (driving, etc.) and the use of alcohol.

Precautions for Use
 By Infants and Children: Safety and effectiveness for use by those under 18 years of age have not been established.
 By Those over 60 Years of Age: It is advisable to use smaller doses (0.125 mg) at first to determine your response. Observe for the possible develop-

ment of lethargy, indifference, fatigue, weakness, unsteadiness, disturbing dreams, nightmares and paradoxical reactions of excitement, agitation, anger, hostility and rage.

▷ **Advisability of Use During Pregnancy**
Pregnancy Category: X (tentative). See Pregnancy Code inside back cover.
Animal studies: Benzodiazepines cause significant birth defects in test animals.
Human studies: Information from adequate studies of pregnant women is not available.
Avoid use during entire pregnancy.

Advisability of Use if Breast-Feeding
Presence of this drug in breast milk: Probably yes.
Avoid drug or refrain from nursing.

Habit-Forming Potential: This drug can produce psychological and/or physical dependence (see Glossary) if used in large doses for an extended period of time. Avoid continual use.

Effects of Overdosage: Marked drowsiness, weakness, feeling of drunkenness, staggering gait, tremor, stupor progressing to deep sleep or coma.

Possible Effects of Long-Term Use: Psychological and/or physical dependence.

Periodic Examinations While Taking This Drug   (at physician's discretion)
Complete blood cell counts during long-term use.

▷ **While Taking This Drug, Observe the Following**
Foods: No restrictions.
Beverages: Avoid excessive intake of caffeine-containing beverages (coffee, tea, cola) within 4 hours of taking this drug. May be taken with milk.
▷ *Alcohol*: Use with extreme caution until the combined effect has been determined. Alcohol may increase the absorption of this drug and add to its depressant effects on the brain. It is advisable to avoid alcohol completely—throughout the day and night—if it is necessary to drive or to engage in any hazardous activity.
Tobacco Smoking: Heavy smoking may reduce the hypnotic action of this drug.
Marijuana Smoking: Increased sedation and significant impairment of intellectual and physical performance.
▷ *Other Drugs*
Triazolam may *increase* the effects of
• digoxin (Lanoxin), and cause digoxin toxicity.
• phenytoin (Dilantin), and cause phenytoin toxicity.
Triazolam may *decrease* the effects of
• levodopa (Sinemet, etc.), and reduce its effectiveness in treating Parkinson's disease.
The following drugs may *increase* the effects of triazolam
• cimetidine (Tagamet).
• disulfiram (Antabuse).

- isoniazid (INH, Rifamate, etc.).
- oral contraceptives.
- valproic acid (Depakene).

The following drugs may *decrease* the effects of triazolam

- rifampin (Rimactane, etc.).
- theophylline (aminophylline, Theo-Dur, etc.).

▷ *Driving, Hazardous Activities*: This drug can impair mental alertness, judgment, physical coordination and reaction time. Avoid hazardous activities accordingly.

Aviation Note: The use of this drug *is a disqualification* for piloting. Consult a designated Aviation Medical Examiner.

Exposure to Sun: No restrictions.

Exposure to Heat: Use caution until the effect of excessive perspiration is determined. Because of reduced urine volume, this drug may accumulate in the body and produce effects of overdosage.

Discontinuation: Avoid sudden discontinuation if this drug has been taken for over 4 weeks without interruption. Dosage should be tapered gradually to prevent a withdrawal syndrome that could include depression, confusion, hallucinations, tremor, seizures, muscle cramping, sweating and vomiting.

TRIFLUOPERAZINE
(tri floo oh PER a zeen)

Introduced: 1958

Class: Strong Tranquilizer, Phenothiazines

Prescription: USA: Yes
Canada: Yes

Controlled Drug: USA: No
Canada: No

Available as Generic: USA: Yes
Canada: Yes

Brand Names: ✤Apo-Trifluoperazine, ✤Novoflurazine, ✤Solazine, Stelazine, Suprazine, ✤Terfluzine

---

BENEFITS versus RISKS

Possible Benefits	*Possible Risks*
EFFECTIVE CONTROL OF ACUTE MENTAL DISORDERS in the majority of patients: beneficial effects on thinking, mood and behavior	SERIOUS TOXIC EFFECTS ON BRAIN with long-term use Liver damage with jaundice (infrequent) Rare blood cell disorders: abnormally low red and white blood cell and platelet counts

▷ **Principal Uses**

As a Single Drug Product: This antipsychotic drug is used primarily to treat psychotic thinking and behavior associated with acute psychoses of unknown nature, mania, paranoid states and acute schizophrenia. It is most effective in those who are withdrawn and apathetic and in those with agitation, delusions and hallucinations.

How This Drug Works: Not completely established. Present theory is that by inhibiting the action of dopamine, this drug acts to correct an imbalance of nerve impulse transmissions that is thought to be responsible for certain mental disorders.

Available Dosage Forms and Strengths
Concentrate — 10 mg per ml
Injection — 2 mg per ml
Tablets — 1 mg, 2 mg, 5 mg, 10 mg

▷ **Usual Adult Dosage Range:**   Initially, 1 or 2 mg twice daily. The dose may be increased by 1 or 2 mg at 3 to 4 day intervals as needed and tolerated. Usual dosage range is 10 to 30 mg daily. The total daily dosage should not exceed 40 mg. **Note: Actual dosage and administration schedule must be determined by the physician for each patient individually.**

▷ **Dosing Instructions:**   May be taken with or following meals to reduce stomach irritation. The tablets may be crushed for administration.

Usual Duration of Use: Continual use on a regular schedule for several weeks is usually necessary to determine this drug's effectiveness in controlling psychotic disorders. If not significantly beneficial within 6 weeks, it should be discontinued. Long-term use (months to years) requires periodic evaluation of response, appropriate dosage adjustment and consideration of continued need.

▷ **This Drug Should Not Be Taken If**
- you are allergic to any of the drugs bearing the brand names listed above.
- you have active liver disease.
- you have cancer of the breast.
- you have a current blood cell or bone marrow disorder.

▷ **Inform Your Physician Before Taking This Drug If**
- you are allergic or abnormally sensitive to any phenothiazine drug (see Drug Class, Section Four).
- you have impaired liver or kidney function.
- you have any type of seizure disorder.
- you have diabetes, glaucoma or heart disease.
- you have a history of lupus erythematosus.
- you are taking any drug with sedative effects.
- you plan to have surgery under general or spinal anesthesia in the near future.

Possible Side-Effects (natural, expected and unavoidable drug actions)

Drowsiness (usually during the first 2 weeks), orthostatic hypotension (see Glossary), blurred vision, dry mouth, nasal congestion, constipation, impaired urination.

Pink or purple coloration of urine, of no significance.

▷ **Possible Adverse Effects** (unusual, unexpected and infrequent reactions)
If any of the following develop, consult your physician promptly.

Mild Adverse Effects

Allergic Reactions: Skin rash, hives, low-grade fever.

Lowering of body temperature, especially in the elderly. (See Hypothermia in Glossary.)

Increased appetite and weight gain.

Breast fullness, tenderness, milk production, menstrual irregularity.

Dizziness, weakness, agitation, insomnia, impaired day and night vision.

Chronic constipation, fecal impaction.

Serious Adverse Effects

Allergic Reactions: Hepatitis with jaundice (see Glossary), severe skin reactions, anaphylactic reaction (see Glossary).

Idiosyncratic Reactions: Inappropriate, prolonged and painful erection of the penis (priapism).

Depression, disorientation, seizures, loss of peripheral vision.

Rapid heart rate, heart rhythm disorders.

Blood cell disorders: significant reduction in all cellular elements of the blood (reduced counts of red cells, white cells and blood platelets).

Nervous system reactions: Parkinson-like disorders (see Glossary), severe restlessness, muscle spasms involving the face and neck, tardive dyskinesia (see Glossary) (10% to 20%).

▷ **Adverse Effects That May Mimic Natural Diseases or Disorders**

Nervous system reactions may suggest true Parkinson's disease.

Liver reactions may suggest viral hepatitis.

Reactions resembling systemic lupus erythematosus may occur.

Natural Diseases or Disorders That May Be Activated by This Drug

Latent epilepsy, glaucoma, diabetes mellitus, prostatism (see Glossary).

CAUTION

1. Many over-the-counter medications (see OTC Drugs in Glossary) for allergies, colds and coughs contain drugs that can interact unfavorably with this drug. Ask your physician or pharmacist for guidance before using any such medications.

2. Antacids that contain aluminum and/or magnesium may prevent the absorption of this drug and reduce its effectiveness.

3. Obtain prompt evaluation of any change or disturbance of vision.

Precautions for Use

By Infants and Children: Use of this drug is not recommended in children under 6 years of age. Do not use this drug in the presence of symptoms suggestive of Reye syndrome (see Glossary). Children with acute infectious diseases ("flulike" infections, chicken pox, measles, etc.) are more prone to develop muscular spasms of the face, back and extremities when this drug is given.

By Those over 60 Years of Age: Small doses are advisable until individual response has been determined. You may be more susceptible to the development of drowsiness, lethargy, constipation, lowering of body temperature (hypothermia) and orthostatic hypotension (see Glossary). This drug may enhance existing prostatism (see Glossary). You may also be more susceptible to the development of Parkinson-like reactions and/or tardive dyskinesia (see discussion of these terms in Glossary). These reactions must be recognized early since they may become unresponsive to treatment and irreversible.

▷ **Advisability of Use During Pregnancy**
Pregnancy Category: C (tentative). See Pregnancy Code inside back cover.
Animal studies: Significant birth defects reported in mouse and rat studies.
Human studies: No increase in birth defects reported in 700 exposures.
Information from adequate studies of pregnant women is not available.
Avoid drug during the first 3 months; avoid during the last month because of possible effects on the newborn infant.

Advisability of Use if Breast-Feeding
Presence of this drug in breast milk: Yes, in minute amounts.
Monitor nursing infant closely and discontinue drug or nursing if adverse effects develop.

Habit-Forming Potential: None.

Effects of Overdosage: Marked drowsiness, weakness, tremor, agitation, unsteadiness, deep sleep, coma, convulsions.

Possible Effects of Long-Term Use: Tardive dyskinesia (see Glossary).

Suggested Periodic Examinations While Taking This Drug   (at physician's discretion)
Complete blood cell counts, especially between the fourth and tenth weeks of treatment.
Liver function tests, electrocardiograms.
Complete eye examinations—eye structures and vision.
Careful inspection of the tongue for early evidence of fine, involuntary, wavelike movements that could indicate the beginning of tardive dyskinesia.

▷ **While Taking This Drug, Observe the Following**
Foods: No restrictions.
Nutritional Support: A riboflavin (vitamin B-2) supplement should be taken with long-term use.
Beverages: No restrictions. May be taken with milk.
▷   *Alcohol*: Avoid completely. Alcohol can increase the sedative action of phenothiazines and accentuate their depressant effects on brain function and blood pressure. Phenothiazines can increase the intoxicating effects of alcohol.

Tobacco Smoking: Possible reduction of drowsiness from drug.

Marijuana Smoking: Moderate increase in drowsiness; accentuation of orthostatic hypotension; increased risk of precipitating latent psychoses, confusing the interpretation of mental status and drug responses.

▷ *Other Drugs*

Trifluoperazine may *increase* the effects of

- all sedative drugs, especially narcotic analgesics, and cause excessive sedation.
- all atropinelike drugs, and cause nervous system toxicity.

Trifluoperazine may *decrease* the effects of

- guanethidine (Ismelin, Esimil), and reduce its effectiveness in lowering blood pressure.

Trifluoperazine *taken concurrently* with

- lithium (Lithobid, Lithotabs) may impair the effectiveness of lithium and cause nervous system toxicity.

The following drugs may *decrease* the effects of trifluoperazine

- antacids containing aluminum and/or magnesium.
- barbiturates (see Drug Class, Section Four).
- benztropine (Cogentin).
- disulfiram (Antabuse).
- trihexyphenidyl (Artane).

▷ *Driving, Hazardous Activities*: This drug can impair mental alertness, judgment and physical coordination. Avoid hazardous activities.

Aviation Note: The use of this drug *is a disqualification* for piloting. Consult a designated Aviation Medical Examiner.

Exposure to Sun: Use caution until sensitivity has been determined. Some phenothiazines can cause photosensitivity (see Glossary).

Exposure to Heat: Use caution and avoid excessive heat as much as possible. This drug may impair the regulation of body temperature and increase the risk of heat stroke.

Exposure to Cold: Use caution and dress warmly. This drug can increase the risk of hypothermia in the elderly.

Discontinuation: After a period of long-term use, do not discontinue this drug suddenly. Gradual withdrawal over 2 to 3 weeks under physician supervision is recommended. Do not discontinue this drug without your physician's knowledge and approval. The relapse rate of schizophrenia after discontinuation is 50% to 60%.

TRIMETHOBENZAMIDE
(tri meth oh BEN za mide)

Introduced: 1959　　**Class:** Antiemetic
Prescription: USA: Yes　　**Controlled Drug:** USA: No
Available as Generic: Yes
Brand Names: Tigan

BENEFITS versus RISKS

Possible Benefits	*Possible Risks*
Possibly effective prevention and control of nausea and vomiting in selected disorders	TOXIC EFFECTS ON BRAIN: disorientation, Parkinson-like tremors, muscle spasms and rigidity, seizures Rare liver damage Rare blood cell disorders: abnormally low white blood cell count

---

▷ **Principal Uses**

As a Single Drug Product: Used exclusively for the control of nausea and vomiting associated with motion sickness, inner ear infections, Meniere's syndrome, surgery and radiation therapy. It is not as effective as the phenothiazines in relieving nausea and preventing vomiting, but it is significantly safer to use for long-term therapy.

How This Drug Works: Not completely established. It is thought that this drug relieves nausea and prevents vomiting by suppressing the transmission of nerve impulses to the vomiting centers in the brain.

Available Dosage Forms and Strengths
    Capsules — 100 mg, 250 mg
    Injection — 100 mg per ml
Suppositories — 100 mg, 200 mg

▷ **Usual Adult Dosage Range:**   250 mg every 4 to 6 hours as needed. The total daily dosage should not exceed 1000 mg. **Note: Actual dosage and administration schedule must be determined by the physician for each patient individually.**

▷ **Dosing Instructions:**   May be taken without regard to food. The capsule may be opened for administration.

Usual Duration of Use: Continual use on a regular schedule for 24 to 48 hours is usually necessary to determine this drug's effectiveness in controlling nausea and vomiting. If this drug is not effective within 3 days, it should be discontinued. Long-term use requires supervision and periodic evaluation by your physician.

▷ **This Drug Should Not Be Taken If**
   • you have had an allergic reaction to it previously.
   • you have any symptoms suggestive of Reye syndrome (see Glossary).
   • you have active liver disease.
   • you have any type of blood cell or bone marrow disorder.

▷ **Inform Your Physician Before Taking This Drug If**
   • you have had any unfavorable reactions to antihistamine drugs in the past.
   • you have impaired liver or kidney function.

- you have a seizure disorder.
- you have any type of parkinsonism.
- you have a history of blood cell or bone marrow disorders, especially one induced by drugs.

Possible Side-Effects   (natural, expected and unavoidable drug actions)
Drowsiness. Temporary drop in blood pressure when given by injection.

▷ **Possible Adverse Effects**   (unusual, unexpected and infrequent reactions)
If any of the following develop, consult your physician promptly.
Mild Adverse Effects
Allergic Reactions: Skin rash.
Headache, dizziness, blurred vision, muscle spasms.
Diarrhea.
Serious Adverse Effects
Nervous system reactions: mental depression, disorientation, seizures, Parkinson-like syndrome (see Glossary).
Liver damage with jaundice (see Glossary).
Blood cell disorder: abnormally low white blood cell count, causing infections, fever, sore throat.

▷ **Adverse Effects That May Mimic Natural Diseases or Disorders**
Liver reaction may suggest viral hepatitis.

Natural Diseases or Disorders That May Be Activated by This Drug
Reye syndrome (see Glossary).

CAUTION
1. The suppository form of this drug contains 2% benzocaine; it should not be used by anyone who is allergic to benzocaine or related local anesthetics.
2. This drug has a toxicity pattern similar to the phenothiazines. It may lower the seizure threshold in epileptic individuals. Observe closely for any change in seizure patterns.

Precautions for Use
By Infants and Children: Do not use this drug in children of any age with symptoms suggestive of Reye syndrome or with illnesses that predispose to Reye syndrome (see Glossary). Children with "flulike" infections, measles, chicken pox, etc. are very susceptible to adverse effects when this drug is given to control nausea or vomiting.
By Those over 60 Years of Age: Observe closely for excessive sedation, weakness, unsteadiness or tendency to fall. Take precautions to prevent injury.

▷ **Advisability of Use During Pregnancy**
Pregnancy Category: B (tentative). See Pregnancy Code inside back cover.
Animal studies: No birth defects reported in rat and rabbit studies.
Human studies: No increase in birth defects reported in 700 exposures to this drug. Information from adequate studies of pregnant women is not available.

Avoid use of drug during the first 3 months if possible. Use it otherwise only if clearly needed. Ask your physician for guidance.

Advisability of Use if Breast-Feeding
Presence of this drug in breast milk: Unknown.
Avoid drug or refrain from nursing.

Habit-Forming Potential: None.

Effects of Overdosage: Drowsiness, weakness, incoordination, muscle spasms in neck and extremities, confusion, disorientation, seizures, coma.

Possible Effects of Long-Term Use: None reported.

Suggested Periodic Examinations While Taking This Drug   (at physician's discretion)
Complete blood cell counts, liver function tests.

▷ **While Taking This Drug, Observe the Following**
  Foods: No restrictions.
  Beverages: No restrictions. May be taken with milk.
▷ *Alcohol*: Avoid completely. Alcohol may increase the depressant effects of this drug on brain function.
  Tobacco Smoking: No interactions expected.
▷ *Other Drugs*
    Trimethobenzamide may *increase* the effects of
    • other drugs with sedative effects, and cause excessive sedation; concurrent use may provoke other reactions of nervous system toxicity: severe spasms of neck and back muscles, seizures and coma.
▷ *Driving, Hazardous Activities*: This drug may cause dizziness and drowsiness. Restrict activities as necessary.
  Aviation Note: The use of this drug *is a disqualification* for piloting. Consult a designated Aviation Medical Examiner.
  Exposure to Sun: No restrictions.

TRIMETHOPRIM
(tri METH oh prim)

Introduced: 1966

Class: Anti-infective

Prescription: USA: Yes
  Canada: Yes

Controlled Drug: USA: No
  Canada: No

Available as Generic: USA: Yes
  Canada: No

Brand Names: Bactrim [CD], Bactrim DS [CD], ✤Coptin [CD], Proloprim, Septra [CD], Septra DS [CD], Trimpex

---

BENEFITS versus RISKS

Possible Benefits	*Possible Risks*
EFFECTIVE TREATMENT OF INFECTIONS due to susceptible microorganisms	Rare blood cell disorders: megaloblastic anemia methemoglobinemia abnormally low white blood cell and platelet counts

---

▷ **Principal Uses**

As a Single Drug Product: Used primarily to treat the initial episode of certain infections of the urinary tract that are not complicated by the presence of kidney stones or obstructions to the normal flow of urine. It is sometimes used to prevent the recurrence of such infections.

As a Combination Drug Product [CD]: This drug is available in combination with sulfamethoxazole; the generic name co-trimoxazole is used in some countries to identify this combination. It is very effective in the treatment of certain urinary tract infections, middle ear infections, chronic bronchitis, acute enteritis and certain types of pneumonia.

How This Drug Works: This drug prevents the growth and multiplication of susceptible infecting organisms by inactivating the enzyme systems that are necessary for the formation of essential nuclear elements and cell proteins.

Available Dosage Forms and Strengths

Tablets — 100 mg, 200 mg
Tablets — 80 mg combined with 400 mg of sulfamethoxazole
Tablets — 160 mg combined with 800 mg of sulfamethoxazole
Oral suspension — 40 mg combined with 200 mg of sulfamethoxazole per 5 ml teaspoonful

▷ **Usual Adult Dosage Range:**   100 mg every 12 hours for 10 days. For certain pneumonias, the same dose is given every 6 hours. The total daily dosage should not exceed 640 mg. **Note: Actual dosage and administration schedule must be determined by the physician for each patient individually.**

▷ **Dosing Instructions:**   May be taken without regard to meals. However, it may also be taken with or following food if necessary to reduce stomach irritation. The tablet may be crushed for administration.

Usual Duration of Use: Continual use on a regular schedule for 7 to 14 days is usually necessary to determine this drug's effectiveness in controlling responsive infections. The actual duration of use will depend upon the nature of the infection.

▷ **This Drug Should Not Be Taken If**
- you have had an allergic reaction to it previously.
- you have an anemia due to folic acid deficiency.

▷ **Inform Your Physician Before Taking This Drug If**
- you have a history of folic acid deficiency.
- you have impaired liver or kidney function.
- you are pregnant or breast-feeding.

Possible Side-Effects   (natural, expected and unavoidable drug actions)
None with short-term use.

▷ **Possible Adverse Effects**   (unusual, unexpected and infrequent reactions)
If any of the following develop, consult your physician promptly.
Mild Adverse Effects
Allergic Reactions: Skin rash (2.9%), itching, drug fever.
Headache, abnormal taste, sore mouth or tongue, loss of appetite, nausea, vomiting, abdominal cramping, diarrhea.
Serious Adverse Effects
Allergic Reactions: Severe dermatitis with peeling of skin.
Blood cell disorders: megaloblastic anemia, methemoglobinemia, abnormally low white blood cell and platelet counts. (All are rare.)

CAUTION
1. Certain strains of bacteria that cause urinary tract infections can develop resistance to this drug. If you do not show significant improvement within 10 days, consult your physician.
2. Comply with your physician's request for periodic blood counts during long-term therapy.

Precautions for Use
By Infants and Children: Safety and effectiveness for use by those under 2 months of age have not been established.
By Those over 60 Years of Age: The natural decline in liver and kidney function may require smaller doses. If you develop itching reactions in the genital or anal areas, report this promptly.

▷ **Advisability of Use During Pregnancy**
Pregnancy Category: C (tentative). See Pregnancy Code inside back cover.
Animal studies: Birth defects due to this drug reported in rat and rabbit studies.
Human studies: Information from adequate studies of pregnant women is not available.
Avoid use of drug during the first 3 months and during the last 2 weeks of pregnancy. Use this drug otherwise only if clearly needed. Ask your physician for guidance.

Advisability of Use if Breast-Feeding
Presence of this drug in breast milk: Yes.
Avoid drug or refrain from nursing.

Habit-Forming Potential: None.

Effects of Overdosage: Headache, dizziness, confusion, depression, nausea, vomiting, bone marrow depression, possible liver toxicity with jaundice.

Possible Effects of Long-Term Use: Impaired production of red and white blood cells and blood platelets.

Suggested Periodic Examinations While Taking This Drug   (at physician's discretion)
Complete blood cell counts.

▷ **While Taking This Drug, Observe the Following**
Foods: No restrictions.
Beverages: No restrictions. May be taken with milk.
▷ *Alcohol*: No interactions expected.
Tobacco Smoking: No interactions expected.
▷ *Other Drugs*
Trimethoprim may *increase* the effects of
  • phenytoin (Dilantin), and cause phenytoin toxicity.
The following drugs may *decrease* the effects of trimethoprim
  • rifampin (Rifadin, Rimactane).
▷ *Driving, Hazardous Activities*: No restrictions.
Aviation Note: The use of this drug is probably not a disqualification for piloting. Consult a designated Aviation Medical Examiner.
Exposure to Sun: No restrictions.

TRIPROLIDINE
(tri PROH li deen)

Introduced: 1958

Class: Antihistamines

Prescription: USA: No
Canada: No

Controlled Drug: USA: No
Canada: No

Available as Generic: USA: Yes
Canada: No

Brand Names: Actidil, Actifed [CD], ♣Actifed-A [CD], Actifed w/Codeine [CD], ♣Actifed DM [CD]

BENEFITS versus RISKS	
Possible Benefits	*Possible Risks*
EFFECTIVE RELIEF OF ALLERGIC RHINITIS AND ALLERGIC SKIN DISORDERS	Mild sedation Atropinelike effects Very rare blood cell disorders

▷ **Principal Uses**
As a Single Drug Product: Used primarily to provide symptomatic relief in allergic and related disorders: seasonal and perennial allergic rhinitis (hay fever), allergic conjunctivitis and vasomotor rhinitis; also in hives and localized swellings (angioedema) of allergic origin.
As a Combination Drug Product [CD]: This drug is combined with a decon-

gestant drug (pseudoephedrine) to enhance its ability to reduce tissue swelling and secretions in allergic and infectious disorders of the upper respiratory tract—hay fever, head colds and sinusitis. It is also combined with decongestants, expectorants and codeine to increase their effectiveness in the symptomatic treatment of allergic and infectious disorders of the lower respiratory tract, often with associated coughing.

How This Drug Works: Antihistamines reduce the intensity of the allergic response by blocking the action of histamine after it has been released from sensitized tissue cells in the eyes, nose, respiratory passages and skin.

Available Dosage Forms and Strengths
    Syrup — 1.25 mg per 5 ml teaspoonful
    Tablets — 2.5 mg

▷ **Usual Adult Dosage Range:**   2.5 mg/4 to 6 hours. The total daily dosage should not exceed 10 mg. **Note: Actual dosage and administration schedule must be determined by the physician for each patient individually.**

▷ **Dosing Instructions:**   Take with food or milk to prevent stomach irritation. The tablet may be crushed for administration.

Usual Duration of Use: Continual use on a regular schedule for 2 to 3 days is usually necessary to determine this drug's effectiveness in relieving the symptoms of allergic rhinitis and dermatosis. It may be necessary to take this drug throughout the entire pollen season, depending upon individual sensitivity. However, antihistamines should not be taken continually (without interruption) for long-term use. Limit their use to periods that require symptomatic relief.

▷ **This Drug Should Not Be Taken If**
   • you have had an allergic reaction to any dosage form of it previously.
   • you are currently undergoing allergy skin tests.
   • you are taking, or have taken within the past 14 days, any monoamine oxidase (MAO) inhibitor drug (see Drug Class, Section Four).

▷ **Inform Your Physician Before Taking This Drug If**
   • you have had any allergic reactions or unfavorable responses to the previous use of antihistamines.
   • you have glaucoma (narrow-angle type) or asthma.
   • you have epilepsy or a seizure disorder.
   • you have difficulty emptying the urinary bladder, especially if due to prostate gland enlargement.
   • you plan to have surgery under general anesthesia in the near future.

Possible Side-Effects   (natural, expected and unavoidable drug actions)
    Drowsiness; sense of weakness; blurred vision; dryness of the nose, mouth and throat; impaired urination.
    Reduced tolerance for contact lenses.

▷ **Possible Adverse Effects**   (unusual, unexpected and infrequent reactions)
    If any of the following develop, consult your physician promptly.

Mild Adverse Effects
Allergic Reactions: Skin rash, hives.
Headache, nervous agitation, dizziness, unsteadiness, confusion, tremor, numbness and tingling, blurred or double vision, ringing in ears.
Palpitation, rapid heart rate, low blood pressure.
Thickening of bronchial secretions in asthma or bronchitis.
Indigestion, nausea, vomiting, diarrhea.
Serious Adverse Effects
Allergic Reactions: Anaphylactic reaction (see Glossary).
Idiosyncratic Reactions: Euphoria, hysteria, depression, nightmares.
Hemolytic anemia (see Glossary).
Abnormally low white blood cell count, causing fever, sore throat, infections.
Abnormally low blood platelet count, causing abnormal bleeding or bruising.

Natural Diseases or Disorders That May Be Activated by This Drug
Latent epilepsy, glaucoma, prostatism (see Glossary).

CAUTION
1. Discontinue this drug 5 days before diagnostic skin testing procedures in order to prevent false negative test results.
2. Do not use this drug if you have active bronchial asthma, bronchitis or pneumonia. It can thicken bronchial mucus and make it more difficult to remove (by absorption or coughing).

Precautions for Use
By Infants and Children: This drug should not be used in premature or full-term newborn infants. Doses for children should be small. The young child is especially sensitive to the effects of antihistamines on the brain and nervous system.
By Those over 60 Years of Age: You may be more susceptible to the development of drowsiness, dizziness and unsteadiness, and to impairment of thinking, judgment and memory. This drug can increase the degree of impaired urination associated with prostate gland enlargement (prostatism). The sedative effects of antihistamines in the elderly can cause a syndrome of underactivity that may be misinterpreted as senility or emotional depression.

▷ Advisability of Use During Pregnancy
Pregnancy Category: B (tentative). See Pregnancy Code inside back cover.
Animal studies: No birth defects due to this drug reported in test animals.
Human studies: Information from adequate studies of pregnant women is not available. However, there have been no reports of birth defects attributed to this drug in over 20 years of wide use.
Use this drug only if clearly needed. Ask your physician for guidance.

Advisability of Use if Breast-Feeding
Presence of this drug in breast milk: Yes.
Avoid drug or refrain from nursing.

Habit-Forming Potential: None.

Effects of Overdosage: Drowsiness; unsteadiness; faintness; marked dryness of mouth, nose and throat; flushing of face; shortness of breath; hallucinations; convulsions; stupor progressing to coma.

Possible Effects of Long-Term Use: Tardive dyskinesia (see Glossary) has been reported in association with the long-term use of several widely used antihistamines. It is advisable to avoid the prolonged, continual use of antihistamines without interruption.

Suggested Periodic Examinations While Taking This Drug   (at physician's discretion)

Complete blood cell counts.

▷ **While Taking This Drug, Observe the Following**
Foods: No restrictions.
Beverages: No restrictions. May be taken with milk.

▷   *Alcohol*: Use with extreme caution until the combined effects have been determined. The combination of antihistamine and alcohol can produce rapid and marked sedation.
Tobacco Smoking: No interactions expected.

▷   *Other Drugs*
Triprolidine may *increase* the effects of
• all sedatives, sleep-inducing drugs, tranquilizers, analgesics and narcotic drugs, and produce oversedation.
Triprolidine *taken concurrently* with
• phenytoin (Dilantin) may cause phenytoin toxicity, and may alter the pattern of seizures. Dosage adjustments may be necessary.
The following drugs may *increase* the effects of triprolidine
• monoamine oxidase (MAO) inhibitor drugs (see Drug Class, Section Four) may prolong the action of antihistamines.

▷   *Driving, Hazardous Activities*: This drug can impair mental alertness, judgment, coordination and reaction time. Avoid hazardous activities until the full sedative effects have been determined.
Aviation Note: The use of this drug *is a disqualification* for piloting. Consult a designated Aviation Medical Examiner.
Exposure to Sun: Use caution. Some drugs of this class can cause photosensitivity (see Glossary).

VALPROIC ACID
(val PROH ik)

Introduced: 1967

Class: Anticonvulsant

Prescription: USA: Yes
Canada: Yes

Controlled Drug: USA: No
Canada: No

Available as Generic: USA: Yes
Canada: No

Brand Names: Depakene, Depakote

```
┌─────────────────────────────────────────────────────────────────┐
│                     BENEFITS versus RISKS                         │
│                                                                   │
│        Possible Benefits              Possible Risks              │
│   EFFECTIVE CONTROL OF           LIVER TOXICITY, infrequent but   │
│     MULTIPLE SEIZURE TYPES:        may be severe                  │
│     ABSENCE SEIZURES, TONIC-     Rare reduction of blood platelets│
│     CLONIC SEIZURES,               and impaired platelet function │
│     MYOCLONIC SEIZURES,            with risk of bleeding          │
│     PSYCHOMOTOR SEIZURES                                          │
│     when used adjunctively with                                   │
│     other antiseizure drugs                                       │
└─────────────────────────────────────────────────────────────────┘
```

▷ **Principal Uses**

As a Single Drug Product: Used effectively in the management of the following types of epilepsy: simple and complex absence seizures (petit mal); tonic-clonic seizures (grand mal); myoclonic seizures; complex partial seizures (psychomotor, temporal lobe epilepsy). It is sometimes used adjunctively with other anticonvulsants as needed.

How This Drug Works: Not completely established. It is thought that by increasing the availability of the nerve impulse transmitter gamma-aminobutyric acid (GABA), this drug suppresses the spread of abnormal electrical discharges that cause seizures.

Available Dosage Forms and Strengths

Capsules — 250 mg

Syrup — 250 mg per 5 ml teaspoonful

Tablets, enteric coated — 125 mg, 250 mg, 500 mg

▷ **Usual Adult Dosage Range:** Initially, 15 mg/kg/24 hours. The dose is increased cautiously by 5 to 10 mg/kg/24 hours every 7 days as needed and tolerated. *The usual daily dose is from 1000 mg to 1600 mg in divided doses*. The total daily dosage should not exceed 60 mg/kg. **Note: Actual dosage and administration schedule must be determined by the physician for each patient individually.**

Dosing Instructions: Preferably taken 1 hour before meals. However, it may be taken with or following food if necessary to prevent stomach irritation. The capsule should not be opened and the tablet should not be crushed for administration. Do not administer the syrup in carbonated beverages. It may be diluted in water or milk.

Usual Duration of Use: Continual use on a regular schedule for 2 weeks is usually necessary to determine this drug's effectiveness in reducing the frequency and severity of seizures. Long-term use (months to years) requires supervision and periodic evaluation by your physician.

▸ **This Drug Should Not Be Taken If**
- you have had an allergic reaction to it previously.
- you have active liver disease.
- you have an active bleeding disorder.

▷ **Inform Your Physician Before Taking This Drug If**
- you have a history of liver disease or impaired liver function.
- you have a history of any type of bleeding disorder.
- you are pregnant or planning pregnancy.
- you have myasthenia gravis.
- you are taking any of the following drugs: anticoagulants; other anticonvulsants; antidepressants, either the tricyclic type or monoamine oxidase (MAO) inhibitors (see Drug Classes, Section Four).
- you plan to have surgery or dental extraction in the near future.

Possible Side-Effects   (natural, expected and unavoidable drug actions)
Drowsiness and lethargy (5%).

▷ **Possible Adverse Effects**   (unusual, unexpected and infrequent reactions)
If any of the following develop, consult your physician promptly.
Mild Adverse Effects
Allergic Reactions: Skin rash (rare).
Headache, dizziness, confusion, unsteadiness, slurred speech.
Nausea, indigestion, stomach cramps, diarrhea.
Temporary loss of scalp hair.
Serious Adverse Effects
Idiosyncratic Reactions: Bizarre behavior, hallucinations.
Drug-induced hepatitis with jaundice (see Glossary).
Drug-induced pancreatitis.
Possible Reye syndrome (see Glossary).
Reduced formation of blood platelets and impaired function of platelets, with increased risk of abnormal bleeding.

▷ **Adverse Effects That May Mimic Natural Diseases or Disorders**
Liver reactions may suggest viral hepatitis.

CAUTION
1. The capsules and tablets should be swallowed whole without alteration to avoid irritation of the mouth and throat.
2. This drug can impair normal blood clotting mechanisms. In the event of injury, dental extraction, or need for surgery, inform your physician or dentist that you are taking this drug.
3. Because this drug can impair the normal function of blood platelets, it is advisable to avoid aspirin (which has the same effect).
4. Over-the-counter drug products that contain antihistamines (allergy and cold remedies, sleep aids) can enhance the sedative effects of this drug.

Precautions for Use
By Infants and Children: The concurrent use of aspirin with this drug can cause abnormal bleeding or bruising. Children with mental retardation, organic brain disease or severe seizure disorders may be at increased risk for severe liver toxicity while taking this drug. Observe closely for the development of fever that could indicate the onset of a drug-induced Reye syndrome (see Glossary). Avoid concurrent use of clonazepam

(Clonopin); the combined use could result in continuous petit mal episodes.

By Those over 60 Years of Age: Start treatment with small doses and increase dosage cautiously. Observe closely for excessive sedation, confusion or unsteadiness that could predispose to falling and injury.

▷ **Advisability of Use During Pregnancy**

Pregnancy Category: D (tentative). See Pregnancy Code inside back cover.

Animal studies: Palate and skeletal birth defects reported in mouse, rat and rabbit studies.

Human studies: Information from adequate studies of pregnant women is not available. There have been several reports of birth defects attributed to the use of this drug during early pregnancy.

Consult your physician regarding the advantages and disadvantages of using this drug. If it is used, it is advisable to keep the dose as low as possible.

Advisability of Use if Breast-Feeding

Presence of this drug in breast milk: Yes, in small amounts.

Monitor nursing infant closely and discontinue drug or nursing if adverse effects develop.

Habit-Forming Potential: None.

Effects of Overdosage: Increased drowsiness, weakness, unsteadiness, confusion, stupor progressing to coma.

Possible Effects of Long-Term Use: None reported.

Suggested Periodic Examinations While Taking This Drug (at physician's discretion)

Complete blood cell counts and baseline liver function tests should be done before treatment is started. During treatment, blood counts should be repeated every month and liver function tests repeated every 2 months.

▷ **While Taking This Drug, Observe the Following**

Foods: No restrictions.

Beverages: Do not administer the syrup in carbonated beverages; this could liberate the valproic acid and irritate the mouth and throat. This drug may be taken with milk.

Alcohol: Use extreme caution until the combined effects have been determined. Alcohol can increase the sedative effect of this drug. Also, this drug can increase the depressant effects of alcohol on brain function.

Tobacco Smoking: No interactions expected.

▷ *Other Drugs*

Valproic acid may *increase* the effects of

- anticoagulants (Coumadin, etc.), and increase the risk of bleeding.
- antidepressants, both monoamine oxidase (MAO) inhibitors and tricyclics, and cause toxicity.
- phenobarbital, and cause barbiturate intoxication.
- phenytoin (Dilantin), and cause phenytoin toxicity.

Valproic acid *taken concurrently* with
- antiplatelet drugs: aspirin, dipyridamole (Persantine), sulfinpyrazone (Anturane) may enhance the inhibition of platelet function and increase the risk of bleeding.

▷ *Driving, Hazardous Activities*: This drug may cause drowsiness, dizziness or confusion. Restrict activities as necessary.

Aviation Note: The use of this drug *is a disqualification* for piloting. Consult a designated Aviation Medical Examiner.

Exposure to Sun: No restrictions.

Discontinuation: **Do not discontinue this drug suddenly.** Abrupt withdrawal can cause repetitive seizures that are difficult to control.

VERAPAMIL
(ver AP a mil)

Introduced: 1967

Class: Antianginal, Calcium Channel Blocker

Prescription: USA: Yes
Canada: Yes

Controlled Drug: USA: No
Canada: No

Available as Generic: No

Brand Names: Calan, Isoptin

BENEFITS versus RISKS

Possible Benefits	*Possible Risks*
EFFECTIVE PREVENTION OF BOTH MAJOR TYPES OF ANGINA	Congestive heart failure Low blood pressure (2.9%) Heart rhythm disturbance Fluid retention (1.7%) Liver damage without jaundice (very rare)

▷ **Principal Uses**

As a Single Drug Product: Used primarily to treat (1) angina pectoris due to coronary artery spasm (Prinzmetal's variant angina) that occurs spontaneously and is not associated with exertion; and (2) classical angina-of-effort (due to atherosclerotic disease of the coronary arteries) in individuals who have not responded to or cannot tolerate the nitrates and "beta-blocker" drugs customarily used to treat this disorder.

How This Drug Works: Not completely established. It is thought that by blocking the normal passage of calcium through certain cell walls (which is necessary for the function of nerve and muscle tissue), this drug slows the spread of electrical activity through the conduction system of the heart and inhibits the contraction of coronary arteries and peripheral arterioles. As a result of these combined effects, this drug

- prevents spontaneous spasm of the coronary arteries (Prinzmetal's type of angina).
- reduces the rate and contraction force of the heart during exertion, thus lowering the oxygen requirement of the heart muscle; this reduces the occurrence of effort-induced angina (classical angina pectoris).
- reduces the degree of contraction of peripheral arterial walls, resulting in their relaxation and consequent lowering of blood pressure. This further reduces the work load of the heart during exertion and contributes to the prevention of angina.

Available Dosage Forms and Strengths

Injection — 5 mg per 2 ml
Tablets — 80 mg, 120 mg
Tablets, film coated — 80 mg, 120 mg

▷ **Usual Adult Dosage Range:** Initially, 80 mg 3 or 4 times daily. The dose may be increased gradually at 1 to 7 day intervals as needed and tolerated. The usual maintenance dose is from 240 mg to 480 mg daily in 3 or 4 divided doses. The total daily dosage should not exceed 480 mg. **Note: Actual dosage and administration schedule must be determined by the physician for each patient individually.**

▷ **Dosing Instructions:** Preferably taken before meals and at bedtime. The tablet may be crushed for administration.

Usual Duration of Use: Continual use on a regular schedule for 2 to 4 weeks is usually necessary to determine this drug's effectiveness in reducing the frequency and severity of angina. For long-term use (months to years), determine the smallest effective dose; this requires supervision and periodic evaluation by your physician.

▷ **This Drug Should Not Be Taken If**
- you have had an allergic reaction to it previously.
- you have active liver disease.
- you have a "sick sinus" syndrome (and do not have an artificial pacemaker).
- you have been told that you have a second-degree or third-degree heart block.
- you have low blood pressure—systolic pressure below 90.

▷ **Inform Your Physician Before Taking This Drug If**
- you have had an unfavorable response to any "calcium blocker" drug in the past.
- you are currently taking any other drugs, especially digitalis or a "beta-blocker" drug (see Drug Class, Section Four).
- you have had a recent stroke or heart attack.
- you have a history of congestive heart failure or heart rhythm disorders.
- you have impaired liver or kidney function.
- you have a history of drug-induced liver damage.

Possible Side-Effects (natural, expected and unavoidable drug actions)
Low blood pressure (2.9%), fluid retention (1.7%).

▷ **Possible Adverse Effects** (unusual, unexpected and infrequent reactions)
If any of the following develop, consult your physician promptly.
Mild Adverse Effects
Allergic Reactions: Skin rash, hives, itching, aching joints.
Headache (1.8%), dizziness (3.6%), fatigue (1.1%).
Nausea (1.6%), indigestion, constipation (6.3%).
Serious Adverse Effects
Serious disturbances of heart rate and/or rhythm, congestive heart failure
(0.9%).
Drug-induced liver damage without jaundice (very rare).

CAUTION
1. Be sure to inform all physicians and dentists you consult that you are
   taking this drug. Note the use of this drug on your card of personal
   identification.
2. You may use nitroglycerin and other nitrate drugs as needed to relieve
   acute episodes of angina pain. However, if you detect that your angina
   attacks are becoming more frequent or intense, notify your physician
   promptly.
3. If this drug is used concurrently with a "beta-blocker" drug, you may
   develop excessively low blood pressure.
4. This drug may cause swelling of the feet and ankles. This may not be
   indicative of either heart or kidney dysfunction.

Precautions for Use
By Infants and Children: Safety and effectiveness for use by those under 12
years of age have not been established.
By Those over 60 Years of Age: You may be more susceptible to the development of weakness, dizziness, fainting and falling. Take necessary precautions to prevent injury. Report promptly any changes in your pattern of
thirst and urination.

▷ **Advisability of Use During Pregnancy**
Pregnancy Category: C (tentative). See Pregnancy Code inside back cover.
Animal studies: Toxic effects on the embryo and retarded growth of the
fetus (but no birth defects) reported in rat studies.
Human studies: Information from adequate studies of pregnant women is
not available.
Avoid this drug during the first 3 months. Use during the last 6 months only
if clearly needed. Ask your physician for guidance.

Advisability of Use if Breast-Feeding
Presence of this drug in breast milk: Possibly yes.
Avoid drug or refrain from nursing.

Habit-Forming Potential: None.

Effects of Overdosage: Flushed and warm skin, sweating, light-headedness,
irritability, rapid heart rate, low blood pressure, loss of consciousness.

Possible Effects of Long-Term Use: None reported.

Suggested Periodic Examinations While Taking This Drug   (at physician's discretion)
> Evaluations of heart function, including electrocardiograms; liver and kidney function tests, with long-term use.

▷ **While Taking This Drug, Observe the Following**
> *Foods*: No restrictions. Avoid excessive salt intake.
> *Beverages*: No restrictions. May be taken with milk.

▷ *Alcohol*: Use with caution until combined effects have been determined. Alcohol may exaggerate the drop in blood pressure experienced by some individuals.
> *Tobacco Smoking*: Nicotine can reduce the effectiveness of this drug. Avoid all forms of tobacco.
> *Marijuana Smoking*: Possible reduced effectiveness of this drug; mild to moderate increase in angina; possible changes in electrocardiogram, confusing interpretation.

▷ *Other Drugs*
> Verapamil may *increase* the effects of
> - carbamazepine (Tegretol), and cause carbamazepine toxicity.
> - digitoxin and digoxin, and cause digitalis toxicity.
>
> Verapamil *taken concurrently* with
> - "beta-blocker" drugs (see Drug Class, Section Four) may affect heart rate and rhythm adversely. Careful monitoring by your physician is necessary if these drugs are taken concurrently.
>
> The following drugs may *increase* the effects of verapamil
> - cimetidine (Tagamet).

▷ *Driving, Hazardous Activities*: Usually no restrictions. This drug may cause dizziness. Restrict activities as necessary.
> *Aviation Note*: Coronary artery disease *is a disqualification* for piloting. Consult a designated Aviation Medical Examiner.
> *Exposure to Sun*: Use caution until sensitivity has been determined. This drug may cause photosensitivity (see Glossary).
> *Exposure to Heat*: Caution advised. Hot environments can exaggerate the blood-pressure-lowering effects of this drug. Observe for light-headedness or weakness.
> *Heavy Exercise or Exertion*: This drug may improve your ability to be more active without resulting angina pain. Use caution and avoid excessive exercise that could impair heart function in the absence of warning pain.
> *Discontinuation*: Do not discontinue this drug abruptly. Consult your physician regarding gradual withdrawal to prevent the development of rebound angina.

VITAMIN C
(VIT a min)

Other Names: Ascorbic Acid

Introduced: 1933   **Class:** Vitamins

Prescription: USA: No   **Controlled Drug:** USA: No
   Canada: No   Canada: No

Available as Generic: Yes

Brand Names: ✿Apo-C, Ascorbicap, Cecon, C-Long, Cetane, Cevalin, Cevi-Bid
   Ce-Vi-Sol, ✿Effer-C, ✿Redoxon

BENEFITS versus RISKS

Possible Benefits	*Possible Risks*
PREVENTION AND TREATMENT OF SCURVY (VITAMIN C DEFICIENCY)	Kidney stone formation (chronic use of large doses)
Effective adjunct in the treatment of some types of anemia	Diarrhea in sensitive individuals (large doses)
Maintenance of an acid urine (large doses)	
Questionable prevention of headcolds	

▷ **Principal Uses**

As a Single Drug Product: Used most commonly at this time in large daily doses to reduce the frequency, severity and duration of headcolds. It is used less frequently to acidify the urine in those individuals who are susceptible to recurrent infections of the urinary tract.

As a Combination Drug Product [CD]: Available in a large variety of combinations that include multiple vitamins and minerals. These preparations are used as nutritional supplements. It is also available in combination with iron to enhance the absorption and utilization of iron in correcting iron deficiency anemia.

How This Drug Works: Not completely established. It is thought that vitamin C plays an essential role in the enzyme activity involved in the formation of collagen (structural material in skin, tendon, cartilage, bone, teeth and connective tissue). It enhances the absorption of iron and contributes to the formation of hemoglobin and red blood cells in the bone marrow. By acidifying the urine, vitamin C creates an environment that is unfavorable for the growth of certain bacteria that commonly infect the urinary tract. This action also enhances the therapeutic effects of some widely used anti-infective drugs.

Note: There is insufficient scientific evidence to establish that vitamin C in large doses is significantly beneficial in the prevention or treatment of the common cold. Individual experience varies greatly. For those who find that the benefits of using vitamin C in large doses clearly outweigh the small risks involved, no significant toxicity is anticipated.

Available Dosage Forms and Strengths

Capsules, prolonged action — 500 mg
Crystals — 4 grams per teaspoonful
Injections — 100 mg per ml, 250 mg per ml, 500 mg per ml
Liquid — 35 mg per 0.6 ml
Powder — 4 grams per teaspoonful
Solution — 100 mg per ml
Syrup — 20 mg per ml, 500 mg per 5 ml teaspoonful
Tablets — 25 mg, 50 mg, 100 mg, 250 mg, 500 mg, 1000 mg, 1500 mg
Tablets, chewable — 100 mg, 250 mg, 500 mg
Tablets, effervescent — 1000 mg
Tablets, prolonged action — 500 mg, 750 mg, 1000 mg, 1500 mg

▷ **Usual Adult Dosage Range:**   As dietary supplement: 50 to 100 mg/day. During chronic dialysis: 100 to 200 mg/day. For correction of deficiency: 100 to 250 mg 1 to 3 times/day. As urinary acidifier: 1 to 3 grams/4 hours.
Recommended Dietary Allowances (RDA) for daily intake:
Children 4 to 6 years of age: 45 mg
Adult males: 60 mg
Adult females: 60 mg
Pregnant females: 80 mg
Breast-feeding females: 100 mg

▷ **Dosing Instructions:**   May be taken without regard to eating. The prolonged-action dosage forms should be taken whole without alteration.

▷ **This Drug Should Not Be Taken If**
- you have had an allergic reaction to a vitamin C drug product previously. Ask your physician for guidance.

▷ **Inform Your Physician Before Taking This Drug If**
- you have a history of kidney stones.
- you have gout.
- you have sickle cell anemia.
- you are taking oral anticoagulants.

Possible Side-Effects   (natural, expected and unavoidable drug actions)
None.

▷ **Possible Adverse Effects**   (unusual, unexpected and infrequent reactions)
If any of the following develop, consult your physician promptly.
Mild Adverse Effects
Diarrhea, with large doses.
Serious Adverse Effects
Idiosyncratic Reactions: Hemolytic anemia (see Glossary).

Formation of cystine, oxalate or urate kidney stones, with large doses. Precipitation of crisis in individuals with sickle cell anemia.

CAUTION

1. Some vitamin C preparations for oral use contain sodium ascorbate as the principal component. For individuals on a low-sodium diet, this intake of sodium could be significant. Consult your physician regarding dosage.
2. It is advisable to avoid large doses of vitamin C while taking sulfonamide ("sulfa") drugs.
3. Large doses of vitamin C may cause a false positive test result for urine sugar when testing with Benedict's solution, and a false negative test result when testing with Clinistix or Tes-Tape.
4. Large doses of vitamin C may cause a false negative test result for blood in the stool (fecal blood) when testing with the Hemoccult slide method.

Precautions for Use

By Those over 60 Years of Age: If you use large doses of vitamin C (1 gram or more) daily, it is advisable to drink 2 quarts of liquids daily to ensure a dilute urine and thus reduce the risk of kidney stone formation. Consult your physician regarding the advisability and safety of a large fluid intake.

▷ **Advisability of Use During Pregnancy**

Pregnancy Category: B (tentative). See Pregnancy Code inside back cover.

Animal studies: No birth defects due to this drug reported.

Human studies: Information from adequate studies of pregnant women is not available.

Adhere to the recommended dose of 80 mg/day. Avoid large doses. An excessive intake during pregnancy can accustom the fetus to larger than normal vitamin C stores; following delivery, the newborn infant can develop a scurvylike condition because of the abrupt reduction of vitamin C intake.

Advisability of Use if Breast-Feeding

Adhere to the recommended dose of 100 mg/day. Avoid large doses.

Habit-Forming Potential: None.

Effects of Overdosage: Diarrhea.

Possible Effects of Long-Term Use: Formation of kidney stones in predisposed individuals.

Suggested Periodic Examinations While Taking This Drug (at physician's discretion)

None required.

▷ **While Taking This Drug, Observe the Following**

Foods: No restrictions.

Beverages: No restrictions.

▷   *Alcohol*: No interactions expected.

Tobacco Smoking: Smoking appears to increase the requirement for vitamin C. The reason for this is not known.

▷ *Other Drugs*

Vitamin C (in large doses) may *increase* the effects of

- aspirin. Vitamin C, taken as ascorbic acid and in large doses, may acidify the urine in some individuals and cause aspirin accumulation to toxic levels.
- sulfonamide drugs (see Drug Class, Section Four).

Vitamin C (in large doses) may *decrease* the effects of

- anticoagulants (Coumadin, etc.), and reduce their protective value.

Exposure to Sun: No restrictions.

Occurrence of Unrelated Illness: Vitamin C requirements are increased during pregnancy, breast-feeding, active peptic ulcer, infections and with over-active thyroid states; also following surgery, injuries and burns. Consult your physician regarding the use of supplementary vitamin C prior to surgery.

WARFARIN
(WAR far in)

Introduced: 1941

Prescription: USA: Yes
Canada: Yes

Available as Generic: USA: Yes
Canada: No

Class: Anticoagulant, Coumarins

Controlled Drug: USA: No
Canada: No

Brand Names: ✦Athrombin-K, Coumadin, Panwarfin, ✦Warfilone

BENEFITS versus RISKS

Possible Benefits
EFFECTIVE PREVENTION OF
  BOTH ARTERIAL AND VENOUS
  THROMBOSIS
EFFECTIVE PREVENTION OF
  EMBOLIZATION IN
  THROMBOEMBOLIC
  DISORDERS

Possible Risks
NARROW TREATMENT RANGE
Dose-related bleeding (5% to 7%)
Skin and soft tissue hemorrhage
  with tissue death (rare)

▷ **Principal Uses**

As a Single Drug Product: Used exclusively for its anticoagulant effect in treating the following conditions: (1) acute thrombosis (clot) or thrombophlebitis of the deep veins; (2) acute pulmonary embolism, resulting from blood clots that originate anywhere in the body; (3) atrial fibrillation, to prevent clotting of blood inside the heart that could result in embolization of small clots to any part of the body; (4) acute myocardial infarction (heart attack), to prevent clotting and embolization; (5) transient ischemic attack (TIA), a temporary reduction of blood flow to a part of the brain; used here to reduce the risk of repeated attacks or possible stroke. Other possible uses include the long-term prevention of recurrent heart attack, and prevention of embolization from the heart in those individuals with artificial heart valves.

How This Drug Works: The coumarin anticoagulants interfere with the production of four essential blood clotting factors by blocking the action of vitamin K. This leads to a deficiency of these clotting factors in circulating blood and inhibits blood clotting mechanisms.

Available Dosage Forms and Strengths
    Injection — 50 mg/vial
    Tablets — 2 mg, 2.5 mg, 5 mg, 7.5 mg, 10 mg

▷ **Usual Adult Dosage Range:**   Initially, 10 to 15 mg daily for 2 to 3 days. A large loading dose is inappropriate and may be hazardous. For maintenance, 2 to 10 mg/day. The dosage is adjusted according to the prothrombin time. **Note: Actual dosage and administration schedule must be determined by the physician for each patient individually.**

▷ **Dosing Instructions:**   Preferably taken when the stomach is empty, and at the same time each day to ensure uniform results. The tablet may be crushed for administration.

Usual Duration of Use: Continual use on a regular schedule for 3 to 5 days is usually necessary to determine this drug's effectiveness in providing significant anticoagulation. An additional 10 to 14 days is required to determine the optimal maintenance dose for each individual. Long-term use (months to years) requires supervision and periodic evaluation by your physician.

▷ **This Drug Should Not Be Taken If**
   • you have had an allergic reaction to it previously.
   • you have an active peptic ulcer or active ulcerative colitis.
   • you have had a recent stroke.

▷ **Inform Your Physician Before Taking This Drug If**
   • you are now taking *any other drugs*, either prescription drugs or over-the-counter drug products.
   • you are pregnant or planning pregnancy.
   • you have a history of a bleeding disorder.
   • you have high blood pressure.
   • you have abnormally heavy or prolonged menstrual bleeding.
   • you have diabetes.
   • you are using an indwelling catheter.
   • you have impaired liver or kidney function.
   • you plan to have surgery or dental extraction in the near future.

Possible Side-Effects   (natural, expected and unavoidable drug actions)
Minor episodes of bleeding may occur even though dosage and prothrombin times are well within the recommended range.

▷ **Possible Adverse Effects**   (unusual, unexpected and infrequent reactions)
If any of the following develop, consult your physician promptly.
Mild Adverse Effects
Allergic Reactions: Skin rash, hives.
Loss of scalp hair.
Loss of appetite, nausea, vomiting, cramping, diarrhea.
Serious Adverse Effects
Allergic Reactions: Drug fever (see Glossary).
Idiosyncratic Reactions: Bleeding into skin and soft tissues causing gangrene of breast, toes and localized areas anywhere (rare).
Abnormal bleeding from nose, gastrointestinal tract, urinary tract or uterus.

▷ **Adverse Effects That May Mimic Natural Diseases or Disorders**
Drug-induced fever may suggest infection.

Natural Diseases or Disorders That May Be Activated by This Drug
Bleeding from "silent" peptic ulcer, intestinal or bladder polyp or tumor.

CAUTION
1. Always carry with you a card of personal identification that includes a statement that *you are taking an anticoagulant drug.*
2. While taking this drug, always consult your physician *before* starting any new drug, changing the dosage schedule of any drug or discontinuing any drug.

Precautions for Use
By Those over 60 Years of Age: Small doses are mandatory until your individual sensitivity has been determined. Observe regularly for indications of excessive drug effects: prolonged bleeding from shaving cuts, bleeding gums, bloody urine, rectal bleeding, excessive bruising.

> **Advisability of Use During Pregnancy**
Pregnancy Category: X. See Pregnancy Code inside back cover.
Animal studies: Fetal hemorrhage and death due to this drug reported in mice.
Human studies: Information from studies of pregnant women indicates fetal defects and fetal hemorrhage due to this drug.
The manufacturers state that this drug is contraindicated during entire pregnancy.

Advisability of Use if Breast-Feeding
Presence of this drug in breast milk: Yes.
Avoid drug or refrain from nursing.

Habit-Forming Potential: None.

Effects of Overdosage: Episodes of bleeding from minor surface bleeding (nose, gums, small lacerations) to major internal bleeding: vomiting blood, bloody urine or stool.

Possible Effects of Long-Term Use: None reported.

Suggested Periodic Examinations While Taking This Drug (at physician's discretion)
Regular determinations of prothrombin time are essential to safe dosage and proper control.
Urine analyses for blood.

▷ **While Taking This Drug, Observe the Following**
Foods: A larger intake than usual of foods rich in vitamin K may reduce the effectiveness of this drug and make larger doses necessary. Foods rich in vitamin K include: asparagus, bacon, beef liver, cabbage, cauliflower, fish, green leafy vegetables.
Beverages: No restrictions. May be taken with milk.
▷ *Alcohol*: Limit alcohol to one drink daily. Note: Heavy users of alcohol with liver damage may be very sensitive to anticoagulants and require smaller than usual doses.
Tobacco Smoking: Heavy smokers may require relatively larger doses of this drug.
▷ *Other Drugs*
Warfarin may *increase* the effects of
• phenytoin (Dilantin).
The following drugs may *increase* the effects of warfarin
• amiodarone.
• androgens.
• cephalosporins.
• chloral hydrate.
• cimetidine.
• clofibrate.
• dextrothyroxine.
• disulfiram.
• glucagon.
• metronidazole.
• phenylbutazone.
• quinidine.
• salicylates.
• sulfinpyrazone.
• sulfonamides.
• thyroid hormones.
The following drugs may *decrease* the effects of warfarin
• barbiturates.
• carbamazepine.
• cholestyramine.
• ethchlorvynol.
• glutethimide.

- griseofulvin.
- rifampin.
- vitamin K.

▷ *Driving, Hazardous Activities*: No restrictions.

Aviation Note: The use of this drug *is a disqualification* for piloting. Consult a designated Aviation Medical Examiner.

Exposure to Sun: No restrictions.

Discontinuation: Do not discontinue this drug abruptly unless abnormal bleeding occurs. Ask your physician for guidance regarding gradual reduction in dosage over a period of 3 to 4 weeks.

DRUG CLASSES

Drug Classes

Throughout the Drug Profiles in Section Three reference is made to various drug classes. The reader may be advised to consult Section Four to become familiar with the drugs which belong to a particular class of drugs that share important characteristics in their chemical composition or in their actions within the body. Often it is important to know that *any* drug (or *all* drugs) within a given class can be expected to behave in a particular way. Such information may be useful in preventing interactions that could reduce the effectiveness of the drugs in use or result in unanticipated and sometimes hazardous adverse effects.

The presentation of each Drug Class is divided into two listings. The upper list contains the more widely recognized brand names of the drugs within the class; the lower list contains the generic names of the class members. In some instances the number of brand names in use is so large that a complete listing is not possible. In such cases, to be certain that you are consulting the correct drug class, determine the generic name of the drug that concerns you and consult the lower list to see if it is included there. The generic name listing is sufficiently complete to serve the scope of this book.

The following page lists the names of all the Drug Classes included in this section.

LIST OF DRUG CLASSES

Amphetaminelike Drugs
Analgesics, Mild
Analgesics, Strong (Narcotic Drugs)
Antiacne Drugs
Antiallergic Drugs
Antianginal Drugs
Antiarthritic/Anti-inflammatory Drugs (Aspirin Substitutes)
Antiasthmatic Drugs (Bronchodilators)
Antibiotics
Anticoagulants
Antidepressants
Antidiabetics, Oral (Sulfonylureas)
Antidiarrheal Drugs
Antiepileptic Drugs (Anticonvulsants)
Antiglaucoma Drugs
Antigout Drugs
Antihistamines
Antihypertensives
Anti-itching Drugs (Antipruritics)
Antimicrobial Drugs (Nonantibiotic)
Anti-motion Sickness/Antinausea Drugs (Antiemetics)
Antiparkinsonism Drugs
Antispasmodics, Synthetic
Appetite Suppressants (Anorexiants)
Atropinelike Drugs
Barbiturates
Benzodiazepines
Beta-Adrenergic Blocking Drugs ("Beta-Blockers")
Calcium Channel Blocking Drugs ("Calcium Blockers")

Cephalosporins
Cholesterol-Reducing Drugs
Cortisonelike Drugs (Adrenocortical Steroids)
Cough Suppressants (Antitussives)
Decongestants
Digitalis Preparations
Diuretics
Female Sex Hormones
Fever-Reducing Drugs (Antipyretics)
Heart Rhythm Regulators (Antiarrhythmic Drugs)
Histamine (H-2) Blocking Drugs ("H-2 Blockers")
Male Sex Hormones (Androgens)
Monoamine Oxidase (MAO) Inhibitor Drugs
Muscle Relaxants
Nitrates
Penicillins
Phenothiazines
Salicylates
Sedatives/Sleep Inducers, Nonbarbiturate (Hypnotics)
Sulfonamides ("Sulfa" Drugs)
Sulfonylureas
Tetracyclines
Thiazide Diuretics
Tranquilizers, Mild (Antianxiety Drugs)
Tranquilizers, Strong (Antipsychotic Drugs)
Vasodilators
Xanthines

AMPHETAMINELIKE DRUGS

BRAND NAMES

Amodex
Benzedrine
Biphetamine
Desoxyn
Dexatrim
Dexedrine

Didrex
Fastin
Ionamin
Obalan
Plegine
Preludin

Ritalin
Tenuate
Tepanil
Tora
Wilpowr

GENERIC NAMES

amphetamine
benzphetamine
dextroamphetamine
diethylpropion
levamphetamine
methamphetamine

methylphenidate
phendimetrazine
phenmetrazine
phentermine
phenylpropanolamine

ANALGESICS, MILD

BRAND NAMES

Anaprox
A.S.A. Preparations
2 Darvocet
Darvon
Datril

Hycodan
Indocin
3 Motrin
Nebs
2 Percodan

Talwin
Taper
Tempra
Tylenol 1
Valadol

GENERIC NAMES

1 acetaminophen
aspirin
codeine
hydrocodone
3 ibuprofen
indomethacin

naproxen
2 oxycodone
paregoric
pentazocine
2 propoxyphene

ANALGESICS, STRONG

(Narcotic Drugs)

BRAND NAMES

Demerol
⦚ Dilaudid
Dolophine
Leritine

GENERIC NAMES

anileridine
⦚ hydromorphone
meperidine
methadone
morphine

ANTIACNE DRUGS

BRAND NAMES

Accutane
Achromycin V
Eryderm
Lucidol
Retin-A

GENERIC NAMES

benzoyl peroxide
erythromycin
isotretinoin
tetracycline
tretinoin

ANTIALLERGIC DRUGS

See: Antihistamines
Cortisonelike Drugs

ANTIANGINAL DRUGS

BRAND NAMES

Calan
Cardizem
Corgard
Inderal
Isoptin
Isordil

Nitrostat
Peritrate
Persantine
Procardia
Tenormin

GENERIC NAMES

beta-blockers (see Class)
diltiazem
dipyridamole

nifedipine
nitrates (see Class)
verapamil

ANTIARTHRITIC/ANTI-INFLAMMATORY DRUGS

(Aspirin Substitutes)

BRAND NAMES

Clinoral
Dolobid
Feldene
Indocin
Meclomen
Motrin

Nalfon
Naprosyn
Orudis
Suprol
Tolectin

GENERIC NAMES

diflunisal
fenoprofen
ibuprofen
indomethacin
ketoprofen
meclofenamate

naproxen
piroxicam
sulindac
suprofen
tolmetin

ANTIASTHMATIC DRUGS

(Bronchodilators)

BRAND NAMES

Aarane
Adrenalin
Alupent
Aminodur
Brethine
Bricanyl
Bronkodyl
Bronkometer
Bronkosol
Bronkotabs

Choledyl
Elixophyllin
Intal
Isuprel
Lufyllin
Medihaler-Epi
Medihaler-Iso
Metaprel
Neothylline
Norisodrine

Proternol
Proventil
Slo-Phyllin
Somophylline
Sus-Phrine
Theolair
Tornalate
Vaponefrin
Ventolin

GENERIC NAMES

albuterol
aminophylline
bitolterol
cromolyn
dyphylline
ephedrine
epinephrine

isoetharine
isoproterenol
metaproterenol
oxtriphylline
terbutaline
theophylline

ANTIBIOTICS

BRAND NAMES

See respective Classes listed under Generic Names

GENERIC NAMES

cephalosporins
chloramphenicol
clindamycin
erythromycins

lincomycin
penicillins
rifampin
tetacyclines

ANTICOAGULANTS

Coumarin Class

BRAND NAMES

Coumadin
Dicumarol
Liquamar
Panwarfin
Sintrom
Tromexan

GENERIC NAMES

acenocoumarol
dicumarol
phenprocoumon
warfarin

Indandione Class

BRAND NAMES

Danilone
Dipaxin
Eridione
Hedulin
Miradon

GENERIC NAMES

anisindione
diphenadione
phenindione

ANTIDEPRESSANTS
Tricyclic Antidepressants

<u>BRAND NAMES</u>

Adapin
Asendin
Aventyl
x Elavil
Endep
Loxitane
Norpramin

x Pamelor
Pertofrane
Presamine
Sinequan
Surmontil
Tofranil
Vivactil

<u>GENERIC NAMES</u>

amitriptyline
amoxapine
desipramine
doxepin
imipramine

loxapine
nortriptyline
protriptyline
trimipramine

Tetracyclic Antidepressants

<u>BRAND NAMES</u>

Ludiomil

<u>GENERIC NAMES</u>

maprotiline

Other Antidepressants

<u>BRAND NAMES</u>

Desyrel

<u>GENERIC NAMES</u>

trazodone

ANTIDIABETICS, ORAL

Sulfonylurea Class

BRAND NAMES

Chloronase

DiaBeta

Diabinese

Dimelor

Dymelor

Euglucon

Glucotrol

Micronase

Mobenol

Orinase

Stabinol

Tolinase

GENERIC NAMES

acetohexamide

chlorpropamide

glipizide

glyburide

tolazamide

tolbutamide

ANTIDIARRHEAL DRUGS

BRAND NAMES

Donnagel

Imodium

Kaopectate

Lomotil

Parepectolin

GENERIC NAMES

atropine

diphenoxylate

kaolin

loperimide

paregoric

pectin

ANTIEPILEPTIC DRUGS

(Anticonvulsants)

BRAND NAMES

Clonopin
Y Depakene
✗ Diamox
Y Dilantin
Luminal

Mysoline
✗ Tegretol
N Valium
✗ Zarontin

GENERIC NAMES

acetazolamide
carbamazepine
clonazepam
/ diazepam
ethosuximide

phenobarbital
2 phenytoin
primidone
valproic acid

ANTIGLAUCOMA DRUGS

BRAND NAMES

Diamox
Glaucon
Isopto-carpine
Timoptic

GENERIC NAMES

acetazolamide
epinephrine
pilocarpine
timolol

ANTIGOUT DRUGS

BRAND NAMES

Anaprox
Anturane
Benemid
Clinoril
✗ Naprosyn
Zyloprim

GENERIC NAMES

allopurinol
colchicine
naproxen
probenecid
sulfinpyrazone
sulindac

ANTIHISTAMINES

BRAND NAMES

Actidil	Dramamine	Optimine
Atarax	Hispril	Periactin
Benadryl	Histadyl	Phenergan
Bonine	Histalon	Pyribenzamine
Chlor-Trimeton	Inhiston	Seldane
Clistin	Marezine	Tavist
Decapryn	Neo-Antergan	Trimeton
Dimetane	Norflex	Vistaril

GENERIC NAMES

azatadine	dimenhydrinate	orphenadrine
brompheniramine	diphenhydramine	pheniramine
carbinoxamine	diphenylpyraline	promethazine
chlorpheniramine	doxylamine	pyrilamine
clemastine	hydroxyzine	terfenidine
cyclizine	meclizine	tripelennamine
cyproheptadine	methapyrilene	triprolidine

ANTIHYPERTENSIVES

BRAND NAMES

Aldomet
Anhydron
Apresoline
Blocadren
Capoten
Catapres
Corgard
Diuril
Enduron
Esbaloid
Esidrix
Eutonyl

Exna
HydroDiuril
Hygroton
Inderal
Inversine
Ismelin
Lasix
Loniten
Lopressor
Lozol
Minipress

Naqua
Naturetin
Normodyne
Renese
Saluron
Sectral
Serpasil
Tenormin
Trandate
Vasotec
Visken

GENERIC NAMES

bendroflumethiazide
benzthiazide
beta-blockers (see
   Class)
bethanidine
captopril
chlorothiazide
chlorthalidone
clonidine

cyclothiazide
enalapril
furosemide
guanethidine
hydralazine
hydrochlorothiazide
hydroflumethiazide
indapamide
mecamylamine

methyclothiazide
methyldopa
minoxidil
pargyline
polythiazide
prazosin
reserpine
trichlormethiazide

ANTI-ITCHING DRUGS

(Antipruritics)

BRAND NAMES

Atarax
Cortaid
Dermolate
Periactin
Temaril
Vistaril

GENERIC NAMES

cortisonelike drugs (see Class)
cyproheptadine
hydroxyzine
trimeprazine

ANTIMICROBIAL DRUGS

(Nonantibiotic)

BRAND NAMES

Bactrim   Macrodantin
Flagyl   NegGram
Furadantin   Septra
Gantrisin

GENERIC NAMES

metronidazole
nalidixic acid
nitrofurantoin
sulfonamides (see Class)
trimethoprim

ANTI-MOTION SICKNESS/ANTINAUSEA DRUGS

(Antiemetics)

BRAND NAMES

Antivert
Atarax
Benadryl
Bonine
Compazine
Dexedrine

Dramamine
Marezine
Phenergan
Thorazine
Tigan
Vistaril

GENERIC NAMES

chlorpromazine
cyclizine
dextroamphetamine
dimenhydrinate
diphenhydramine
hydroxyzine

meclizine
prochlorperazine
promethazine
scopolamine
trimethobenzamide

ANTIPARKINSONISM DRUGS

BRAND NAMES

Akineton
Artane
Bendopa
Biodopa
Cogentin
Disipal
Dopar

Kemadrin
Larodopa
ʀ Levodopa
Norflex
Pagitane
Parda
Parlodel

Parsidol
Phenoxene
Pipanol
Sinemet
Symmetrel
Tremin

GENERIC NAMES

amantadine
benztropine
biperiden
bromocriptine
chlorphenoxamine
cycrimine

ethopropazine
levodopa
orphenadrine
procyclidine
trihexyphenidyl

ANTISPASMODICS, SYNTHETIC

BRAND NAMES

Antrenyl
Banthine
Bentyl
Cantil
Darbid

Nacton
Pamine
Pathilon
Prantal
Pro-Banthine

Quarzan
Robinul
Tral
Trocinate

GENERIC NAMES

clidinium
dicyclomine
diphemanil
glycopyrrolate
hexocyclium

isopropamide
mepenzolate
methantheline
methscopolamine
oxyphenonium

poldine
propantheline
thiphenamil
tridihexethyl

APPETITE SUPPRESSANTS

(Anorexiants)

BRAND NAMES

Dexedrine
Dietac
Fastin
Ionamin
Plegine
Pondimin

Preludin
Pre-Sate
Sanorex
Tenuate
Tepanil

GENERIC NAMES

chlorphentermine
dextroamphetamine
diethylpropion
fenfluramine
mazindol

phendimetrazine
phenmetrazine
phentermine
phenylpropanolamine

ATROPINELIKE DRUGS

The drugs included in the following groups may exhibit atropinelike (anticholinergic) action. This can be important in the management of certain diseases and in potential interactions with other drugs used concurrently.

All drugs containing:

atropine   Antidepressants, tricyclic
belladonna   Antihistamines (some)
hyoscyamine   Antiparkinsonism Drugs (some)
scopolamine   Antispasmodics, Synthetic
                            Muscle Relaxants (some)

BARBITURATES

BRAND NAMES

Alurate   Mebaral
Amytal   Nembutal
Butisol   Sandoptal
Lotusate   Seconal
Luminal   Sombulex

GENERIC NAMES

amobarbital   mephobarbital
aprobarbital   pentobarbital
butabarbital   phenobarbital
butalbital   secobarbital
hexobarbital   talbutal

BENZODIAZEPINES

BRAND NAMES

Ativan	Paxipam
Centrax	Restoril
Clonopin	Serax
Dalmane	Tranxene
Halcion	Valium
Libritabs	Verstran
Librium	Xanax

GENERIC NAMES

alprazolam	halazepam
chlordiazepoxide	lorazepam
clonazepam	oxazepam
clorazepate	prazepam
diazepam	temazepam
flurazepam	triazolam

BETA-ADRENERGIC BLOCKING DRUGS

("Beta-Blockers")

BRAND NAMES

Blocadren	Sectral
Corgard	Tenormin
Inderal	Trandate
Lopressor	Visken
Normodyne	

GENERIC NAMES

acebutolol	nadolol
atenolol	pindolol
labetalol	propranolol
metoprolol	timolol

CALCIUM CHANNEL BLOCKING DRUGS

("Calcium Blockers")

BRAND NAMES

Calan
Cardizem
Isoptin
Procardia

GENERIC NAMES

diltiazem
nifedipine
verapamil

CEPHALOSPORINS

BRAND NAMES

Anspor
Ceclor
Ceporex
Duricef

Keflex
Novolexin
Ultracef
Velosef

GENERIC NAMES

cefaclor
cefadroxil
cephalexin
cephradine

CHOLESTEROL-REDUCING DRUGS

BRAND NAMES

Atromid S
Choloxin
Colestid
Cytellin

Lorelco
Nicobid
Questran

GENERIC NAMES

cholestyramine
clofibrate
colestipol
dextrothyroxine

nicotinic acid (niacin)
probucol
sitosterols

CORTISONELIKE DRUGS

(Adrenocortical Steroids)

BRAND NAMES

Aristocort
Colisone
Cortef
Cortril
Decadron
Delta-Cortef
Deltasone
Deltra
Deronil
Dexameth

Dexamethadrone
Dexasone
Gammacorten
Hexadrol
Hydeltra
Hydrocortone
Inflamase
Kenacort
Maxidex
Medrol

Meticorten
Novadex
Novapred
Paracort
Prednis
Servisone
Sterane
Valisone
Vanceril
Wescopred

GENERIC NAMES

beclomethasone
betamethasone
cortisone
dexamethasone
hydrocortisone

methylprednisolone
prednisolone
prednisone
triamcinolone

COUGH SUPPRESSANTS

(Antitussives)

BRAND NAMES

Benylin
Benylin DM
Dilaudid
Hycodan

Phenergan
Tessalon
Tussionex

GENERIC NAMES

benzonatate
codeine
dextromethorphan
diphenhydramine

hydrocodone
hydromorphone
promethazine

DECONGESTANTS

BRAND NAMES

Afrin
Gluco-Fedrin
Neo-Synephrine
Novafed
Otrivin

Privine
Propadrine
Sudafed
Tyzine

GENERIC NAMES

ephedrine
naphazoline
oxymetazoline
phenylephrine

phenylpropanolamine
pseudoephedrine
tetrahydrozoline
xylometazoline

DIGITALIS PREPARATIONS

BRAND NAMES

Crystodigin	Lanoxicaps
Digifortis	Lanoxin
Digiglusin	Purodigin
Gitaligin	

GENERIC NAMES

digitalis	digoxin
digitoxin	gitalin

DIURETICS

BRAND NAMES

Aldactone	Hygroton
Bumex	Lasix
⋈ Diamox	Lozol
Diulo	Midamor
⋈ Diuril	Zaroxolyn
Dyrenium	(See Thiazide Brand
Edecrin	Names)

GENERIC NAMES

acetazolamide	indapamide
amiloride	metolazone
bumetanide	spironolactone
chlorthalidone	thiazides (see Class)
ethacrynic acid	triamterene
furosemide	

FEMALE SEX HORMONES

BRAND NAMES

Estrogens	*Progestogens*
Delestrogen	Amen
DES	Curretab
Estinyl	Megace
Estrace	Micronor
Estrovis	Norlutin
Evex	Ovrette
Feminone	Provera
Ogen	
Premarin	
TACE	

GENERIC NAMES

Estrogens	*Progestogens*
chlorotrianisene	medroxyprogesterone
diethylstilbestrol	megestrol
estradiol	norethindrone
estrogens, conjugated	norgestrel
estrogens, esterified	
estropipate	
ethinyl estradiol	
quinestrol	

FEVER-REDUCING DRUGS

(Antipyretics)

BRAND NAMES

Anaprox	Naprosyn
Clinoril	Ponstel
Indocin	Rufen
Motrin	Tolectin
Nalfon	Tylenol

GENERIC NAMES

acetaminophen	ibuprofen	naproxen
aspirin	indomethacin	sulindac
fenoprofen	mefenamic acid	tolmetin

HEART RHYTHM REGULATORS

(Antiarrhythmic Drugs)

BRAND NAMES

Calan
Crystodigin
Inderal
Isoptin
Lanoxin
Mexitil
Norpace
Procan SR

Pronestyl
Purodigin
Quinaglute
Quinidex
Quinora
Tambocor
Tonocard

GENERIC NAMES

digitoxin
digoxin
disopyramide
flecainide
mexiletine

procainamide
propranolol
quinidine
tocainide
verapamil

HISTAMINE (H-2) BLOCKING DRUGS

("H-2 Blockers")

BRAND NAMES

Tagamet
Zantac

GENERIC NAMES

cimetidine
ranitidine

MALE SEX HORMONES

(Androgens)

<u>BRAND NAMES</u>

Android   Oratestin
Android F   Ora-Testryl
Depo-Testosterone   Oreton
Halotestin   Oreton Methyl
Metandren   Testred

<u>GENERIC NAMES</u>

fluoxymesterone
methyltestosterone
testosterone

MONOAMINE OXIDASE (MAO) INHIBITOR DRUGS

<u>BRAND NAMES</u>

Actomol   Marsilid
Catron   Nardil
Drazine   Niamid
Eutonyl   Parnate
Furoxone   Tersavid
Marplan

<u>GENERIC NAMES</u>

furazolidone   phenelzine
iproniazid   pheniprazine
isocarboxazid   phenoxypropazine
mebanazine   piohydrazine
nialamide   tranylcypromine
pargyline

MUSCLE RELAXANTS

BRAND NAMES

Equanil
Flexeril
Lioresal
Norflex
Paraflex
Parafon Forte

Rela
Robaxin
Skelaxin
Soma
Valium

GENERIC NAMES

baclofen
carisoprodol
chlorzoxazone
cyclobenzaprine
diazepam

meprobamate
metaxalone
methocarbamol
orphenadrine

NITRATES

BRAND NAMES

Cardilate
Isordil
Laserdil
Neo-Corovas

Nitro-Bid
Nitroglyn
Nitrospan
Nitrostat

Peritrate
SK-Petn
Sorbide
Sorbitrate

GENERIC NAMES

erythrityl tetranitrate
isosorbide dinitrate
nitroglycerin
pentaerythritol tetranitrate

PENICILLINS

BRAND NAMES

Alpen	Omnipen	Principen
Amcill	Orbenin	Prostaphlin
Amoxil	Pathocil	Spectrobid
Bactocil	Penbritin	Tegopen
Dynapen	Pentids	Unipen
Geocillin	Pen-Vee K	V-Cillin K
Geopen	Polycillin	Veracillin
Larotid	Polymox	

GENERIC NAMES

amoxicillin	dicloxacillin
ampicillin	nafcillin
bacampicillin	oxacillin
carbenicillin	penicillin G
cloxacillin	penicillin V

PHENOTHIAZINES

BRAND NAMES

Chlor-PZ	Proketazine	Tacaryl
Compazine	Prolixin	Temaril
Largon	Promatar	Thorazine
Levoprome	Quide	Tindal
Mellaril	Repoise	Torecan
Parsidol	Serentil	Trilafon
Permitil	Sparine	Vesprin
Phenergan	Stelazine	

GENERIC NAMES

acetophenazine	methdilazine	propiomazine
butaperazine	methotrimeprazine	thiethylperazine
carphenazine	perphenazine	thioridazine
chlorpromazine	piperacetazine	trifluoperazine
ethopropazine	procholorperazine	triflupromazine
fluphenazine	promazine	trimeprazine
mesoridazine	promethazine	

SALICYLATES

BRAND NAMES

Arthropan   Empirin
Bufferin   Magan
Causalin   Neocylate
Ecotrin   Uracel

GENERIC NAMES

aspirin
choline salicylate
magnesium salicylate
potassium salicylate
sodium salicylate

SEDATIVES/SLEEP INDUCERS, NONBARBITURATE

(Hypnotics)

BRAND NAMES

Carbrital   Halcion   Restoril
Dalmane   Noctec   Somnafac
Doriden   Noludar   Sopor
Dorimide   Parest   Valmid
Felsules   Placidyl

GENERIC NAMES

carbromal   glutethimide
chloral hydrate   methyprylon
ethchlorvynol   temazepam
ethinamate   triazolam
flurazepam

SULFONAMIDES

("Sulfa" Drugs)

BRAND NAMES

Azulfidine
Coco-Diazine
Cosulfa
Dagenan
Diamox
Elkosin

Gantanol
Gantrisin
Kynex
Madribon
Midicel
Neotrizine

Sonilyn
Suladyne
Thiosulfil
Triple Sulfas
Urobiotic

GENERIC NAMES

acetazolamide
sulfachlorpyridazine
sulfadiazine
sulfadimethoxine
sulfamerazine

sulfamethazine
sulfamethizole
sulfamethoxazole
sulfamethoxy-
    pyridazine

sulfapyridine
sulfasalazine
sulfisomidine
sulfisoxazole
trisulfapyrimidines

SULFONYLUREAS

BRAND NAMES

Chloronase
DiaBeta
Diabinese
Dimelor
Dymelor
Euglucon
Glucotrol

Micronase
Mobenol
Novobutamide
Orinase
Tolbutone
Tolinase

GENERIC NAMES

acetohexamide
chlorpropamide
glipizide
glyburide
tolazamide
tolbutamide

TETRACYCLINES

BRAND NAMES

Achromycin
Aureomycin
Declomycin
Minocin
Panmycin

Rondomycin
Steclin
Sumycin
Terramycin
Tetrachel

Tetracyn
Vectrin
Velacycline
Vibramycin

GENERIC NAMES

chlortetracycline
demeclocycline
doxycycline
methacycline

minocycline
oxytetracycline
rolitetracycline
tetracycline

THIAZIDE DIURETICS

BRAND NAMES

Anhydron
Chemhydrazide
Diucardin
Diuchlor
Diuril
Duretic
Edemol
Enduron
Esidrix
Exna

Hydrazide
Hydrid
Hydrite
Hydro-Aquil
Hydrodiuretex
HydroDiuril
Hydrosaluret
Hydrozide
Metahydrin

Naqua
Naturetin
Neocodema
Novohydrazide
Oretic
Renese
Saluron
Thiuretic
Urozide

GENERIC NAMES

bendroflumethiazide
benzthiazide
chlorothiazide
cyclothiazide
hydrochlorothiazide

hydroflumethiazide
methyclothiazide
polythiazide
trichlormethiazide

TRANQUILIZERS, MILD

(Antianxiety Drugs)

BRAND NAMES

6 Atarax
3 Buspar
Deprol
Equanil
Fenarol
2 Librium

Miltown
Paxipam
Serax
Trancopal
4 Tranxene

Tybatran
Ultran
Valium *1*
Vistaril
Xanax *5*

GENERIC NAMES

5 alprazolam
benactyzine
3 buspirone
2 chlordiazepoxide
chlormezanone
4 clorazepate
1 diazepam

halazepam
6 hydroxyzine. *HCl*
meprobamate
oxazepam
phenaglycodol
tybamate

TRANQUILIZERS, STRONG

(Antipsychotic Drugs)

BRAND NAMES

Carbolith
Eskalith
Haldol
Lithane
Lithonate

Lithotabs
Loxitane
Moban
Navane
Sandril

Serpasil
Taractan
(See Phenothiazines,
    Brand Names)

GENERIC NAMES

chlorprothixene
haloperidol
lithium
loxapine
molindone

phenothiazines (see
    Class)
reserpine
thiothixene

VASODILATORS

BRAND NAMES

Arlidin
Cerespan
Cyclospasmol
Ethatab

Pavabid
Vasodilan
Vasospan

GENERIC NAMES

cyclandelate
ethaverine
isoxsuprine
nylidrin
papaverine

XANTHINES

BRAND NAMES

Aminodur
Bronkodyl
Choledyl
Droxine
Elixophylline

Quibron-T
Slo-Phyllin
Theo-Dur
Theolixir
Theovent

GENERIC NAMES

aminophylline
dyphylline
oxtriphylline
theophylline

A GLOSSARY
OF
DRUG-RELATED TERMS

Glossary

Addiction The traditional term used to identify the irresistible craving for and compulsive use of habit-forming drugs. The more recent preference for the term *dependence* has served to clarify the distinction between habituation and addiction. Drugs capable of producing addiction do so by interacting with the biochemistry of the brain in such a way that they assume a working role. This physical incorporation of the drug into the fundamental processes of brain tissue function is responsible for the agony of the "withdrawal syndrome"—the intense mental and physical pain experienced by the addict when intake of the drug is stopped abruptly. Thus addiction is a *physical dependence*. (See DEPENDENCE for a further account of physical and psychological dependence.)

Adverse Effect or Reaction An abnormal, unexpected, infrequent and usually unpredictable injurious response to a drug. Used in this restrictive sense, the term *adverse reaction* does *not* include effects of a drug which are normally a part of its pharmacological action, even though such effects may be undesirable and unintended. (See SIDE-EFFECT.) Adverse reactions are of three basic types: those due to drug *allergy*, those caused by individual *idiosyncrasy* and those representing *toxic* effects of drugs on tissue structure and function (see ALLERGY, IDIOSYNCRASY and TOXICITY).

Allergy (Drug) An abnormal mechanism of drug response that occurs in individuals who produce injurious antibodies* that react with foreign substances—in this instance, a drug. The person who is allergic by nature and has a history of hay fever, asthma, hives or eczema is more likely to develop drug allergies. Allergic reactions to drugs take many forms: skin

---

*Antibodies are special tissue proteins that combine with substances foreign to the body. Protective antibodies destroy bacteria and neutralize toxins. Injurious antibodies, reacting with foreign substances, cause the release of histamine, the principal chemical responsible for allergic reactions.

eruptions of various kinds, fever, swollen glands, painful joints, jaundice, interference with breathing, acute collapse of circulation, etc. Drug allergies can develop gradually over a long period of time, or they can appear with dramatic suddenness and require life-saving intervention.

Analgesic A drug that is used primarily to relieve pain. Analgesics are of three basic types: (1) Simple, nonnarcotic analgesics that relieve pain by suppressing the local production of prostaglandins and related substances; examples are acetaminophen, aspirin and the large group of nonsteroidal anti-inflammatory drugs known as aspirin substitutes (Motrin, Advil, Naprosyn, etc.). (2) Narcotic analgesics or opioids ("like opium" derivatives) that relieve pain by suppressing its perception in the brain; examples are morphine, codeine and hydrocodone (natural derivatives of opium), and meperidine or pentazocine (synthetic drug products). (3) Local anesthetics that prevent or relieve pain by rendering sensory nerve endings insensitive to painful stimulation; an example is the urinary tract analgesic phenazopyridine (Pyridium).

Anaphylactic (Anaphylactoid) Reaction A group of symptoms which represent (or resemble) a sometimes overwhelming and dangerous allergic reaction due to extreme hypersensitivity to a drug. Anaphylactic reactions, whether mild, moderate or severe, often involve several body systems. Mild symptoms consist of itching, hives, nasal congestion, nausea, abdominal cramping and/or diarrhea. Sometimes these precede more severe symptoms such as choking, shortness of breath and sudden loss of consciousness (usually referred to as anaphylactic shock).

Characteristic features of anaphylactic reaction must be kept in mind. It can result from a very small dose of drug; it develops suddenly, usually within a few minutes after taking the drug; it can be rapidly progressive and can lead to fatal collapse in a short time if not reversed by appropriate treatment. A developing anaphylactic reaction is a true medical emergency. Any adverse effect that appears within 20 minutes after taking a drug should be considered the early manifestation of a possible anaphylactic reaction. Obtain medical attention immediately! (See ALLERGY, DRUG and HYPERSENSITIVITY.)

Antihypertensive A drug used to lower excessively high blood pressure. The term *hypertension* denotes blood pressure above the normal range. It does not refer to excessive nervous or emotional tension. The term *antihypertensive* is sometimes used erroneously as if it had the same meaning as *antianxiety* (or tranquilizing) drug action.

Today there are more than 100 drug products in use for treating hypertension. Those most frequently prescribed for long-term use fall into three major groups:

drugs that increase urine production (the diuretics)
drugs that relax blood vessel walls
drugs that reduce the activity of the sympathetic nervous system.

Regardless of their mode of action, all these drugs share an ability to lower the blood pressure. It is important to remember that many other drugs can interact with antihypertensive drugs: some add to their effect and cause excessive reduction in blood pressure; others interfere with their action and reduce their effectiveness. Anyone who is taking medications for hypertension should consult with his or her physician whenever drugs are prescribed for the treatment of other conditions as well.

Antipyretic A drug that is used to treat fever because of its ability to lower body temperature that is elevated above the normal. Antipyretics relieve fever through their effects on the temperature regulating center in the hypothalamus of the brain. Their actions cause dilation of the blood vessels (capillary beds) in the skin, bringing overheated blood to the surface for cooling; in addition, the sweat glands are stimulated to provide copious perspiration that cools the body further through evaporation. An antipyretic drug may also be analgesic (acetaminophen), or analgesic and anti-inflammatory (aspirin).

Aplastic Anemia A form of bone marrow failure in which the production of all 3 types of blood cells is seriously impaired (also known as pancytopenia). Aplastic anemia can occur spontaneously from unknown causes, but about one-half of reported cases are induced by certain drugs or chemicals. The symptoms reflect the consequences of inadequate supplies of all 3 blood cell types: deficiency of red blood cells (anemia) results in fatigue, weakness and pallor; deficiency of white blood cells (leukopenia) predisposes to infections; deficiency of blood platelets (thrombocytopenia) leads to spontaneous bruising and hemorrhage. Treatment is difficult and the outcome unpredictable. Even with the best of care, approximately 50% of cases end fatally.

These drugs and chemicals are known to be capable of inducing aplastic anemia:

acetazolamide
anticancer drugs
aspirin
benzene (solvent)
carbamazepine
carbon tetrachloride (solvent)
chlordane (insecticide)
chlordiazepoxide
chloromycetin
chlorothiazide
chlorpheniramine
chlorpromazine
chlorpropamide
colchicine
DDT (insecticide)
indomethacin
lithium
mephenytoin

meprobamate
methimazole
oxyphenbutazone
penicillin
phenacetin
phenylbutazone
phenytoin
primidone
promazine
quinacrine
sulfonamides
tetracyclines
thiouracil
tolbutamide
triflupromazine
trimethadione
tripelennamine

Although aplastic anemia is a rare consequence of drug treatment (3 in 100,000 users of quinacrine, for example), anyone taking a drug capable of inducing it should have complete blood cell counts periodically if the drug is to be used over an extended period of time.

Bioavailability The measurable characteristics of a drug product (usually a tablet or a capsule) that represent how rapidly the active drug ingredient is absorbed into the bloodstream and to what extent it is absorbed. Two types of measurements—(1) blood levels of the drug at certain time intervals after administration, and (2) the duration of the drug's presence in the blood—indicate how much of the drug is available for biological activity and for how long.

Another method of determining a drug product's bioavailability is to measure (1) the cumulative amount of the drug (or any breakdown product after transformation) that is excreted in the urine, and (2) the rate of drug accumulation in the urine.

The two major factors that govern a drug product's bioavailability are the chemical and physical characteristics (the formulation) of the dosage form given, and the functional state of the digestive system of the individual who takes it. A drug product that disintegrates rapidly in a normally functioning stomach and small intestine produces blood levels of the absorbed drug quite promptly. Such a drug product can be demonstrated to possess good bioavailability.

Specially designed laboratory tests are now available to evaluate a drug product's potential bioavailability when taken by the "average" individual.

Bioequivalence It is generally accepted that the ability of a drug product to produce its intended therapeutic effect is directly related to its bioavailability. When a particular drug is marketed by several manufacturers, often in a variety of dosage forms, it is critically important that the drug product selected for use be one that possesses the bioavailability necessary to be effective therapeutically. Substantial variations occur among manufacturers in the formulation of their drug products. Although the principal drug ingredient of products from different firms may be identical chemically, it cannot be assumed that these products possess equal bioavailability and are therefore equal therapeutically.

The bioavailability of any drug product is governed to a large extent by the physical characteristics of its formulation; these in turn determine how rapidly and how completely the drug product disintegrates and releases its active drug component(s) for absorption into the bloodstream. Drug products that contain the same principal drug ingredient but are combined with different inert additives, are coated with different substances or are enclosed in capsules of different composition may or may not possess the same bioavailability. Those that do are said to be bioequivalent, and can be relied upon to be equally effective in achieving therapeutic results.

If you consider having your prescription filled with the generic equivalent of a brand name drug product, ask your physician *and* pharmacist for guidance. This decision requires professional judgment in each case. In many treatment situations, reasonable differences in the bioavailability patterns among drug products are acceptable. In some situations, however, because of the serious nature of the illness, or because it is mandatory that blood levels of the drug be maintained within a narrowly defined range, it is essential to use the drug product that has been demonstrated to possess reliable bioavailability.

Blood Platelets The smallest of the three types of blood cells produced by the bone marrow. Platelets are normally present in very large numbers. Their primary function is to assist the process of normal blood clotting so as to prevent excessive bruising and bleeding in the event of injury. When present in proper numbers and functioning normally, platelets preserve the retaining power of the walls of the smaller blood vessels. By initiating appropriate clotting processes in the blood, platelets seal small points of leakage in the vessel walls, thereby preventing spontaneous bruising or bleeding (that which is unprovoked by trauma).

Certain drugs and chemicals may reduce the number of available blood platelets to abnormally low levels. Some of these drugs act by suppressing platelet formation; other drugs hasten their destruction. When the number of functioning platelets falls below a critical level, blood begins to leak through the thin walls of smaller vessels. The outward evidence of this leakage is the spontaneous appearance of scattered bruises in the skin of the thighs and legs. This is referred to as purpura. Bleeding may occur anywhere in the body, internally as well as superficially into the tissues immediately beneath the skin.

Bone Marrow Depression A serious reduction in the ability of the bone marrow to carry on its normal production of blood cells. This can occur as an adverse reaction to the toxic effect of certain drugs and chemicals on bone marrow components. When functioning normally, the bone marrow produces the majority of the body's blood cells. These consist of three types: the red blood cells (erythrocytes), the white blood cells (leukocytes) and the blood platelets (thrombocytes). Each type of cell performs one or more specific functions, all of which are indispensable to the maintenance of life and health.

Drugs that are capable of depressing bone marrow activity can impair the production of all types of blood cells simultaneously or of only one type selectively. Periodic examinations of the blood can reveal significant changes in the structure and number of the blood cells that indicate a possible drug effect on bone marrow activity.

Impairment of the production of red blood cells leads to anemia, a condition of abnormally low red cells and hemoglobin. This causes weakness, loss of energy and stamina, intolerance of cold environments and shortness of breath on physical exertion. A reduction in the formation of white blood cells can impair the body's immunity and lower its resistance to infection. These changes may result in the development of fever, sore throat or pneumonia. When the formation of blood platelets is suppressed to abnormally low levels, the blood loses its ability to quickly seal small points of leakage in blood vessel walls. This may lead to episodes of unusual and abnormal spontaneous bruising or to prolonged bleeding in the event of injury.

Any of these symptoms can occur in the presence of bone marrow depression. They should alert both patient and physician to the need for prompt studies of blood and bone marrow.

Brand Name The registered trade name given to a drug product by its manufacturer. Many drugs are marketed by more than one manufacturer or distributor. Each company adopts a distinctive trade name to distinguish its brand of the generic drug from that of its competitors. Thus a brand name designates a proprietary drug—one that is protected by patent or copyright. Generally brand names are shorter, easier to pronounce and more readily remembered than their generic counterparts.

Cause-and-Effect Relationship A possible causative association between a drug and an observed biologic event—most commonly a side-effect or an adverse effect. Knowledge of a drug's full spectrum of effects (wanted and unwanted) is highly desirable when weighing its benefits and risks in any treatment situation. However, it is often impossible to establish with certainty that a particular drug is the primary agent responsible for a suspected adverse effect. In the evaluation of every cause-and-effect relationship, therefore, meticulous consideration must be given to such factors as the time sequence of drug administration and possible reaction, the use of multiple drugs, possible interactions among these drugs, the effects of the disease under treatment, the physiological and psychological characteristics of the patient and the possible influence of unrecognized disorders and malfunctions.

The majority of adverse drug reactions occur sporadically, unpredictably and infrequently in the general population. A *definite* cause-and-effect relationship between drug and reaction is established when (1) the adverse effect immediately follows administration of the drug; or (2) the adverse effect disappears after the drug is discontinued (dechallenge) and promptly reappears when the drug is used again (rechallenge); or (3) the adverse effects are clearly the expected and predictable toxic consequences of drug overdosage.

In contrast to the obvious "causative" (definite) relationship, there exists a large gray area of "probable," "possible" and "coincidental" associations that are clouded by varying degrees of uncertainty. These classifications usually apply to alleged drug reactions that require a relatively long time to develop, are of low incidence and for which there are no clear-cut objective means of demonstrating a causal mechanism that links drug and reaction. Clarification of cause-and-effect relationships in these uncertain groups requires carefully designed observation over a long period of time, followed by sophisticated statistical analysis. Occasionally the public is alerted to a newly found "relationship" based upon suggestive but incomplete data. Though early warning is clearly in the public interest, such announcements should make clear whether the presumed relationship is based upon definitive criteria or is simply inferred because the use of a drug and an observed event were found to occur together within an appropriate time frame.

The most competent techniques for evaluating cause-and-effect relationships of adverse drug reactions have been devised by the Division of

Tissue Reactions to Drugs, a research unit of the Armed Forces Institute of Pathology. Based upon a highly critical examination of all available evidence, the Division's study of 2800 drug-related deaths yielded the following levels of certainty regarding cause-and-effect relationship:

No association	5.0%
Coincidental	14.5%
Possible	33.0%
Probable	30.0%
Causative	17.5%

It is significant that expert evaluation of 2800 drug-related cases concluded that only 47.5% could be substantiated as definitely or probably causative.

Contraindication A condition or disease that precludes the use of a particular drug. Some cointraindications are *absolute*, meaning that the use of the drug would expose the patient to extreme hazard and therefore cannot be justified. Other contraindications are *relative*, meaning that the condition or disease does not entirely bar the use of the drug but requires that, before the decision to use the drug is made, special consideration be given to factors which could aggravate existing disease, interfere with current treatment or produce new injury.

Dependence The preferred term used to identify the drug-dependent states of *psychological dependence* (or *habituation*), and *physical dependence* (or *addiction*). In addition, a third kind of drug-dependence can be included under this term. This might be called *functional dependence*—the need to use a drug continuously in order to sustain a particular body function, the impairment of which causes annoying symptoms of varying degree and significance.

Psychological dependence is a form of neurotic behavior. Its principal characteristic is an obsession to satisfy a particular desire, be it one of self-gratification or one of escape from some real or imagined distress. Psychological dependence is a very human trait that is seen often in many socially acceptable patterns and practices such as entertainment, gambling, sports and collecting. A common form of this dependence in today's culture is the increasing reliance upon drugs to help in coping with the everyday problems of living: pills for frustration, disappointment, nervous stomach, tension headache and insomnia. The 20 million smokers of marijuana have found it to be a drug that eases their stress, one whose effectiveness fosters habit (psychological dependence) but not addiction.

Physical dependence, which is true addiction, includes two elements: habituation and tolerance. Addicting drugs provide relief from anguish and pain swiftly and effectively; they also induce a physiological tolerance that requires increasing dosage or repeated use if they are to remain effective. These two features foster the continued need for the drug and lead to its becoming a functioning component in the biochemistry of the brain. As this occurs, the drug assumes an "essential" role in ongoing chemical processes. (Thus some authorities prefer the term *chemical dependence*.) Sudden removal of the drug from the system causes a major upheaval in body chemistry and provokes a withdrawal syndrome—the intense mental and physical pain experienced by the addict when intake of the drug is stopped abruptly—that is the hallmark of addiction.

Functional dependence differs significantly from both psychological and physical dependence. It occurs when a drug effectively relieves an annoying or distressing condition and the particular body function involved becomes increasingly dependent upon the action of the drug to provide a sense of well-being. Drugs which are capable of inducing functional dependence are used primarily for the relief of symptoms. They do not act on the brain to produce alteration of mood or consciousness as do those drugs with potential for either psychological or physical dependence. The most familiar example of functional dependence is the "laxative habit." Some types of constipation are made worse by the wrong choice of laxative, and natural function gradually fades as the colon becomes more and more dependent upon the action of certain laxative drugs.

Disulfiramlike (Antabuselike) Reaction The symptoms that result from the interaction of alcohol and any drug that is capable of provoking the pattern of response typical of the "Antabuse effect." The interacting drug interrupts the normal decomposition of alcohol by the liver and thereby permits the accumulation of a toxic by-product that enters the bloodstream. When sufficient levels of both alcohol and drug are present in the blood the reaction occurs. It consists of intense flushing and warming of the face, a severe throbbing headache, shortness of breath, chest pains, nausea, repeated vomiting, sweating and weakness. If the amount of alcohol ingested has been large enough, the reaction may progress to blurred vision, vertigo, confusion, marked drop in blood pressure and loss of consciousness. Severe reactions may lead to convulsions and death. The reaction can last from 30 minutes to several hours, depending upon the amount of alcohol in the body. As the symptoms subside, the individual is exhausted and usually sleeps for several hours.

Diuretic A drug that alters kidney function to increase the volume of urine. Diuretics use several different mechanisms to increase urine volume, and these, in turn, have different effects on body chemistry. Diuretics are used primarily to (1) remove excess water from the body (as in congestive heart failure and some types of liver and kidney disease), and (2) treat hypertension by promoting the excretion of sodium from the body.

Dosage Forms and Strengths This information category in the individual Drug Profiles (Section Three) uses several abbreviations to designate measurements of weight and volume. These are:

mcg = microgram = 1,000,000th of a gram (weight)
mg   = milligram   = 1000th of a gram (weight)
ml   = milliliter   = 1000th of a liter (volume)
gm   = gram   = 1000 milligrams (weight)

There are approximately 65 mg in 1 grain.
There are approximately 5 ml in 1 teaspoonful.
There are approximately 15 ml in 1 tablespoonful.
There are approximately 30 ml in 1 ounce.
1 milliliter of water weighs 1 gram.
There are approximately 454 grams in 1 pound.

Drug, Drug Product Terms often used interchangeably to designate a medicine (in any of its dosage forms) used in medical practice. Strictly speaking, the term *drug* refers to the single chemical entity that provokes a specific response when placed within a biological system—the "active" ingredient. A *drug product* is the manufactured dosage form—tablet, capsule, elixir, etc.—that contains the active drug intermixed with inactive ingredients to provide for convenient administration.

Drug products which contain only one active ingredient are referred to as single entity drugs. Drug products with two or more active ingredients are called combination drugs (designed [CD] in the lists of brand names in the Drug Profiles, Section Three).

Drug Class A group of drugs that are similar in chemistry, method of action and use in treatment. Because of their common characteristics, many drugs within a class will produce the same side-effects and have similar potential for provoking related adverse reactions and interactions. However, significant variations among members within a drug class can occur. This sometimes allows the physician an important degree of selectivity in choosing a drug if certain beneficial actions are desired or particular side-effects are to be minimized.

Examples: Antihistamines, phentothiazines, tetracyclines (see Section Four).

Drug Fever The elevation of body temperature that occurs as an unwanted manifestation of drug action. Drugs can induce fever by several mechanisms; these include allergic reactions, drug-induced tissue damage, acceleration of tissue metabolism, constriction of blood vessels in the skin with resulting decrease in loss of body heat and direct action on the temperature-regulating center in the brain.

The most common form of drug fever is that associated with allergic reactions. It may be the only allergic manifestation apparent, or it may be part of a complex of allergic symptoms that can include skin rash, hives, joint swelling and pain, enlarged lymph glands, hemolytic anemia or hepatitis. The fever usually appears about 7 to 10 days after starting the drug and may vary from low-grade to alarmingly high levels. It may be sustained or intermittent, but it usually persists for as long as the drug is taken. In previously sensitized individuals drug fever may occur within 1 or 2 hours after taking the first dose of medication.

While many drugs are capable of producing fever, the following are more commonly responsible:

allopurinol	novobiocin
antihistamines	para-aminosalicylic acid
atropinelike drugs	penicillin
barbiturates	pentazocine
coumarin anticoagulants	phenytoin
hydralazine	procainamide
iodides	propylthiouracil
isoniazid	quinidine
methyldopa	rifampin
nadalol	sulfonamides

Extension Effect An unwanted but predictable drug response that is a logical consequence of mild to moderate overdosage. An extension effect is an exaggeration of the drug's normal pharmacological action; it can be thought of as a mild form of dose-related toxicity (see OVERDOSAGE and TOXICITY).

Example: The continued "hangover" of drowsiness and mental sluggishness that persists after arising in the morning is a common extension effect of a long-acting sleep-inducing drug (hypnotic) taken the night before.

Example: The persistent intestinal cramping and diarrhea that result from too generous a dose of laxative are extension effects of the drug's anticipated action.

Generic Name The official, common or public name used to designate an active drug entity, whether in pure form or in dosage form. Generic names are coined by committees of officially appointed drug experts and are approved by governmental agencies for national and international use. Thus they are nonproprietary. Many drug products are marketed under the generic name of the principal active ingredient and bear no brand name of the manufacturer.

While the total number of prescriptions written in the United States in 1985 increased by 1.1%, prescriptions specifying the *generic name* of the drug increased by 13%. Generically written prescriptions now account for 12.9% of all new prescriptions written in the United States. The drugs most commonly prescribed by generic name are listed below, ranked in descending order of the number of new prescriptions issued.

amoxicillin	erythromycin
penicillin VK	hydrochlorothiazide
ampicillin	phenobarbital
tetracycline	acetaminophen/codeine
prednisone	hydrocortisone

Habituation A form of drug dependence based upon strong psychological gratification rather than the physical (chemical) dependence of addiction. The habitual use of drugs that alter mood or relieve minor discomforts results from a compulsive need to feel pleasure and satisfaction or to escape the manifestations of emotional distress. The abrupt cessation of habituating drugs does not produce the withdrawal syndrome seen in addiction. Thus habituation is a *psychological dependence.* (See DEPENDENCE for a further account of psychological and physical dependence.)

Hemolytic Anemia A form of anemia (deficient red blood cells and hemoglobin) resulting from the premature destruction (hemolysis) of circulating red blood cells. Several mechanisms can be responsible for the development of hemolytic anemia; among these is the action of certain drugs and chemicals. Some individuals are susceptible to hemolytic anemia because of a genetic deficiency in the makeup of their red blood cells. If such people are given certain antimalarial drugs, sulfa drugs or numerous other drugs, some of their red cells will disintegrate on contact with the drug. (About 10% of American blacks have this genetic trait.)

Another type of drug-induced hemolytic anemia is a form of drug allergy. Many drugs in wide use (including quinidine, methyldopa, levodopa and chlorpromazine) are known to cause hemolytic destruction of red cells as a hypersensitivity (allergic) reaction.

Hemolytic anemia can occur abruptly (with evident symptoms) or silently. The acute form lasts about 7 days and is characterized by fever, pallor, weakness, dark-colored urine and varying degrees of jaundice (yellow coloration of eyes and skin). When drug-induced hemolytic anemia is mild, involving the destruction of only a small number of red blood cells, there may be no symptoms to indicate its presence. Such episodes are detected only by means of laboratory studies (see IDIOSYNCRASY and ALLERGY, DRUG).

Hepatitislike Reaction Changes in the liver, induced by certain drugs, which closely resemble those produced by viral hepatitis. The symptoms of drug-induced hepatitis and virus-induced hepatitis are often so similar that the correct cause cannot be established without precise laboratory studies.

Hepatitis due to drugs may be a form of drug allergy (as in reaction to many of the phenothiazines), or it may represent a toxic adverse effect (as in reaction to some of the monoamine oxidase inhibitor drugs). Liver reactions of significance usually result in jaundice and represent serious adverse effects (see JAUNDICE).

Hypersensitivity A term subject to varying usages for many years. One common use has been to identify the trait of overresponsiveness to drug action, that is, an intolerance to even small doses. Used in this sense, the term indicates that the nature of the response is appropriate but the degree of response is exaggerated.

The term is more widely used today to identify a state of allergy. To have a *hypersensitivity* to a drug is to be *allergic* to it (see ALLERGY, DRUG).

Some individuals develop cross-hypersensitivity. This means that once a person has developed an allergy to a certain drug, that person will experience an allergic reaction to other drugs which are closely related in chemical composition.

Example: The patient was known to be *hypersensitive* by nature, having a history of seasonal hay fever and asthma since childhood. His *allergy* to tetracycline developed after his third course of treatment. This drug *hypersensitivity* manifested itself as a diffuse, measleslike rash.

Hypnotic A drug that is used primarily to induce sleep. There are several classes of drugs that have hypnotic effects: antihistamines, barbiturates, benzodiazepines and several unrelated compounds. Within the past 15 years the benzodiazepines, because of their relative safety and lower potential for inducing dependence, have largely replaced the barbiturates as the most commonly used hypnotics. The body usually develops a tolerance to the hypnotic effect after several weeks of continual use. To maintain their effectiveness, hypnotics should be used intermittently for short periods of time.

Hypoglycemia A condition in which the amount of glucose (a sugar) in the blood is below the normal range. Since normal brain function is dependent upon an adequate supply of glucose, reducing the level of glucose in the blood below a critical point will cause serious impairment of brain activity. The resulting symptoms are characteristic of the hypoglycemic state. Early indications are headache, a sensation resembling mild drunkenness and an inability to think clearly. These may be accompanied by hunger. As the level of blood glucose continues to fall, nervousness and confusion develop. Varying degrees of weakness, numbness, trembling, sweating and rapid heart action follow. If sugar is not provided at this point and the blood glucose level drops further, impaired speech, incoordination and unconsciousness, with or without convulsions, will follow.

Hypoglycemia in any stage requires prompt recognition and treatment. Because of the potential for injury to the brain, the mechanisms and management of hypoglycemia should be understood by all who use drugs capable of producing it.

Hypothermia A state of the body characterized by an unexpected decline of internal body temperature to levels significantly below the norm of 98.6 degrees F or 37 degrees C. By definition, hypothermia means a body temperature of less than 95 degrees F or 35 degrees C. The elderly and debilitated are more prone to develop hypothermia if clothed inadequately and exposed to cool environments. Most episodes are initiated by room temperatures below 65 degrees F or 18.3 degrees C. The condition often develops suddenly, can mimic a stroke and has a mortality rate of 50%. Some drugs, such as phenothiazines, barbiturates and benzodiazepines, are conducive to the development of hypothermia in susceptible individuals.

Idiosyncrasy An abnormal mechanism of drug response that occurs in individuals who have a peculiar defect in their body chemistry (often hereditary) which produces an effect totally unrelated to the drug's normal pharmacological action. Idiosyncrasy is not a form of allergy. The actual chemical defects responsible for certain idiosyncratic drug reactions are well understood; others are not.

Example: Approximately 100 million people in the world (including 10% of American blacks) have a specific enzyme deficiency in their red blood cells that causes these cells to disintegrate when exposed to drugs such as sulfonamides (Gantrisin, Kynex), nitrofurantoin (Furadantin, Macrodantin), probenecid (Benemid), quinine and quinidine. As a result of this reaction, these drugs (and others) can cause a significant anemia in susceptible individuals.

Example: Approximately 5% of the population of the United States is susceptible to the development of glaucoma on prolonged use of cortisone-related drugs (see Cortisone Drug Class in Section Four).

Immunosuppressive A drug that significantly impairs (suppresses) the functions of the body's immune system. In some instances, immunosuppression is an intended drug effect as in the use of cyclosporine to prevent the immune system from rejecting a transplanted heart or kidney. In other instances, it is an unwanted side-effect as in the long-term use of cortisone-like drugs (to control chronic asthma) that suppresses the immune system sufficiently to permit reactivation of a dormant tuberculosis. Immunosuppressant drugs are being used to treat several chronic disorders that are thought to be autoimmune diseases, notably advanced rheumatoid arthritis, ulcerative colitis and systemic lupus erythematosus.

Interaction An unwanted change in the body's response to a drug that results when a second drug that is capable of altering the action of the first is administered at the same time. Some drug interactions can enhance the effect of either drug, producing an overresponse similar to overdosage. Other interactions may reduce drug effectiveness and cause inadequate response. A third type of interaction can produce a seemingly unrelated toxic response with no associated increase or decrease in the pharmacological actions of the interacting drugs.

Theoretically, many drugs can interact with one another, but in reality drug interactions are comparatively infrequent. Many interactions can be anticipated, and the physician can make appropriate adjustments in dosage to prevent or minimize unintended fluctuations in drug response.

Jaundice A yellow coloration of the skin (and the white portion of the eyes) that occurs when excessive bile pigments accumulate in the blood as a result of impaired liver function. Jaundice can be produced by several mechanisms. It may occur as a manifestation of a wide variety of diseases, or it may represent an adverse reaction to a particular drug. At times it is difficult to distinguish between disease-induced jaundice and drug-induced jaundice.

Jaundice due to a drug is always a serious adverse effect. Anyone taking a drug that is capable of causing jaundice should watch closely for any significant change in the color of urine or feces. Dark discoloration of the urine and paleness (lack of color) of the stool may be early indications of a developing jaundice. Should either of these symptoms occur, it is advisable to discontinue the drug and notify the prescribing physician promptly. Diagnostic tests are available to clarify the nature of the jaundice.

Lupus Erythematosus (LE) A serious disease of unknown cause that occurs in two forms, one limited to the skin (discoid LE) and the other involving several body systems (systemic LE). Both forms occur predominantly in young women. About 5% of cases of the discoid form convert to the systemic form. Basically, systemic LE is a disorder of the body's immune system which may result in chronic, progressive inflammation and destruction of the connective tissue framework of the skin, blood vessels, joints, brain, heart muscle, lungs and kidneys. Altered proteins in the blood lead to the formation of antibodies which react with certain organ tissues to produce the inflammation and destruction characteristic of the disease. A reduction in the number of white blood cells and blood platelets often occurs. The course of systemic LE is usually quite protracted and unpredictable. While no cure is known, satisfactory management may be achieved in some cases by the judicious use of cortisonelike drugs.

Several drugs in wide use are capable of initiating a form of systemic LE quite similar to that which occurs spontaneously. (More than 100 cases due to the use of procainamide have been reported.) Suggestive symptoms may appear as early as 2 weeks or as late as 8 years after starting the responsible drug. The initial symptoms usually consist of low-grade fever, skin rashes of various kinds, aching muscles and multiple joint pains. Chest pains (pleurisy) are fairly common. Enlargement of the lymph glands occurs less frequently. Symptoms usually subside following discontinuation of the responsible drug, but laboratory evidence of the reaction may persist for many months.

Drugs known to induce systemic LE include:

chlorpromazine	phenothiazines (some)
clofibrate	phenylbutazone
hydralazine	phenytoin
isoniazid	practolol
oral contraceptives	procainamide
penicillamine	thiouracil
phenolphthalein	

Orthostatic Hypotension A type of low blood pressure that is related to body position or posture (also called postural hypotension). The individual who is subject to orthostatic hypotension may have a normal blood pressure while lying down, but on sitting upright or standing he will experience sudden sensations of lightheadedness, dizziness and a feeling of impending faint that compel him to return quickly to a lying position. These symptoms are manifestations of inadequate blood flow (oxygen supply) to the brain due to an abnormal delay in the rise in blood pressure that always occurs as the body adjusts the circulation to the erect position.

Many drugs (especially the stronger antihypertensives) may cause orthostatic hypotension. Individuals who experience this drug effect should report it to their physician so that appropriate dosage adjustment can be made to minimize it. Failure to correct or to compensate for these sudden drops in blood pressure can lead to severe falls and injury.

The tendency to orthostatic hypotension can be reduced by avoiding sudden standing, prolonged standing, vigorous exercise and exposure to hot environments. Alcoholic beverages should be used cautiously until their combined effect with the drug in use has been determined.

Overdosage The meaning of this term should not be limited to the concept of doses that clearly exceed the normal dosage range recommended by the manufacturer. The optimal dose of many drugs (that amount which gives the greatest benefit with least distress) varies greatly from person to person. What may be an average dose for the majority of individuals will be an overdose for some and an underdose for others. Numerous factors, such as age, body size, nutritional status and liver and kidney function, have significant influence on dosage requirements. Drugs with narrow safety margins often produce indications of overdosage if something delays the regular elimination of the customary daily dose. In this instance, overdosage results from accumulation of prescribed daily doses. Massive overdosage—as occurs with accidental ingestion of drugs by children or with suicidal intention by adults—is referred to as poisoning.

Over-the-Counter (OTC) Drugs Drug products that can be purchased without prescription. Many are available in food stores, variety stores and newsstands as well as in conventional drug stores. Because of the unrestricted availability of these drugs, many people do not look upon OTC medicines as drugs. But drugs they are! And like the more potent drug products that are sold only on prescription, they are chemicals that are capable of a wide variety of actions on biological systems. Within the last 30 years, many OTC drugs have assumed greater importance because of their ability to interact unfavorably with some widely used prescription drugs. Serious problems in drug management can arise when (1) the patient fails to inform the physician of the OTC drug(s) he is taking ("because they really aren't drugs") and (2) the physician fails to specify that his question about what medicines are being taken currently *includes all OTC drugs*. During any course of treatment, whether medical or surgical, the patient should consult with the physician regarding any OTC drug that he wishes to take.

The major classes of OTC drugs for internal use include:

allergy medicines (antihistamines)	laxatives
antacids	menstrual aids
antiworm medicines	motion sickness remedies
aspirin and aspirin combinations	pain relievers
aspirin substitutes	reducing aids
asthma aids	salt substitutes
cold medicines (decongestants)	sedatives and tranquilizers
cough medicines	sleeping pills
diarrhea remedies	stimulants (caffeine)
digestion aids	sugar substitutes (saccharin)
diuretics	tonics
iron preparations	vitamins

Paradoxical Reaction An unexpected drug response that is not consistent with the known pharmacology of the drug and may in fact be the opposite of the intended and anticipated response. Such reactions are due to individual sensitivity or variability and can occur in any age group. They are seen more commonly, however, in children and the elderly.

Example: An 80-year-old man was admitted to a nursing home following the death of his wife. He had difficulty adjusting to his new environment and was restless, agitated and irritable. He was given a trial of the tranquilizer diazepam (Valium) to relax him, starting with small doses. On the second day of medication he became confused and erratic in behavior. The dose of diazepam was increased. On the third day he began to wander aimlessly, talked incessantly in a loud voice and displayed anger and hostility when attempts were made to help him. Suspecting the possibility of a paradoxical reaction, the diazepam was discontinued. All behavioral disturbances gradually subsided within 3 days.

Parkinson-like Disorders (Parkinsonism) A group of symptoms that resembles those caused by Parkinson's disease, a chronic disorder of the nervous system also known as shaking palsy. The characteristic features of parkinsonism include a fixed, emotionless facial expression (masklike in appearance), a prominent trembling of the hands, arms or legs and stiffness of the extremities that limits movement and produces a rigid posture and gait.

Parkinsonism is a fairly common adverse effect that occurs in about 15% of all patients who take large doses of strong tranquilizers (notably the phenothiazines) or use them over an extended period of time. If recognized early, the Parkinson-like features will lessen or disappear with reduced dosage or change in medication. In some instances, however, Parkinson-like changes may become permanent, requiring appropriate medication for their control.

Peripheral Neuritis (Peripheral Neuropathy) A group of symptoms that results from injury to nerve tissue in the extremities. A variety of drugs and chemicals are capable of inducing changes in nerve structure or function. The characteristic pattern consists of a sensation of numbness and tingling that usually begins in the fingers and toes and is accompanied by an altered sensation to touch and vague discomfort ranging from aching sensations to burning pain. Severe forms of peripheral neuritis may include loss of muscular strength and coordination.

A relatively common form of peripheral neuritis is that seen with the long-term use of isoniazid in the treatment of tuberculosis. If Vitamin B-6 (pyridoxine) is not given concurrently with isoniazid, peripheral neuritis may occur in sensitive individuals. Vitamin B-6 can be both preventive and curative in this form of drug-induced peripheral neuritis.

Since peripheral neuritis can also occur as a late complication following many viral infections, care must be taken to avoid assigning a cause-and-effect relationship to a drug which is not responsible for the nerve injury (see CAUSE-AND-EFFECT RELATIONSHIP).

Pharmacology The medical science that relates to the development and use of medicinal drugs, their composition and action in animals and man. Used in its broadest sense, pharmacology embraces the related sciences of medicinal chemistry, experimental therapeutics and toxicology.

Example: The widely used sulfonylurea drugs (Diabinese, Dymelor, Orinase, Tolinase) are effective in the treatment of some forms of diabetes because of the accidental discovery that some of their parent "sulfa" drugs produced hypoglycemia (low blood sugar) during their early therapeutic trials as anti-infectives. Subsequent investigation of the mechanisms of action (*pharmacology*) of these drugs revealed that they are capable of stimulating the pancreas to release more insulin.

Pharmacological studies on another group of "sulfa" related drugs— the thiazide diuretics—revealed that they could induce the kidney to excrete more water and salt in the urine. This drug action is of great value in treating high blood pressure and heart failure.

Photosensitivity A drug-induced change in the skin that results in the development of a rash or exaggerated sunburn on exposure to the sun or ultraviolet lamps. The reaction is confined to uncovered areas of skin, providing a clue to the nature of its cause. (See Table 3 in Section Six.)

Porphyria The porphyrias are a group of hereditary disorders characterized by excessive production of prophyrins, essential respiratory pigments of the body. (One porphyrin is a component of hemoglobin, the pigment of red blood cells.) Two forms of porphyria—acute intermittent porphyria and cutaneous porphyria—can be activated by the use of certain drugs. Acute intermittent porphyria involves damage to the nervous system; an acute attack can include fever, rapid heart rate, vomiting, pain in the abdomen and legs, hallucinations, seizures, paralysis and coma. Twenty-three drugs (or drug classes) can induce an acute attack; among these are the barbiturates, "sulfa" drugs, chlordiazepoxide (Librium), chlorpropamide (Diabinese), methyldopa (Aldomet) and phenytoin (Dilantin). Cutaneous porphyria involves damage to the skin and liver. An episode can include reddening and blistering of the skin, followed by crust formation, scarring and excessive hair growth; repeated liver damage can lead to cirrhosis. This form of porphyria can be precipitated by chloroquine, estrogen, oral contraceptives and excessive iron.

Prostatism This term refers to the difficulties associated with an enlarged prostate gland. As the prostate enlarges (a natural development in aging men), it constricts the urethra (outflow passage) where it joins the urinary bladder and impedes urination. This causes a reduction in the size and force of the urinary stream, hesitancy in starting the flow of urine, interruption of urination and incomplete emptying of the bladder. Atropine and drugs with atropinelike effects can impair the bladder's ability to compensate for the obstructing prostate gland, thus intensifying all of the above symptoms.

Raynaud's Phenomenon This term refers to intermittent episodes of reduced blood flow into the fingers or toes, with resulting paleness, discomfort, numbness and tingling. It is due to an exaggerated constriction of the small arteries that supply blood to the digits. Characteristically an attack is precipitated either by emotional stress or exposure to cold. It can occur as part of a systemic disorder (lupus erythematosus, scleroderma), or it can occur without apparent cause (Raynaud's disease). Some widely used drugs, notably beta-adrenergic blockers and products that contain ergotamine, are conducive to the development of Raynaud-like symptoms in predisposed individuals.

Reye (Reye's) Syndrome An acute, often fatal, childhood illness characterized by swelling of the brain and toxic degeneration of the liver. It usually develops during recovery from a flulike infection, measles or chickenpox. Symptoms include fever, headache, delirium, loss of consciousness and seizures. It is one of the 10 major causes of death in children aged 1 to 10 years. Evidence to date suggests that the syndrome may be due to the combined effects of viral infection and chemical toxins (possibly drugs) in a genetically predisposed child. Drugs that have been used just prior to the onset of symptoms include acetaminophen, aspirin, antibiotics and antiemetics (drugs to control nausea and vomiting). Although it has not been definitely established that drugs actually cause Reye syndrome, it is thought that they may contribute to its development or adversely affect its course. Current recommendations are to avoid the use of acetaminophen, aspirin and antiemetic drugs in children with flulike infections, chickenpox or measles.

Secondary Effect A by-product or complication of drug use which does not occur as part of the drug's primary pharmacological activity. Secondary effects are unwanted consequences and may therefore be classified as adverse effects.

Example: The reactivation of dormant tuberculosis can be a *secondary effect* of long-term cortisone administration for arthritis. Cortisone and related drugs (see Drug Class, Section Four) suppress natural immunity and lower resistance to infection.

Example: The cramping of leg muscles can be a *secondary effect* of diuretic (urine-producing) drug treatment for high blood pressure. Excessive loss of potassium through increased urination renders the muscle vulnerable to painful spasm during exercise.

Side-Effect A normal, expected and predictable response to a drug that accompanies the principal (intended) response sought in treatment. Side-effects are part of a drug's pharmacological activity and thus are unavoidable. Most side-effects are undesirable. The majority cause minor annoyance and inconvenience; some may cause serious problems in managing certain diseases; a few can be hazardous.

Example: The drug propantheline (Pro-Banthine) is used to treat peptic ulcer because one of the consequences of its pharmacological action is the reduction of acid formation in the stomach (an intended effect). Other consequences can include blurring of near vision, dryness of the mouth and constipation. These are *side-effects.*

Superinfection (Suprainfection) The development of a second infection that is superimposed upon an initial infection currently under treatment. The superinfection is caused by organisms that are not susceptible to the killing action of the drug(s) used to treat the original (primary) infection. Superinfections usually occur during or immediately following treatment with a broad spectrum antibiotic—one that is capable of altering the customary balance of bacterial populations in various parts of the body. The disturbance of this balance permits the overgrowth of organisms that normally exist in numbers too small to cause disease. The superinfection may also require treatment, using those drugs that are effective against the offending organism.

Example: Recurrent infections of the kidney and bladder often require repeated courses of treatment with a variety of anti-infective drugs. When these are taken by mouth they can suppress the normally dominant types of bacteria present in the colon and rectum, encouraging the overgrowth of yeast organisms which are capable of causing *colitis.* When this occurs, colitis is a *superinfection.*

Tardive Dyskinesia A late-developing, drug-induced disorder of the nervous system characterized by involuntary bizarre movements of the jaws, lips and tongue. It occurs after long-term treatment with the more potent drugs used in the management of serious mental illness. While it may occur in any age group, it is more common in the middle-aged and the elderly. Older, chronically ill women are particularly susceptible to this adverse drug effect. Once developed, the pattern of uncontrollable chewing, lip puckering and repetitive tongue protruding (fly-catching movement) appears to be irreversible. No consistently satisfactory treatment or cure is available. To date, there is no way of identifying beforehand the individual who may develop this distressing reaction to drug treatment, and there is no known prevention. Fortunately, the persistent dyskinesia (abnormal movement) is not accompanied by further impairment of mental function or deterioration of intelligence. It is ironic, however, that the patient who shows significant improvement in his mental illness but is unfortunate enough to develop tardive dyskinesia may have to remain hospitalized because of a reaction to a drug that was given to make it possible for him to leave the hospital.

Tolerance An adaptation by the body that lessens responsiveness to a drug on continuous administration. Body tissues become accustomed to the drug's presence and react to it less vigorously. Tolerance can be beneficial or harmful in treatment.

Examples: Beneficial tolerance occurs when the hay fever sufferer finds that the side-effect of drowsiness gradually disappears after 4 or 5 days of continuous use of antihistamines.

Harmful tolerance occurs when the patient with "shingles" (herpes zoster) finds that the usual dose of codeine is no longer sufficient to relieve pain and that the need for increasing dosage creates a risk of physical dependence or addiction.

Toxicity The capacity of a drug to dangerously impair body functions or to damage body tissues. Most drug toxicity is related to total dosage: the larger the overdose, the greater the toxic effects. Some drugs, however, can produce toxic reactions when used in normal doses. Such adverse effects are not due to allergy or idiosyncrasy; in many instances their mechanisms are not fully understood. Toxic effects due to overdosage are generally a harmful extension of the drug's normal pharmacological actions and—to some extent—are predictable and preventable. Toxic reactions which occur with normal dosage are unrelated to the drug's known pharmacology and for the most part are unpredictable and unexplainable.

Tyramine A chemical present in many common foods and beverages that causes no difficulties to body functioning under normal circumstances. The main pharmacological action of tyramine is to raise the blood pressure. Normally, enzymes present in many body tissues neutralize this action of tyramine in the quantities in which it is consumed in the average diet. The principal enzyme responsible for neutralizing the blood-pressure-elevating action of tyramine (and chemicals related to it) is monoamine oxidase (MAO). Monoamine oxidase serves an important regulatory function that helps to balance several of the chemical processes in the body that control certain activities of the nervous system. Stabilization of the blood pressure is one of these activities. If the action of monoamine oxidase is blocked, chemical substances like tyramine function unopposed, and relatively small amounts can cause alarming and dangerous elevations of blood pressure.

Several drugs in use today are capable of blocking the action of monoamine oxidase. These drugs are commonly referred to as monoamine oxidase inhibitors (see Drug Class, Section Four). If an individual is taking one of these drugs and his diet includes foods or beverages that contain a significant amount of tyramine, he may experience a sudden increase in blood pressure. Before this interaction of food and drug was understood, several deaths due to brain hemorrhage occurred in persons taking MAO inhibitor drugs as a result of an extreme elevation of blood pressure following a meal of tyramine-rich foods.

It should be noted also that MAO inhibitor drugs can interact with many other drugs and cause serious adverse effects. Consult your physician before taking *any* drug concurrently with one that can inhibit the action of monoamine oxidase.

Any protein-containing food that has undergone partial decomposition may present a hazard because of its increased tyramine content. The following foods and beverages have been reported to contain varying amounts of tyramine. Unless their tyramine content is known to be insignificant, they should be avoided altogether while taking a MAO inhibitor drug. Consult your physician about the advisability of using any of the foods or beverages on these lists if you are taking such drugs.

FOODS	BEVERAGES
Aged cheeses of all kinds*	Beer (unpasteurized)
Avocado	Chianti wine
Banana skins	Sherry wine
Beef liver (unless fresh and used at once)	Sour cream
"Bovril" extract	Vermouth
Broad bean pods	
Chicken liver (unless fresh and used at once)	
Chocolate	
Figs, canned	
Fish, canned	
Fish, dried and salted	
Herring, pickled	
"Marmite" extract	
Meat extracts	
Meat tenderizers	
Raisins	
Raspberries	
Soy sauce	
Yeast extracts	

NOTE: *Any* high-protein food that is aged or has undergone breakdown by putrefaction probably contains tyramine and could produce a hypertensive crisis in anyone taking MAO inhibiting drugs.

*Cottage cheese, cream cheese and processed cheese are safe to eat.

TABLES OF DRUG INFORMATION

TABLE 1

Your Drugs and Behavior

In addition to producing side-effects that can alter mood and disturb emotional stability, some drugs are capable of inducing unexpected and unpredictable patterns of abnormal thinking and behavior. Such responses are relatively infrequent, but the nature and degree of mental disturbance can, at times, be quite alarming and potentially dangerous for both patient and family. It is now well recognized that such paradoxical responses are often of an idiosyncratic nature, and that the individual with a history of a serious mental or emotional disorder is more likely to experience bizarre reactions involving disturbed behavior.

It is often difficult to judge whether a particular aberration of thought or behavior is primarily a feature of the disorder under treatment or an effect of one (or more) drugs the patient may be taking at the time. If in doubt, it is advisable to discontinue any drug with potential for such side-effects and observe for changes during a drug-free period.

Drugs reported to impair *concentration* and/or *memory*

antihistamines*
antiparkinsonism drugs*
barbiturates*
benzodiazepines*
isoniazid

monoamine oxidase inhibitor drugs*
phenytoin
primidone
scopolamine

Drugs reported to cause *confusion, delirium* or *disorientation*

acetazolamide
aminophylline
antidepressants*
antihistamines*
atropinelike drugs*
barbiturates*
benzodiazepines*
bromides
carbamazepine
chloroquine
cimetidine
cortisonelike drugs*
cycloserine
digitalis

digitoxin
digoxin
disulfiram
ethchlorvynol
ethinamate
fenfluramine
glutethimide
isoniazid
levodopa
meprobamate
para-aminosalicylic acid
phenelzine
phenothiazines*
phenytoin

*See Drug Class, Section Four.

Drugs reported to cause *confusion, delirium* or *disorientation* (cont.)

piperazine
primidone
propranolol

reserpine
scopolamine

Drugs reported to cause *paranoid thinking*

bromides
cortisonelike drugs*
diphenhydramine

disulfiram
isoniazid
levodopa

Drugs reported to cause *schizophreniclike behavior*

amphetamines*
ephedrine
fenfluramine

phenmetrazine
phenylpropanolamine

Drugs reported to cause *maniclike behavior*

antidepressants*
cortisonelike drugs*

levodopa
monoamine oxidase inhibitor drugs*

Less apparent—but no less important—are the mood-altering *side-effects* of some drugs which are prescribed primarily for altogether unrelated conditions, with no intention of modifying emotional status. In keeping with the wide variation of individual response to the primary and intended effects of drugs, it is to be expected that the emotional and behavioral secondary effects will also be quite unpredictable and will vary enormously from person to person. However, the following experiences have been observed with sufficient frequency to establish recognizable patterns.

Drugs reported to cause *nervousness* (anxiety and irritability)

amantadine
amphetaminelike drugs* (appetite
   suppressants)
antihistamines*
caffeine
chlorphenesin
cortisonelike drugs*
ephedrine
epinephrine
isoproterenol

levodopa
liothyronine (in excessive dosage)
methylphenidate
methysergide
monoamine oxidase inhibitor drugs*
nylidrin
oral contraceptives
theophylline
thyroid (in excessive dosage)
thyroxine (in excessive dosage)

*See Drug Class, Section Four.

Drugs reported to cause *emotional depression*

amantadine
amphetamine* (on withdrawal)
benzodiazepines*
carbamazepine
chloramphenicol
cortisonelike drugs*
cycloserine
digitalis
digitoxin
digoxin
diphenoxylate
estrogens
ethionamide
fenfluramine (on withdrawal)
fluphenazine
guanethidine

haloperidol
indomethacin
isoniazid
levodopa
methsuximide
methyldopa
methysergide
metoprolol
oral contraceptives
phenylbutazone
procainamide
progesterones
propranolol
reserpine
sulfonamides*
vitamin D (in excessive dosage)

Drugs reported to cause *euphoria*

amantadine
aminophylline
amphetamines
antihistamines* (some)
antispasmodics, synthetic*
aspirin
barbiturates*
benzphetamine
chloral hydrate
clorazepate
codeine
cortisonelike drugs*
diethylpropion
diphenoxylate

ethosuximide
flurazepam
haloperidol
levodopa
meprobamate
methysergide
monoamine oxidase inhibitor drugs*
morphine
pargyline
pentazocine
phenmetrazine
propoxyphene
scopalamine
tybamate

Drugs reported to cause *excitement*

acetazolamide
amantadine
amphetaminelike drugs*
antidepressants*
antihistamines*
atropinelike drugs*

barbiturates* (paradoxical response)
benzodiazepines* (paradoxical response)
cortisonelike drugs
cycloserine
diethylpropion

*See Drug Class, Section Four.

Drugs reported to cause *excitement* (cont.)

digitalis
ephedrine
epinephrine
ethinamate (paradoxical response)
ethionamide
glutethimide (paradoxical response)
isoniazid
isoproterenol
levodopa

meperidine and MAO inhibitor
   drugs*
methyldopa and MAO inhibitor
   drugs*
methyprylon (paradoxical response)
nalidixic acid
orphenadrine
quinine
scopolamine

*See Drug Class, Section Four.

TABLE 2

Your Drugs and Vision

Approximately 3.5% of all adverse drug effects involve impairment of vision or damage to structures of the eye. Some effects, such as blurring of vision or double vision, may occur shortly after starting a drug. These quickly disappear with adjustment of dosage. More subtle and serious effects, such as the development of cataracts or damage to the retina or optic nerve, may not occur until a drug has been in continuous use for an extended period of time. Some of these changes are irreversible. If you are taking a drug that can affect the eye in any way, you are urged to report promptly any eye discomfort or change in vision so that appropriate evaluation can be made and corrective action taken as soon as possible.

Drugs reported to cause *blurring of vision*

acetazolamide
antiarthritic/anti-inflammatory drugs
antidepressants*
antihistamines*
atropinelike drugs*
chlorthalidone
cortisonelike drugs*

diethylstilbestrol
fenfluramine
oral contraceptives
phenytoin
sulfonamides*
tetracyclines*
thiazide diuretics*

Drugs reported to cause *double vision*

antidepressants*
antidiabetic drugs*
antihistamines*
aspirin
barbiturates*
benzodiazepines*
bromides
carbamazepine
carisoprodol
chloroquine
chlorprothixene
clomiphene
colchicine
colistin
cortisonelike drugs*
digitalis
digitoxin

digoxin
ethionamide
ethosuximide
guanethidine
hydroxychloroquine
indomethacin
isoniazid
levodopa
mephenesin
methocarbamol
methsuximide
morphine
nalidixic acid
nitrofurantoin
oral contraceptives
orphenadrine
oxyphenbutazone

*See Drug Class, Section Four.

Drugs reported to cause *double vision* (cont.)

pentazocine
phenothiazines*
phensuximide
phenylbutazone
phenytoin
primidone

propranolol
quinidine
sedatives/sleep inducers*
thiothixene
tranquilizers*

Drugs reported to cause *farsightedness*

ergot
penicillamine

sulfonamides* (possibly)
tolbutamide (possibly)

Drugs reported to cause *nearsightedness*

acetazolamide
aspirin
carbachol
chlorthalidone
codeine
cortisonelike drugs*
ethosuximide
methsuximide
morphine

oral contraceptives
penicillamine
phenothiazines*
phensuximide
spironolactone
sulfonamides*
tetracyclines*
thiazide diuretics*

Drugs reported to *alter color vision*

acetaminophen
amodiaquine
amyl nitrite
aspirin
atropine
barbiturates*
belladonna
chloramphenicol
chloroquine
chlorpromazine
chlortetracycline
cortisonelike drugs*
digitalis
digitoxin
digoxin
disulfiram

epinephrine
ergotamine
erythromycin
ethchlorvynol
ethionamide
fluphenazine
furosemide
hydroxychloroquine
indomethacin
isocarboxazid
isoniazid
mephenamic acid
mesoridazine
methysergide
nalidixic acid
oral contraceptives

*See Drug Class, Section Four.

Drugs reported to alter color vision (cont.)

oxyphenbutazone
paramethadione
pargyline
penicillamine
pentylenetetrazol
perphenazine
phenacetin
phenylbutazone
primidone
prochlorperazine
promazine
promethazine
quinacrine

quinidine
quinine
reserpine
sodium salicylate
streptomycin
sulfonamides*
thioridazine
tranylcypromine
trifluoperazine
triflupromazine
trimeprazine
trimethadione

Drugs reported to cause sensitivity to light (photophobia)

antidiabetic drugs*
atropinelike drugs*
bromides
chloraquine
clomiphene
digitoxin
doxepin
ethambutol
ethionamide
ethosuximide
hydroxychloroquine

mephenytoin
methsuximide
monoamine oxidase inhibitor drugs*
nalidixic acid
oral contraceptives
paramethadione
phenothiazines*
quinidine
quinine
tetracyclines*
trimethadione

Drugs reported to cause halos around lights

amyl nitrite
chloroquine
cortisonelike drugs*
digitalis
digitoxin
digoxin
hydrochloroquine

nitroglycerin
oral contraceptives
paramethadione
phenothiazines*
quinacrine
trimethadione

Drugs reported to cause visual hallucinations

amantadine
amphetaminelike drugs*

amyl nitrite
antihistamines*

*See Drug Class, Section Four.

Drugs reported to cause *visual hallucinations* (cont.)

aspirin
atropinelike drugs*
barbiturates*
benzodiazepines*
bromides
carbamazepine
cephalexin
cephaloglycin
chloroquine
cycloserine
digitalis
digoxin
disulfiram
ephedrine
furosemide
griseofulvin
haloperidol
hydroxychloroquine
indomethacin
isosorbide
levodopa
nialamide
oxyphenbutazone
pargyline
pentazocine
phenothiazines*
phenylbutazone
phenytoin
primidone
propranolol
quinine
sedatives/sleep inducers*
sulfonamides*
tetracyclines*
tricyclic antidepressants*
tripelennamine

Drugs reported to impair the use of *contact lenses*

brompheniramine
carbinoxamine
chlorpheniramine
cyclizine
cyproheptadine
dexbrompheniramine
dexchlorpheniramine
dimethindene
diphenhydramine
diphenpyraline
furosemide
oral contraceptives
terfenadine
tripelennamine

Drugs reported to cause *cataracts* or *lens deposits*

allopurinol
busulfan
chlorpromazine
chlorprothixene
cortisonelike drugs*
fluphenazine
mesoridazine
methotrimeprazine
perphenazine
phenmetrazine
pilocarpine
prochlorperazine
promazine
promethazine
thioridazine
thiothixene
trifluoperazine
triflupromazine
trimeprazine

*See Drug Class, Section Four.

TABLE 3

Your Drugs and the Sun: Photosensitivity

Some drugs are capable of sensitizing the skin of some individuals to the action of ultraviolet light. This can cause uncovered areas of the skin to react with a rash or exaggerated burn on exposure to sun or ultraviolet lamps. If you are taking any of the following drugs, ask your physician for guidance and use caution with regard to sun exposure.

acetohexamide
amitriptyline
amoxapine
barbiturates
bendroflumethiazide
carbamazepine
chlordiazepoxide
chloroquine
chlorothiazide
chlorpromazine
chlorpropamide
chlortetracycline
chlorthalidone
clindamycin
cyproheptadine
demeclocycline
desipramine
diethylstilbestrol
diltiazem
diphenhydramine
doxepin
doxycycline
estrogen
fluphenazine
glyburide
gold preparations
griseofulvin
hydrochlorothiazide
hydroflumethiazide
imipramine
isotretinoin

lincomycin
maprotiline
mesoridazine
methacycline
methotrexate
nalidixic acid
nortriptyline
oral contraceptives
oxyphenbutazone
oxytetracycline
perphenazine
phenobarbital
phenylbutazone
phenytoin
prochlorperazine
promazine
promethazine
protriptyline
pyrazinamide
sulfonamides
tetracycline
thioridazine
tolazamide
tolbutamide
tranylcypromine
triamterene
trifluoperazine
trimeprazine
trimipramine
triprolidine

TABLE 4

Your Drugs and Sexuality

It is now well established that certain drugs have the potential for affecting sexual functions in a variety of unintended ways. Many commonly prescribed drugs can cause both obvious and subtle effects on one or more aspects of sexual expression. Patients are usually unaware that changes in sexual performance or response may be related to medications they are taking. If they should suspect it, they are often reluctant to discuss the possible association with their physician. In some situations, the sexual dysfunction may be a natural consequence of the disorder under treatment—or of a concurrent and undetected disorder—possibilities often overlooked by both practitioner and patient. It is well known that disorders such as diabetes, kidney failure, hypertension, depression and alcoholism may reduce libido and cause failure of erection. In addition, many of the drugs commonly used to treat these conditions may have the ability to augment a subclinical sexual dysfunction through unavoidable pharmacological activity. Such situations require the closest cooperation between therapist and patient in order to correctly assess the possible cause-and-effect relationships and to modify the treatment program appropriately.

Possible Drug Effects on Male Sexuality

1. Increased libido
   androgens (replacement therapy in deficiency states)
   baclofen (Lioresal)
   chlordiazepoxide (Librium) (antianxiety effect)
   diazepam (Valium) (antianxiety effect)
   haloperidol (Haldol)
   levodopa (Larodopa, Sinemet) (may be an indirect effect due to improved sense of well-being)

2. Decreased libido
   antihistamines
   barbiturates
   chlordiazepoxide (Librium) (sedative effect)
   chlorpromazine (Thorazine) 10% to 20% of users
   cimetidine (Tagamet)
   clofibrate (Atromid-S)
   clonidine (Catapres) 10% to 20% of users
   danazol (Danocrine)
   diazepam (Valium) (sedative effect)
   disulfiram (Antabuse)
   estrogens (therapy for prostatic cancer)

fenfluramine (Pondimin)
heroin
licorice
medroxyprogesterone (Provera)
methyldopa (Aldomet) 10% to 15% of users
perhexilene (Pexid)
prazosin (Minipress) 15% of users
propranolol (Inderal) rarely
reserpine (Serpasil, Ser-Ap-Es)
spironolactone (Aldactone)
tricyclic antidepressants (TAD's)

3. Impaired erection (Impotence)
anticholinergics
antihistamines
baclofen (Lioresal)
barbiturates (when abused)
chlordiazepoxide (Librium) (in high dosage)
chlorpromazine (Thorazine)
cimetidine (Tagamet)
clofibrate (Atromid-S)
clonidine (Catapres) 10% to 20% of users
cocaine
diazepam (Valium) (in high dosage)
digitalis and its glycosides
disopyramide (Norpace)
disulfiram (Antabuse) (uncertain)
estrogens (therapy for prostatic cancer)
ethacrynic acid (Edecrin) 5% of users
ethionamide (Trecator-SC)
fenfluramine (Pondimin)
furosemide (Lasix) 5% of users
guanethidine (Ismelin)
haloperidol (Haldol) 10% to 20% of users
heroin
hydroxyprogesterone (therapy for prostatic cancer)
licorice
lithium (Lithonate)
marijuana
mesoridazine (Serentil)
methantheline (Banthine)
methyldopa (Aldomet) 10% to 15% of users
monoamine oxidase inhibitors (MAOI's) 10% to 15% of users
perhexilene (Pexid)
prazosin (Minipres) infrequently
propranolol (Inderal) infrequently

reserpine (Serpasil, Ser-Ap-Es)
spironolactone (Aldactone)
thiazide diuretics, 5% of users
thioridazine (Mellaril)
tricyclic antidepressants (TAD's)

4. Impaired ejaculation
anticholinergics
barbiturates (when abused)
chlorpromazine (Thorazine)
clonidine (Catapres)
estrogens (therapy for prostatic cancer)
guanethidine (Ismelin)
heroin
mesoridazine (Serentil)
methyldopa (Aldomet)
monoamine oxidase inhibitors (MAOI's)
phenoxybenzamine (Dibenzyline)
phentolamine (Regitine)
reserpine (Serpasil, Ser-Ap-Es)
thiazide diuretics
thioridazine (Mellaril)
tricyclic antidepressants (TAD's)

5. Decreased testosterone
adrenocorticotropic hormone (ACTH)
barbiturates
digoxin (Lanoxin)
haloperidol (Haldol)
   increased testosterone with low dosage
   decreased testosterone with high dosage
lithium (Lithonate)
marijuana
medroxyprogesterone (Provera)
monoamine oxidase inhibitors (MAOI's)
spironolactone (Aldactone)

6. Impaired spermatogenesis (reduced fertility)
adrenocorticosteroids (prednisone, etc.)
androgens (moderate to high dosage, extended use)
antimalarials
aspirin (abusive, chronic use)
chlorambucil (Leukeran)
cimetidine (Tagamet)
colchicine
co-trimoxazole (Bactrim, Septra)

cyclophosphamide (Cytoxan)
estrogens (therapy for prostatic cancer)
marijuana
medroxyprogesterone (Provera)
methotrexate
monoamine oxidase inhibitors (MAOI's)
niridazole (Ambilhar)
nitrofurantoin (Furadantin)
spironolactone (Aldactone)
sulfasalazine (Azulfidine)
testosterone (moderate to high dosage, extended use)
vitamin C (in doses of 1 gram or more)

7. Testicular disorders
    Swelling
        tricyclic antidepressants (TAD's)
    Inflammation
        oxyphenbutazone (Tandearil)
    Atrophy
        androgens (moderate to high dosage, extended use)
        chlorpromazine (Thorazine)
        cyclophosphamide (Cytoxan) (in prepubescent boys)
        spironolactone (Aldactone)

8. Penile disorders
    Priapism
        cocaine
        heparin
        phenothiazines
    Peyronie's disease
        metoprolol (Lopressor)

9. Gynecomastia (excessive development of the male breast)
    androgens (partial conversion to estrogen)
    BCNU
    busulfan (Myleran)
    chlormadinone
    chlorpromazine (Thorazine)
    chlortetracycline (Aureomycin)
    cimetidine (Tagamet)
    clonidine (Catapres) (infrequently)
    diethylstilbestrol (DES)
    digitalis and its glycosides
    estrogens (therapy for prostatic cancer)
    ethionamide (Trecator-SC)
    griseofulvin (Fulvicin, etc.)

> haloperidol (Haldol)
> heroin
> human chorionic gonadotropin
> isoniazid (INH, Nydrazid)
> marijuana
> mestranol
> methyldopa (Aldomet)
> phenelzine (Nardil)
> reserpine (Serpasil, Ser-Ap-Es)
> spironolactone (Aldactone)
> thioridazine (Mellaril)
> tricyclic antidepressants (TAD's)
> vincristine (Oncovin)

10. Feminization (loss of libido, impotence, gynecomastia, testicular atrophy)
    conjugated estrogens (Premarin, etc.)

11. Precocious puberty
    anabolic steroids
    androgens
    isoniazid (INH)

Possible Drug Effects on Female Sexuality

1. Increased libido
   androgens
   chlordiazepoxide (Librium) (antianxiety effect)
   diazepam (Valium) (antianxiety effect)
   mazindol (Sanorex)
   oral contraceptives (freedom from fear of pregnancy)

2. Decreased libido
   See list of drug effects on male sexuality. Some of these *may* have
   potential for reducing libido in the female. The literature is sparse on
   this subject.

3. Impaired arousal and orgasm
   anticholinergics
   clonidine (Catapres)
   methyldopa (Aldomet)
   monoamine oxidase inhibitors (MAOI's)
   tricyclic antidepressants (TAD's)

4. Breast enlargement
   penicillamine
   tricyclic antidepressants (TAD's)

5. Galactorrhea (spontaneous flow of milk)
   amphetamine
   chlorpromazine (Thorazine)
   cimetidine (Tagamet)
   haloperidol (Haldol)
   heroin
   methyldopa (Aldomet)
   metoclopramide (Reglan)
   oral contraceptives
   phenothiazines
   reserpine (Serpasil, Ser-Ap-Es)
   sulpiride (Equilid)
   tricyclic antidepressants (TAD's)

6. Ovarian failure (reduced fertility)
   anesthetic gases (operating room staff)
   cyclophosphamide (Cytoxan)
   cytostatic drugs
   danazol (Danacrine)
   medroxyprogesterone (Provera)

7. Altered menstruation (menstrual disorders)
   adrenocorticosteroids (prednisone, etc.)
   androgens
   barbiturates (when abused)
   chlorambucil (Leukeran)
   chlorpromazine (Thorazine)
   cyclophosphamide (Cytoxan)
   danazol (Danocrine)
   estrogens
   ethionamide (Trecator-SC)
   haloperidol (Haldol)
   heroin
   isoniazid (INH, Nydrazid)
   marijuana
   medroxyprogesterone (Provera)
   oral contraceptives
   phenothiazines
   progestins
   radioisotopes
   rifampin (Rifadin, Rifamate, Rimactane)
   spironolactone (Aldactone)
   testosterone
   thioridazine (Mellaril)
   vitamin A (in excessive dosage)

8. Virilization (acne, hirsutism, lowering of voice, enlargement of clitoris)
anabolic drugs
androgens
haloperidol (Haldol)
oral contraceptives (lowering of voice)

9. Precocious puberty
estrogens (in hair lotions)
isoniazid (INH, Nydrazid)

TABLE 5

Your Drugs and Alcohol

Beverages containing alcohol may interact unfavorably with a wide variety of drugs. The most important (and most familiar) interaction occurs when the depressant action on the brain of sedatives, sleep-inducing drugs, tranquilizers and narcotic drugs is intensified by alcohol. Alcohol may also reduce the effectiveness of some drugs, and it can interact with certain other drugs to produce toxic effects. Some drugs may increase the intoxicating effects of alcohol, producing further impairment of mental alertness, judgment, physical coordination and reaction time.

While drug interactions with alcohol are generally predictable, the intensity and significance of these interactions can vary greatly from one individual to another and from one occasion to another. This is because many factors influence what happens when drugs and alcohol interact. These factors include individual variations in sensitivity to drugs (including alcohol), the chemistry and quantity of the drug, the type and amount of alcohol consumed and the sequence in which drug and alcohol are taken. If you need to use any of the drugs listed in the following tables, you should ask your physician for guidance concerning the use of alcohol.

Drugs with which it is advisable to avoid alcohol completely

Drug name or class	Possible interaction with alcohol
amphetamines	excessive rise in blood pressure with alcoholic beverages containing tyramine**
barbiturates*	excessive sedation
bromides	confusion, delirium, increased intoxication
calcium carbamide	disulfiramlike reaction**
carbamazepine	excessive sedation
chlorprothixene	excessive sedation
chlorzoxazone	excessive sedation
disulfiram	disulfiram reaction**
ergotamine	reduced effectiveness of ergotamine
fenfluramine	excessive stimulation of nervous system with some beers and wines
furazolidone	disulfiramlike reaction**
haloperidol	excessive sedation

*See Drug Class, Section Four.
**See Glossary.

Drug name or class	Possible interaction with alcohol
MAO inhibitor drugs*	excessive rise in blood pressure with alcoholic beverages containing tyramine**
meperidine	excessive sedation
meprobamate	excessive sedation
methotrexate	increased liver toxicity and excessive sedation
metronidazole	disulfiramlike reaction**
narcotic drugs	excessive sedation
oxyphenbutazone	increased stomach irritation and/or bleeding
pentazocine	excessive sedation
pethidine	excessive sedation
phenothiazines*	excessive sedation
phenylbutazone	increased stomach irritation and/or bleeding
procarbazine	disulfiramlike reaction**
propoxyphene	excessive sedation
reserpine	excessive sedation, orthostatic hypotension**

sleep-inducing drugs (hypnotics)
  carbromal
  chloral hydrate
  ethchlorvynol
  ethinamate
  glutethimide
  flurazepam
  methaqualone
  methyprylon
  temazepam
  triazolam
	excessive sedation

thiothixene	excessive sedation
tricyclic antidepressants*	excessive sedation, increased intoxication
trimethobenzamide	excessive sedation

Drugs with which alcohol should be used only in small amounts (use cautiously until combined effects have been determined)

Drug name or class	Possible interaction with alcohol
acetaminophen (Tylenol, etc.)	increased liver toxicity
amantadine	excessive lowering of blood pressure

*See Drug Class, Section Four.
**See Glossary.

Drug name or class	Possible interaction with alcohol
antiarthritic/anti-inflammatory drugs	increased stomach irritation and/or bleeding
anticoagulants (coumarins)*	increased anticoagulant effect
antidiabetic drugs (sulfonylureas)*	increased antidiabetic effect, excessive hypoglycemia**
antihistamines*	excessive sedation
antihypertensives*	excessive orthostatic hypotension**
aspirin (large doses or continuous use)	increased stomach irritation and/or bleeding
benzodiazepines*	excessive sedation
carisoprodol	increased alcoholic intoxication
diethylpropion	excessive nervous system stimulation with alcoholic beverages containing tyramine**
dihydroergotoxine	excessive lowering of blood pressure
diphenoxylate	excessive sedation
dipyridamole	excessive lowering of blood pressure
diuretics*	excessive orthostatic hypotension**
ethionamide	confusion, delirium, psychotic behavior
fenoprofen	increased stomach irritation and/or bleeding
griseofulvin	flushing and rapid heart action
ibuprofen	increased stomach irritation and/or bleeding
indomethacin	increased stomach irritation and/or bleeding
insulin	excessive hypoglycemia**
iron	excessive absorption of iron
isoniazid	decreased effectiveness of isoniazid, increased incidence of hepatitis
lithium	increased confusion and delirium (avoid all alcohol if any indication of lithium overdosage)
methocarbamol	excessive sedation
methotrimeprazine	excessive sedation
methylphenidate	excessive nervous system stimulation with alcoholic beverages containing tyramine**
metoprolol	excessive orthostatic hypotension**
nalidixic acid	increased alcoholic intoxication
naproxen	increased stomach irritation and/or bleeding

*See Drug Class, Section Four.
**See Glossary.

Drug name or class	Possible interaction with alcohol
nicotinic acid	possible orthostatic hypotension**
nitrates* (vasodilators)	possible orthostatic hypotension**
nylidrin	increased stomach irritation
orphenadrine	excessive sedation
phenelzine	increased alcoholic intoxication
phenoxybenzamine	possible orthostatic hypotension**
phentermine	excessive nervous system stimulation with alcoholic beverages containing tyramine**
phenytoin	decreased effect of phenytoin
pilocarpine	prolongation of alcohol effect
prazosin	excessive lowering of blood pressure
primidone	excessive sedation
propranolol	excessive orthostatic hypotension**
sulfonamides*	increased alcoholic intoxication
sulindac	increased stomach irritation and/or bleeding
tolmetin	increased stomach irritation and/or bleeding
tranquilizers (mild) chlordiazepoxide clorazepate diazepam hydroxyzine meprobamate oxazepam phenaglycodol tybamate	excessive sedation
tranylcypromine	increased alcoholic intoxication

Drugs capable of producing a disulfiramlike reaction** when used concurrently with alcohol

antidiabetic drugs (sulfonylureas)*	nifuroxine
calcium carbamide	nitrofurantoin
chloral hydrate	procarbazine
chloramphenicol	quinacrine
disulfiram	sulfonamides*
furazolidone	tinidazole
metronidazole	tolazoline

*See Drug Class, Section Four.
**See Glossary.

TABLE 6

High-Potassium Foods

Diuretic drugs that cause loss of potassium from the body are often used to treat conditions that also require a reduced intake of sodium. The high-potassium foods listed below have been selected for their compatibility with a sodium restricted diet (500 to 1000 mg of sodium daily).

Beverages

orange juice	tea
prune juice	tomato juice
skim milk	whole milk

Breads and Cereals

brown rice	oatmeal
cornbread	shredded wheat
griddle cakes	waffles
muffins	

Fruits

apricot	mango
avocado	orange
banana	papaya
fig	prune
honeydew melon	

Meats

beef	liver
chicken	pork
codfish	rockfish
flounder	salmon
haddock	turkey
halibut	veal

Vegetables

baked beans	radishes
lima beans	squash
mushrooms	sweet potato
navy beans	tomato
parsnips	white potato

SOURCES

Sources

The following sources were consulted in the compilation and revision of this book:

Adverse Drug Reaction Bulletin. Edited by D. M. Davies. Newcastle upon Tyne, England: Regional Postgraduate Institute for Medicine and Dentistry, 1986.

AMA Department of Drugs, *AMA Drug Evaluations*, 5th ed. Chicago: American Medical Association, 1983.

Andreoli, T. E., Carpenter, C. C. J., Plum, F., Smith, L. H., eds., *Cecil Essentials of Medicine*. Philadelphia: W. B. Saunders Co., 1986.

Atkinson, A. J., Ambre, J. J., *Kalman and Clark's Drug Assay, The Strategy of Therapeutic Drug Monitoring*, 2nd ed. New York: Masson Publishing USA, 1985.

Avery, G. S., ed., *Drug Treatment*, 2nd ed. Sydney, Australia: ADIS Press, 1980.

Bevan, J. A., ed., *Essentials of Pharmacology*. Hagerstown, Maryland: Harper & Row, 1976.

Billups, N. F., ed., *American Drug Index 1986*. Philadelphia: J. B. Lippincott Co., 1986.

Branch, W. T., *Office Practice of Medicine*. Philadelphia: W. B. Saunders Co., 1982.

Briggs, G. G., Bodendorfer, T. W., Freeman, R. K., Yaffee, S. J., *Drugs in Pregnancy and Lactation*. Baltimore: Williams & Wilkins, 1983.

Canadian Pharmaceutical Association, *Compendium of Pharmaceuticals and Specialties*, 21st ed. Ottawa: Canadian Pharmaceutical Association, 1986.

Cape, Ronald, *Aging: Its Complex Management*. Hagerstown, Maryland: Harper & Row, 1978.

Clin-Alert. Louisville, Kentucky: Science Editors, Inc., 1986.

Davies, D. M., ed., *Textbook of Adverse Drug Reactions*, 2nd ed. New York: Oxford University Press, 1981.

Drug Interaction Facts. Edited by R. J. Mangini. St. Louis: Facts and Comparisons Division, J. B. Lippincott Co., 1986.

Drug Interactions Newsletter. Edited by P. D. Hansten, J. R. Horn. Spokane, Washington: Applied Therapeutics, Inc., 1986.

Drug Newsletter. Edited by G. H. Schwach, B. R. Olin. St. Louis: Facts and Comparisons Division, J. B. Lippincott Co., 1986.

Drug Therapy, Clinical Therapeutics for Physicians. New York: Biomedical Information Corporation, 1986.

Dukes, M. N. G., ed., *Meyler's Side Effects of Drugs,* 9th ed. Amsterdam: Excerpta Medica, 1980.

Facts and Comparisons. Edited by B. R. Olin. St. Louis: Facts and Comparisons Division, J. B. Lippincott Co., 1986.

F.D.A. Drug Bulletin. Rockville, Maryland: Department of Health and Human Services, Food and Drug Administration.

Fraunfelder, F. T., *Drug-Induced Ocular Side Effects and Drug Interactions.* Philadelphia: Lea & Febiger, 1976.

Goodman, L. S., Gilman, A., eds., *The Pharmacological Basis of Therapeutics,* 6th ed. New York: Macmillan, 1980.

Greenberger, N. J., Arvanitakis, C., Hurwitz, A., *Drug Treatment of Gastrointestinal Disorders.* New York: Churchill Livingstone, 1978.

Hansten, P. D., *Drug Interactions,* 5th ed. Philadelphia: Lea & Febiger, 1985.

Heinonen, O. P., Slone, D., Shapiro, S., *Birth Defects and Drugs in Pregnancy.* Littleton, Massachusetts: PSG Publishing Co., 1977.

Hollister, L. E., *Clinical Pharmacology of Psychotherapeutic Drugs,* 2nd ed. New York: Churchill Livingstone, 1983.

Huff, B. B., ed., *The Physicians' Desk Reference,* 40th ed. Oradell, New Jersey: Medical Economics Company, 1986.

International Drug Therapy Newsletter. Edited by F. J. Ayd. Baltimore: Ayd Medical Communications, 1986.

Jefferson, J. W., Greist, J. H., *Primer of Lithium Therapy.* Baltimore: Williams & Wilkens, 1977.

Journal of the American Medical Association. Edited by G. D. Lundberg. Chicago: American Medical Association, 1986.

Kolodny, R. C., Masters, W. H., Johnson, V. E., *Textbook of Sexual Medicine.* Boston: Little, Brown and Co., 1979.

Lawrence, R. A., *Breast-Feeding.* St. Louis: Mosby, 1980.

Long, J. W., *Clinical Management of Prescription Drugs.* Philadelphia: Harper & Row, 1984.

McEvoy, G. K., ed., *American Hospital Formulary Service, Drug Information 86.* Bethesda, Maryland: American Society of Hospital Pharmacists, 1986.

The Medical Letter on Drugs and Therapeutics. Edited by H. Aaron. New Rochelle, New York: The Medical Letter, Inc., 1986.

Melmon, K. L., Morrelli, H. F., *Clinical Pharmacology,* 2nd ed. New York: Macmillan, 1978.

Meyler, L., Herxheimer, A., eds., *Side-Effects of Drugs,* Vol. 8. Amsterdam: Excerpta Medica, 1975.

Mohler, S. R., *Medication and Flying: A Pilot's Guide.* Boston: Boston Publishing Co., 1982.

The New England Journal of Medicine. Edited by A. S. Relman. Boston: The Massachusetts Medical Society, 1986.

Pharmacotherapy, The Journal of Human Pharmacology and Drug Therapy. Edited by R. T. Scheife. Boston: Pharmacotherapy Publications, Inc., 1986.

Postgraduate Medicine, The Journal of Applied Medicine for the Primary Care Physician. Minneapolis, MN: McGraw-Hill, Inc., 1986.

Rakel, R. E., ed., *Conn's Current Therapy 1986.* Philadelphia: W. B. Saunders Co., 1986.

Rational Drug Therapy, Pharmacology for Physicians. Bethesda, Maryland: American Society for Pharmacology and Experimental Therapeutics, 1986.

Reynolds, J. E. F., ed. *Martindale, The Extra Pharmacopoeia,* 28th ed. London: The Pharmaceutical Press, 1982.

Rodman, M. J., Smith, D. W., *Clinical Pharmacology in Nursing*. Philadelphia: J. B. Lippincott Co., 1984.

Schardein, J. L., *Drugs As Teratogens*. Cleveland: CRC Press, 1976.

Shepard, T. H., *Catalog of Teratogenic Agents*, 3rd ed. Baltimore: Johns Hopkins University Press, 1980.

Tuchmann-Duplessis, H., *Drug Effects on the Fetus*. Sydney, Australia: ADIS Press, 1975.

USAN 1986 and the USP Dictionary of Drug Names. Edited by M. C. Griffiths. Rockville, Maryland: United States Pharmacopeial Convention, Inc., 1986.

USP Dispensing Information 1986, Vol. 1, Drug Information for the Health Care Provider. Rockville, Maryland: United States Pharmacopeial Convention, 1986.

Utian, W. H., *Menopause in Modern Perspective*. New York: Appleton-Century-Crofts, 1980.

Wartak, J., *Drug Dosage and Administration*. Baltimore: University Park Press, 1983.

Worley, R. J., ed., *Clinical Obstetrics and Gynecology*, Vol. 24, No. 1: *Menopause*. Hagerstown, Maryland: Harper & Row, 1981.

INDEX

Index

This index contains all the brand and generic drug names included in Section Three and the names and alternative names of the disorders and conditions for which drug management is described in Section Two.

Brand names of drugs appear in italic type and are capitalized.

Each brand name is followed by the generic name of its Drug Profile in Section Three.

The symbol [CD] indicates that the brand name represents a combination drug that contains the generic drug components listed below it. To be fully familiar with any combination drug [CD], it is necessary to read the Drug Profile of each of the components listed. The brand name of a combination drug *may* or *may not* appear in the brand name list of each Drug Profile that is cited in the index as a component of a particular combination drug. The index listing of component drugs for any combination drug product represents the manufacturer's formulation of that brand at the time this information was compiled for publication.

The symbol ♣ before the brand name of a combination drug indicates that the brand name is used both in the United States and Canada, but that the ingredients in the combination product in each country differ. The Canadian drug is marked with the symbol ♣ to distinguish it from the American drug which has the same name.

A generic name with no page designation indicates an active component of a combination drug for which there is no Profile in Section Three. It is included to alert you to its presence, should you wish to consult your physician regarding its significance.

Index

*The symbol [CD] indicates that the brand name given is a combination drug consisting of generic drug components listed below it. If there is no page numbering following the name of the generic drug component, there is no Drug Profile for that ingredient in this book.

*The symbol [CD] indicates that the brand name given is a combination drug consisting of generic drug components listed below it. If there is no page numbering following the name of the generic drug component, there is no Drug Profile for that ingredient in this book.

*The symbol [CD] indicates that the brand name given is a combination drug consisting of generic drug components listed below it. If there is no page numbering following the name of the generic drug component, there is no Drug Profile for that ingredient in this book.

Brethine, terbutaline, 717
Brevicon, oral contraceptives, 556
Bricanyl, terbutaline, 717
Bricanyl Spacer, terbutaline, 717
Bristamycin, erythromycin, 356
bromocriptine, 190
Bromo-Seltzer [CD]
  CONTAINS
  acetaminophen, 121
  citric acid*
  sodium bicarbonate, 687
brompheniramine, 194
bronchial asthma. *See* asthma
Brondecon [CD]
  CONTAINS
  guaifenesin*
  theophylline, 727
Bronkaid Mistometer, epinephrine, 346
Bronkaid Tablets [CD]
  CONTAINS
  ephedrine*
  guaifenesin*
  theophylline, 727
Bronkodyl, theophylline, 727
Bronkolixir [CD]
  CONTAINS
  ephedrine*
  guaifenesin*
  phenobarbital, 591
  theophylline, 727
Bronkotabs [CD]
  CONTAINS
  ephedrine*
  guaifenesin*
  phenobarbital, 591
  theophylline, 727

Bufferin [CD]
  CONTAINS
  aluminum glycinate*
  aspirin, 157
  magnesium carbonate, 461
Bufferin, Arthritis Strength [CD]
  CONTAINS
  aluminum glycinate*
  aspirin, 157
  magnesium carbonate, 461
Bufferin, Extra Strength [CD]
  CONTAINS
  aluminum glycinate*
  aspirin, 157
  magnesium carbonate, 461
Bufferin w/Codeine [CD]
  CONTAINS
  aluminum glycinate*
  aspirin, 157
  codeine, 280
  magnesium carbonate, 461
bumetanide, 198
Bumex, bumetanide, 198
Buspar, buspirone, 201
buspirone, 201
butalbital, 203
Butazolidin, phenylbutazone, 596
Butibel [CD]
  CONTAINS
  atropine, 166
  butabarbital*

C

Cafergot [CD]
  CONTAINS
  caffeine, 207
  ergotamine, 353

*The symbol [CD] indicates that the brand name given is a combination drug consisting of generic drug components listed below it. If there is no page numbering following the name of the generic drug component, there is no Drug Profile for that ingredient in this book.

*The symbol [CD] indicates that the brand name given is a combination drug consisting of generic drug components listed below it. If there is no page numbering following the name of the generic drug component, there is no Drug Profile for that ingredient in this book.

---

*The symbol [CD] indicates that the brand name given is a combination drug consisting of generic drug components listed below it. If there is no page numbering following the name of the generic drug component, there is no Drug Profile for that ingredient in this book.

*The symbol [CD] indicates that the brand name given is a combination drug consisting of generic drug components listed below it. If there is no page numbering following the name of the generic drug component, there is no Drug Profile for that ingredient in this book.

*The symbol [CD] indicates that the brand name given is a combination drug consisting of generic drug components listed below it. If there is no page numbering following the name of the generic drug component, there is no Drug Profile for that ingredient in this book.

*The symbol [CD] indicates that the brand name given is a combination drug consisting of generic drug components listed below it. If there is no page numbering following the name of the generic drug component, there is no Drug Profile for that ingredient in this book.

*The symbol [CD] indicates that the brand name given is a combination drug consisting of generic drug components listed below it. If there is no page numbering following the name of the generic drug component, there is no Drug Profile for that ingredient in this book.

*The symbol [CD] indicates that the brand name given is a combination drug consisting of generic drug components listed below it. If there is no page numbering following the name of the generic drug component, there is no Drug Profile for that ingredient in this book.

*The symbol [CD] indicates that the brand name given is a combination drug consisting of generic drug components listed below it. If there is no page numbering following the name of the generic drug component, there is no Drug Profile for that ingredient in this book.

*The symbol [CD] indicates that the brand name given is a combination drug consisting of generic drug components listed below it. If there is no page numbering following the name of the generic drug component, there is no Drug Profile for that ingredient in this book.

*The symbol [CD] indicates that the brand name given is a combination drug consisting of generic drug components listed below it. If there is no page numbering following the name of the generic drug component, there is no Drug Profile for that ingredient in this book.

---

*The symbol [CD] indicates that the brand name given is a combination drug consisting of generic drug components listed below it. If there is no page numbering following the name of the generic drug component, there is no Drug Profile for that ingredient in this book.

*The symbol [CD] indicates that the brand name given is a combination drug consisting of generic drug components listed below it. If there is no page numbering following the name of the generic drug component, there is no Drug Profile for that ingredient in this book.

*The symbol [CD] indicates that the brand name given is a combination drug consisting of generic drug components listed below it. If there is no page numbering following the name of the generic drug component, there is no Drug Profile for that ingredient in this book.

*The symbol [CD] indicates that the brand name given is a combination drug consisting of generic drug components listed below it. If there is no page numbering following the name of the generic drug component, there is no Drug Profile for that ingredient in this book.

The symbol [CD] indicates that the brand name given is a combination drug consisting of generic drug components listed below it. If there is no page numbering following the name of the generic drug component, there is no Drug Profile for that ingredient in this book.

About the Author

James W. Long, M.D., was born in Allentown, Pennsylvania. He received his pre-medical education from the University of Maryland and his medical degree from the George Washington University School of Medicine in Washington, D.C. For twenty years he was in the private practice of internal medicine in the Washington metropolitan area, and for over thirty-five years he was a member of the faculty of the George Washington University School of Medicine. He has served with the Food and Drug Administration, the National Library of Medicine, and the Bureau of Health Manpower of the National Institutes of Health. Prior to his retirement, Dr. Long was director of Health Services for the National Science Foundation in Washington. He lives in Oxford, Maryland.

Dr. Long's involvement in drug information activities includes service on the H.E.W. Task Force on Prescription Drugs, on the F.D.A. Task Force on Adverse Drug Reactions, as a delegate-at-large to the U.S. Pharmacopeial Convention, as Editorial Consultant for *Hospital Formulary*, as a director of the Drug Information Association, and as a member of the Toxicology Information Program Committee of the National Research Council/National Academy of Sciences. He was consultant to the Food and Drug Administration, serving as advisor to their staff on the development of Patient Package Inserts. He is also the author of numerous articles in professional journals. *The Essential Guide to Prescription Drugs* is an outgrowth of his conviction that the general public needs and is entitled to practical drug information which is the equivalent of the professional "package insert." He believes the patient can be reasonably certain of using medications with the least risk and the greatest benefit only when the patient has all the relevant information about the drugs he or she is taking.

Schedules of Controlled Drugs*

Schedule I: Non-medicinal substances with high abuse potential and dependence liability. Used for research purposes only. Examples: heroin, marijuana, LSD. Not legally available for medicinal use by prescription.

Schedule II: Medicinal drugs in current use that have the highest abuse potential and dependence liability. Examples: opium derivatives (morphine, codeine, etc.), meperidine (Demerol), amphetamines (Dexedrine), short-acting barbiturates (Amytal, Nembutal, Seconal). A written prescription is required. Telephoned prescribing is prohibited. No refills are allowed.

Schedule III: Medicinal drugs with abuse potential and dependence liability less than Schedule II drugs but greater than Schedule IV or V drugs. Examples: codeine, hydrocodone and paregoric in combination wth one or more non-narcotic drugs, some hypnotics (Doriden, Noludar), some appetite suppressants (Didrex, Tenuate, Sanorex). A telephoned prescription is permitted, to be converted to written form by the dispensing pharmacist. Prescriptions must be renewed every 6 months. Refills are limited to 5.

Schedule IV: Medicinal drugs with less abuse potential and dependence liability than Schedule III drugs. Examples: pentazocine (Talwin), propoxyphene (Darvon), all benzodiazepines (Librium, Valium, etc.), certain hypnotics (Placidyl, Noctec, Valmid, etc.). Prescription requirements are the same as for Schedule III.

Schedule V: Medicinal drugs with the lowest abuse potential and dependence liability. Examples: diphenoxylate (Lomotil), loperamide (Imodium). Drugs requiring a prescription are handled the same as any non-scheduled prescription drug. Some non-prescription drugs can be sold only with approval of the pharmacist; the buyer is required to sign a log of purchase at the time the drug is dispensed. Examples: codeine and hydrocodone in combination with other active, non-narcotic drugs, sold in preparations that contain limited quantities for control of cough and diarrhea.

*Under jurisdiction of the Controlled Substances Act of 1970.